M000274896

HARRISON'S
Nephrology and Acid-Base Disorders

Derived from Harrison's Principles of Internal Medicine, 17th Edition

Editors

ANTHONY S. FAUCI, MD
Chief, Laboratory of Immunoregulation;
Director, National Institute of Allergy and Infectious Diseases,
National Institutes of Health, Bethesda

DENNIS L. KASPER, MD
William Ellery Channing Professor of Medicine, Professor of
Microbiology and Molecular Genetics, Harvard Medical School;
Director, Channing Laboratory, Department of Medicine,
Brigham and Women's Hospital, Boston

DAN L. LONGO, MD
Scientific Director, National Institute on Aging,
National Institutes of Health, Bethesda and Baltimore

EUGENE BRAUNWALD, MD
Distinguished Hersey Professor of Medicine,
Harvard Medical School; Chairman, TIMI Study Group,
Brigham and Women's Hospital, Boston

STEPHEN L. HAUSER, MD
Robert A. Fishman Distinguished
Professor and Chairman,
Department of Neurology,
University of California, San Francisco

J. LARRY JAMESON, MD, PhD
Professor of Medicine;
Vice President for Medical Affairs and Lewis
Landsberg Dean,
Northwestern University Feinberg School of
Medicine, Chicago

JOSEPH LOSCALZO, MD, PhD
Hersey Professor of Theory and Practice of Medicine,
Harvard Medical School; Chairman, Department of Medicine;
Physician-in-Chief, Brigham and Women's Hospital, Boston

HARRISON'S
Nephrology and Acid-Base Disorders

Editors

J. Larry Jameson, MD, PhD
Professor of Medicine;
Vice President for Medical Affairs and Lewis Landsberg Dean,
Northwestern University Feinberg School of Medicine, Chicago

Joseph Loscalzo, MD, PhD
Hersey Professor of Theory and Practice of Medicine,
Harvard Medical School; Chairman, Department of Medicine;
Physician–in–Chief, Brigham and Women's Hospital, Boston

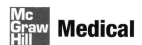

New York   Chicago   San Francisco   Lisbon   London   Madrid
Mexico City   Milan   New Delhi   San Juan   Seoul   Singapore   Sydney   Toronto

The McGraw·Hill Companies

Harrison's Nephrology and Acid-Base Disorders

Copyright © 2010 by The McGraw-Hill Companies, Inc. All rights reserved. Printed in China. Except as permitted under the United States Copyright Act of 1976, no part of this publication may be reproduced or distributed in any form or by any means, or stored in a data base or retrieval system, without prior written permission of the publisher.

Dr. Fauci's and Dr. Longo's works were performed outside the scope of their employment as U.S. government employees. These works represent their personal and professional views and not necessarily those of the U.S. government.

1 2 3 4 5 6 7 8 9 0   CTP/CTP   14 13 12 11 10

ISBN 978-0-07-166339-7
MHID 0-07-166339-8

This book was set in Bembo by Glyph International. The editors were James Shanahan and Kim J. Davis. The production supervisor was Catherine H. Saggese. Project management was provided by Arushi Chawla of Glyph International. The cover design was by Thomas DePierro. Cover, section, and chapter opener illustrations © MedicalRF.com. All rights reserved.

China Translation & Printing Services Ltd. was the printer and binder.

Library of Congress Cataloging-in-Publication Data

Harrison's nephrology and acid-base disorders / editors, J. Larry Jameson, Joseph Loscalzo.
   p. ; cm.
   Compilation of chapters related to kidney function from Harrison's principles of internal medicine.
   Includes bibliographical references and index.
   ISBN-13: 978-0-07-166339-7 (pbk. : alk. paper)
   ISBN-10: 0-07-166339-8 (pbk. : alk. paper)
   1. Nephrology.   2. Kidneys—Diseases.   3. Acid-base imbalances.
I. Jameson, J. Larry.   II. Loscalzo, Joseph.   III. Harrison, Tinsley Randolph,
1900-1978.   IV. Harrison's principles of internal medicine.   V. Title: Nephrology
and acid-base disorders.
   [DNLM: 1. Kidney Diseases.   2. Acid-Base Imbalance.
3. Kidney—pathology. WJ 300 H323   2010]
RC902.A3H37   2010
616.6'1—dc22
                                                                2009033437

McGraw-Hill books are available at special quantity discounts to use as premiums and sales promotions, or for use in corporate training programs. To contact a representative please e-mail us at bulksales@mcgraw-hill.com.

CONTENTS

CONTRIBUTORS

Numbers in brackets refer to the chapter(s) written or co-written by the contributor.

JOHN R. ASPLIN, MD
Clinical Associate, Department of Medicine, University of Chicago; Medical Director, Litholink Corporation, Chicago [9]

KAMAL F. BADR, MD
Professor and Dean, School of Medicine, Lebanese American University, Byblos, Lebanon [18]

JOANNE M. BARGMAN, MD
Professor of Medicine, University of Toronto; Director, Peritoneal Dialysis Program, and Co-Director, Combined Renal-Rheumatology Lupus Clinic, University Health Network, Toronto [11]

GERALD BLOOMFIELD, MD, MPH
Department of Internal Medicine, The Johns Hopkins University School of Medicine, Baltimore [Review and Self-Assessment]

BARRY M. BRENNER, MD, AM, DSc (Hon), DMSc (Hon), DIPL (Hon)
Samuel A. Levine Professor of Medicine, Harvard Medical School; Director Emeritus, Renal Division, Brigham and Women's Hospital, Boston [3, 6, 17, 18, 21]

CYNTHIA D. BROWN, MD
Department of Internal Medicine, The Johns Hopkins University School of Medicine, Baltimore [Review and Self-Assessment]

CHARLES B. CARPENTER, MD
Professor of Medicine, Harvard Medical School; Senior Physician, Brigham and Women's Hospital, Boston [13]

LAN X. CHEN, MD
Clinical Assistant Professor of Medicine, University of Pennsylvania, Penn Presbyterian Medical Center and Philadelphia Veteran Affairs Medical Center, Philadelphia [8]

GLENN M. CHERTOW, MD
Professor of Medicine, Epidemiology and Biostatistics, University of California, San Francisco School of Medicine; Director, Clinical Services, Division of Nephrology, University of California, San Francisco Medical Center, San Francisco [10, 12]

FREDRIC L. COE, MD
Professor of Medicine, University of Chicago, Chicago [9]

BRADLEY M. DENKER, MD
Associate Professor of Medicine, Harvard Medical School; Physician, Brigham and Women's Hospital; Chief of Nephrology, Harvard Vanguard Medical Associates, Boston [3]

THOMAS D. DUBOSE, Jr., MD
Tinsley R. Harrison Professor and Chair of Internal Medicine; Professor of Physiology and Pharmacology, Wake Forest University School of Medicine, Winston-Salem [5]

MURRAY J. FAVUS, MD
Professor of Medicine, Interim Head, Endocrine Section; Director, Bone Section, University of Chicago Pritzker School of Medicine, Chicago [9]

ROBERT FINBERG, MD
Professor and Chair, Department of Medicine, University of Massachusetts Medical School, Worcester [14]

JOYCE FINGEROTH, MD
Associate Professor of Medicine, Harvard Medical School, Boston [14]

DANIEL J. FINK, MD, MPH†
Associate Professor of Clinical Pathology, College of Physicians and Surgeons, Columbia University, New York [Appendix]

AGNES B. FOGO, MD
Professor of Pathology, Medicine and Pediatrics; Director, Renal/EM Division, Department of Pathology, Vanderbilt University Medical Center, Nashville [4]

ALFRED L. GEORGE, Jr., MD
Grant W. Liddle Professor of Medicine and Pharmacology; Chief, Division of Genetic Medicine, Department of Medicine, Vanderbilt University, Nashville [1]

RAYMOND C. HARRIS, Jr., MD
Ann and Roscoe R. Robinson Professor of Medicine; Chief, Division of Nephrology and Hypertension, Department of Medicine, Vanderbilt University, Nashville [2]

SUNDEEP KHOSLA, MD
Professor of Medicine and Physiology, Mayo Clinic College of Medicine, Rochester [7]

THEODORE A. KOTCHEN, MD
Associate Dean for Clinical Research; Director, General Clinical Research Center, Medical College of Wisconsin, Wisconsin [19]

ALEXANDER KRATZ, MD, PhD, MPH
Assistant Professor of Clinical Pathology, Columbia University College of Physicians and Surgeons; Associate Director, Core Laboratory, Columbia University Medical Center, New York-Presbyterian Hospital; Director, Allen Pavilion Laboratory, New York [Appendix]

JULIA B. LEWIS, MD
Professor of Medicine, Division of Nephrology and Hypertension, Department of Medicine, Vanderbilt University School of Medicine, Nashville [15]

KATHLEEN D. LIU, MD, PhD, MCR
Assistant Professor, Division of Nephrology, San Francisco [10, 12]

EDGAR L. MILFORD, MD
Associate Professor of Medicine, Harvard Medical School; Director, Tissue Typing Laboratory, Brigham and Women's Hospital, Boston [13]

---

†Deceased.

ROBERT J. MOTZER, MD
Attending Physician, Department of Medicine, Memorial
Sloan-Kettering Cancer Center; Professor of Medicine, Weill
Medical College of Cornell University, New York [22]

ERIC G. NEILSON, MD
Hugh J. Morgan Professor of Medicine and Cell Biology,
Physician-in-Chief, Vanderbilt University Hospital; Chairman,
Department of Medicine, Vanderbilt University School of
Medicine, Nashville [1, 2, 4, 15]

PARUL S. PATEL, MD
Transplant Neurologist, California Pacific Medical Center,
San Francisco [16]

MICHAEL A. PESCE, PhD
Clinical Professor of Pathology, Columbia University
College of Physicians and Surgeons; Director of Specialty
Laboratory, New York Presbyterian Hospital, Columbia
University Medical Center, New York [Appendix]

DAVID J. SALANT, MD
Professor of Medicine, Pathology, and Laboratory Medicine,
Boston University School of Medicine; Chief, Section of
Nephrology, Boston Medical Center, Boston [16]

MOHAMED H. SAYEGH, MD
Director, Warren E. Grupe and John P. Morill Chair in
Transplantation Medicine; Professor of Medicine and
Pediatrics, Harvard Medical School, Boston [13]

HOWARD I. SCHER, MD
Professor of Medicine, Weill Medical College of Cornell
University; D. Wayne Calloway Chair in Urologic
Oncology; Chief, Genitourinary Oncology Service,
Memorial Sloan-Kettering Cancer Center, New York [22]

JOSHUA SCHIFFER, MD
Department of Internal Medicine, The Johns Hopkins University
School of Medicine, Baltimore [Review and Self-Assessment]

H. RALPH SCHUMACHER, MD
Professor of Medicine, University of Pennsylvania School of
Medicine, Philadelphia [8]

JULIAN L. SEIFTER, MD
Physician, Brigham and Women's Hospital;
Associate Professor of Medicine, Harvard Medical School,
Boston [21]

GARY G. SINGER, MD
Assistant Professor of Clinical Medicine,
Washington University School of Medicine,
St. Louis [6]

KARL SKORECKI, MD
Annie Chutick Professor in Medicine (Nephrology);
Director, Rappaport Research Institute,
Director of Medical and Research Development,
Rambam Medical Health Care Campus, Haifa,
Israel [11]

ADAM SPIVAK, MD
Department of Internal Medicine, The Johns Hopkins University
School of Medicine, Baltimore [Review and Self-Assessment]

WALTER E. STAMM, MD
Professor of Medicine; Head, Division of Allergy and Infectious
Diseases, University of Washington School of Medicine,
Seattle [20]

CHARLES WIENER, MD
Professor of Medicine and Physiology; Vice Chair, Department of
Medicine; Director, Osler Medical Training Program, The Johns
Hopkins University School of Medicine, Baltimore [Review and
Self-Assessment]

ROBERT L. WORTMANN, MD
Dartmouth-Hitchcock Medical Center, Lebanon [8]

ALAN S. L. YU, MB, BChir
Associate Professor of Medicine, Physiology and Biophysics,
University of Southern California Keck School of Medicine,
Los Angeles [17]

PREFACE

The Editors of *Harrison's Principles of Internal Medicine* refer to it as the "Mother Book," a description that confers respect but also acknowledges its size and its ancestral status among the growing list of Harrison's products, which now include *Harrison's Manual of Medicine, Harrison's Online,* and *Harrison's Practice,* an online, highly structured reference for point-of-care use and continuing education. This book, *Harrison's Nephrology and Acid-Base Disorders,* is a compilation of chapters related to kidney function.

Our readers consistently note the sophistication of the material in the specialty sections of *Harrison's.* Our goal was to bring this information to our audience in a more compact and usable form. Because the topic is more focused, it is possible to enhance the presentation of the material by enlarging the text and the tables. We have also included a Review and Self-Assessment section that includes questions and answers to provoke reflection and to provide additional teaching points.

Renal dysfunction, electrolyte, and acid-base disorders are among the most common problems faced by the clinician. Indeed, hyponatremia is consistently the most frequently searched term for readers of *Harrison's Online.* Unlike some specialties, there is no specific renal exam. Instead, the specialty relies heavily on laboratory tests, urinalyses, and characteristics of urinary sediments. Evaluation and management of renal disease also requires a broad knowledge of physiology and pathology since the kidney is involved in many systemic disorders. Thus, this book considers a broad spectrum of topics including acid-base and electrolyte disorders, vascular injury to the kidney, as well as specific diseases of the kidney.

Kidney disorders, such as glomerulonephritis, can be a primary cause for clinical presentation. More commonly, however, the kidney is affected secondary to other medical problems such as diabetes, shock, or complications from dye administration or medications. As such, renal dysfunction may be manifest by azotemia, hypertension, proteinuria, or an abnormal urinary sediment, and it may herald the presence of an underlying medical disorder. Renal insufficiency may also appear late in the course of chronic conditions such as diabetes, lupus, or scleroderma and significantly alter a patient's quality of life. Fortunately, intervention can often reverse or delay renal insufficiency. And, when this is not possible, dialysis and renal transplant provide life-saving therapies.

Understanding normal and abnormal renal function provides a strong foundation for diagnosis and clinical management. Therefore, topics such as acidosis and alkalosis, fluid and electrolyte disorders, and hypercalcemia are covered here. These basic topics are useful in all fields of medicine and represent a frequent source of renal consultation.

The first section of the book, "Introduction to the Renal System," provides a systems overview, beginning with renal development, function, and physiology, as well as providing an overview of how the kidney responds to injury. The integration of pathophysiology with clinical management is a hallmark of *Harrison's,* and can be found throughout each of the subsequent disease-oriented chapters. The book is divided into seven main sections that reflect the scope of nephrology: (I) Introduction to the Renal System; (II) Alterations of Renal Function and Electrolytes; (III) Acute and Chronic Renal Failure; (IV) Glomerular and Tubular Disorders; (V) Renal Vascular Disease; (VI) Urinary Tract Infections and Obstruction; and (VII) Cancer of the Kidney and Urinary Tract.

While *Harrison's Nephrology and Acid-Base Disorders* is classic in its organization, readers will sense the impact of the scientific advances as they explore the individual chapters in each section. Genetics and molecular biology are transforming the field of nephrology, whether illuminating the genetic basis of a tubular disorder or explaining the regenerative capacity of the kidney. Recent clinical studies involving common diseases like chronic kidney disease, hypertensive vascular disease, and urinary tract infections provide powerful evidence for medical decision making and treatment. These rapid changes in nephrology are exciting for new students of medicine and underscore the need for practicing physicians to continuously update their knowledge base and clinical skills.

Our access to information through web-based journals and databases is remarkably efficient. While these sources of information are invaluable, the daunting body of data creates an even greater need for synthesis and for highlighting important facts. Thus, the preparation of these chapters is a special craft that requires the ability to distill core information from the ever-expanding knowledge base. The editors are therefore indebted to our authors, a group of internationally recognized authorities who are masters at providing a comprehensive overview while being able to distill a topic into a concise and interesting chapter. We are grateful to Emily Cowan for assisting with research and preparation of this book. Our colleagues at McGraw-Hill continue to innovate in healthcare publishing. This new product was championed by Jim Shanahan and impeccably produced by Kim Davis.

We hope you find this book useful in your effort to achieve continuous learning on behalf of your patients.

J. Larry Jameson, MD, PhD
Joseph Loscalzo, MD, PhD

NOTICE

Medicine is an ever-changing science. As new research and clinical experience broaden our knowledge, changes in treatment and drug therapy are required. The authors and the publisher of this work have checked with sources believed to be reliable in their efforts to provide information that is complete and generally in accord with the standards accepted at the time of publication. However, in view of the possibility of human error or changes in medical sciences, neither the authors nor the publisher nor any other party who has been involved in the preparation or publication of this work warrants that the information contained herein is in every respect accurate or complete, and they disclaim all responsibility for any errors or omissions or for the results obtained from use of the information contained in this work. Readers are encouraged to confirm the information contained herein with other sources. For example, and in particular, readers are advised to check the product information sheet included in the package of each drug they plan to administer to be certain that the information contained in this work is accurate and that changes have not been made in the recommended dose or in the contraindications for administration. This recommendation is of particular importance in connection with new or infrequently used drugs.

Review and self-assessment questions and answers were taken from Wiener C, Fauci AS, Braunwald E, Kasper DL, Hauser SL, Longo DL, Jameson JL, Loscalzo J (editors) Bloomfield G, Brown CD, Schiffer J, Spivak A (contributing editors). *Harrison's Principles of Internal Medicine Self-Assessment and Board Review*, 17th ed. New York, McGraw-Hill, 2008, ISBN 978-0-07-149619-3.

 The global icons call greater attention to key epidemiologic and clinical differences in the practice of medicine throughout the world.

 The genetic icons identify a clinical issue with an explicit genetic relationship.

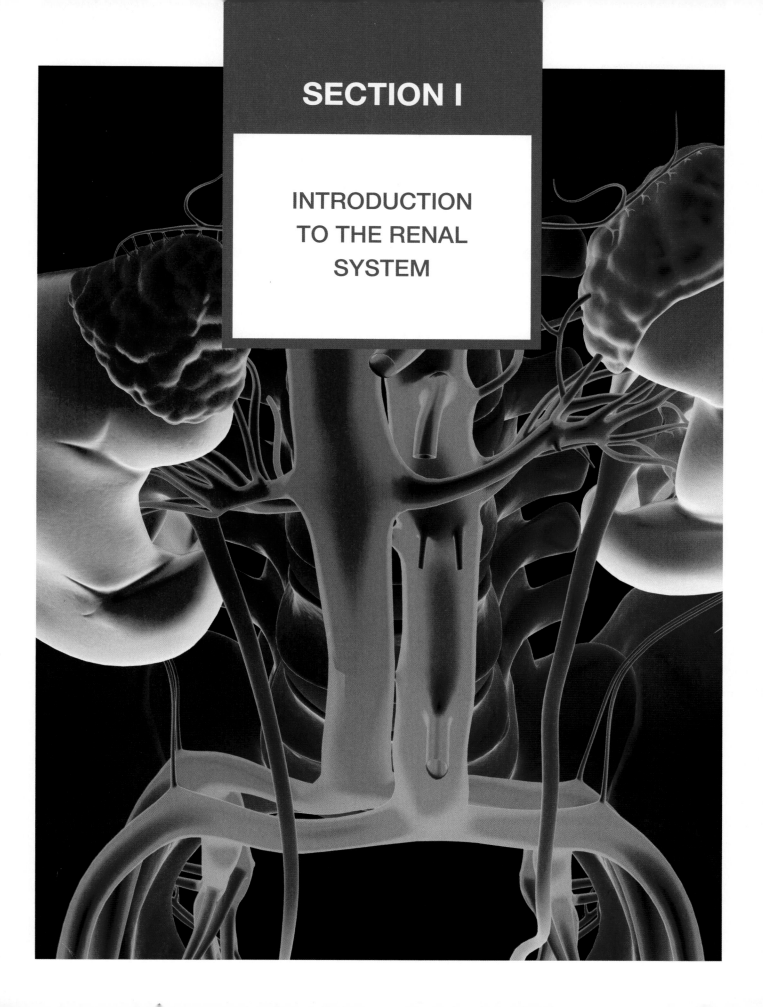

SECTION I

INTRODUCTION TO THE RENAL SYSTEM

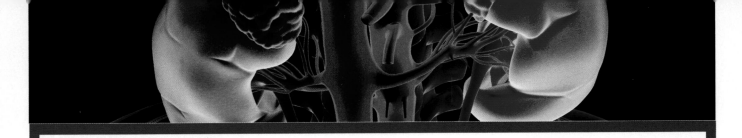

CHAPTER 1
BASIC BIOLOGY OF THE KIDNEY

Alfred L. George, Jr. ■ Eric G. Neilson

The kidney is one of the most highly differentiated organs in the body. Nearly 30 different cell types can be found in the renal interstitium or along segmented nephrons, blood vessels, and filtering capillaries at the conclusion of embryological development. This panoply of cells modulates a variety of complex physiologic processes. Endocrine functions, the regulation of blood pressure and intraglomerular hemodynamics, solute and water transport, acid–base balance, and removal of fuel or drug metabolites are all accomplished by intricate mechanisms of renal response. This breadth of physiology hinges on the clever ingenuity of nephron architecture that evolved as complex organisms came out of water to live on land.

EMBRYOLOGICAL DEVELOPMENT

The kidney develops from within the intermediate mesoderm under the timed or sequential control of a growing number of genes, described in **Fig. 1-1**. The transcription of these genes is guided by morphogenic cues that invite ureteric buds to penetrate the metanephric blastema, where they induce primary mesenchymal cells to form early nephrons. This induction involves a number of complex signaling pathways mediated by c-Met, fibroblast growth factor, transforming growth factor β, glial cell–derived neurotrophic factor, hepatocyte growth factor, epithelial growth factor, and

the Wnt family of proteins. The ureteric buds derive from the posterior nephric ducts and mature into collecting ducts that eventually funnel to a renal pelvis and ureter. Induced mesenchyme undergoes mesenchymal-epithelial transitions to form comma-shaped bodies at the proximal end of each ureteric bud. These lead to the formation of S-shaped nephrons that cleft and enjoin with penetrating endothelial cells derived from sprouting angioblasts. Under the influence of vascular endothelial growth factor A, these penetrating cells form capillaries with surrounding mesangial cells that differentiate into a glomerular filter for plasma water and solute. The ureteric buds branch, and each branch produces a new set of nephrons. The number of branching events ultimately determines the total number of nephrons in each kidney. There are approximately 900,000 glomeruli in each kidney in normal-birth-weight adults and as few as 225,000 in low-birth-weight adults. In the latter case, a failure to complete the last one or two rounds of branching leads to smaller kidneys and increased risk for hypertension and cardiovascular disease later in life.

Glomeruli evolved as complex capillary filters with fenestrated endothelia. Outlining each capillary is a basement membrane covered by epithelial podocytes. Podocytes attach by special foot processes and share a slit-pore membrane with their neighbor. The slit-pore membrane is formed by the interaction of nephrin, annexin-4, CD2AP, FAT, ZO-1, P-cadherin, podocin, and neph 1–3 proteins. These glomerular capillaries seat

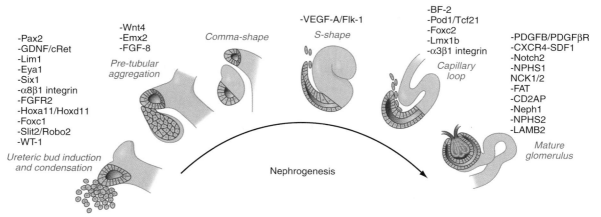

FIGURE 1-1

Genes controlling renal nephrogenesis. A growing number of genes have been identified at various stages of glomerulotubular development in mammalian kidney. The genes listed have been tested in various genetically modified mice, and their location corresponds to the classical stages of kidney development postulated by Saxen in 1987. GDNF, giant cell line–derived neutrophilic factor; FGFR2, fibroblast growth factor receptor 2; WT-1, Wilms tumor gene 1; FGF-8, fibroblast growth factor 8; VEGF–A/ Flk-1, vascular endothelial growth factor–A/fetal liver kinase-1; PDGFB, platelet-derived growth factor B; PDGFβR, PDGFβ receptor; SDF-1, stromal-derived factor 1; NPHS1, nephrin; NCK1/2, NCK-adaptor protein; CD2AP, CD2-associated protein; NPHS2, podocin; LAMB2, laminin beta-2.

in a mesangial matrix shrouded by parietal and proximal tubular epithelia forming Bowman's capsule. Mesangial cells have an embryonic lineage consistent with arteriolar or juxtaglomerular cells and contain contractile actin-myosin fibers. These cells make contact with glomerular capillary loops, and their matrix holds them in condensed arrangement. Between nephrons lies the renal interstitium. This region forms the functional space surrounding glomeruli and their downstream tubules, which are home to resident and trafficking cells, such as fibroblasts, dendritic cells, occasional lymphocytes, and lipid-laden macrophages. The cortical and medullary capillaries, which siphon off solute and water following tubular reclamation of glomerular filtrate, are also part of the interstitial fabric as well as a web of connective tissue that supports the kidney's emblematic architecture of folding tubules. The relational precision of these structures determines the unique physiology of the kidney.

Each nephron segments during embryological development into a proximal tubule, descending and ascending limbs of the loop of Henle, distal tubule, and the collecting duct. These classic tubular segments have subsegments recognized by highly unique epithelia serving regional physiology. All nephrons have the same structural components, but there are two types whose structure depends on their location within the kidney. The majority of nephrons are cortical, with glomeruli located in the mid- to outer cortex. Fewer nephrons are juxtamedullary, with glomeruli at the boundary of the cortex and outer medulla. Cortical nephrons have short loops of Henle, whereas juxtamedullary nephrons have long loops of Henle. There are critical differences in blood supply as well. The peritubular capillaries surrounding cortical nephrons are shared among adjacent nephrons. By contrast, juxtamedullary nephrons use separate capillaries called *vasa recta*. Cortical nephrons perform most of the glomerular filtration because there are more of them and because their afferent arterioles are larger than their respective efferent arterioles. The juxtamedullary nephrons, with longer loops of Henle, create a hyperosmolar gradient that allows for the production of concentrated urine. How developmental instructions specify the differentiation of all these unique epithelia among various tubular segments is still unknown.

DETERMINANTS AND REGULATION OF GLOMERULAR FILTRATION

Renal blood flow drains approximately 20% of the cardiac output, or 1000 mL/min. Blood reaches each nephron through the afferent arteriole leading into a glomerular capillary where large amounts of fluid and solutes are filtered as tubular fluid. The distal ends of the glomerular capillaries coalesce to form an efferent arteriole leading to the first segment of a second capillary network (peritubular capillaries) surrounding the cortical tubules (**Fig. 1-2A**). Thus, the cortical nephron has two capillary beds arranged in series separated by the efferent arteriole that regulates the hydrostatic pressure in both capillary beds. The peritubular capillaries empty into small venous branches, which coalesce into larger veins to eventually form the renal vein.

The hydrostatic pressure gradient across the glomerular capillary wall is the primary driving force for glomerular filtration. Oncotic pressure within the capillary lumen, determined by the concentration of unfiltered plasma proteins, partially offsets the hydrostatic pressure gradient and opposes filtration. As the oncotic pressure rises along the length of the glomerular capillary, the driving force for filtration falls to zero before reaching the efferent arteriole. Approximately 20% of the renal plasma flow is filtered into Bowman's space, and the ratio of glomerular filtration rate (GFR) to renal plasma flow determines the filtration fraction. Several factors, mostly hemodynamic, contribute to the regulation of filtration under physiologic conditions.

Although glomerular filtration is affected by renal artery pressure, this relationship is not linear across the range of physiologic blood pressures. Autoregulation of glomerular filtration is the result of three major factors that modulate either afferent or efferent arteriolar tone: these include an autonomous vasoreactive (myogenic) reflex in the afferent arteriole, *tubuloglomerular feedback*, and angiotensin II–mediated vasoconstriction of the efferent arteriole. The myogenic reflex is a first line of defense against fluctuations in renal blood flow. Acute changes in renal perfusion pressure evoke reflex constriction or dilatation of the afferent arteriole in response to increased or decreased pressure, respectively. This phenomenon helps protect the glomerular capillary from sudden elevations in systolic pressure.

Tubuloglomerular feedback changes the rate of filtration and tubular flow by reflex vasoconstriction or dilatation of the afferent arteriole. Tubuloglomerular feedback is mediated by specialized cells in the thick ascending limb of the loop of Henle called the *macula densa* that act as sensors of solute concentration and flow of tubular fluid. With high tubular flow rates, a proxy for an inappropriately high filtration rate, there is increased solute delivery to the macula densa (**Fig. 1-2B**), which evokes vasoconstriction of the afferent arteriole causing the GFR to return to normal. One component of the soluble signal from the macula densa is adenosine triphosphate (ATP), which is released by the cells during increased NaCl reabsorption. ATP is metabolized in the extracellular space by ecto-59-nucleotidase to generate adenosine, a potent vasoconstrictor of the afferent arteriole. Direct release of adenosine by macula densa cells also occurs. During conditions associated with a fall in filtration rate, reduced solute delivery to the macula densa attenuates the tubuloglomerular response, allowing afferent arteriolar dilatation and restoring glomerular filtration to normal levels. Loop diuretics block tubuloglomerular feedback by interfering with NaCl reabsorption by macula densa cells. Angiotensin II and reactive oxygen

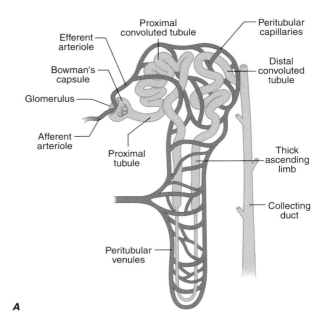

A

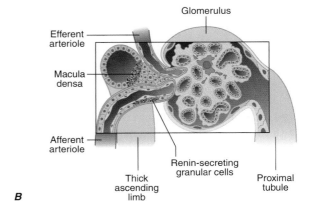

B

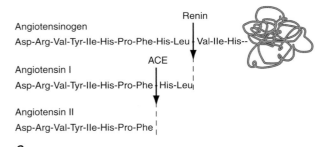

C

FIGURE 1-2

Renal microcirculation and the renin-angiotensin system.
A. Diagram illustrating relationships of the nephron with glomerular and peritubular capillaries. **B.** Expanded view of the glomerulus with its juxtaglomerular apparatus including the macula densa and adjacent afferent arteriole. **C.** Proteolytic processing steps in the generation of angiotensin II.

species enhance, while nitric oxide blunts tubuloglomerular feedback.

The third component underlying autoregulation of filtration rate involves angiotensin II. During states of reduced renal blood flow, renin is released from granular cells within the wall of the afferent arteriole near the macula densa in a region called the juxtaglomerular apparatus (Fig. 1-2B). Renin, a proteolytic enzyme, catalyzes the conversion of angiotensinogen to angiotensin I, which is subsequently converted to angiotensin II by angiotensin-converting enzyme (ACE) (Fig. 1-2C). Angiotensin II evokes vasoconstriction of the efferent arteriole, and the resulting increased glomerular hydrostatic pressure elevates filtration to normal levels.

MECHANISMS OF RENAL TUBULAR TRANSPORT

The renal tubules are composed of highly differentiated epithelia that vary dramatically in morphology and function along the nephron (Fig. 1-3). The cells lining the various tubular segments form monolayers connected to one another by a specialized region of the adjacent lateral membranes called the *tight junction*. Tight junctions form an occlusive barrier that separates the lumen of the tubule from the interstitial spaces surrounding the tubule. These specialized junctions also divide the cell membrane into discrete domains: the apical membrane faces the tubular lumen, and the basolateral membrane faces the interstitium. This physical separation of membranes allows cells to allocate membrane proteins and lipids asymmetrically to different regions of the membrane. Owing to this feature, renal epithelial cells are said to be *polarized*. The asymmetrical assignment of membrane proteins, especially proteins mediating transport processes, provides the structural machinery for directional movement of fluid and solutes by the nephron.

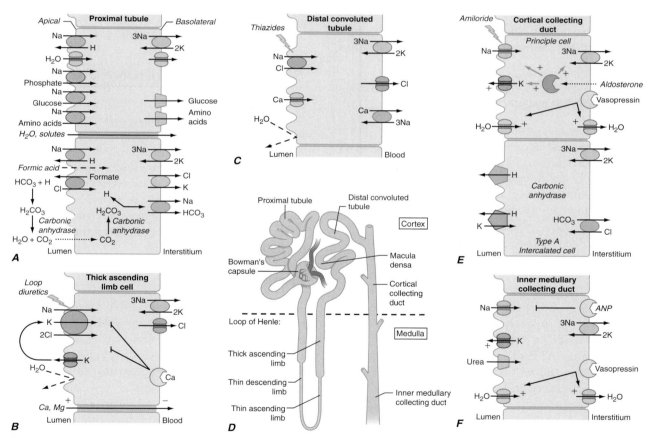

FIGURE 1-3

Transport activities of the major nephron segments. Representative cells from five major tubular segments are illustrated with the lumen side (apical membrane) facing left and interstitial side (basolateral membrane) facing right. **A.** Proximal tubular cells. **B.** Typical cell in the thick ascending limb of the loop of Henle. **C.** Distal convoluted tubular cell. **D.** Overview of entire nephron. **E.** Cortical collecting duct cells. **F.** Typical cell in the inner medullary collecting duct. The major membrane transporters, channels, and pumps are drawn with arrows indicating the direction of solute or water movement. For some events, the stoichiometry of transport is indicated by numerals preceding the solute. Targets for major diuretic agents are labeled. The actions of hormones are illustrated by arrows with plus signs for stimulatory effects and lines with perpendicular ends for inhibitory events. Dotted lines indicate free diffusion across cell membranes. The dashed line indicates water impermeability of cell membranes in the thick ascending limb and distal convoluted tubule.

EPITHELIAL SOLUTE TRANSPORT

There are two types of epithelial transport. The movement of fluid and solutes sequentially across the apical and basolateral cell membranes (or vice versa) mediated by transporters, channels, or pumps is called *cellular transport*. By contrast, movement of fluid and solutes through the narrow passageway between adjacent cells is called *paracellular transport*. Paracellular transport occurs through tight junctions, indicating that they are not completely "tight." Indeed, some epithelial cell layers allow rather robust paracellular transport to occur (*leaky epithelia*), whereas other epithelia have more effective tight junctions (*tight epithelia*). In addition, because the ability of ions to flow through the paracellular pathway determines the electrical resistance across the epithelial monolayer, leaky and tight epithelia are also referred to as low- and high-resistance epithelia, respectively. The proximal tubule contains leaky epithelia, whereas distal nephron segments, such as the collecting duct, contain tight epithelia. Leaky epithelia are best suited for bulk fluid reabsorption, whereas tight epithelia allow for more refined control and regulation of transport.

MEMBRANE TRANSPORT

Cell membranes are composed of hydrophobic lipids that repel water and aqueous solutes. The movement of solutes and water across cell membranes is made possible by discrete classes of integral membrane proteins, including channels, pumps, and transporters. These different components mediate specific types of transport activities, including *active transport* (pumps), *passive transport* (channels), *facilitated diffusion* (transporters), and *secondary active transport* (co-transporters). Different cell types in the mammalian nephron are endowed with distinct combinations of proteins that serve specific transport functions. Active transport requires metabolic energy generated by the hydrolysis of ATP. The classes of protein that mediate active transport ("pumps") are ion-translocating ATPases, including the ubiquitous Na^+/K^+-ATPase, the H^+-ATPases, and Ca^{2+}-ATPases. Active transport can create asymmetrical ion concentrations across a cell membrane and can move ions against a chemical gradient. The potential energy stored in a concentration gradient of an ion such as Na^+ can be utilized to drive transport through other mechanisms (secondary active transport). Pumps are often *electrogenic*, meaning they can create an asymmetrical distribution of electrostatic charges across the membrane and establish a voltage or membrane potential. The movement of solutes through a membrane protein by simple diffusion is called passive transport. This activity is mediated by channels created by selectively permeable membrane proteins, and it allows solute or water to move across a

membrane driven by favorable *concentration gradients* or *electrochemical potential*. Examples in the kidney include water channels (aquaporins), K^+ channels, epithelial Na^+ channels, and Cl^- channels. Facilitated diffusion is a specialized type of passive transport mediated by simple transporters called *carriers* or *uniporters*. For example, a family of hexose transporters (GLUTs 1–13) mediates glucose uptake by cells. These transporters are driven by the concentration gradient for glucose, which is highest in extracellular fluids and lowest in the cytoplasm due to rapid metabolism. Many transporters operate by translocating two or more ions/solutes in concert either in the same direction (*symporters* or *co-transporters*) or in opposite directions (*antiporters* or *exchangers*) across the cell membrane. The movement of two or more ions/solutes may produce no net change in the balance of electrostatic charges across the membrane (*electroneutral*), or a transport event may alter the balance of charges (*electrogenic*). Several inherited disorders of renal tubular solute and water transport occur as a consequence of mutations in genes encoding a variety of channels, transporter proteins, and their regulators (**Table 1-1**)

SEGMENTAL NEPHRON FUNCTIONS

Each anatomic segment of the nephron has unique characteristics and specialized functions that enable selective transport of solutes and water (Fig. 1-3). Through sequential events of reabsorption and secretion along the nephron, tubular fluid is progressively conditioned into final urine for excretion. Knowledge of the major tubular mechanisms responsible for solute and water transport is critical for understanding hormonal regulation of kidney function and the pharmacologic manipulation of renal excretion.

PROXIMAL TUBULE

The proximal tubule is responsible for reabsorbing ~60% of filtered NaCl and water, as well as ~90% of filtered bicarbonate and most critical nutrients such as glucose and amino acids. The proximal tubule utilizes both cellular and paracellular transport mechanisms. The apical membrane of proximal tubular cells has an expanded surface area available for reabsorptive work created by a dense array of microvilli called the *brush border*, and comparatively leaky tight junctions further enable high-capacity fluid reabsorption.

Solute and water pass through these tight junctions to enter the lateral intercellular space where absorption by the peritubular capillaries occurs. Bulk fluid reabsorption by the proximal tubule is driven by high oncotic pressure and low hydrostatic pressure within the peritubular capillaries. Physiologic adjustments in GFR made by changing efferent arteriolar tone cause proportional changes in reabsorption, a phenomenon known as

TABLE 1-1

7

INHERITED DISORDERS AFFECTING RENAL TUBULAR ION AND SOLUTE TRANSPORT

DISEASE OR SYNDROME	GENE	OMIMA[a]
Disorders Involving the Proximal Tubule		
Proximal renal tubular acidosis	Sodium bicarbonate co-transporter (*SLC4A4*, 4q21)	604278
Faconi-Bickel syndrome	Glucose transporter-2 (*SLC2A2* 3q26.1-q26.3)	227810
Isolated renal glycosuria	Sodium glucose co-transporter (*SLC5A2*,16p11.2)	233100
Cystinuria, type I	Cystine, dibasic and neutral amino acid transporter (*SLC3A1*, 2p16.3)	220100
Cystinuria, non-type I	Amino acid transporter, light subunit (*SLC7A9*, 19q13.1)	600918
Lysinuric protein intolerance	Amino acid transporter (*SLC7A7*, 4q11.2)	222700
Hereditary hypophosphatemic rickets with hypercalcemia	Sodium phosphate co-transporter (*SLC34A3*, 9q34)	241530
Renal hypouricemia	Urate-anion exchanger (*SLC22A12*, 11q13)	220150
Dent's disease	Chloride channel, ClC-5 (*CLCN5*, Xp11.22)	300009
X-linked recessive nephrolithiasis with renal failure	Chloride channel, ClC-5 (*CLCN5*, Xp11.22)	310468
X-linked recessive hypophosphatemic rickets	Chloride channel, ClC-5 (*CLCN5*, Xp11.22)	307800
Disorders Involving the Loop of Henle		
Bartter's syndrome, type 1	Sodium potassium-chloride co-transporter (*SLC12A1*,15q15-q21)	241200
Bartter's syndrome, type 2	Potassium channel, ROMK (*KCNJ1*, 11q24)	601678
Bartter's syndrome, type 3	Chloride channel, ClC-Kb (*CLCNKB*, 1p36)	602023
Bartter's syndrome with sensorineural deafness	Chloride channel accessory subunit, barttin (*BSND*, 1p31)	602522
Autosomal dominant hypocalcemia with Bartter-like syndrome	Calcium-sensing receptor (*CASR*, 3q13.3-q21)	601199
Familial hypocalciuric hypercalcemia	Calcium-sensing receptor (*CASR*, 3q13.3-q21)	145980
Primary hypomagnesemia	Claudin-16 or paracellin-1 (*CLDN16* or *PCLN1*, 3q27)	248250
Isolated renal magnesium loss	Sodium potassium ATPase, γ_1-subunit (*ATP1G1*, 11q23)	154020
Primary hypomagnesemia with secondary hypocalcemia	Melastatin-related transient receptor potential cation channel 6 (*TRPM6*, 9q22)	602014
Disorders Involving the Distal Tubule and Collecting Duct		
Gitelman's syndrome	Sodium-chloride co-transporter (*SLC12A3*, 16q13)	263800
Pseudoaldosteronism (Liddle's syndrome)	Epithelial sodium channel β and γ subunits (*SCNN1B*, *SCNN1G*, 16p13-p12)	177200
Recessive pseudohypoaldosteronism type 1	Epithelial sodium channel, α, β, and γ subunits (*SCNN1A*, 12p13; *SCNN1B*, *SCNN1G*, 16p13-p12)	264350
Pseudohypoaldosteronism type 2 (Gordon's hyperkalemia-hypertension syndrome)	Kinases WNK-1, WNK-4 (*WNK1*, 12p13; *WNK4*, 17q21-q22)	145260

(Continued)

TABLE 1-1 (CONTINUED)

INHERITED DISORDERS AFFECTING RENAL TUBULAR ION AND SOLUTE TRANSPORT		
DISEASE OR SYNDROME	**GENE**	**OMIMa**
Disorders Involving the Distal Tubule and Collecting Duct		
X-linked nephrogenic diabetes insipidus	Vasopressin V_2 receptor (AVPR2, Xq28)	304800
Nephrogenic diabetes insipidus (autosomal)	Water channel, aquaporin-2 (AQP2, 12q13)	125800
Distal renal tubular acidosis, autosomal dominant	Anion exchanger-1 (SLC4A1, 17q21-q22)	179800
Distal renal tubular acidosis, autosomal recessive	Anion exchanger-1 (SLC4A1, 17q21-q22)	602722
Distal renal tubular acidosis with neural deafness	Proton ATPase, β1 subunit (ATP6B1, 2cen-q13)	192132
Distal renal tubular acidosis with normal hearing	Proton ATPase, 116-kD subunit (ATP6N1B, 7q33-q34)	602722

aOnline Mendelian Inheritance in Man database (http://www.ncbi.nlm.nih.gov/Omim).

glomerulotubular balance. For example, vasoconstriction of the efferent arteriole by angiotensin II will increase glomerular capillary hydrostatic pressure but lower pressure in the peritubular capillaries. At the same time, increased GFR and filtration fraction cause a rise in oncotic pressure near the end of the glomerular capillary. These changes, a lowered hydrostatic and increased oncotic pressure, increase the driving force for fluid absorption by the peritubular capillaries.

Cellular transport of most solutes by the proximal tubule is coupled to the Na^+ concentration gradient established by the activity of a basolateral Na^+/K^+-ATPase (Fig. 1-3A). This active transport mechanism maintains a steep Na^+ gradient by keeping intracellular Na^+ concentrations low. Solute reabsorption is coupled to the Na^+ gradient by Na^+-dependent co-transporters such as Na^+-glucose and the Na^+-phosphate. In addition to the paracellular route, water reabsorption also occurs through the cellular pathway enabled by constitutively active water channels (aquaporin-1) present on both apical and basolateral membranes. In addition, small, local *osmotic gradients* close to plasma membranes generated by cellular Na^+ reabsorption are likely responsible for driving directional water movement across proximal tubule cells.

Proximal tubular cells reclaim bicarbonate by a mechanism dependent on carbonic anhydrases. Filtered bicarbonate is first titrated by protons delivered to the lumen by Na^+/H^+ exchange. The resulting carbonic acid is metabolized by brush border carbonic anhydrase to water and carbon dioxide. Dissolved carbon dioxide then diffuses into the cell, where it is enzymatically hydrated by cytoplasmic carbonic anhydrase to reform carbonic acid. Finally, intracellular carbonic acid dissociates into free protons and bicarbonate anions, and bicarbonate exits

the cell through a basolateral Na^+/HCO_3^- co-transporter. This process is saturable, resulting in renal bicarbonate excretion when plasma levels exceed the physiologically normal range (24–26 meq/L). Carbonic anhydrase inhibitors such as acetazolamide, a class of weak diuretic agents, block proximal tubule reabsorption of bicarbonate and are useful for alkalinizing the urine.

Chloride is poorly reabsorbed throughout the first segment of the proximal tubule, and a rise in Cl^- concentration counterbalances the removal of bicarbonate anion from tubular fluid. In later proximal tubular segments, cellular Cl^- reabsorption is initiated by apical exchange of cellular formate for higher luminal concentrations of Cl^-. Once in the lumen, formate anions are titrated by H^+ (provided by Na^+/H^+ exchange) to generate neutral formic acid, which can diffuse passively across the apical membrane back into the cell where it dissociates a proton and is recycled. Basolateral Cl^- exit is mediated by a K^+/Cl^- co-transporter.

Reabsorption of glucose is nearly complete by the end of the proximal tubule. Cellular transport of glucose is mediated by apical Na^+-glucose co-transport coupled with basolateral, facilitated diffusion by a glucose transporter. This process is also saturable, leading to glycosuria when plasma levels exceed 180–200 mg/dL, as seen in untreated diabetes mellitus.

The proximal tubule possesses specific transporters capable of secreting a variety of organic acids (carboxylate anions) and bases (mostly primary amine cations). Organic anions transported by these systems include urate, ketoacid anions, and several protein-bound drugs not filtered at the glomerulus (penicillins, cephalosporins, and salicylates). Probenecid inhibits renal organic anion secretion and can be clinically useful for raising plasma concentrations of certain drugs like penicillin and oseltamivir. Organic cations secreted by the proximal tubule include various biogenic amine neurotransmitters (dopamine, acetylcholine, epinephrine, norepinephrine, and histamine) and creatinine. Certain drugs like cimetidine and trimethoprim compete with endogenous compounds for transport by the organic cation pathways. These drugs elevate levels of serum creatinine, but this change does not reflect changes in the GFR.

The proximal tubule, through distinct classes of Na^+-dependent and Na^+-independent transport systems, reabsorbs amino acids efficiently. These transporters are specific for different groups of amino acids. For example, cystine, lysine, arginine, and ornithine are transported by a system comprising two proteins encoded by the *SLC3A1* and *SLC7A9* genes. Mutations in either *SLC3A1* or *SLC7A9* impair reabsorption of these amino acids and cause the disease cystinuria. Peptide hormones, such as insulin and growth hormone, β_2-microglobulin, and other small proteins, are taken up by the proximal tubule through a process of absorptive endocytosis and are degraded in acidified endocytic vesicles or lysosomes. Acidification of these vesicles depends on a "proton pump" (vacuolar H^+-ATPase) and a Cl^- channel. Impaired acidification of endocytic vesicles because of mutations in a Cl^- channel gene (*CLCN5*) causes low-molecular-weight proteinuria in Dent's disease. Renal ammoniagenesis from glutamine in the proximal tubule provides a major tubular fluid buffer to ensure excretion of secreted H^+ ion as NH_4^+ by the collecting duct. Cellular K^+ levels inversely modulate ammoniagenesis, and in the setting of high serum K^+ from hypoaldosteronism, reduced ammoniagenesis facilitates the appearance of type IV renal tubular acidosis.

LOOP OF HENLE

The loop of Henle consists of three major segments: descending thin limb, ascending thin limb, and ascending thick limb. These divisions are based on cellular morphology and anatomic location, but also correlate well with specialization of function. Approximately 15–25% of filtered NaCl is reabsorbed in the loop of Henle, mainly by the thick ascending limb. The loop of Henle has a critically important role in urinary concentrating ability by contributing to the generation of a hypertonic medullary interstitium in a process called *countercurrent multiplication*. The loop of Henle is the site of action for the most potent class of diuretic agents (loop diuretics) and contributes to reabsorption of calcium and magnesium ions.

The descending thin limb is highly water permeable owing to dense expression of constitutively active aquaporin-1 water channels. By contrast, water permeability is negligible in the ascending limb. In the thick ascending limb, there is a high level of secondary active salt transport

enabled by the $Na^+/K^+/2Cl^-$ co-transporter on the apical membrane in series with basolateral Cl^- channels and Na^+/K^+-ATPase (Fig. 1-3B). The $Na^+/K^+/2Cl^-$ co-transporter is the primary target for loop diuretics. Tubular fluid K^+ is the limiting substrate for this co-transporter (tubular concentration of K^+ is similar to plasma, about 4 meq/L), but it is maintained by K^+ recycling through an apical potassium channel. An inherited disorder of the thick ascending limb, Bartter's syndrome, results in a salt-wasting renal disease associated with hypokalemia and metabolic alkalosis. Loss-of-function mutations in one of four distinct genes encoding components of the $Na^+/K^+/2Cl^-$ co-transporter (*NKCC2*), apical K^+ channel (*KCNJ1*), or basolateral Cl^- channel (*CLCNKB, BSND*) can cause the syndrome.

Potassium recycling also contributes to a positive electrostatic charge in the lumen relative to the interstitium, which promotes divalent cation (Mg^{2+} and Ca^{2+}) reabsorption through the paracellular pathway. A Ca^{2+}-sensing, G-protein coupled receptor (CaSR) on basolateral membranes regulates NaCl reabsorption in the thick ascending limb through dual signaling mechanisms utilizing either cyclic adenosine monophosphate (AMP) or eicosanoids. This receptor enables a steep relationship between plasma Ca^{2+} levels and renal Ca^{2+} excretion. Loss-of-function mutations in CaSR cause familial hypercalcemic hypocalciuria because of a blunted response of the thick ascending limb to exocellular Ca^{2+}. Mutations in *CLDN16* encoding paracellin-1, a transmembrane protein located within the tight junction complex, leads to familial hypomagnesemia with hypercalcuria and nephrocalcinosis, suggesting that the ion conductance of the paracellular pathway in the thick limb is regulated. Mutations in *TRPM6* encoding an Mg^{2+} permeable ion channel also cause familial hypomagnesemia with hypocalcemia. A molecular complex of TRPM6 and TRPM7 proteins is critical for Mg^{2+} reabsorption in the thick ascending limb of Henle.

The loop of Henle contributes to urine concentrating ability by establishing a *hypertonic medullary interstitium*, which promotes water reabsorption by a more distal nephron segment, the inner medullary collecting duct. *Countercurrent multiplication* produces a hypertonic medullary interstitium using two countercurrent systems: the loop of Henle (opposing descending and ascending limbs) and the vasa recta (medullary peritubular capillaries enveloping the loop). The countercurrent flow in these two systems helps maintain the hypertonic environment of the inner medulla, but NaCl reabsorption by the thick ascending limb is the primary initiating event. Reabsorption of NaCl without water dilutes the tubular fluid and adds new osmoles to the interstitial fluid surrounding the thick ascending limb. Because the descending thin limb is highly water permeable, osmotic equilibrium occurs between the descending-limb tubular fluid and the interstitial space, leading to progressive solute trapping in the inner medulla. Maximum medullary interstitial osmolality also requires partial recycling of urea from the collecting duct.

DISTAL CONVOLUTED TUBULE

The distal convoluted tubule reabsorbs ~5% of the filtered NaCl. This segment is composed of a tight epithelium with little water permeability. The major NaCl transporting pathway utilizes an apical membrane, electroneutral thiazide-sensitive Na^+/Cl^- co-transporter in tandem with basolateral Na^+/K^+-ATPase and Cl^- channels (Fig. 1-3C). Apical Ca^{2+}-selective channels (TRPV5) and basolateral Na^+/Ca^{2+} exchange mediate calcium reabsorption in the distal convoluted tubule. Ca^{2+} reabsorption is inversely related to Na^+ reabsorption and is stimulated by parathyroid hormone. Blocking apical Na^+/Cl^- co-transport will reduce intracellular Na^+, favoring increased basolateral Na^+/Ca^{2+} exchange and passive apical Ca^{2+} entry. Loss-of-function mutations of SLC12A3 encoding the apical Na^+/Cl^- co-transporter cause Gitelman's syndrome, a salt-wasting disorder associated with hypokalemic alkalosis and hypocalciuria. Mutations in genes encoding WNK kinases, WNK-1 and WNK-4, cause pseudohypoaldosteronism type II or Gordon's syndrome characterized by familial hypertension with hyperkalemia. WNK kinases influence the activity of several tubular ion transporters. Mutations in this disorder lead to overactivity of the apical Na^+/Cl^- co-transporter in the distal convoluted tubule as the primary stimulus for increased salt reabsorption, extracellular volume expansion, and hypertension. Hyperkalemia may be caused by diminished activity of apical K^+ channels in the collecting duct, a primary route for K^+ secretion.

COLLECTING DUCT

The collecting duct regulates the final composition of the urine. The two major divisions, the cortical collecting duct and inner medullary collecting duct, contribute to reabsorbing ~4–5% of filtered Na^+ and are important for hormonal regulation of salt and water balance. The cortical collecting duct contains a *high-resistance epithelia* with two cell types. Principal cells are the main Na^+ reabsorbing cells and the site of action of aldosterone, K^+-sparing diuretics, and spironolactone. The other cells are type A and B intercalated cells. Type A intercalated cells mediate acid secretion and bicarbonate reabsorption. Type B intercalated cells mediate bicarbonate secretion and acid reabsorption.

Virtually all transport is mediated through the cellular pathway for both principal cells and intercalated cells. In principal cells, passive apical Na^+ entry occurs through the amiloride-sensitive, epithelial Na^+ channel with basolateral exit via the Na^+/K^+-ATPase (Fig. 1-3E). This Na^+ reabsorptive process is tightly regulated by aldosterone.

Aldosterone enters the cell across the basolateral membrane, binds to a cytoplasmic mineralocorticoid receptor, and then translocates into the nucleus, where it modulates gene transcription, resulting in increased sodium reabsorption. Activating mutations in this epithelial Na^+ channel increase Na^+ reclamation and produce hypokalemia, hypertension, and metabolic alkalosis (Liddle's syndrome). The potassium-sparing diuretics amiloride and triamterene block the epithelial Na^+ channel causing reduced Na^+ reabsorption.

Principal cells secrete K^+ through an apical membrane potassium channel. Two forces govern the secretion of K^+. First, the high intracellular K^+ concentration generated by Na^+/K^+-ATPase creates a favorable concentration gradient for K^+ secretion into tubular fluid. Second, with reabsorption of Na^+ without an accompanying anion, the tubular lumen becomes negative relative to the cell interior, creating a favorable electrical gradient for secretion of cations. When Na^+ reabsorption is blocked, the electrical component of the driving force for K^+ secretion is blunted. K^+ secretion is also promoted by fast tubular fluid flow rates (which might occur during volume expansion or diuretics acting "upstream" of the cortical collecting duct), and the presence of relatively nonreabsorbable anions (including bicarbonate and penicillins) that contribute to the lumen-negative potential. Principal cells also participate in water reabsorption by increased water permeability in response to vasopressin; this effect is explained more fully below for the inner medullary collecting duct.

Intercalated cells do not participate in Na^+ reabsorption but instead mediate acid-base secretion. These cells perform two types of transport: active H^+ transport mediated by H^+-ATPase ("proton pump") and Cl^-/HCO_3^- exchanger. Intercalated cells arrange the two transport mechanisms on opposite membranes to enable either acid or base secretion. Type A intercalated cells have an apical proton pump that mediates acid secretion and a basolateral anion exchanger for mediating bicarbonate reabsorption (Fig. 1-3E). By contrast, type B intercalated cells have the anion exchanger on the apical membrane to mediate bicarbonate secretion while the proton pump resides on the basolateral membrane to enable acid reabsorption. Under conditions of acidemia, the kidney preferentially uses type A intercalated cells to secrete the excess H^+ and generate more HCO_3^-. The opposite is true in states of bicarbonate excess with alkalemia where the type B intercalated cells predominate. An extracellular protein called *hensin* mediates this adaptation.

Inner medullary collecting duct cells share many similarities with principal cells of the cortical collecting duct. They have apical Na^+ and K^+ channels that mediate Na^+ reabsorption and K^+ secretion, respectively (Fig. 1-3F). Inner medullary collecting duct cells also have vasopressin-regulated water channels (aquaporin-2 on the apical membrane, aquaporin-3 and -4 on the basolateral membrane). The antidiuretic hormone vasopressin binds to the V_2 receptor on the basolateral membrane and triggers an intracellular signaling cascade through G-protein–mediated activation of adenylyl cyclase, resulting in an increase in levels of cyclic AMP. This signaling cascade ultimately stimulates the insertion of water channels into the apical membrane of the inner medullary collecting duct cells to promote increased water permeability. This increase in permeability enables water reabsorption and production of concentrated urine. In the absence of vasopressin, inner medullary collecting duct cells are water impermeable, and urine remains dilute. Thus, the nephron separates NaCl from water so that considerations of volume or tonicity can determine whether to retain or excrete water.

Sodium reabsorption by inner medullary collecting duct cells is also inhibited by the natriuretic peptides called *atrial natriuretic peptide* or *renal natriuretic peptide* (urodilatin); the same gene encodes both peptides but uses different posttranslational processing of a common pre-prohormone to generate different proteins. Atrial natriuretic peptides are secreted by atrial myocytes in response to volume expansion, whereas urodilatin is secreted by renal tubular epithelia. Natriuretic peptides interact with either apical (urodilatin) or basolateral (atrial natriuretic peptides) receptors on inner medullary collecting duct cells to stimulate guanylyl cyclase and increase levels of cytoplasmic cyclic guanosine monophosphate (cGMP). This effect in turn reduces the activity of the apical Na^+ channel in these cells and attenuates net Na^+ reabsorption producing natriuresis. The inner medullary collecting duct is permeable to urea, allowing urea to diffuse into the interstitium, where it contributes to the hypertonicity of the medullary interstitium. Urea is recycled by diffusing from the interstitium into the descending and ascending limbs of the loop of Henle.

HORMONAL REGULATION OF SODIUM AND WATER BALANCE

The balance of solute and water in the body is determined by the amounts ingested, distributed to various fluid compartments, and excreted by skin, bowel, and kidneys. *Tonicity*, the osmolar state determining the volume behavior of cells in a solution, is regulated by water balance (**Fig. 1-4A**), and *extracellular blood volume* is regulated by Na^+ balance (**Fig. 1-4B**). The kidney is a critical modulator for both of these physiologic processes.

WATER BALANCE

Tonicity depends on the variable concentration of *effective osmoles* inside and outside the cell that cause water to move in either direction across its membrane. Classic

effective osmoles, like Na^+, K^+, and their anions, are solutes trapped on either side of a cell membrane, where they collectively partition and obligate water to move and find equilibrium in proportion to retained solute; Na^+/K^+-ATPase keeps most K^+ inside cells and most Na^+ outside. Normal tonicity (~280 mosmol/L) is rigorously defended by osmoregulatory mechanisms that control water balance to protect tissues from inadvertent *dehydration* (cell shrinkage) or *water intoxication* (cell swelling), both of which are deleterious to cell function (Fig. 1-4A).

The mechanisms that control osmoregulation are distinct from those governing extracellular volume, although there is some shared physiology in both processes. While cellular concentrations of K^+ have a determinant role in reaching any level of tonicity, the routine surrogate marker for assessing clinical tonicity is the concentration of serum Na^+. Any reduction in total body water, which raises the Na^+ concentration, triggers a brisk sense of thirst and conservation of water by decreasing renal water excretion mediated by release of vasopressin from the posterior pituitary. Conversely, a decrease in plasma Na^+ concentration triggers an increase in renal water excretion by suppressing the secretion of vasopressin. While all cells expressing mechanosensitive TRPV4 channels respond to changes in tonicity by altering their volume and Ca^{2+} concentration, only TRPV4$^+$ neuronal cells connected to the supraoptic and paraventricular nuclei in the hypothalamus are *osmoreceptive*; that is, they alone, because of their neural connectivity, modulate the release of vasopressin by the posterior lobe of the pituitary gland. Secretion is stimulated primarily by changing tonicity and secondarily by other nonosmotic signals, such as variable blood volume, stress, pain, and some drugs. The release of vasopressin by the posterior pituitary increases linearly as plasma tonicity rises above normal, although this varies depending on the perception of extracellular volume (one form of cross-talk between mechanisms that adjudicate blood volume and osmoregulation). Changing the intake or excretion of water provides a means for adjusting plasma tonicity; thus, osmoregulation governs water balance.

The kidneys play a vital role in maintaining water balance through their regulation of renal water excretion. The ability to concentrate urine to an osmolality exceeding that of plasma enables water conservation, while the ability to produce urine more dilute than plasma promotes excretion of excess water. Cell membranes are composed of lipids and other hydrophobic substances that are intrinsically impermeable to water. In order for water to enter or exit a cell, the cell membrane must express water channel aquaporins. In the kidney, aquaporin-1 is constitutively active in all water-permeable segments of the proximal and distal tubules, while aquaporins-2, -3, and -4 are regulated by vasopressin in the

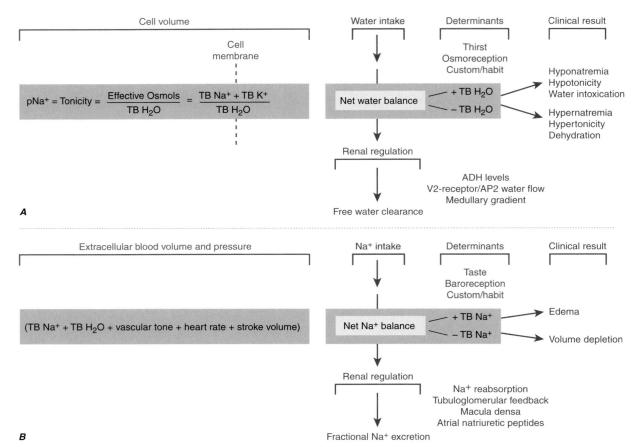

FIGURE 1-4

Determinants of sodium and water balance. A. Plasma Na$^+$ concentration is a surrogate marker for plasma tonicity, the volume behavior of cells in a solution. Tonicity is determined by the number of effective osmols in the body divided by the total body H$_2$O (TB H$_2$O), which translates simply into the total body Na (TB Na$^+$) and anions outside the cell separated from the total body K (TB K$^+$) inside the cell by the cell membrane. Net water balance is determined by the integrated functions of thirst, osmoreception, Na reabsorption, vasopressin release, and the strength of the medullary gradient in the kidney, keeping tonicity within a narrow range of osmolality around 280 mosmol. When water metabolism is disturbed and total-body water increases, hyponatremia, hypotonicity, and water intoxication occurs; when total-body water decreases, hypernatremia, hypertonicity, and dehydration occurs. **B.** Extracellular blood volume and pressure are an integrated function of total body Na$^+$ (TB Na$^+$), total body H$_2$O (TB H$_2$O), vascular tone, heart rate, and stroke volume that modulates volume and pressure in the vascular tree of the body. This extracellular blood volume is determined by net Na balance under the control of taste, baroreception, habit, Na$^+$ reabsorption, macula densa/tubuloglomerular feedback, and natriuretic peptides. When Na$^+$ metabolism is disturbed and total body Na$^+$ increases, edema occurs; when total body Na$^+$ is decreased, volume depletion occurs. ADH, antidiuretic hormone; AP2, aquaporin-2.

collecting duct. Vasopressin interacts with the V$_2$ receptor on basolateral membranes of collecting duct cells and signals the insertion of new water channels into apical membranes to promote water permeability. Net water reabsorption is ultimately driven by the osmotic gradient between dilute tubular fluid and a hypertonic medullary interstitium.

SODIUM BALANCE

The perception of *extracellular blood volume* is determined, in part, by the integration of arterial tone, cardiac stroke volume, heart rate, and the water and solute content of the extracellular volume. Na$^+$ and its anions are the most abundant extracellular effective osmoles, and together they support a blood volume around which pressure is generated. Under normal conditions, this volume is regulated by sodium balance (Fig. 1-4B), and the balance between daily Na$^+$ intake and excretion is under the influence of *baroreceptors* in regional blood vessels and vascular hormone-sensors modulated by atrial natriuretic peptides, the renin-angiotensin-aldosterone system, Ca^{2+} signaling, adenosine, vasopressin, and the neural adrenergic axis. If Na$^+$ intake exceeds Na$^+$ excretion (positive Na$^+$ balance), then an increase in blood volume will trigger a proportional increase in urinary

Na$^+$ excretion. Conversely, when Na$^+$ intake is less than urinary excretion (negative Na$^+$ balance), blood volume will decrease and trigger enhanced renal Na$^+$ reabsorption, leading to decreased urinary Na$^+$ excretion.

The renin-angiotensin-aldosterone system is the best-understood hormonal system modulating renal Na$^+$ excretion. Renin is synthesized and secreted by granular cells in the wall of the afferent arteriole. Its secretion is controlled by several factors, including β$_1$-adrenergic stimulation to the afferent arteriole, input from the macula densa, and prostaglandins. Renin and ACE activity eventually produce angiotensin II, which directly or indirectly promotes renal Na$^+$ and water reabsorption. Stimulation of proximal tubular Na$^+$/H$^+$ exchange by angiotensin II directly increases Na$^+$ reabsorption. Angiotensin II also promotes Na$^+$ reabsorption along the collecting duct by stimulating aldosterone secretion by the adrenal cortex. Constriction of the efferent glomerular arteriole by angiotensin II indirectly increases the filtration fraction and raises peritubular capillary oncotic pressure to promote Na$^+$ reabsorption. Finally, angiotensin II inhibits renin secretion through a negative feedback loop.

Aldosterone is synthesized and secreted by granulosa cells in the adrenal cortex. It binds to cytoplasmic mineralocorticoid receptors in principal cells of the collecting duct that increase the activity of the apical membrane Na$^+$ channel, apical membrane K$^+$ channel, and basolateral Na$^+$/K$^+$-ATPase. These effects are mediated in part by aldosterone-stimulated transcription of the gene encoding serum/glucocorticoid-induced kinase 1 (SGK1). The activity of the epithelial Na$^+$ channel is increased by SGK1-mediated phosphorylation of Nedd4-2, a protein that promotes recycling of the Na$^+$ channel from the plasma membrane. Phosphorylated Nedd4-2 has impaired interactions with the epithelial Na$^+$ channel, leading to increased channel density at the plasma membrane and increased capacity for Na$^+$ reabsorption by the collecting duct.

Chronic overexpression of aldosterone causes a decrease in urinary Na$^+$ excretion lasting only a few days, after which Na$^+$ excretion returns to previous levels. This phenomenon, called *aldosterone escape*, is explained by decreased proximal tubular Na$^+$ reabsorption following blood volume expansion. Excess Na$^+$ that is not reabsorbed by the proximal tubule overwhelms the reabsorptive capacity of more distal nephron segments. This escape may be facilitated by atrial natriuretic peptides, which lose their effectiveness in the clinical settings of heart failure, nephrotic syndrome, and cirrhosis, leading to severe Na$^+$ retention and volume overload.

FURTHER READINGS

BALLERMANN BJ: Glomerular endothelial cell differentiation. Kidney Int 67:1668, 2005

DRESSLER GR: Epigenetics, development, and the kidney. J Am Soc Nephrol 19:2060, 2008

FOGELGREN B et al: Deficiency in Six2 during prenatal development is associated with reduced nephron number, chronic renal failure, and hypertension in Br/+ adult mice. Am J Physiol Renal Physiol 296:F1166, 2009

GIEBISCH G et al: New aspects of renal potassium transport. Pflugers Arch 446:289, 2003

KOPAN R et al: Molecular insights into segmentation along the proximal-distal axis of the nephron. J Am Soc Nephrol 18:2014, 2007

KRAMER BK et al: Mechanisms of disease: The kidney-specific chloride channels ClCKA and ClCKB, the Barttin subunit, and their clinical relevance. Nat Clin Pract Nephrol 4:38, 2008

RIBES D et al: Transcriptional control of epithelial differentiation during kidney development. J Am Soc Nephrol 14:S9, 2003

SAUTER A et al: Development of renin expression in the mouse kidney. Kidney Int 73:43, 2008

SCHRIER RW, ECDER T: Gibbs memorial lecture: Unifying hypothesis of body fluid volume regulation. Mt Sinai J Med 68:350, 2001

TAKABATAKE Y et al: The CXCL12 (SDF-1)/CXCR4 axis is essential for the development of renal vasculature. J Am Soc Nephrol 20:1714, 2009

WAGNER CA et al: Renal acid-base transport: Old and new players. Nephron Physiol 103:1, 2006

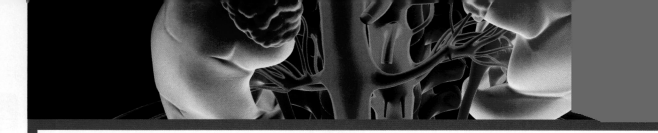

CHAPTER 2

ADAPTATION OF THE KIDNEY TO RENAL INJURY

Raymond C. Harris, Jr. ■ Eric G. Neilson

The size of a kidney and the number of nephrons formed late in embryological development depend on the frequency with which the ureteric bud undergoes branching morphogenesis. Humans have between 225,000 and 900,000 nephrons in each kidney, a number that mathematically hinges on whether ureteric branching goes to completion or is prematurely terminated by one or two cycles. Although the signaling mechanism regulating cycle number is unknown, these final rounds of branching likely determine how well the kidney will adapt to the physiologic demands of blood pressure and body size, various environmental stresses, or unwanted inflammation leading to chronic renal failure.

One of the intriguing generalities made in the course of studying chronic renal failure is that residual nephrons hyperfunction to compensate for the loss of those nephrons falling to primary disease. This compensation depends on adaptive changes produced by renal hypertrophy and adjustments in *tubuloglomerular feedback* and *glomerulotubular balance*, as advanced in the *intact nephron hypothesis* by Neal Bricker in 1969. Some physiologic adaptations to nephron loss also produce unintended clinical consequences explained by Bricker's *trade-off hypothesis* in 1972, and eventually some adaptations accelerate the deterioration of residual nephrons,

as described by Barry Brenner in his *hyperfiltration hypothesis* in 1982. These three important notions regarding chronic renal failure form a conceptual foundation for understanding common pathophysiology leading to uremia.

COMMON MECHANISMS OF PROGRESSIVE RENAL DISEASE

When the initial complement of nephrons is reduced by a sentinel event, like unilateral nephrectomy, the remaining kidney adapts by enlarging and increasing its glomerular filtration rate (GFR). If the kidneys were initially normal, the GFR usually returns to 80% of normal for two kidneys. The remaining kidney grows by *compensatory renal hypertrophy* with very little cellular proliferation. This unique event is accomplished by increasing the size of each cell along the nephron, which is accommodated by the elasticity or growth of interstitial spaces and the renal capsule. The mechanism of this compensatory renal hypertrophy is only partially understood, but the signals for the remaining kidney to hypertrophy may rest with the local expression of angiotensin II; transforming growth factor β (TGF-β); p27[kip1], a cell cycle protein that prevents tubular cells exposed to angiotensin II from proliferating; and epidermal growth factor (EGF), which induces the mammalian target of rapamycin (mTOR) to engage a transcriptome supporting new protein synthesis.

Hyperfiltration during pregnancy, or in humans born with one kidney or who lose one to trauma or transplantation, generally leads to no ill consequences. By contrast, experimental animals who undergo resection of 80% of their renal mass, or humans who have persistent injury that destroys a comparable amount of renal tissue, progress to end-stage disease (**Fig. 2-1**). Clearly there is a critical amount of primary nephron loss that produces a maladaptive deterioration in the remaining nephrons. This maladaptive response is referred to clinically as *renal progression*, and the pathologic correlate of renal progression is *relentless tubular atrophy* and *tissue fibrosis*. The mechanism for this maladaptive response has been the focus of intense investigation. A unified theory of renal progression is just starting to emerge, and, most importantly, this progression follows a final common pathway regardless of whether renal injury begins in glomeruli or within the tubulointerstitium.

There are six mechanisms that hypothetically unify this final common pathway. If injury begins in glomeruli, these sequential steps build on each other: (1) Persistent glomerular injury produces local hypertension in capillary tufts, increases their single-nephron GFR, and engenders protein leak into the tubular fluid. (2) Significant glomerular proteinuria, accompanied by increases in the local production of angiotensin II, facilitates (3) a downstream cytokine bath that induces an accumulation of interstitial mononuclear cells. (4) The initial appearance of interstitial neutrophils is quickly replaced by gathering macrophages and T lymphocytes that form a nephritogenic immune response producing interstitial nephritis. (5) Some tubular epithelia respond to this inflammation by disaggregating from their basement membrane and adjacent sister cells to undergo *epithelial-mesenchymal transitions* forming new interstitial fibroblasts. (6) Finally, surviving fibroblasts lay down a collagenous matrix that disrupts adjacent capillaries and tubular nephrons, eventually leaving an acellular scar. The details of these complex events are outlined in **Fig. 2-2**.

Significant ablation of renal mass results in *hyperfiltration* characterized by an increase in the rate of *single-nephron glomerular filtration*. The remaining nephrons lose their ability to autoregulate, and systemic hypertension is transmitted to the glomerulus. Both the hyperfiltration and *intraglomerular hypertension* stimulate the eventual appearance of glomerulosclerosis. Angiotensin II acts as an essential mediator of increased *intraglomerular capillary pressure* by selectively increasing efferent arteriolar vasoconstriction relative to afferent arteriolar tone. Angiotensin II impairs glomerular size-selectivity, induces protein ultrafiltration, and increases intracellular Ca^{2+} in podocytes, which alters podocyte function. Diverse vasoconstrictor mechanisms, including blockade of nitric oxide synthase and activation of angiotensin II and thromboxane receptors, can also induce oxidative stress in surrounding renal tissue. Finally, the effects of aldosterone on increasing renal vascular resistance and glomerular capillary pressure, or stimulating plasminogen activator inhibitor-1, facilitate fibrogenesis and complement the detrimental activity of angiotensin II.

On occasion, inflammation that begins in the renal interstitium disables tubular reclamation of filtered protein, producing mild nonselective proteinuria. Renal inflammation that initially damages glomerular capillaries often spreads to the tubulointerstitium in association with heavier proteinuria. Many clinical observations support the association of worsening *glomerular proteinuria* with renal progression. The simplest explanation for this expansion is that increasingly severe proteinuria triggers a downstream inflammatory cascade around epithelia that line the nephron, producing interstitial nephritis, fibrosis, and tubular atrophy. As albumin is an abundant polyanion in plasma and can bind a variety of cytokines, chemokines, and lipid mediators, it might be that these small molecules carried by albumin initiate the tubular inflammation brought on by proteinuria. Furthermore, glomerular injury either adds activated mediators to the proteinuric filtrate or alters the balance of cytokine inhibitors and activators such that attainment of a critical level of activated cytokines eventually damages downstream tubular epithelia.

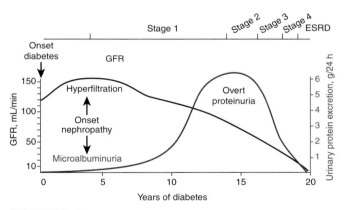

FIGURE 2-1

Progression of chronic renal injury. Although various types of renal injury have their own unique rates of progression, one of the best understood is that associated with Type 1 diabetic nephropathy. Notice the early increase in glomerular filtration rate (GFR), followed by inexorable decline associated with increasing proteinuria. Also indicated is the National Kidney Foundation K/DOQI classification of the stages of chronic kidney disease. ESRD, end-stage renal disease.

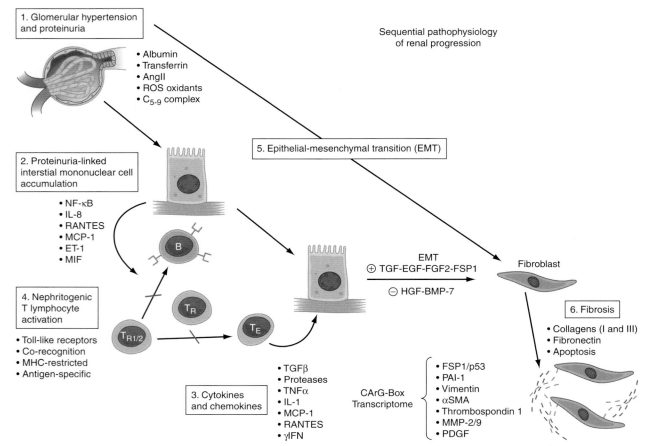

Sequential pathophysiology
of renal progression

1. Glomerular hypertension
and proteinuria

• Albumin
• Transferrin
• AngII
• ROS oxidants
• C$_{5-9}$ complex

2. Proteinuria-linked
interstial mononuclear cell
accumulation

• NF-κB
• IL-8
• RANTES
• MCP-1
• ET-1
• MIF

4. Nephritogenic
T lymphocyte
activation

• Toll-like receptors
• Co-recognition
• MHC-restricted
• Antigen-specific

3. Cytokines
and chemokines

• TGFβ
• Proteases
• TNFα
• IL-1
• MCP-1
• RANTES
• γIFN

5. Epithelial-mesenchymal transition (EMT)

EMT
⊕ TGF-EGF-FGF2-FSP1
⊖ HGF-BMP-7

Fibroblast

6. Fibrosis

• Collagens (I and III)
• Fibronectin
• Apoptosis

CArG-Box
Transcriptome

• FSP1/p53
• PAI-1
• Vimentin
• αSMA
• Thrombospondin 1
• MMP-2/9
• PDGF

FIGURE 2-2

Mechanisms of renal progression. The general mechanisms of renal progression advance sequentially through six
stages that include hyperfiltration, proteinuria, cytokine bath,
mononuclear cell infiltration, epithelial-mesenchymal transition, and fibrosis. *(Modified from Harris and Neilson.)*

Tubular epithelia bathed in these complex mixtures
of proteinuric cytokines respond by increasing their
secretion of chemokines and relocating nuclear factor
κB to the nucleus to induce proinflammatory release of
TGF-β, platelet-derived growth factor B (PDGF-BB),
and fibroblast growth factor 2 (FGF-2). Inflammatory
cells are drawn into the renal interstitium by this
cytokine milieu. This interstitial spreading reduces the
likelihood that the kidney will survive. The immunologic mechanisms for spreading include loss of tolerance
to parenchymal self, immune deposits that share cross-
reactive epitopes in either compartment, or glomerular
injury that reveals a new interstitial epitope. Drugs,
infection, and metabolic defects may also induce
autoimmunity through Toll-like receptors that bind to
moieties with an immunologically distinct molecular
pattern. Bacterial and viral ligands do so, but, interestingly, so do Tamm-Horsfall protein, bacterial CpG
repeats, and RNA that is released nonspecifically from
injured tubular cells. Dendritic cells and macrophages
are subsequently activated, and circulating T cells engage
in the formal cellular immunologic response.

Nephritogenic interstitial T cells are a mix of CD4$^+$
helper and CD8$^+$ cytotoxic lymphocytes. Presumptive
evidence of antigen-driven T cells found by examining
the DNA sequence of T-cell receptors suggests a polyclonal expansion that responds to multiple epitopes.
Some experimental interstitial lesions are histologically
analogous to a cutaneous delayed-type hypersensitivity
reaction, and more intense reactions sometimes induce
granuloma formation. The cytotoxic activity of antigen-
reactive T cells probably accounts for tubular cell
destruction and atrophy. Cytotoxic T cells synthesize
proteins with serine esterase activity as well as pore-
forming proteins, which can affect membrane damage
much like the activated membrane attack complex of
the complement cascade. Such enzymatic activity provides a structural explanation for target cell lysis.

One long-term consequence of tubular epithelia
exposed to cytokines is the profibrotic activation of
epithelial-mesenchymal transition. Persistent cytokine
activity during renal inflammation and disruption of
underlying basement membrane by local proteases initiates the process of transition. Rather than collapsing into

the tubular lumens and dying, some epithelia become fibroblasts while translocating back into the interstitial space behind deteriorating tubules through holes in the ruptured basement membrane. Wnt proteins, integrin-linked kinases, insulin-like growth factors, EGF, FGF-2, and TGF-β are among the classic modulators of epithelial-mesenchymal transition. Fibroblasts that deposit collagen during fibrogenesis also replicate locally at sites of persistent inflammation. Estimates indicate that half of the total fibroblasts found in fibrotic renal tissues are products of the proliferation of newly transitioned or preexisting fibroblasts. Fibroblasts are stimulated to multiply by activation of cognate cell-surface receptors for PDGF and TGF-β.

Tubulointerstitial scars are composed principally of fibronectin, collagen types I and III, and tenascin, but other glycoproteins such as thrombospondin, SPARC, osteopontin, and proteoglycan may be also important. Although tubular epithelia can synthesize collagens I and III and are modulated by a variety of growth factors, these epithelia disappear through transition and tubular atrophy, leaving fibroblasts as the major contributor to matrix production. After fibroblasts acquire a synthetic phenotype, expand their population, and locally migrate around areas of inflammation, they begin to deposit fibronectin, which provides a scaffold for interstitial collagens. When fibroblasts outdistance their survival factors, they die from apoptosis, leaving an acellular scar.

Angiotensin II incrementally vasoconstricts the efferent arteriole, and studies in animals and humans demonstrate that interruption of the renin-angiotensin system with either angiotensin-converting inhibitors or angiotensin II receptor blockers will decrease intraglomerular capillary pressure, decrease proteinuria, and slow the rate of nephron destruction. The vasoconstrictive agent, endothelin, has also been implicated in hyperfiltration, and increases in afferent vasodilatation have been attributed, at least in part, to local prostaglandins and release of endothelium-derived nitric oxide. Finally, hyperfiltration may be mediated in part by a resetting of the kidney's intrinsic autoregulatory mechanism of glomerular filtration by a *tubuloglomerular feedback system*. This feedback originates from the macula densa and modulates renal blood flow and glomerular filtration (Chap. 1).

Even with the loss of functioning nephrons, there is some continued maintenance of *glomerulotubular balance*, by which the residual tubules adapt to increases in single-nephron glomerular filtration with appropriate alterations in reabsorption or excretion of filtered water and solutes in order to maintain homeostasis. Glomerulotubular balance results both from tubular hypertrophy and from regulatory adjustments in tubular oncotic pressure or solute transport along the proximal tubule. Some studies have indicated that these alterations in tubule size and function may themselves be maladaptive and, as a trade-off, predispose to further tubule injury.

RESPONSE TO REDUCTION IN NUMBERS OF FUNCTIONING NEPHRONS

The response to the loss of functioning nephrons produces an increase in renal blood flow with glomerular hyperfiltration. Hyperfiltration is the result of increased vasoconstriction in postglomerular efferent arterioles relative to preglomerular afferent arterioles, increasing the intraglomerular capillary pressure and filtration fraction. The discovery of this intraglomerular hypertension and the demonstration that maneuvers decrease its effect abrogates further expression of glomerular and tubulointerstitial injury led to the formulation of the hyperfiltration hypothesis. The hypothesis explains why residual nephrons in the setting of persistent disease will first stabilize or increase the rate of glomerular filtration, only to succumb later to inexorable deterioration and progression to renal failure. Persistent intraglomerular hypertension is critical to this transition.

Although the hormonal and metabolic factors mediating hyperfiltration are not fully understood, a number of vasoconstrictive and vasodilatory substances have been implicated, chief among them being angiotensin II.

TUBULAR FUNCTION IN CHRONIC RENAL FAILURE

SODIUM

Na^+ ions are reclaimed along most of the nephron by various transport mechanisms (Chap. 1). This transport function and its contribution to extracellular blood volume is usually maintained near normal until limitations from advanced renal disease can no longer keep up with dietary Na^+ intake. Prior to this point in the spectrum of renal progression, increasing the fractional excretion of Na^+ in final urine at reduced rates of glomerular filtration provides a mechanism of early adaptation. Na^+ excretion increases predominantly by decreasing Na^+ reabsorption in the loop of Henle and distal nephron. Increases in the osmotic obligation of residual nephrons lower the concentration of Na^+ in tubular fluid, and increased excretion of inorganic and organic anions obligates more Na^+ excretion. In addition, hormonal influences, notably increased expression of atrial natriuretic peptides that increase distal Na^+ excretion, as well as levels of GFR, play an important role in maintaining adequate Na^+ excretion. Although many details of these adjustments are only understood conceptually, it is an example of a trade-off by which initial adjustments following the loss of functioning nephrons lead to compensatory responses that maintain homeostasis. Eventually, with advancing nephron loss, the atrial natriuretic peptides lose their effectiveness, and Na^+ retention results in intravascular volume expansion, edema, and worsening hypertension.

URINARY DILUTION AND CONCENTRATION

Patients with progressive renal injury gradually lose the capacity either to dilute or concentrate their urine, and urine osmolality becomes relatively fixed around 350 mosmol/L (specific gravity approximating 1.010). Although the ability of a single nephron to excrete water free of solute may not be impaired, the reduced number of functioning nephrons obligates increased fractional solute excretion by residual nephrons, and this greater obligation impairs the ability to dilute tubular fluid maximally. Similarly, urinary concentrating ability falls due to the need for more water to hydrate the increased solute load. Tubulointerstitial damage also creates insensitivity to the antidiuretic effects of vasopressin along the collecting duct or loss of the medullary gradient, which eventually disturbs control of variation in urine osmolality. Patients with moderate degrees of chronic renal failure often complain of *nocturia* as a manifestation of this fixed urine osmolality and are prone to extracellular volume depletion if they do not keep up with the persistent loss of Na^+, or hypotonicity if they drink too much water.

POTASSIUM

Renal excretion is a major pathway for reducing excess total-body K^+. Normally, the kidney excretes 90% of dietary K^+, while 10% is excreted in the stool, with a trivial amount lost to sweat. Although the colon possesses some capacity to increase K^+ excretion—up to 30% of ingested K^+ may be excreted in the stool of patients with worsening renal failure—the majority of the K^+ load continues to be excreted by the kidneys due to elevation in levels of serum K^+ that increase this filtered load. Aldosterone also regulates collecting duct Na^+ reabsorption and K^+ secretion. Aldosterone is released from the adrenal cortex not only in response to the renin-angiotensin system but also in direct response to elevated levels of serum K^+, and for a while a compensatory increase in the capacity of the collecting duct to secrete K^+ keeps up with renal progression. As serum K^+ levels rise with renal failure, circulating levels of aldosterone also increase

over what is required to maintain normal levels of blood volume.

ACID-BASE REGULATION

The kidneys excrete 1 meq/kg per day of noncarbonic H^+ ion on a normal diet. To do this, all of the filtered HCO_3^{2-} needs to be reabsorbed proximally so that H^+ pumps in the intercalated cells of the collecting duct can secrete H^+ ions that are subsequently trapped by urinary buffers, particularly phosphates and ammonia (Chap. 1). While remaining nephrons increase their solute load with loss of renal mass, the ability to maintain total-body H^+ excretion is often impaired by the gradual loss of H^+ pumps or with reductions in ammoniagenesis leading to development of a non-delta acidosis. Although hypertrophy of the proximal tubules initially increases their ability to reabsorb filtered HCO_3^{2-} and increase ammoniagenesis, with progressive loss of nephrons this compensation is eventually overwhelmed. In addition, with advancing renal failure, ammoniagenesis is further inhibited by elevation in levels of serum K^+, producing type IV renal tubular acidosis. Once the GFR falls below 25 mL/min, organic acids accumulate, producing a delta metabolic acidosis. Hyperkalemia can also inhibit tubular HCO_3^{2-} reabsorption, as can extracellular volume expansion and elevated levels of parathyroid hormone (PTH). Eventually, as the kidneys fail, the level of serum HCO_3^{2-} falls severely, reflecting the exhaustion of all body buffer systems, including bone.

CALCIUM AND PHOSPHATE

The kidney and gut play an important role in the regulation of serum levels of Ca^{2+} and PO_4^{2-}. With decreasing renal function and the appearance of tubulointerstitial nephritis, the expression of α_1-hydroxylase by the proximal tubule is reduced, lowering levels of calcitriol and Ca^{2+} absorption by the gut. Loss of nephron mass with progressive renal failure also gradually reduces the excretion of PO_4^{2-} and Ca^{2+}, and elevations in serum PO_4^{2-} further lower serum levels of Ca^{2+}, causing sustained secretion of PTH. Unregulated increases in levels of PTH cause Ca^{2+} mobilization from bone, Ca^{2+}/PO_4^{2-} precipitation in tissues, abnormal bone remodeling, decreases in tubular bicarbonate reabsorption, and increases in renal PO_4^{2-} excretion. While elevated serum levels of PTH initially maintain serum PO_4^{2-} near normal, with progressive nephron destruction the capacity for renal PO_4^{2-} excretion is overwhelmed, the serum PO_4^{2-} elevates, and bone is progressively demineralized from secondary hyperparathyroidism. These adaptations evoke another classic functional trade-off (**Fig. 2-3**).

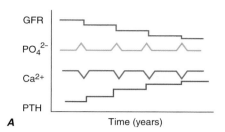

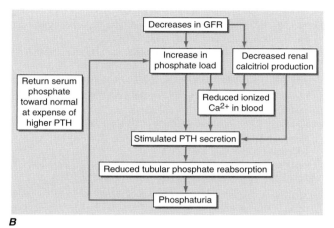

A

B

FIGURE 2-3

The "trade-off hypothesis" for Ca²⁺/PO₄²⁻ homeostasis with progressively declining renal function. A. How adaptation to maintain Ca²⁺/PO₄²⁻ homeostasis leads to increasing levels of parathyroid hormone ("classic" presentation from E Slatopolsky, NS Bricker: The role of phosphorous restriction in the prevention of secondary hyperparathyroidism in chronic renal disease. Kidney Int 4:141, 1973). **B.** Current understanding of the underlying mechanisms for this Ca²⁺/PO₄²⁻ trade-off. GFR, glomerular filtration rate; PTH, parathyroid hormone.

MODIFIERS INFLUENCING THE PROGRESSION OF RENAL DISEASE

Well-described risk factors for the progressive loss of renal function include systemic hypertension, diabetes, and activation of the renin-angiotensin-aldosterone system (Table 2-1). Poor glucose control will aggravate renal progression in both diabetic and nondiabetic renal disease. Angiotensin II produces intraglomerular hypertension and stimulates fibrogenesis. Aldosterone also serves as an independent fibrogenic mediator of progressive nephron loss apart from its role in modulating Na⁺ and K⁺ homeostasis.

Lifestyle choices also have an impact on the progression of renal disease. Cigarette smoking has been shown to either predispose or accelerate the progression of nephron loss. Whether the effect of cigarettes is related to systemic hemodynamic alterations or specific damage to the renal microvasculature and/or tubules is unclear. Lipid oxidation associated with obesity or central adiposity can

TABLE 2-1

19

CHAPTER 2

Adaptation of the Kidney to Renal Injury

POTENTIAL MODIFIERS OF RENAL DISEASE PROGRESSION	
Hypertension	Hyperlipidemia
RAS activation	Abnormal calcium/phosphorus
Angiotensin II	homeostasis
Aldosterone	Cigarette smoking
Diabetes	Intrinsic paucity in nephron number
Obesity	Prematurity/low birth weight
Excessive dietary	Genetic predisposition
protein	Undefined genetic factors

also accelerate cardiovascular disease and progressive renal damage. Recent epidemiologic studies confirm an association between high-protein diets and progression of renal disease. Progressive nephron loss in experimental animals, and possibly in humans, can be slowed by adherence to a low-protein diet. Although a large multicenter trial, the Modification of Diet in Renal Disease, did not provide conclusive evidence that dietary protein restriction could retard progression to renal failure, secondary analyses and a number of meta-analyses suggest a renoprotective effect from supervised low-protein diets in the range of 0.6–0.75 g/kg per day. Abnormal Ca²⁺ and PO₄²⁻ metabolism in chronic kidney disease also plays a role in renal progression, and administration of calcitriol or its analogues can attenuate progression in a variety of models of chronic kidney disease.

An intrinsic paucity in the number of functioning nephrons predisposes to the development of renal disease. A reduced number of nephrons can lead to permanent hypertension, either through direct renal damage or hyperfiltration producing glomerulosclerosis, or by primary induction of systemic hypertension that further exacerbates glomerular barotrauma. Younger individuals with hypertension who died suddenly as a result of trauma have 47% fewer glomeruli per kidney than age-matched controls.

A consequence of low birth weight is a relative deficit in the number of total nephrons; low birth weight is associated in adulthood with more hypertension and renal failure, among other abnormalities. In this regard, in addition to or instead of a genetic predisposition to development of a specific disease or condition such as low birth weight, different epigenetic phenomena may produce varying clinical phenotypes from a single genotype, depending on maternal exposure to different environmental stimuli during gestation, a phenomenon known as *developmental plasticity*. A specific clinical phenotype can also be selected in response to an adverse environmental exposure during critical periods of intrauterine development, also known as *fetal programming*. In the United States there is at least a twofold increased incidence of low birth weight among African Americans compared with Caucasians, much but not all of which can be attributed to maternal age, health, or socioeconomic status.

As in other conditions producing nephron loss, the glomeruli of low-birth-weight individuals are enlarged and associated with early hyperfiltration to maintain normal levels of renal function. With time, the resulting intraglomerular hypertension may initiate a progressive decline in residual hyperfunctioning nephrons, ultimately accelerating renal failure. In African Americans, as well as other populations at increased risk for kidney failure, such as Pima Indians and Australian aborigines, large glomeruli are seen at early stages of kidney disease. An association between low birth weight and the development of albuminuria and nephropathy has been reported for both diabetic and nondiabetic renal disease.

FURTHER READINGS

BRENNER BM: Remission of renal disease: Recounting the challenge, acquiring the goal. J Clin Invest 110:1753, 2002

CHRISTENSEN EI et al: Interstitial fibrosis: Tubular hypothesis versus glomerular hypothesis. Kidney Int 74:1233, 2008

HARRIS RC, NEILSON EG: Towards a unified theory of renal progression. Ann Rev Med 57:365, 2006

ISEKI K: Factors influencing the development of end-stage renal disease. Clin Exp Nephrol 9:5, 2005

KNIGHT SF et al: Endothelial dysfunction and the development of renal injury in spontaneously hypertensive rats fed a high-fat diet. Hypertension 51:352, 2008

LIAO TD et al: Role of inflammation in the development of renal damage and dysfunction in angiotensin II–induced hypertension. Hypertension 52:256, 2008

LLACH F: Secondary hyperparathyroidism in renal failure: The trade-off hypothesis revisited. Am J Kidney Dis 25:663, 1995

LUYCKX VA, BRENNER BM: Low birth weight, nephron number, and kidney disease. Kidney Int 68:S68, 2005

MEYER TW: Tubular injury in glomerular disease. Kidney Int 63:774, 2003

PHOON RK et al: T-bet deficiency attenuates renal injury in experimental crescentic glomerulonephritis. J Am Soc Nephrol 19:477, 2008

SATAKE A et al: Protective effect of 17beta-estradiol on ischemic acute renal failure through the PI3K/Akt/eNOS pathway. Kidney Int 73:308, 2008

SLATOPOLSKY E et al: Calcium, phosphorus and vitamin D disorders in uremia. Contrib Nephrol 149:261, 2005

WONG MG et al: Peritubular ischemia contributes more to tubular damage than proteinuria in immune-mediated glomerulonephritis. J Am Soc Nephrol 19:290, 2008

ZANDI-NEJAD K et al: Adult hypertension and kidney disease: The role of fetal programming. Hypertension 47:502, 2006

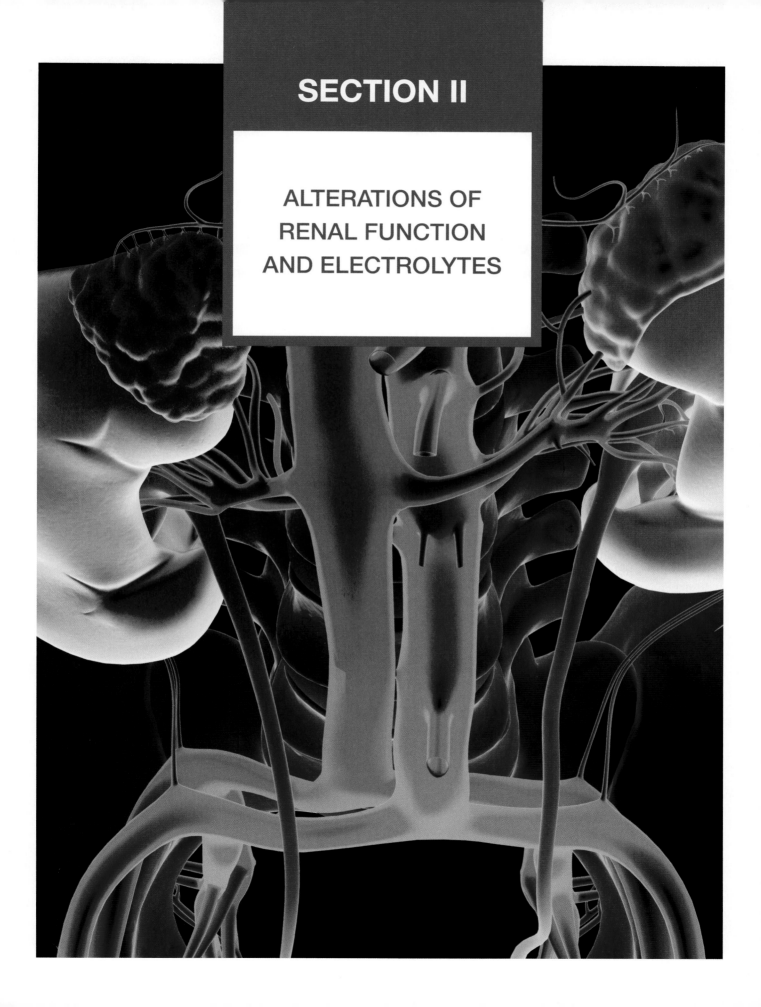

SECTION II

ALTERATIONS OF RENAL FUNCTION AND ELECTROLYTES

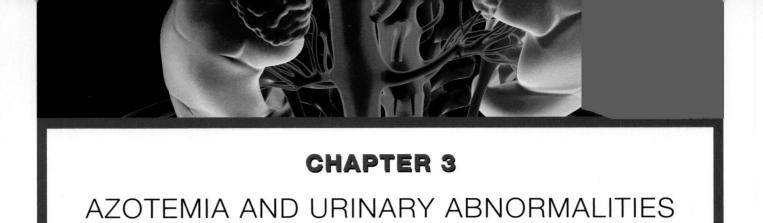

CHAPTER 3

AZOTEMIA AND URINARY ABNORMALITIES

Bradley M. Denker ■ Barry M. Brenner

Normal kidney functions occur through numerous cellular processes to maintain body homeostasis. Disturbances in any of these functions can lead to a constellation of abnormalities that may be detrimental to survival. The clinical manifestations of these disorders will depend upon the pathophysiology of the renal injury and will often be initially identified as a complex of symptoms, abnormal physical findings, and laboratory changes that together make possible the identification of specific syndromes. These renal syndromes (Table 3-1) may arise as the consequence of a systemic illness or can occur as a primary renal disease. Nephrologic syndromes usually consist of several elements that reflect the underlying pathologic processes. The duration and severity of the disease will affect these findings and typically include one or more of the following: (1) disturbances in urine volume (oliguria, anuria, polyuria); (2) abnormalities of urine sediment [red blood cells (RBC); white blood cells, casts, and crystals]; (3) abnormal excretion of serum proteins (proteinuria); (4) reduction in glomerular filtration rate (GFR) (azotemia); (5) presence of hypertension and/or expanded total body fluid volume (edema); (6) electrolyte abnormalities; or (7) in some syndromes, fever/pain. The combination of these findings should permit identification of one of the major nephrologic syndromes (Table 3-1) and will allow differential diagnoses to be narrowed and the appropriate diagnostic evaluation and therapeutic course to be determined. Each of these

syndromes and their associated diseases are discussed in more detail in subsequent chapters. This chapter focuses on several aspects of renal abnormalities that are critically important to distinguishing among these processes: (1) reduction in GFR leading to azotemia, (2) alterations of the urinary sediment and/or protein excretion, and (3) abnormalities of urinary volume.

AZOTEMIA

ASSESSMENT OF GLOMERULAR FILTRATION RATE

Monitoring the GFR is important in both the hospital and outpatient settings, and several different methodologies are available. In most acute clinical circumstances a measured GFR is not available, and the serum creatinine level is used to estimate the GFR in order to supply appropriate doses of renally excreted drugs and to follow short-term changes in GFR. Serum creatinine is the most widely used marker for GFR, and the GFR is directly related to the urine creatinine excretion and inversely to the serum creatinine (U_{Cr}/P_{Cr}). The creatinine clearance is calculated from these measurements for a defined time period (usually 24 h) and is expressed in mL/min. Based upon this relationship and some important caveats, the GFR will fall in roughly inverse proportion to the rise in P_{Cr}. Failure to account for

TABLE 3-1 23

INITIAL CLINICAL AND LABORATORY DATA BASE FOR DEFINING MAJOR SYNDROMES IN NEPHROLOGY

SYNDROMES	IMPORTANT CLUES TO DIAGNOSIS	FINDINGS THAT ARE COMMON
Acute or rapidly progressive renal failure	Anuria Oliguria Documented recent decline in GFR	Hypertension, hematuria Proteinuria, pyuria Casts, edema
Acute nephritis	Hematuria, RBC casts Azotemia, oliguria Edema, hypertension	Proteinuria Pyuria Circulatory congestion
Chronic renal failure	Azotemia for >3 months Prolonged symptoms or signs of uremia Symptoms or signs of renal osteodystrophy Kidneys reduced in size bilaterally Broad casts in urinary sediment	Proteinuria Casts Polyuria, nocturia Edema, hypertension Electrolyte disorders
Nephrotic syndrome	Proteinuria >3.5 g per 1.73 m² per 24 h Hypoalbuminemia Edema Hyperlipidemia	Casts Lipiduria
Asymptomatic urinary abnormalities	Hematuria Proteinuria (below nephrotic range) Sterile pyuria, casts	
Urinary tract infection/ pyelonephritis	Bacteriuria >10⁵ colonies per milliliter Other infectious agent documented in urine Pyuria, leukocyte casts Frequency, urgency Bladder tenderness, flank tenderness	Hematuria Mild azotemia Mild proteinuria Fever
Renal tubule defects	Electrolyte disorders Polyuria, nocturia Renal calcification Large kidneys Renal transport defects	Hematuria "Tubular" proteinuria (<1 g/24 h) Enuresis
Hypertension	Systolic/diastolic hypertension	Proteinuria Casts Azotemia
Nephrolithiasis	Previous history of stone passage or removal Previous history of stone seen by x-ray Renal colic	Hematuria Pyuria Frequency, urgency
Urinary tract obstruction	Azotemia, oliguria, anuria Polyuria, nocturia, urinary retention Slowing of urinary stream Large prostate, large kidneys Flank tenderness, full bladder after voiding	Hematuria Pyuria Enuresis, dysuria

Note: GFR, glomerular filtration rate; RBC, red blood cell.

GFR reductions in drug dosing can lead to significant morbidity and mortality from drug toxicities (e.g., digoxin, aminoglycosides). In the outpatient setting, the serum creatinine is often used as a surrogate for GFR (although much less accurate). In patients with chronic progressive renal disease there is an approximately linear relationship between $1/P_{Cr}$ and time. The slope of this line will remain constant for an individual patient, and when values are obtained that do not fall on this line, an investigation for a superimposed acute process (e.g., volume depletion, drug reaction) should be initiated. It should be emphasized that the signs and symptoms of uremia will develop at significantly different levels of serum creatinine depending upon the patient (weight, age, and sex), the underlying renal disease, existence of concurrent diseases, and true GFR. In general, patients do not develop symptomatic uremia until renal insufficiency is usually quite severe (GFR <15 mL/min).

A reduced GFR leads to retention of nitrogenous waste products (azotemia) such as urea and creatinine.

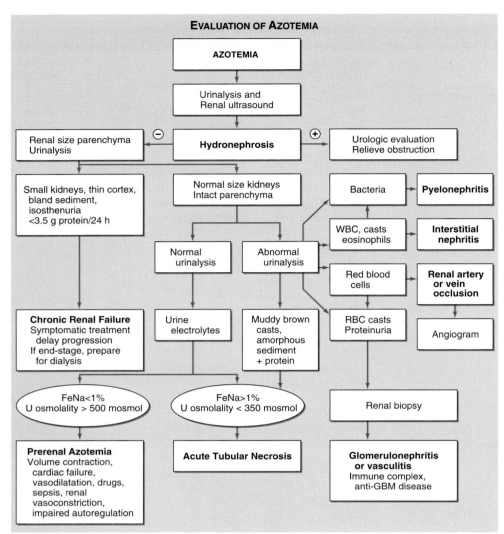

EVALUATION OF AZOTEMIA

FIGURE 3-1

Approach to the patient with azotemia. WBC, white blood cell; RBC, red blood cell; GBM, glomerular basement membrane.

Azotemia may result from reduced renal perfusion, intrinsic renal disease, or postrenal processes (ureteral obstruction; Fig. 3-1). Precise determination of GFR is problematic as both commonly measured indices (urea and creatinine) have characteristics that affect their accuracy as markers of clearance. Urea clearance may significantly underestimate GFR because of tubule urea reabsorption. Creatinine is derived from muscle metabolism of creatine, and its generation varies little from day to day. Creatinine is useful for estimating GFR because it is a small, freely filtered solute. However, serum creatinine levels can increase acutely from dietary ingestion of cooked meat, and creatinine can be secreted into the proximal tubule through an organic cation pathway, leading to overestimation of the GFR. There are many clinical settings where a creatinine clearance is not available, and decisions concerning drug dosing must be made based on the serum creatinine. Two formulas are widely used to estimate GFR: (1) Cockcroft-Gault,

which accounts for age and muscle mass (this value should be multiplied by 0.85 for women, since a lower fraction of the body weight is composed of muscle):

$$\text{Creatinine clearance (mL/min)} = \frac{(140 - \text{age}) \times \text{lean body weight (kg)}}{\text{plasma creatinine (mg/dL)} \times 72}$$

and (2) MDRD (modification of diet in renal disease):

$$\text{GFR (mL/min per 1.73 m}^2) = 186.3 \times P_{Cr} \, (e^{-1.154}) \times \text{age} \, (e^{-0.203}) \times (0.742 \text{ if female}) \times (1.21 \text{ if black}).$$

Although more cumbersome than Cockcroft-Gault, the MDRD equation is felt to be more accurate, and numerous websites are available for making the calculation (*www.kidney.org/professionals/kdoqi/gfr_calculator.cfm*).

The gradual loss of muscle from chronic illness, chronic use of glucocorticoids, or malnutrition can mask significant changes in GFR with small or imperceptible changes in serum creatinine concentration. More accurate determinations of GFR are available using inulin clearance or radionuclide-labeled markers such as ^{125}I-iothalamate or ethylenediaminetetraacetic acid (EDTA). These methods are highly accurate due to precise quantitation and the absence of any renal reabsorption/secretion and should be used to follow GFR in patients in whom creatinine is not likely to be a reliable indicator (patients with decreased muscle mass secondary to age, malnutrition, concurrent illnesses). (See also Table 11-2.) Cystatin C is a member of the cystatin superfamily of cysteine protease inhibitors and is produced at a relatively constant rate from all nucleated cells. Cystatin C production is not affected by diet or nutritional status and may provide a more sensitive indicator of GFR than the plasma creatinine concentration. However, it remains to be validated in many clinical settings.

Approach to the Patient:
AZOTEMIA

Once it has been established that GFR is reduced, the physician must decide if this represents acute or chronic renal injury. The clinical situation, history, and laboratory data often make this an easy distinction. However, the laboratory abnormalities characteristic of chronic renal failure, including anemia, hypocalcemia, and hyperphosphatemia, are often also present in patients presenting with acute renal failure. Radiographic evidence of renal osteodystrophy (Chap. 11) would be seen only in chronic renal failure but is a very late finding, and these patients are usually on dialysis. The urinalysis and renal ultrasound can occasionally facilitate distinguishing acute from chronic renal failure. An approach to the evaluation of azotemic patients is shown in Fig. 3-1. Patients with advanced chronic renal insufficiency often have some proteinuria, nonconcentrated urine (isosthenuria; isoosmotic with plasma), and small kidneys on ultrasound, characterized by increased echogenicity and cortical thinning. Treatment should be directed toward slowing the progression of renal disease and providing symptomatic relief for edema, acidosis, anemia, and hyperphosphatemia, as discussed in Chap. 11. Acute renal failure (Chap. 10) can result from processes affecting renal blood flow (prerenal azotemia), intrinsic renal diseases (affecting small vessels, glomeruli, or tubules), or postrenal processes (obstruction to urine flow in ureters, bladder, or urethra) (Chap. 21).

PRERENAL FAILURE   Decreased renal perfusion accounts for 40–80% of acute renal failure and, if appropriately

treated, is readily reversible. The etiologies of prerenal azotemia include any cause of decreased circulating blood volume (gastrointestinal hemorrhage, burns, diarrhea, diuretics), volume sequestration (pancreatitis, peritonitis, rhabdomyolysis), or decreased effective arterial volume (cardiogenic shock, sepsis). Renal perfusion can also be affected by reductions in cardiac output from peripheral vasodilatation (sepsis, drugs) or profound renal vasoconstriction [severe heart failure, hepatorenal syndrome, drugs such as nonsteroidal anti-inflammatory drugs (NSAIDs)]. True, or "effective," arterial hypovolemia leads to a fall in mean arterial pressure, which in turn triggers a series of neural and humoral responses that include activation of the sympathetic nervous and renin-angiotensin-aldosterone systems and antidiuretic hormone ADH release. GFR is maintained by prostaglandin-mediated relaxation of afferent arterioles and angiotensin II–mediated constriction of efferent arterioles. Once the mean arterial pressure falls below 80 mmHg, there is a steep decline in GFR.

Blockade of prostaglandin production by NSAIDs can result in severe vasoconstriction and acute renal failure. Angiotensin-converting enzyme (ACE) inhibitors decrease efferent arteriolar tone and in turn decrease glomerular capillary perfusion pressure. Patients on NSAIDs and/or ACE inhibitors are most susceptible to hemodynamically mediated acute renal failure when blood volume is reduced for any reason. Patients with bilateral renal artery stenosis (or stenosis in a solitary kidney) are dependent upon efferent arteriolar vasoconstriction for maintenance of glomerular filtration pressure and are particularly susceptible to precipitous decline in GFR when given ACE inhibitors.

Prolonged renal hypoperfusion can lead to acute tubular necrosis (ATN; an intrinsic renal disease). The urinalysis and urinary electrolytes can be useful in distinguishing prerenal azotemia from ATN (Table 3-2). The urine of patients with prerenal azotemia can be predicted from the stimulatory actions of norepinephrine, angiotensin II, ADH, and low tubule fluid flow rate on salt and water reabsorption. In prerenal conditions, the tubules are intact leading to a concentrated urine (>500 mosmol), avid Na retention (urine Na concentration <20 mM/L; fractional excretion of Na <1%), U_{Cr}/P_{Cr} >40 (Table 3-2). The prerenal urine sediment is usually normal or has occasional hyaline and granular casts, while the sediment of ATN is usually filled with cellular debris and dark (muddy brown) granular casts.

POSTRENAL AZOTEMIA   Urinary tract obstruction accounts for <5% of cases of acute renal failure, but it

TABLE 3-2

LABORATORY FINDINGS IN ACUTE RENAL FAILURE

INDEX	PRERENAL AZOTEMIA	OLIGURIC ACUTE RENAL FAILURE
BUN/P$_{Cr}$ ratio	>20:1	10–15:1
Urine sodium (U$_{Na}$), meq/L	<20	>40
Urine osmolality, mosmol/L H$_2$O	>500	<350
Fractional excretion of sodium $$FE_{Na} = \frac{U_{Na} \times P_{Cr} \times 100}{P_{Na} \times U_{Cr}}$$	<1%	>2%
Urine/plasma creatinine (U$_{Cr}$/P$_{Cr}$)	>40	<20

Note: BUN, blood urea nitrogen; P$_{Cr}$, plasma creatinine; U$_{Na}$, urine sodium concentration; P$_{Na}$, plasma sodium concentration; U$_{Cr}$, urine creatinine concentration.

is usually reversible and must be ruled out early in the evaluation (Fig. 3-1). Since a single kidney is capable of adequate clearance, acute renal failure from obstruction requires obstruction at the urethra or bladder outlet, bilateral ureteral obstruction, or unilateral obstruction in a patient with a single functioning kidney. Obstruction is usually diagnosed by the presence of ureteral and renal pelvic dilatation on renal ultrasound. However, early in the course of obstruction or if the ureters are unable to dilate (such as encasement by pelvic tumors or periureteral), the ultrasound examination may be negative.

The specific urologic conditions that cause obstruction are discussed in Chap. 21.

INTRINSIC RENAL DISEASE When prerenal and postrenal azotemia have been excluded as etiologies of renal failure, an intrinsic parenchymal renal disease is present. Intrinsic renal disease can arise from processes involving large renal vessels, intrarenal microvasculature and glomeruli, or tubulointerstitium. Ischemic and toxic ATN account for ~90% of acute intrinsic renal failure. As outlined in Fig. 3-1, the clinical setting and urinalysis are helpful in separating the possible etiologies of acute intrinsic renal failure. Prerenal azotemia and ATN are part of a spectrum of renal hypoperfusion; evidence of structural tubule injury is present in ATN, whereas prompt reversibility occurs with prerenal azotemia upon restoration of adequate renal perfusion. Thus, ATN can often be distinguished from prerenal azotemia by urinalysis and urine electrolyte composition (Table 3-2 and Fig. 3-1). Ischemic ATN is observed most frequently in patients who have undergone major surgery, trauma, severe hypovolemia, overwhelming sepsis, or extensive burns. Nephrotoxic ATN complicates the administration of many common medications, usually by inducing a combination of intrarenal vasoconstriction, direct

tubule toxicity, and/or tubule obstruction. The kidney is vulnerable to toxic injury by virtue of its rich blood supply (25% of cardiac output) and its ability to concentrate and metabolize toxins. A diligent search for hypotension and nephrotoxins will usually uncover the specific etiology of ATN. Discontinuation of nephrotoxins and stabilizing blood pressure will often suffice without the need for dialysis while the tubules recover.

An extensive list of potential drugs and toxins implicated in ATN can be found in Chap. 10.

Processes that involve the tubules and interstitium can lead to acute renal failure. These include drug-induced interstitial nephritis (especially antibiotics, NSAIDs, and diuretics), severe infections (both bacterial and viral), systemic diseases (e.g., systemic lupus erythematosus), or infiltrative disorders (e.g., sarcoid, lymphoma, or leukemia). A list of drugs associated with allergic interstitial nephritis can be found in Chap. 17. The urinalysis usually shows mild to moderate proteinuria, hematuria, and pyuria (~75% of cases) and occasionally white blood cell casts. The finding of RBC casts in interstitial nephritis has been reported but should prompt a search for glomerular diseases (Fig. 3-1). Occasionally renal biopsy will be needed to distinguish among these possibilities. The finding of eosinophils in the urine is suggestive of allergic interstitial nephritis or atheroembolic renal disease and is optimally observed by using a Hansel stain. The absence of eosinophiluria, however, does not exclude these possible etiologies.

Occlusion of large renal vessels including arteries and veins is an uncommon cause of acute renal failure. A significant reduction in GFR by this mechanism suggests bilateral processes or a unilateral process in a patient with a single functioning kidney. Renal arteries can be occluded with atheroemboli, thromboemboli, in situ thrombosis, aortic dissection, or vasculitis. Atheroembolic renal failure can occur spontaneously but is most often associated with recent aortic instrumentation. The emboli are cholesterol rich and lodge in medium and small renal arteries, leading to an eosinophil-rich inflammatory reaction. Patients with atheroembolic acute renal failure often have a normal urinalysis, but the urine may contain eosinophils and casts. The diagnosis can be confirmed by renal biopsy, but this is often unnecessary when other stigmata of atheroemboli are present (livedo reticularis, distal peripheral infarcts, eosinophilia). Renal artery thrombosis may lead to mild proteinuria and hematuria, whereas renal vein thrombosis typically induces heavy proteinuria and hematuria.

These vascular complications often require angiography for confirmation and are discussed in Chap. 18.

Diseases of glomeruli (glomerulonephritis or vasculitis) and the renal microvasculature (hemolytic uremic syndromes, thrombotic thrombocytopenic purpura, or malignant hypertension) usually present with various combinations of glomerular injury: proteinuria, hematuria, reduced GFR, and alterations of Na excretion leading to hypertension, edema, and circulatory congestion (acute nephritic syndrome). These findings may occur as primary renal diseases or as renal manifestations of systemic diseases. The clinical setting and other laboratory data will help distinguish primary renal from systemic diseases. The finding of RBC casts in the urine is an indication for early renal biopsy (Fig. 3-1) as the pathologic pattern has important implications for diagnosis, prognosis, and treatment. Hematuria without RBC casts can also be an indication of glomerular disease, and this evaluation is summarized in **Fig. 3-2**.

A detailed discussion of glomerulonephritis and diseases of the microvasculature can be found in Chap. 15.

OLIGURIA AND ANURIA   *Oliguria* refers to a 24-h urine output of <500 mL, and *anuria* is the complete absence of urine formation (<50 mL). Anuria can be caused by total urinary tract obstruction, total renal artery or vein occlusion, and shock (manifested by severe hypotension and intense renal vasoconstriction). Cortical necrosis, ATN, and rapidly progressive glomerulonephritis can occasionally cause anuria. Oliguria can accompany any cause of acute renal failure and carries a more serious prognosis for renal recovery in all conditions except prerenal azotemia. *Nonoliguria* refers to urine output >500 mL/d in patients with acute or chronic azotemia. With nonoliguric ATN, disturbances of potassium and hydrogen balance are less severe than in oliguric patients, and recovery to normal renal function is usually more rapid.

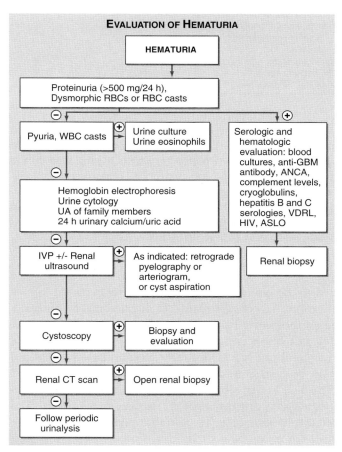

FIGURE 3-2

Approach to the patient with hematuria. RBC, red blood cell; WBC, white blood cell; GBM, glomerular basement membrane; ANCA, antineutrophil cytoplasmic antibody; VDRL, venereal disease research laboratory; ASLO, antistreptolysin O; UA, urinalysis; IVP, intravenous pyelography; CT, computed tomography.

ABNORMALITIES OF THE URINE

PROTEINURIA

The evaluation of proteinuria is shown schematically in **Fig. 3-3** and is typically initiated after detection of proteinuria by dipstick examination. The dipstick measurement detects mostly albumin and gives false-positive results when pH is >7.0 and the urine is very concentrated or contaminated with blood. A very dilute urine may obscure significant proteinuria on dipstick examination, and proteinuria that is not predominantly albumin will be missed. This is particularly important for the detection of Bence-Jones proteins in the urine of patients with multiple myeloma. Tests to measure total urine concentration accurately rely on precipitation with sulfosalicylic or trichloracetic acids. Currently, ultrasensitive dipsticks are available to measure microalbuminuria (30–300 mg/d), an early marker of glomerular disease that has been shown to predict glomerular injury in early diabetic nephropathy (Fig. 3-3).

The magnitude of proteinuria and the protein composition of the urine depend upon the mechanism of renal injury leading to protein losses. Both charge and size selectivity normally prevent virtually all plasma albumin, globulins, and other large-molecular-weight proteins from crossing the glomerular wall. However, if this barrier is disrupted, there can be leakage of plasma proteins into the urine (glomerular proteinuria; Fig. 3-3). Smaller proteins (<20 kDa) are freely filtered but are readily reabsorbed by the proximal tubule. Normal individuals excrete <150 mg/d of total protein and <30 mg/d

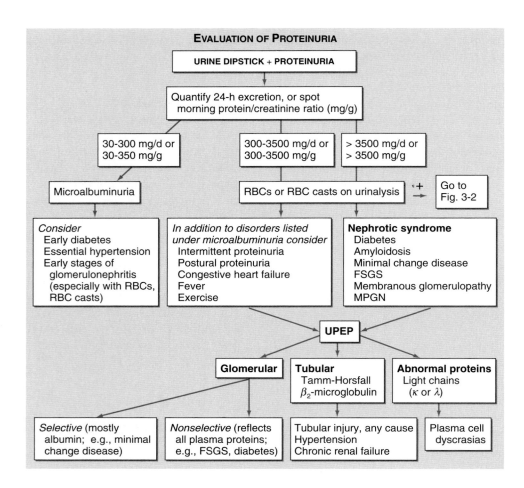

EVALUATION OF PROTEINURIA

URINE DIPSTICK + PROTEINURIA

Quantify 24-h excretion, or spot
morning protein/creatinine ratio (mg/g)

| 30-300 mg/d or | 300-3500 mg/d or | > 3500 mg/d or |
| 30-350 mg/g | 300-3500 mg/g | > 3500 mg/g |

Microalbuminuria

RBCs or RBC casts on urinalysis · + → Go to Fig. 3-2

Consider
Early diabetes
Essential hypertension
Early stages of
  glomerulonephritis
  (especially with RBCs,
  RBC casts)

*In addition to disorders listed
under microalbuminuria consider*
Intermittent proteinuria
Postural proteinuria
Congestive heart failure
Fever
Exercise

Nephrotic syndrome
Diabetes
Amyloidosis
Minimal change disease
FSGS
Membranous glomerulopathy
MPGN

UPEP

Glomerular

Tubular
Tamm-Horsfall
β_2-microglobulin

Abnormal proteins
Light chains
(κ or λ)

Selective (mostly
albumin; e.g., minimal
change disease)

Nonselective (reflects
all plasma proteins;
e.g., FSGS, diabetes)

Tubular injury, any cause
Hypertension
Chronic renal failure

Plasma cell
dyscrasias

FIGURE 3-3

Approach to the patient with proteinuria. Investigation of proteinuria is often initiated by a positive dipstick on routine urinalysis. Conventional dipsticks detect predominantly albumin and cannot detect urinary albumin levels of 30–300 mg/d. However, more exact determination of proteinuria should employ a 24-h urine collection or a spot morning protein/creatinine ratio (mg/g). The pattern of proteinuria on UPEP (urine protein electrophoresis) can be classified as "glomerular," "tubular," or "abnormal" depending upon the origin of the urine proteins. Glomerular proteinuria is due to abnormal glomerular permeability. "Tubular proteins" such as Tamm-Horsfall are normally produced by the renal tubule and shed into the urine. Abnormal circulating proteins such as kappa or lambda light chains are readily filtered because of their small size. RBC, red blood cell; FSGS, focal segmental glomerulosclerosis; MPGN, membranoproliferative glomerulonephritis.

of albumin. The remainder of the protein in the urine is secreted by the tubules (Tamm-Horsfall, IgA, and urokinase) or represents small amounts of filtered β_2-microglobulin, apoproteins, enzymes, and peptide hormones. Another mechanism of proteinuria occurs when there is excessive production of an abnormal protein that exceeds the capacity of the tubule for reabsorption. This most commonly occurs with plasma cell dyscrasias such as multiple myeloma, amyloidosis, and lymphomas that are associated with monoclonal production of immunoglobulin light chains.

The normal glomerular endothelial cell forms a barrier composed of pores of ~100 nm that hold back blood cells but offer little impediment to passage of most proteins. The glomerular basement membrane traps most large proteins (>100 kDa), while the foot processes of epithelial cells (podocytes) cover the urinary side of the glomerular basement membrane and produce a series of narrow channels (slit diaphragms) to normally allow molecular passage of small solutes and water but not proteins. Some glomerular diseases, such as minimal change disease, cause fusion of glomerular epithelial cell foot processes, resulting in predominantly "selective" (Fig. 3-3) loss of albumin. Other glomerular diseases can present with disruption of the basement membrane and slit diaphragms (e.g., by immune complex deposition), resulting in losses of albumin and other plasma proteins. The fusion of foot processes causes increased pressure across the capillary basement membrane, resulting in areas with larger pore sizes. The combination of increased pressure and larger pores results in significant proteinuria ("nonselective"; Fig. 3-3).

When the total daily excretion of protein is >3.5 g, there is often associated hypoalbuminemia, hyperlipidemia, and edema (nephrotic syndrome; Fig. 3-3). However, total daily urinary protein excretion >3.5 g can occur without the other features of the nephrotic syndrome in a variety of other renal diseases (Fig. 3-3). Plasma cell dyscrasias (multiple myeloma) can be associated with large amounts of excreted light chains in the urine, which may not be detected by dipstick (which detects mostly albumin). The light chains produced from these disorders are filtered by the glomerulus and overwhelm the reabsorptive capacity of the proximal tubule. A sulfosalicylic acid precipitate that is out of proportion to the dipstick estimate is suggestive of light chains (Bence Jones protein), and light chains typically redissolve upon warming of the precipitate. Renal failure from these disorders occurs through a variety of mechanisms including tubule obstruction (cast nephropathy) and light chain deposition.

Hypoalbuminemia in nephrotic syndrome occurs through excessive urinary losses and increased proximal tubule catabolism of filtered albumin. Hepatic rates of albumin synthesis are increased, although not to levels sufficient to prevent hypoalbuminemia. Edema forms from renal sodium retention and from reduced plasma oncotic pressure, which favors fluid movement from capillaries to interstitium. The mechanisms designed to correct the decrease in effective intravascular volume contribute to edema formation in some patients. These mechanisms include activation of the renin-angiotensin system, antidiuretic hormone, and the sympathetic nervous system, all of which promote excessive renal salt and water reabsorption.

The severity of edema correlates with the degree of hypoalbuminemia and is modified by other factors such as heart disease or peripheral vascular disease. The diminished plasma oncotic pressure and urinary losses of regulatory proteins appear to stimulate hepatic lipoprotein synthesis. The resulting hyperlipidemia results in lipid bodies (fatty casts, oval fat bodies) in the urine. Other proteins are lost in the urine, leading to a variety of metabolic disturbances. These include thyroxine-binding globulin, cholecalciferol-binding protein, transferrin, and metal-binding proteins. A hypercoagulable state frequently accompanies severe nephrotic syndrome due to urinary losses of antithrombin III, reduced serum levels of proteins S and C, hyperfibrinogenemia, and enhanced platelet aggregation. Some patients develop severe IgG deficiency with resulting defects in immunity. Many diseases (some listed in Fig. 3-3) and drugs can cause the nephrotic syndrome, and a complete list can be found in Chap. 15.

HEMATURIA, PYURIA, AND CASTS

Isolated hematuria without proteinuria, other cells, or casts is often indicative of bleeding from the urinary tract. Normal red blood cell excretion is up to 2 million RBCs per day. Hematuria is defined as two to five RBCs per high-power field (HPF) and can be detected by dipstick. Common causes of isolated hematuria include stones, neoplasms, tuberculosis, trauma, and prostatitis. Gross hematuria with blood clots is almost never indicative of glomerular bleeding; rather, it suggests a postrenal source in the urinary collecting system. Evaluation of patients presenting with microscopic hematuria is outlined in Fig. 3-2. A single urinalysis with hematuria is common and can result from menstruation, viral illness, allergy, exercise, or mild trauma. Annual urinalysis of servicemen over a 10-year period showed an incidence of 38%. However, persistent or significant hematuria (>three RBCs/HPF on three urinalyses, or a single urinalysis with >100 RBCs, or gross hematuria) identified significant renal or urologic lesions in 9.1%. Even patients who are chronically anticoagulated should be investigated as outlined in Fig. 3-2. The suspicion for urogenital neoplasms in patients with isolated painless hematuria (nondysmorphic RBCs) increases with age. Neoplasms are rare in the pediatric population, and isolated hematuria is more likely to be "idiopathic" or associated with a congenital anomaly. Hematuria with pyuria and bacteriuria is typical of infection and should be treated with antibiotics after appropriate cultures. Acute cystitis or urethritis in women can cause gross hematuria. Hypercalciuria and hyperuricosuria are also risk factors for unexplained isolated hematuria in both children and adults. In some of these patients (50–60%), reducing calcium and uric acid excretion through dietary interventions can eliminate the microscopic hematuria.

Isolated microscopic hematuria can be a manifestation of glomerular diseases. The RBCs of glomerular origin are often dysmorphic when examined by phase-contrast microscopy. Irregular shapes of RBCs may also occur due to pH and osmolarity changes produced along the distal nephron. There is, however, significant observer variability in detecting dysmorphic RBCs. The most common etiologies of isolated glomerular hematuria are IgA nephropathy, hereditary nephritis, and thin basement membrane disease. IgA nephropathy and hereditary nephritis can lead to episodic gross hematuria. A family history of renal failure is often present in patients with hereditary nephritis, and patients with thin basement membrane disease often have other family members with microscopic hematuria. A renal biopsy is needed for the definitive diagnosis of these disorders, which are discussed in more detail in Chap. 15. Hematuria with dysmorphic RBCs, RBC casts, and protein excretion >500 mg/d is virtually diagnostic of glomerulonephritis. RBC casts form as RBCs that enter the tubule fluid become trapped in a cylindrical mold of gelled Tamm-Horsfall protein. Even in the absence of azotemia, these patients should undergo serologic evaluation and renal biopsy as outlined in Fig. 3-2.

Isolated pyuria is unusual since inflammatory reactions in the kidney or collecting system are also associated with hematuria. The presence of bacteria suggests infection, and white blood cell casts with bacteria are indicative of pyelonephritis. White blood cells and/or white blood cell casts may also be seen in tubulointerstitial processes such as interstitial nephritis, systemic lupus erythematosus, and transplant rejection. In chronic renal diseases, degenerated cellular casts called *waxy casts* can be seen in the urine. *Broad casts* are thought to arise in the dilated tubules of enlarged nephrons that have undergone compensatory hypertrophy in response to reduced renal mass (i.e., chronic renal failure). A mixture of broad casts typically seen with chronic renal failure together with cellular casts and RBCs may be seen in smoldering processes such as chronic glomerulonephritis.

ABNORMALITIES OF URINE VOLUME

The volume of urine produced varies depending upon the fluid intake, renal function, and physiologic demands of the individual. See "Azotemia," for discussion of decreased (oliguria) or absent urine production (anuria).

The physiology of water formation and renal water conservation are discussed in Chap. 2.

POLYURIA

By history, it is often difficult for patients to distinguish urinary frequency (often of small volumes) from polyuria (>3 L/d), and a 24-h urine collection is needed for evaluation (**Fig. 3-4**). Polyuria results from two potential mechanisms: (1) excretion of nonabsorbable solutes (such as glucose) or (2) excretion of water (usually from a defect in ADH production or renal responsiveness). To distinguish a solute diuresis from a water diuresis and to determine if the diuresis is appropriate for the clinical circumstances, a urine osmolality is measured. The average person excretes between 600 and 800 mosmol of solutes per day, primarily as urea and electrolytes. If the urine output is >3 L/d and the urine is dilute (<250 mosmol/L), then total mosmol excretion is normal and a water diuresis is present. This circumstance could arise from polydipsia, inadequate secretion of vasopressin (central diabetes insipidus), or failure of renal tubules to respond to vasopressin (nephrogenic diabetes insipidus). If the urine volume is >3 L/d and urine osmolality is >300 mosmol/L, then a solute diuresis is clearly present and a search for the responsible solute(s) is mandatory.

Excessive filtration of a poorly reabsorbed solute such as glucose, mannitol, or urea can depress reabsorption of NaCl and water in the proximal tubule and lead to enhanced excretion in the urine. Poorly controlled diabetes mellitus with glucosuria is the most common cause of a solute diuresis, leading to volume depletion and serum hypertonicity. Since the urine Na concentration is

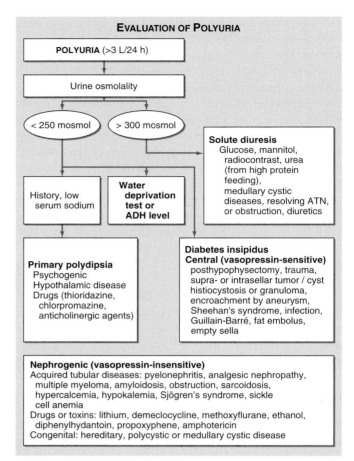

FIGURE 3-4

Approach to the patient with polyuria. ATN, acute tubular necrosis; ADH, antidiuretic hormone.

less than that of blood, more water than Na is lost, causing hypernatremia and hypertonicity. Common iatrogenic solute diuresis occurs from mannitol administration, radiocontrast media, and high-protein feedings (enterally or parenterally), leading to increased urea production and excretion. Less commonly, excessive Na loss may occur from cystic renal diseases, Bartter's syndrome, or during the course of a tubulointerstitial process (such as resolving ATN). In these so-called salt-wasting disorders, the tubule damage results in direct impairment of Na reabsorption and indirectly reduces the responsiveness of the tubule to aldosterone. Usually, the Na losses are mild, and the obligatory urine output is <2 L/d (resolving ATN and postobstructive diuresis are exceptions and may be associated with significant natriuresis and polyuria).

Formation of large volumes of dilute urine represent polydipsic states or diabetes insipidus. Primary polydipsia can result from habit, psychiatric disorders, neurologic lesions, or medications. During deliberate polydipsia, extracellular fluid volume is normal or expanded and plasma vasopressin levels are reduced because serum osmolality tends to be near the lower limits of normal.

Central diabetes insipidus may be idiopathic in origin or secondary to a variety of hypothalamic conditions including posthypophysectomy or trauma or neoplastic, inflammatory, vascular, or infectious hypothalamic diseases. Idiopathic central diabetes insipidus is associated with selective destruction of the vasopressin-secreting neurons in the supraoptic and paraventricular nuclei and can be inherited as an autosomal dominant trait or occur spontaneously. Nephrogenic diabetes insipidus can occur in a variety of clinical situations as summarized in Fig. 3-4.

A plasma vasopressin level is recommended as the best method for distinguishing between central and nephrogenic diabetes insipidus. Alternatively, a water deprivation test plus exogenous vasopressin may also distinguish primary polydipsia from central and nephrogenic diabetes insipidus.

FURTHER READINGS

ANDERSON S et al: Renal and systemic manifestations of glomerular disease, in *Brenner & Rector's The Kidney,* 7th ed, BM Brenner (ed). Philadelphia, Saunders, 2004, pp 1927–1954

BERL T, VERBALIS J: Pathophysiology of water metabolism, in *Brenner & Rector's The Kidney,* 7th ed, BM Brenner (ed). Philadelphia, Saunders, 2004, pp 857–920

BOMBACK AS et al: Change in proteinuria after adding aldosterone blockers to ACE inhibitors or angiotensin receptor blockers in CKD: A systematic review. Am J Kidney Dis 51:199, 2008

DE ZEEUW D: Targeting proteinuria as a valid surrogate for individualized kidney protective therapy. Am J Kidney Dis 51:713, 2008

FOGAZZI GB et al: Urinalysis: Core curriculum 2008. Am J Kidney Dis 51:1052, 2008

KASISKE BL, KEANE WE: Laboratory assessment of renal disease: Clearance, urinalysis and renal biopsy, in *Brenner & Rector's The Kidney,* 7th ed, BM Brenner (ed). Philadelphia, Saunders, 2004, pp 1107–1150

KHADRA MH et al: A prospective analysis of 1,930 patients with hematuria to evaluate current diagnostic practice. J Urol 163:524, 2000

RODRIGO E et al: Measurement of renal function in pre-ESRD patients. Kidney Int Suppl 80:11, 2002

SASAKI S: Nephrogenic diabetes insipidus: Update of genetic and clinical aspects. Nephrol Dial Transplant 19:1351, 2004

SHRIER RW et al: Acute renal failure: Definitions, diagnosis, pathogenesis and therapy. J Clin Invest 114:5, 2004

TAM LS et al: Are spot urine samples adequate for assessment of proteinuria in patients with lupus nephritis? Nat Clin Pract Nephrol 4:72, 2008

Azotemia and Urinary Abnormalities

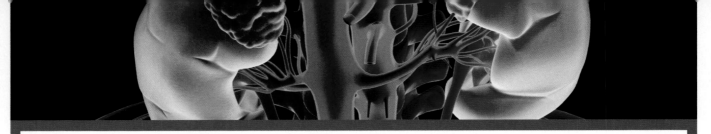

CHAPTER 4
ATLAS OF URINARY SEDIMENTS
AND RENAL BIOPSIES

Agnes B. Fogo ■ Eric G. Neilson

Key diagnostic features of selected diseases in renal biopsy and urinalysis are illustrated, with light, immunofluorescence, and electron microscopic images. Common urinalysis findings are also documented.

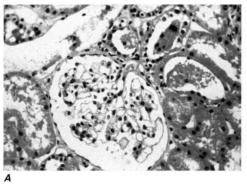

FIGURE 4-1
Minimal change disease. In minimal change disease, light microscopy is unremarkable (**A**), while electron microscopy reveals podocyte injury evidenced by complete foot process effacement (**B**). (ABF/Vanderbilt Collection.)

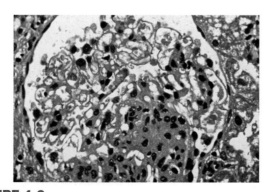

FIGURE 4-2
Focal segmental glomerulosclerosis. There is a well-defined segmental increase in matrix and obliteration of capillary loops, the sine qua non of segmental sclerosis. (EGN/UPenn Collection.)

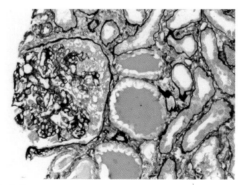

FIGURE 4-3
Collapsing glomerulopathy. There is segmental collapse of the glomerular capillary loops and overlying podocyte hyperplasia. This lesion may be idiopathic or associated with HIV infection and has a particularly poor prognosis. (ABF/Vanderbilt Collection.)

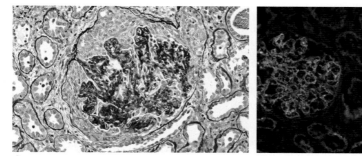
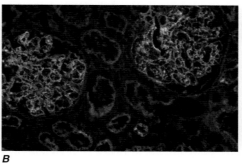
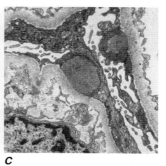

A **B** **C**

FIGURE 4-4

Postinfectious (poststreptococcal) glomerulonephritis. The glomerular tuft shows proliferative changes with numerous PMNs, with a crescentic reaction in severe cases (**A**). These deposits localize in the mesangium and along the capillary wall in a subepithelial pattern and stain dominantly for C3 and to a lesser extent for IgG (**B**). Subepithelial hump-shaped deposits are seen by electron microscopy (**C**). *(ABF/Vanderbilt Collection.)*

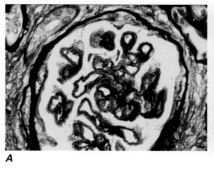
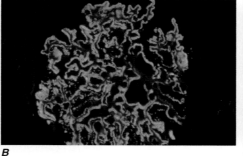
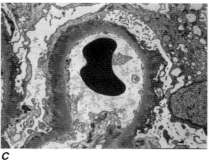

A **B** **C**

FIGURE 4-5

Membranous glomerulopathy. Membranous glomerulopathy is due to subepithelial deposits, with resulting basement membrane reaction, resulting in the appearance of spike-like projections on silver stain (**A**). The deposits are directly visualized by fluorescent anti-IgG, revealing diffuse granular capillary loop staining (**B**). By electron microscopy, the subepithelial location of the deposits and early surrounding basement membrane reaction is evident, with overlying foot process effacement (**C**). *(ABF/Vanderbilt Collection.)*

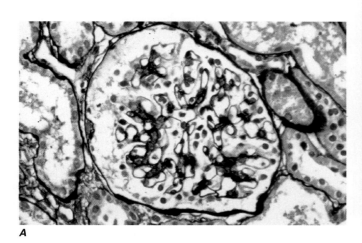
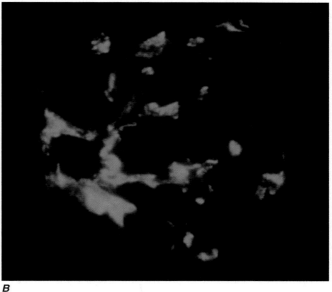

A **B**

FIGURE 4-6

IgA nephropathy. There is variable mesangial expansion due to mesangial deposits, with some cases also showing endocapillary proliferation or segmental sclerosis (**A**). By immunofluorescence, deposits are evident (**B**). *(ABF/Vanderbilt Collection.)*

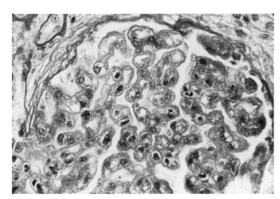

FIGURE 4-7

Membranoproliferative glomerulonephritis. There is mesangial expansion and endocapillary proliferation resulting in the "tram-track" sign of cellular interposition along the glomerular basement membrane. *(EGN/UPenn Collection.)*

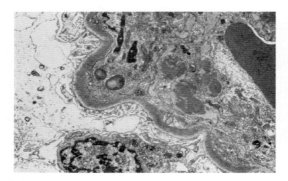

FIGURE 4-8

Dense deposit disease (membranoproliferative glomerulonephritis type II). By light microscopy, there is a membranoproliferative pattern. By electron microscopy, there is a dense transformation of the glomerular basement membrane with round, globular deposits within the mesangium. By immunofluorescence, only C3 staining is usually present. *(ABF/Vanderbilt Collection.)*

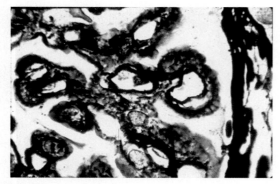

FIGURE 4-9

Membranoproliferative glomerulonephritis. This specimen shows pink subepithelial deposits with spike reaction and the "tram-track" sign of reduplication of glomerular basement membrane, resulting from subendothelial deposits, as may be seen in mixed membranous and proliferative lupus nephritis (ISN/RPS class V and IV) or membranoproliferative glomerulonephritis type III. *(EGN/UPenn Collection.)*

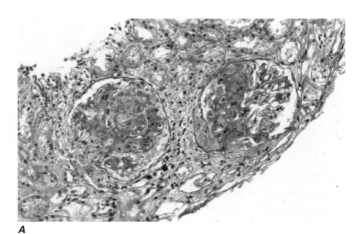

A

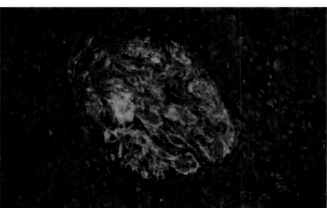

B

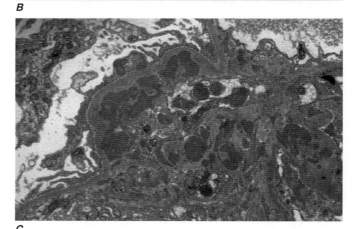

C

FIGURE 4-10

Lupus nephritis. Proliferative lupus nephritis, ISN/RPS class III or IV, manifests as endocapillary proliferation, which may result in segmental necrosis due to deposits, particularly in the subendothelial area (**A**). By immunofluorescence, chunky irregular mesangial and capillary loop deposits are evident, with some of the peripheral loop deposits having a smooth, molded outer contour due to their subendothelial location. These deposits typically stain for all three immunoglobulins, IgG, IgA, IgM, and both C3 and C1q (**B**). By electron microscopy, subendothelial, mesangial, and rare subepithelial dense immune complex deposits are evident, along with extensive foot process effacement (**C**). *(ABF/Vanderbilt Collection.)*

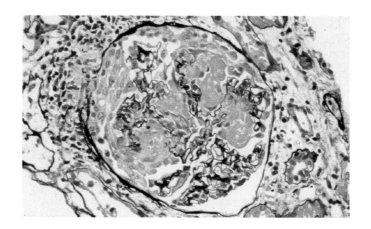

FIGURE 4-11

Wegener's granulomatosis. This pauci-immune necrotizing crescentic glomerulonephritis shows numerous breaks in the glomerular basement membrane with associated segmental fibrinoid necrosis, and a crescent formed by proliferation of the parietal epithelium. Note that the uninvolved segment of the glomerulus (at ~5 o'clock) shows no evidence of proliferation or immune complexes. *(ABF/Vanderbilt Collection.)*

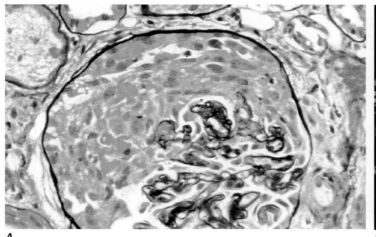

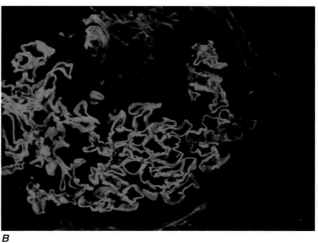

A

B

FIGURE 4-12

Anti-GBM antibody-mediated glomerulonephritis. There is segmental necrosis with a break of the glomerular basement membrane and a cellular crescent (**A**), and immunofluorescence for IgG shows linear staining of the glomerular basement membrane with a small crescent at ~1 o'clock (**B**). *(ABF/Vanderbilt Collection.)*

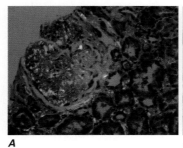

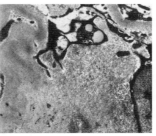

A

B

FIGURE 4-13

Amyloidosis. Amyloidosis shows amorphous, acellular expansion of the mesangium, with material often also infiltrating glomerular basement membranes, vessels, and in the interstitium, with apple-green birefringence by polarized Congo red stain (**A**). The deposits are composed of randomly organized 9- to 11-nm fibrils by electron microscopy (**B**). *(ABF/Vanderbilt Collection.)*

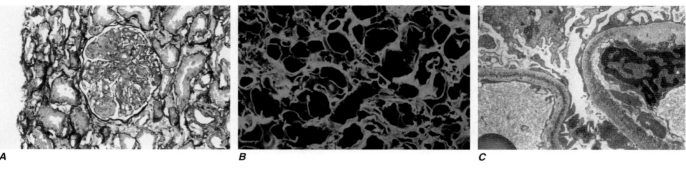

A   B   C

FIGURE 4-14

Light chain deposition disease. There is mesangial expansion, often nodular by light microscopy (**A**), with immunofluorescence showing monoclonal staining, more commonly with kappa than lambda light chain, of tubules (**B**) and glomerular tufts. By electron microscopy (**C**), the deposits show an amorphous granular appearance and line the inside of the glomerular basement membrane and are also found along the tubular basement membranes. (*ABF/Vanderbilt Collection.*)

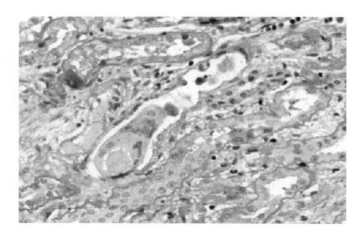

FIGURE 4-15

Light chain cast nephropathy (myeloma kidney). Monoclonal light chains precipitate in tubules and result in a syncytial giant cell reaction (**left**) surrounding the cast, and a surrounding chronic interstitial nephritis with tubulointerstitial fibrosis. (*ABF/Vanderbilt Collection.*)

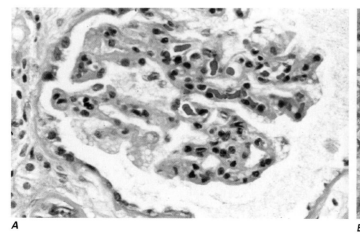

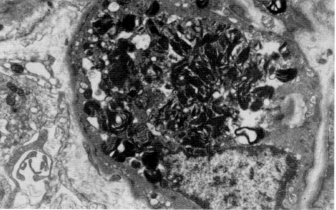

A   B

FIGURE 4-16

Fabry's disease. Due to deficiency of α-galactosidase, there is abnormal accumulation of glycolipids, resulting in foamy podocytes by light microscopy (**A**). These deposits can be directly visualized by electron microscopy (**B**), where the glycosphingolipid appears as whorled so-called myeloid bodies, particularly in the podocytes. (*ABF/Vanderbilt Collection.*)

CHAPTER 4

Atlas of Urinary Sediments and Renal Biopsies

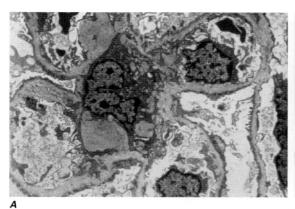

A

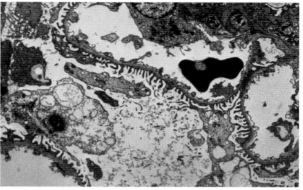

B

FIGURE 4-17

Alport's syndrome and thin glomerular basement membrane lesion. In Alport's syndrome, there is irregular thinning alternating with thickened so-called basket-weaving abnormal organization of the glomerular basement membrane (**A**).

In benign familial hematuria, or in early cases of Alport's syndrome or female carriers, only extensive thinning of the GBM is seen by electron microscopy (**B**). *(ABF/Vanderbilt Collection.)*

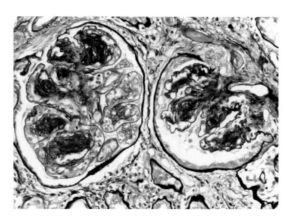

FIGURE 4-18

Diabetic nephropathy. There is nodular mesangial expansion, so-called Kimmelstiel-Wilson nodules, with increased mesangial matrix and cellularity, microaneurysm formation in the glomerulus on the left, and prominent glomerular basement

membranes without evidence of immune deposits and arteriolar hyalinosis of both afferent and efferent arterioles. *(ABF/Vanderbilt Collection.)*

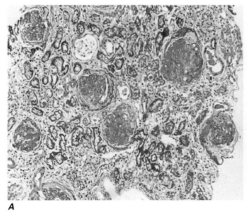

A

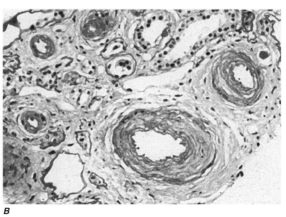

B

FIGURE 4-19

Arterionephrosclerosis. Hypertension-associated injury often manifests extensive global sclerosis of glomeruli, with accompanying and proportional tubulointerstitial fibrosis and pericapsular fibrosis, and there may be segmental sclerosis (**A**).

The vessels show disproportionately severe changes of intimal fibrosis, medial hypertrophy, and arteriolar hyaline deposits (**B**). *(ABF/Vanderbilt Collection.)*

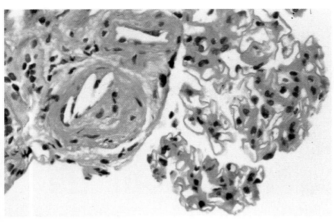

FIGURE 4-20
Cholesterol emboli. Cholesterol emboli cause cleft-like spaces where the lipid has been extracted during processing, with smooth outer contours, and surrounding fibrotic and mononuclear cell reaction in these arterioles. *(ABF/Vanderbilt Collection.)*

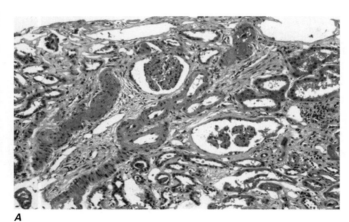

A

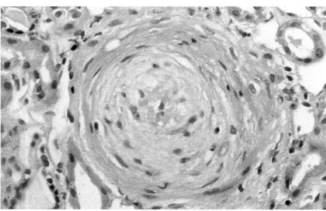

B

FIGURE 4-22
Progressive systemic sclerosis. Acutely, there is fibrinoid necrosis of interlobular and larger vessels, with intervening normal vessels and ischemic change in the glomeruli (*A*). Chronically, this injury leads to intimal proliferation, the so-called onion-skinning appearance (*B*). *(ABF/Vanderbilt Collection.)*

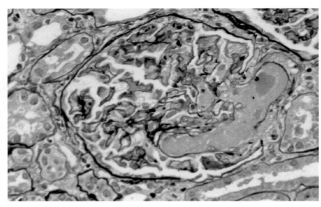

FIGURE 4-21
Hemolytic uremic syndrome. There are characteristic intra-glomerular fibrin thrombi, with a chunky pink appearance. The remaining portion of the capillary tuft shows corrugation of the glomerular basement membrane due to ischemia. *(ABF/Vanderbilt Collection.)*

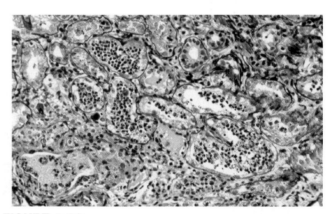

FIGURE 4-23
Acute pyelonephritis. There are characteristic intratubular plugs and casts of PMNs with inflammation extending into the surrounding interstitium, and accompanying tubular injury. *(ABF/Vanderbilt Collection.)*

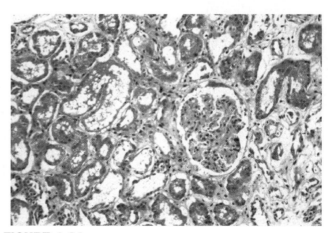

FIGURE 4-24
Acute tubular necrosis. There is extensive flattening of the tubular epithelium and loss of the brush border, with mild interstitial edema. *(ABF/Vanderbilt Collection.)*

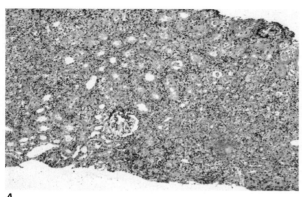

A

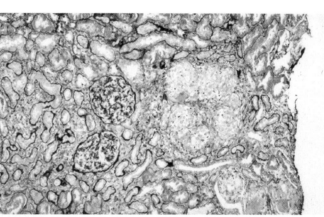

B

FIGURE 4-25

Acute interstitial nephritis. There is extensive interstitial lymphocytic infiltrate with mild edema and associated tubular injury (**A**), which is frequently associated with interstitial eosinophils (**B**) when caused by a drug hypersensitivity reaction. *(ABF/Vanderbilt Collection.)*

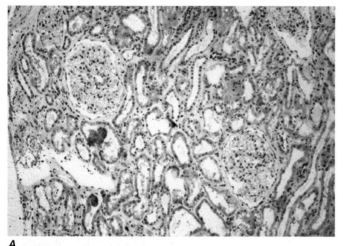

A

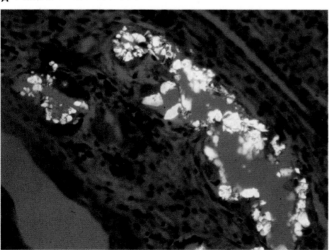

B

FIGURE 4-26

Oxalosis. Calcium oxalate crystals have caused extensive tubular injury, with flattening and regeneration of tubular epithelium (**A**). Crystals are well visualized as sheaves when viewed under polarized light (**B**). *(ABF/Vanderbilt Collection.)*

FIGURE 4-27

Sarcoidosis. There is chronic interstitial nephritis with numerous, confluent, non-necrotizing granulomas. The glomeruli are unremarkable, but there is moderate tubular interstitial fibrosis. *(ABF/Vanderbilt Collection.)*

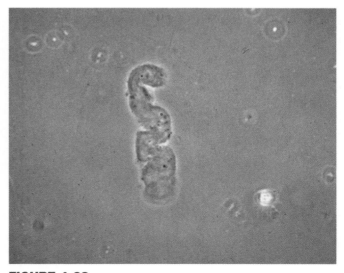

FIGURE 4-28

Hyaline cast. *(ABF/Vanderbilt Collection.)*

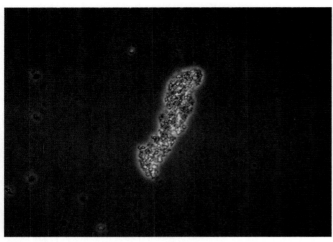

FIGURE 4-29
Coarse granular cast. *(ABF/Vanderbilt Collection.)*

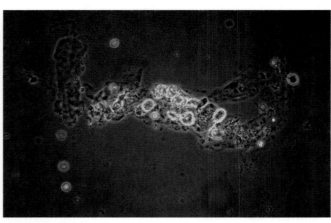

FIGURE 4-32
WBC cast. *(ABF/Vanderbilt Collection.)*

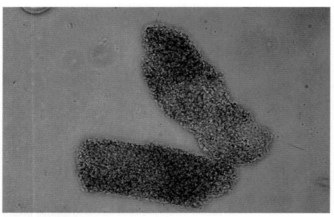

FIGURE 4-30
Fine granular cast. *(ABF/Vanderbilt Collection.)*

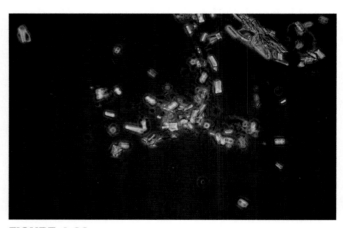

FIGURE 4-33
Triple phosphate crystals. *(ABF/Vanderbilt Collection.)*

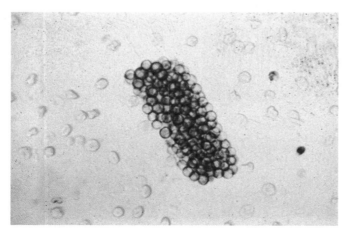

FIGURE 4-31
Red blood cell cast. *(ABF/Vanderbilt Collection.)*

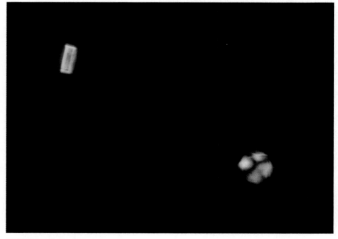

FIGURE 4-34
"Maltese cross" formation in an oval fat body. *(ABF/ Vanderbilt Collection.)*

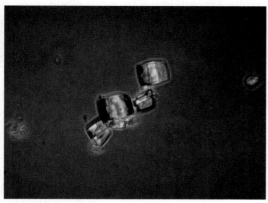

FIGURE 4-35
Uric acid crystals. *(ABF/Vanderbilt Collection.)*

FURTHER READINGS

ABBOTT KC et al: A new supine anterolateral approach to percutaneous ultrasound-guided renal biopsy. Nat Clin Pract Nephrol 4:244, 2008

COHEN SD et al: Renal biopsy is necessary for the diagnosis of HIV-associated renal diseases. Nat Clin Pract Nephrol 5:22, 2009

JENNETTE JC et al: How can the safety and diagnostic yield of percutaneous renal biopsies be optimized? Nat Clin Pract Nephrol 4:126, 2008

SEDOR JR: Tissue proteomics: A new investigative tool for renal biopsy analysis. Kidney Int 75:876, 2009

CHAPTER 4

Atlas of Urinary Sediments and Renal Biopsies

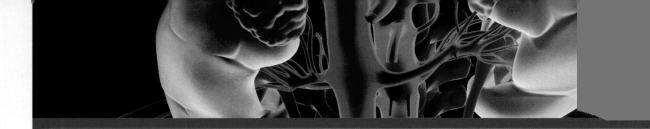

CHAPTER 5

ACIDOSIS AND ALKALOSIS

Thomas D. DuBose, Jr.

NORMAL ACID-BASE HOMEOSTASIS

Systemic arterial pH is maintained between 7.35 and 7.45 by extracellular and intracellular chemical buffering together with respiratory and renal regulatory mechanisms. The control of arterial CO_2 tension (Pa_{CO_2}) by the central nervous system and respiratory systems and the control of the plasma bicarbonate by the kidneys stabilize the arterial pH by excretion or retention of acid or alkali. The metabolic and respiratory components that regulate systemic pH are described by the Henderson-Hasselbalch equation:

$$pH = 6.1 + \log \frac{HCO_3^-}{Pa_{CO_2} \times 0.0301}$$

Under most circumstances, CO_2 production and excretion are matched, and the usual steady-state Pa_{CO_2} is maintained at 40 mmHg. Underexcretion of CO_2 produces hypercapnia, and overexcretion causes hypocapnia. Nevertheless, production and excretion are again matched at a new steady-state Pa_{CO_2}. Therefore, the Pa_{CO_2} is regulated primarily by neural respiratory factors and is not subject to regulation by the rate of CO_2 production. Hypercapnia is usually the result of hypoventilation rather than of increased CO_2 production. Increases or decreases in Pa_{CO_2} represent derangements of neural respiratory control or are due to compensatory changes in response to a primary alteration in the plasma $[HCO_3^-]$.

The kidneys regulate plasma $[HCO_3^-]$ through three main processes: (1) "reabsorption" of filtered HCO_3^-, (2) formation of titratable acid, and (3) excretion of NH_4^+ in the urine. The kidney filters ~4000 mmol of HCO_3^- per day. To reabsorb the filtered load of HCO_3^-, the renal tubules must therefore secrete 4000 mmol of hydrogen ions. Between 80 and 90% of HCO_3^- is reabsorbed in the proximal tubule. The distal nephron reabsorbs the remainder and secretes protons, as generated from metabolism, to defend systemic pH. While this quantity of protons, 40–60 mmol/d, is small, it must be secreted to prevent chronic positive H^+ balance and metabolic acidosis. This quantity of secreted protons is represented in the urine as titratable acid and NH_4^+. Metabolic acidosis in the face of normal renal function increases NH_4^+ production and excretion. NH_4^+ production and excretion are impaired in chronic renal failure, hyperkalemia, and renal tubular acidosis.

In sum, these regulatory responses, including chemical buffering, the regulation of Pa_{CO_2} by the respiratory system, and the regulation of $[HCO_3^-]$ by the kidneys, act in concert to maintain a systemic arterial pH between 7.35 and 7.45.

DIAGNOSIS OF GENERAL TYPES OF DISTURBANCES

The most common clinical disturbances are simple acid-base disorders, i.e., metabolic acidosis or alkalosis or respiratory acidosis or alkalosis. Since compensation is not complete, the pH is abnormal in simple disturbances. More complicated clinical situations can give rise to mixed acid-base disturbances.

SIMPLE ACID-BASE DISORDERS

Primary respiratory disturbances (primary changes in Pa_{CO_2}) invoke compensatory metabolic responses (secondary changes in $[HCO_3^-]$), and primary metabolic disturbances elicit predictable compensatory respiratory responses. Physiologic compensation can be predicted from the relationships displayed in (Table 5-1). Metabolic acidosis due to an increase in endogenous acids (e.g., ketoacidosis) lowers extracellular fluid $[HCO_3^-]$ and decreases extracellular pH. This stimulates the medullary chemoreceptors to increase ventilation and to return the ratio of $[HCO_3^-]$ to Pa_{CO_2}, and thus pH, toward normal, although not to normal. The degree of respiratory compensation expected in a simple form of metabolic acidosis can be predicted from the relationship: $Pa_{CO_2} = (1.5 \times [HCO_3^-]) + 8 \pm 2$, i.e., the Pa_{CO_2} is expected to decrease 1.25 mmHg for each mmol per liter decrease in $[HCO_3^-]$. Thus, a patient with metabolic acidosis and $[HCO_3^-]$ of 12 mmol/L would be expected to have a Pa_{CO_2} between 24 and 28 mmHg. Values for Pa_{CO_2} <24 or >28 mmHg define a mixed disturbance (metabolic acidosis and respiratory alkalosis or metabolic alkalosis and respiratory acidosis, respectively). Another way to judge the appropriateness of the response in $[HCO_3^-]$ or Pa_{CO_2} is to use an acid-base nomogram (Fig. 5-1). While the shaded areas of the nomogram show the 95% confidence limits for normal compensation in simple disturbances, finding acid-base values within the shaded area does not necessarily rule out a mixed disturbance. Imposition of one disorder over another may result in values lying within the area of a third. Thus, the nomogram, while convenient, is not a substitute for the equations in Table 5-1.

MIXED ACID-BASE DISORDERS

Mixed acid-base disorders—defined as independently coexisting disorders, not merely compensatory responses—are often seen in patients in critical care units and can

TABLE 5-1

PREDICTION OF COMPENSATORY RESPONSES ON SIMPLE ACID-BASE DISTURBANCES AND PATTERN OF CHANGES

DISORDER	PREDICTION OF COMPENSATION	RANGE OF VALUES		
		PH	HCO$_3^-$	Pa$_{CO_2}$
Metabolic acidosis	$Pa_{CO_2} = (1.5 \times HCO_3^-) + 8 \pm 2$ *or* Pa_{CO_2} will ↓ 1.25 mmHg per mmol/L ↓ in $[HCO_3^-]$ *or* $Pa_{CO_2} = [HCO_3^-] + 15$	Low	Low	Low
Metabolic alkalosis	Pa_{CO_2} will ↑ 0.75 mmHg per mmol/L ↑ in $[HCO_3^-]$ *or* Pa_{CO_2} will ↑ 6 mmHg per 10 mmol/L ↑ in $[HCO_3^-]$ *or* $Pa_{CO_2} = [HCO_3^-] + 15$	High	High	High
Respiratory alkalosis Acute Chronic	 $[HCO_3^-]$ will ↓ 0.2 mmol/L per mmHg ↓ in Pa_{CO_2} $[HCO_3^-]$ will ↓ 0.4 mmol/L per mmHg ↓ in Pa_{CO_2}	High	Low	Low
Respiratory acidosis Acute Chronic	 $[HCO_3^-]$ will ↑ 0.1 mmol/L per mmHg ↑ in Pa_{CO_2} $[HCO_3^-]$ will ↑ 0.4 mmol/L per mmHg ↑ in Pa_{CO_2}	Low	High	High

SECTION II

Alterations of Renal Function and Electrolytes

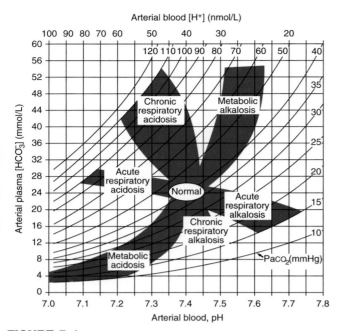

Arterial blood [H⁺] (nmol/L)

FIGURE 5-1

Acid-base nomogram. Shown are the 90% confidence limits (range of values) of the normal respiratory and metabolic compensations for primary acid-base disturbances. *(From DuBose, used with permission.)*

lead to dangerous extremes of pH (Table 5-2). A patient with diabetic ketoacidosis (metabolic acidosis) may develop an independent respiratory problem leading to respiratory acidosis or alkalosis. Patients with underlying pulmonary disease may not respond to metabolic acidosis with an appropriate ventilatory response because of insufficient respiratory reserve. Such imposition of respiratory acidosis on metabolic acidosis can lead to severe acidemia and a poor outcome. When metabolic acidosis and metabolic alkalosis coexist in the same patient, the pH may be normal or near normal. When the pH is normal, an elevated anion gap (AG) denotes the presence of a metabolic acidosis. A discrepancy in the ΔAG (prevailing minus normal AG) and the ΔHCO_3^- (normal minus prevailing HCO_3^-) indicates the presence of a mixed high–gap acidosis—metabolic alkalosis (see example later in the chapter). A diabetic patient with ketoacidosis may have renal dysfunction resulting in simultaneous metabolic acidosis. Patients who have ingested an overdose of drug combinations such as sedatives and salicylates may have mixed disturbances as a result of the acid-base response to the individual drugs (metabolic acidosis mixed with respiratory acidosis or respiratory alkalosis, respectively). Even more complex are triple acid-base disturbances. For example, patients with metabolic acidosis due to alcoholic ketoacidosis may develop metabolic alkalosis due to vomiting and superimposed respiratory alkalosis due to the hyperventilation of hepatic dysfunction or alcohol withdrawal.

TABLE 5-2

EXAMPLES OF MIXED ACID-BASE DISORDERS

Mixed Metabolic and Respiratory

Metabolic acidosis—respiratory alkalosis
  Key: High- or normal-AG metabolic acidosis; prevailing $Paco_2$ *below* predicted value (Table 5-1)
  Example: Na⁺, 140; K⁺, 4.0; Cl⁻, 106; HCO_3^-, 14; AG, 20; $Paco_2$, 24; pH, 7.39 (lactic acidosis, sepsis in ICU)

Metabolic acidosis—respiratory acidosis
  Key: High- or normal-AG metabolic acidosis; prevailing $Paco_2$ *above* predicted value (Table 5-1)
  Example: Na⁺, 140; K⁺, 4.0; Cl⁻, 102; HCO_3^-, 18; AG, 20; $Paco_2$, 38; pH, 7.30 (severe pneumonia, pulmonary edema)

Metabolic alkalosis—respiratory alkalosis
  Key: $Paco_2$ does not increase as predicted; pH higher than expected
  Example: Na⁺, 140; K⁺, 4.0; Cl⁻, 91; HCO_3^-, 33; AG, 16; $Paco_2$, 38; pH, 7.55 (liver disease and diuretics)

Metabolic alkalosis—respiratory acidosis
  Key: $Paco_2$ higher than predicted; pH normal
  Example: Na⁺, 140; K⁺, 3.5; Cl⁻, 88; HCO_3^-, 42; AG, 10; $Paco_2$, 67; pH, 7.42 (COPD on diuretics)

Mixed Metabolic Disorders

Metabolic acidosis—metabolic alkalosis
  Key: Only detectable with high-AG acidosis; ΔAG $\gg$ ΔHCO_3^-
  Example: Na⁺, 140; K⁺, 3.0; Cl⁻, 95; HCO_3^-, 25; AG, 20; $Paco_2$, 40; pH, 7.42 (uremia with vomiting)

Metabolic acidosis—metabolic acidosis
  Key: Mixed high-AG—normal-AG acidosis; ΔHCO_3^- accounted for by combined change in ΔAG and ΔCl⁻
  Example: Na⁺, 135; K⁺, 3.0; Cl⁻, 110; HCO_3^-, 10; AG, 15; $Paco_2$, 25; pH, 7.20 (diarrhea and lactic acidosis, toluene toxicity, treatment of diabetic ketoacidosis)

Note: AG, anion gap; ICU, intensive care unit; COPD, chronic obstructive pulmonary disease.

Approach to the Patient:
ACID-BASE DISORDERS

A stepwise approach to the diagnosis of acid-base disorders follows (Table 5-3). Care should be taken when measuring blood gases to obtain the arterial blood sample without using excessive heparin. Blood for electrolytes and arterial blood gases should be drawn simultaneously prior to therapy, since an increase in $[HCO_3^-]$ occurs with metabolic alkalosis and respiratory acidosis. Conversely, a decrease in $[HCO_3^-]$ occurs in metabolic acidosis and respiratory alkalosis. In the determination of arterial blood gases by the clinical laboratory, both pH and $Paco_2$ are measured, and the $[HCO_3^-]$ is calculated from the

TABLE 5-3

STEPS IN ACID-BASE DIAGNOSIS
1. Obtain arterial blood gas (ABG) and electrolytes simultaneously.
2. Compare [HCO_3^-] on ABG and electrolytes to verify accuracy.
3. Calculate anion gap (AG).
4. Know four causes of high-AG acidosis (ketoacidosis, lactic acid acidosis, renal failure, and toxins).
5. Know two causes of hyperchloremic or nongap acidosis (bicarbonate loss from GI tract, renal tubular acidosis).
6. Estimate compensatory response (Table 5-1).
7. Compare ΔAG and ΔHCO_3^-.
8. Compare change in [Cl^-] with change in [Na^+].

Henderson-Hasselbalch equation. This calculated value should be compared with the measured [HCO_3^-] (total CO_2) on the electrolyte panel. These two values should agree within 2 mmol/L. If they do not, the values may not have been drawn simultaneously, a laboratory error may be present, or an error could have been made in calculating the [HCO_3^-]. After verifying the blood acid-base values, one can then identify the precise acid-base disorder.

CALCULATE THE ANION GAP All evaluations of acid-base disorders should include a simple calculation of the AG; it represents those unmeasured anions in plasma (normally 10 to 12 mmol/L) and is calculated as follows: $AG = Na^+ - (Cl^- + HCO_3^-)$. The unmeasured anions include anionic proteins, phosphate, sulfate, and organic anions. When acid anions, such as acetoacetate and lactate, accumulate in extracellular fluid, the AG increases, causing a high-AG acidosis. An increase in the AG is most often due to an increase in unmeasured anions and less commonly is due to a decrease in unmeasured cations (calcium, magnesium, potassium). In addition, the AG may increase with an increase in anionic albumin, because of either increased albumin concentration or alkalosis, which alters albumin charge. A decrease in the AG can be due to (1) an increase in unmeasured cations; (2) the addition to the blood of abnormal cations, such as lithium (lithium intoxication) or cationic immunoglobulins (plasma cell dyscrasias); (3) a reduction in the major plasma anion albumin concentration (nephrotic syndrome); (4) a decrease in the effective anionic charge on albumin by acidosis; or (5) hyperviscosity and severe hyperlipidemia, which can lead to an underestimation of sodium and chloride concentrations. A fall in serum albumin by 1 g/dL from the normal value (4.5 g/dL) decreases the anion gap by 2.5 meq/L. Know the common causes of a high-AG acidosis (Table 5-3).

In the face of a normal serum albumin, a high AG is usually due to non-chloride-containing acids that contain inorganic (phosphate, sulfate), organic (ketoacids, lactate, uremic organic anions), exogenous (salicylate or ingested toxins with organic acid production), or unidentified anions. The high AG is significant even if an additional acid-base disorder is superimposed to modify the [HCO_3^-] independently. Simultaneous metabolic acidosis of the high-AG variety plus either chronic respiratory acidosis or metabolic alkalosis represents such a situation in which [HCO_3^-] may be normal or even high (Table 5-2). Compare the change in [HCO_3^-] (ΔHCO_3^-) and the change in the AG (ΔAG).

Similarly, normal values for [HCO_3^-], $PaCO_2$, and pH do not ensure the absence of an acid-base disturbance. For instance, an alcoholic who has been vomiting may develop a metabolic alkalosis with a pH of 7.55, $PaCO_2$ of 48 mmHg, [HCO_3^-] of 40 mmol/L, [Na^+] of 135, [Cl^-] of 80, and [K^+] of 2.8. If such a patient were then to develop a superimposed alcoholic ketoacidosis with a β-hydroxybutyrate concentration of 15 mM, arterial pH would fall to 7.40, [HCO_3^-] to 25 mmol/L, and the $PaCO_2$ to 40 mmHg. Although these blood gases are normal, the AG is elevated at 30 mmol/L, indicating a mixed metabolic alkalosis and metabolic acidosis. A mixture of high-gap acidosis and metabolic alkalosis is recognized easily by comparing the differences (Δ values) in the normal to prevailing patient values. In this example, the ΔHCO_3^- is 0 (25 − 25 mmol/L) but the ΔAG is 20 (30 − 10 mmol/L). Therefore, 20 mmol/L is unaccounted for in the Δ / Δ value (ΔAG to ΔHCO_3^-).

METABOLIC ACIDOSIS

Metabolic acidosis can occur because of an increase in endogenous acid production (such as lactate and ketoacids), loss of bicarbonate (as in diarrhea), or accumulation of endogenous acids (as in renal failure). Metabolic acidosis has profound effects on the respiratory, cardiac, and nervous systems. The fall in blood pH is accompanied by a characteristic increase in ventilation, especially the tidal volume (Kussmaul respiration). Intrinsic cardiac contractility may be depressed, but inotropic function can be normal because of catecholamine release. Both peripheral arterial vasodilation and central venoconstriction can be present; the decrease in central and pulmonary vascular compliance predisposes to pulmonary edema with even minimal volume overload. Central nervous system function is depressed, with headache, lethargy, stupor, and, in some cases, even coma. Glucose intolerance may also occur.

There are two major categories of clinical metabolic acidosis: high-AG and normal-AG, or hyperchloremic acidosis (Tables 5-3 and 5-4).

TABLE 5-4

CAUSES OF HIGH-ANION-GAP METABOLIC ACIDOSIS	
Lactic acidosis	Toxins
Ketoacidosis	Ethylene glycol
Diabetic	Methanol
Alcoholic	Salicylates
Starvation	Propylene glycol
	Pyroglutamic acid
	Renal failure (acute and chronic)

℞ **Treatment:**
METABOLIC ACIDOSIS

Treatment of metabolic acidosis with alkali should be reserved for severe acidemia except when the patient has no "potential HCO_3^-" in plasma. Potential $[HCO_3^-]$ can be estimated from the increment (Δ) in the AG (ΔAG = patient's AG – 10). It must be determined if the acid anion in plasma is metabolizable (i.e., β-hydroxybutyrate, acetoacetate, and lactate) or nonmetabolizable (anions that accumulate in chronic renal failure and after toxin ingestion). The latter requires return of renal function to replenish the $[HCO_3^-]$ deficit, a slow and often unpredictable process. Consequently, patients with a normal AG acidosis (hyperchloremic acidosis), a slightly elevated AG (mixed hyperchloremic and AG acidosis), or an AG attributable to a nonmetabolizable anion in the face of renal failure should receive alkali therapy, either PO (NaHCO₃ or Shohl's solution) or IV (NaHCO₃), in an amount necessary to slowly increase the plasma $[HCO_3^-]$ into the 20–22 mmol/L range.

Controversy exists, however, in regard to the use of alkali in patients with a pure AG acidosis owing to accumulation of a metabolizable organic acid anion (ketoacidosis or lactic acidosis). In general, severe acidosis (pH < 7.20) warrants the IV administration of 50–100 meq of NaHCO₃, over 30–45 min, during the initial 1–2 h of therapy. Provision of such modest quantities of alkali in this situation seems to provide an added measure of safety, but it is essential to monitor plasma electrolytes during the course of therapy, since the $[K^+]$ may decline as pH rises. The goal is to increase the $[HCO_3^-]$ to 10 meq/L and the pH to 7.15, not to increase these values to normal.

HIGH-ANION-GAP ACIDOSES

Approach to the Patient:
HIGH-ANION-GAP ACIDOSES

There are four principal causes of a high–AG acidosis: (1) lactic acidosis, (2) ketoacidosis, (3) ingested toxins, and (4) acute and chronic renal failure (Table 5-4). Initial screening to differentiate the high–AG acidoses should include (1) a probe of the history for evidence of drug and toxin ingestion and measurement of arterial blood gas to detect coexistent respiratory alkalosis (salicylates); (2) determination of whether diabetes mellitus is present (diabetic ketoacidosis); (3) a search for evidence of alcoholism or increased levels of β-hydroxybutyrate (alcoholic ketoacidosis); (4) observation for clinical signs of uremia and determination of the blood urea nitrogen (BUN) and creatinine (uremic acidosis); (5) inspection of the urine for oxalate crystals (ethylene glycol); and (6) recognition of the numerous clinical settings in which lactate levels may be increased (hypotension, shock, cardiac failure, leukemia, cancer, and drug or toxin ingestion).

Lactic Acidosis

An increase in plasma L-lactate may be secondary to poor tissue perfusion (type A)—circulatory insufficiency (shock, cardiac failure), severe anemia, mitochondrial enzyme defects, and inhibitors (carbon monoxide, cyanide); or to aerobic disorders (type B)—malignancies, nucleoside analogue reverse transcriptase inhibitors in HIV, diabetes mellitus, renal or hepatic failure, thiamine deficiency, severe infections (cholera, malaria), seizures, or drugs/toxins (biguanides, ethanol, methanol, propylene glycol, isoniazid, and fructose). Propylene glycol may be used as a vehicle for IV medications including lorazepam, and toxicity has been reported in several settings. Unrecognized bowel ischemia or infarction in a patient with severe atherosclerosis or cardiac decompensation receiving vasopressors is a common cause of lactic acidosis. Pyroglutamic acidemia has been reported in critically ill patients receiving acetaminophen, which is associated with depletion of glutathione. D-Lactic acid acidosis, which may be associated with jejunoileal bypass, short bowel syndrome, or intestinal obstruction, is due to formation of D-lactate by gut bacteria.

Approach to the Patient:
LACTIC ACID ACIDOSIS

The underlying condition that disrupts lactate metabolism must first be corrected; tissue perfusion must be restored when inadequate. Vasoconstrictors should be avoided, if possible, since they may worsen tissue perfusion. Alkali therapy is generally advocated for acute, severe acidemia (pH < 7.15) to improve cardiac function and lactate utilization. However, NaHCO₃ therapy may paradoxically depress cardiac performance and exacerbate acidosis by enhancing lactate production (HCO_3^- stimulates phosphofructokinase). While the use of alkali in moderate lactic acidosis is controversial, it is generally agreed that attempts to return the pH or [HCO$_3^-$] to normal by administration of exogenous NaHCO$_3$ are deleterious. A reasonable approach is to infuse sufficient NaHCO$_3$ to raise the arterial pH to no more than 7.2 over 30–40 min.

NaHCO$_3$ therapy can cause fluid overload and hypertension because the amount required can be massive when accumulation of lactic acid is relentless. Fluid administration is poorly tolerated because of central venoconstriction, especially in the oliguric patient. When the underlying cause of the lactic acidosis can be remedied, blood lactate will be converted to HCO$_3^-$ and may result in an overshoot alkalosis.

Ketoacidosis

▇▇▇ Diabetic Ketoacidosis (DKA)

This condition is caused by increased fatty acid metabolism and the accumulation of ketoacids (acetoacetate and β-hydroxybutyrate). DKA usually occurs in insulin-dependent diabetes mellitus in association with cessation of insulin or an intercurrent illness, such as an infection, gastroenteritis, pancreatitis, or myocardial infarction, which increases insulin requirements temporarily and acutely. The accumulation of ketoacids accounts for the increment in the AG and is accompanied most often by hyperglycemia [glucose > 17 mmol/L (300 mg/dL)]. The relationship between the ΔAG and ΔHCO$_3^-$ is ~1:1 in DKA but may decrease in the well-hydrated patient with preservation of renal function. Ketoacid excretion in the urine reduces the anion gap in this situation. It should be noted that since insulin prevents production of ketones, bicarbonate therapy is rarely needed except with extreme acidemia (pH < 7.1), and then in only limited amounts. Patients with DKA are typically volume depleted and require fluid resuscitation with isotonic saline. Volume overexpansion is not uncommon, however, after IV fluid administration, and contributes to the development of a hyperchloremic acidosis during treatment of DKA because volume expansion increases urinary ketoacid anion excretion (loss of potential bicarbonate).

▇▇▇ Alcoholic Ketoacidosis (AKA)

Chronic alcoholics can develop ketoacidosis when alcohol consumption is abruptly curtailed and nutrition is poor. AKA is usually associated with binge drinking, vomiting, abdominal pain, starvation, and volume depletion. The glucose concentration is variable, and acidosis may be severe because of elevated ketones, predominantly β-hydroxybutyrate. Hypoperfusion may enhance lactic acid production, chronic respiratory alkalosis may accompany liver disease, and metabolic alkalosis can result from vomiting (refer to the relationship between ΔAG and ΔHCO$_3^-$). Thus, mixed acid–base disorders are common in AKA. As the circulation is restored by administration of isotonic saline, the preferential accumulation of β-hydroxybutyrate is then shifted to acetoacetate. This explains the common clinical observation of an increasingly positive nitroprusside reaction as the patient improves. The nitroprusside ketone reaction (Acetest) can detect acetoacetic acid but not β-hydroxybutyrate, so that the degree of ketosis and ketonuria can not only change with therapy, but can be underestimated initially. Patients with AKA usually present with relatively normal renal function, as opposed to DKA where renal function is often compromised because of volume depletion (osmotic diuresis) or diabetic nephropathy. The AKA patient with normal renal function may excrete relatively large quantities of ketoacids in the urine, therefore, and may have a relatively normal AG and a discrepancy in the ΔAG/ΔHCO$_3^-$ relationship. Typically, insulin levels are low, and concentrations of triglyceride, cortisol, glucagon, and growth hormone are increased.

℞ Treatment: ALCOHOLIC KETOACIDOSIS

Extracellular fluid deficits almost always accompany AKA and should be repleted by IV administration of saline and glucose (5% dextrose in 0.9% NaCl). Hypophosphatemia, hypokalemia, and hypomagnesemia may coexist and should be corrected. Hypophosphatemia usually emerges 12–24 h after admission, may be exacerbated by glucose infusion, and, if severe, may induce rhabdomyolysis. Upper gastrointestinal hemorrhage, pancreatitis, and pneumonia may accompany this disorder.

Drug- and Toxin-Induced Acidosis

▇▇▇ Salicylates

Salicylate intoxication in adults usually causes respiratory alkalosis or a mixture of high-AG metabolic acidosis and respiratory alkalosis. Only a portion of the AG is due to salicylates. Lactic acid production is also often increased.

℞ Treatment: SALICYLATE-INDUCED ACIDOSIS

Vigorous gastric lavage with isotonic saline (not NaHCO$_3$) should be initiated immediately followed by administration of activated charcoal per NG tube. In the acidotic patient, to facilitate removal of salicylate, intravenous NaHCO$_3$ is administered in amounts adequate to alkalinize the urine and to maintain urine output (urine pH > 7.5). While this form of therapy is straightforward in acidotic patients, a coexisting respiratory alkalosis may make this approach hazardous. Alkalemic patients should not receive $NaHCO_3^-$. Acetazolamide may be administered in the face of alkalemia, when an alkaline diuresis cannot be achieved, or to ameliorate volume overload associated with $NaHCO_3^-$ administration, but this drug can cause systemic metabolic acidosis if HCO_3^- is not replaced. Hypokalemia should be anticipated with an alkaline diuresis and should be treated promptly and aggressively. Glucose-containing fluids should be administered because of the danger of hypoglycemia. Excessive insensible fluid losses may cause severe volume depletion and hypernatremia. If renal failure prevents rapid clearance of salicylate, hemodialysis can be performed against a bicarbonate dialysate.

Alcohols

Under most physiologic conditions, sodium, urea, and glucose generate the osmotic pressure of blood. Plasma osmolality is calculated according to the following expression: $P_{osm} = 2Na^+ + Glu + BUN$ (all in mmol/L), or, using conventional laboratory values in which glucose and BUN are expressed in milligrams per deciliter: $P_{osm} = 2Na^+ + Glu/18 + BUN/2.8$. The calculated and determined osmolality should agree within 10–15 mmol/kg H_2O. When the measured osmolality exceeds the calculated osmolality by >15–20 mmol/kg H_2O, one of two circumstances prevails. Either the serum sodium is spuriously low, as with hyperlipidemia or hyperproteinemia (pseudohyponatremia), or osmolytes other than sodium salts, glucose, or urea have accumulated in plasma. Examples include mannitol, radiocontrast media, isopropyl alcohol, ethylene glycol, propylene glycol, ethanol, methanol, and acetone. In this situation, the difference between the calculated osmolality and the measured osmolality (*osmolar gap*) is proportional to the concentration of the unmeasured solute. With an appropriate clinical history and index of suspicion, identification of an osmolar gap is helpful in identifying the presence of poison-associated AG acidosis. Three alcohols may cause fatal intoxications: ethylene glycol, methanol, and isopropyl alcohol. All cause an elevated osmolar gap, but only the first two cause a high-AG acidosis.

Ethylene Glycol

Ingestion of ethylene glycol (commonly used in antifreeze) leads to a metabolic acidosis and severe damage to the central nervous system, heart, lungs, and kidneys. The increased AG and osmolar gap are attributable to ethylene glycol and its metabolites, oxalic acid, glycolic acid, and other organic acids. Lactic acid production increases secondary to inhibition of the tricarboxylic acid cycle and altered intracellular redox state. Diagnosis is facilitated by recognizing oxalate crystals in the urine, the presence of an osmolar gap in serum, and a high-AG acidosis.

If antifreeze containing a fluorescent dye is ingested, a Wood's lamp applied to the urine may be revealing. Treatment should not be delayed while awaiting measurement of ethylene glycol levels in this setting.

℞ Treatment:
ETHYLENE GLYCOL–INDUCED ACIDOSIS

This includes the prompt institution of a saline or osmotic diuresis, thiamine and pyridoxine supplements, fomepizole or ethanol, and hemodialysis. The IV administration of the alcohol dehydrogenase inhibitor fomepizole (4-methylpyrazole; 7 mg/kg as a loading dose) or ethanol IV to achieve a level of 22 mmol/L (100 mg/dL) serves to lessen toxicity because they compete with ethylene glycol for metabolism by alcohol dehydrogenase. Fomepizole, although expensive, offers the advantages of a predictable decline in ethylene glycol levels without excessive obtundation during ethyl alcohol infusion.

Methanol

The ingestion of methanol (wood alcohol) causes metabolic acidosis, and its metabolites formaldehyde and formic acid cause severe optic nerve and central nervous system damage. Lactic acid, ketoacids, and other unidentified organic acids may contribute to the acidosis. Due to its low molecular weight (32 Da), an osmolar gap is usually present.

℞ Treatment:
METHANOL–INDUCED ACIDOSIS

This is similar to that for ethylene glycol intoxication, including general supportive measures, fomepizole or ethanol administration, and hemodialysis.

Isopropyl Alcohol

Ingested isopropanol is absorbed rapidly and may be fatal when as little as 150 mL of rubbing alcohol, solvent, or deicer is consumed. A plasma level >400 mg/dL is life threatening. Isopropyl alcohol differs from ethylene glycol and methanol in that the parent compound, not the metabolites, causes toxicity, and acidosis is not present because acetone is rapidly excreted.

℞ Treatment:
ISOPROPYL ALCOHOL TOXICITY

Isopropanol alcohol toxicity is treated by watchful waiting and supportive therapy; IV fluids, pressors, ventilatory support if needed; and occasionally hemodialysis for prolonged coma or levels >400 mg/dL.

Renal Failure

(See also Chaps. 10 and 11.) The hyperchloremic acidosis of moderate renal insufficiency is eventually converted to the high-AG acidosis of advanced renal failure. Poor filtration and reabsorption of organic anions contribute to the pathogenesis. As renal disease progresses, the number of functioning nephrons eventually becomes insufficient to keep pace with net acid production. Uremic acidosis is characterized, therefore, by a reduced rate of NH_4^+ production and excretion, primarily due to decreased renal mass. $[HCO_3^-]$ rarely falls to <15 mmol/L, and the AG is rarely >20 mmol/L. The acid retained in chronic renal disease is buffered by alkaline salts from bone. Despite significant retention of acid (up to 20 mmol/d), the serum $[HCO_3^-]$ does not decrease further, indicating participation of buffers outside the extracellular compartment. Chronic metabolic acidosis results in significant loss of bone mass due to reduction in bone calcium carbonate. Chronic acidosis also increases urinary calcium excretion, proportional to cumulative acid retention.

℞ **Treatment:**
RENAL FAILURE

Because of the association of renal failure acidosis with muscle catabolism and bone disease, both uremic acidosis and the hyperchloremic acidosis of renal failure require oral alkali replacement to maintain the $[HCO_3^-]$ between 20 and 24 mmol/L. This can be accomplished with relatively modest amounts of alkali (1.0–1.5 mmol/kg body weight per day). Sodium citrate (Shohl's solution) or $NaHCO_3$ tablets (650-mg tablets contain 7.8 meq) are equally effective alkalinizing salts. Citrate enhances the absorption of aluminum from the gastrointestinal tract and should never be given together with aluminum-containing antacids because of the risk of aluminum intoxication. When hyperkalemia is present, furosemide (60–80 mg/d) should be added.

Hyperchloremic (Nongap) Metabolic Acidoses

Alkali can be lost from the gastrointestinal tract in diarrhea or from the kidneys (renal tubular acidosis, RTA). In these disorders (Table 5-5), reciprocal changes in $[Cl^-]$ and $[HCO_3^-]$ result in a normal AG. In pure hyperchloremic acidosis, therefore, the increase in $[Cl^-]$ above the normal value approximates the decrease in $[HCO_3^-]$. The absence of such a relationship suggests a mixed disturbance.

Approach to the Patient:
HYPERCHLOREMIC METABOLIC ACIDOSES

In diarrhea, stools contain a higher $[HCO_3^-]$ and decomposed HCO_3^- than plasma so that metabolic

TABLE 5-5

CAUSES OF NON-ANION-GAP ACIDOSIS
I. Gastrointestinal bicarbonate loss
A. Diarrhea
B. External pancreatic or small-bowel drainage
C. Ureterosigmoidostomy, jejunal loop, ileal loop
D. Drugs
1. Calcium chloride (acidifying agent)
2. Magnesium sulfate (diarrhea)
3. Cholestyramine (bile acid diarrhea)
II. Renal acidosis
A. Hypokalemia
1. Proximal RTA (type 2)
2. Distal (classic) RTA (type 1)
B. Hyperkalemia
1. Generalized distal nephron dysfunction (type 4 RTA)
a. Mineralocorticoid deficiency
b. Mineralocorticoid resistance (autosomal dominant PHA I)
c. Voltage defect (autosomal dominant PHA I and PHA II)
d. Tubulointerstitial disease
III. Drug-induced hyperkalemia (with renal insufficiency)
A. Potassium-sparing diuretics (amiloride, triamterene, spironolactone)
B. Trimethoprim
C. Pentamidine
D. ACE-Is and ARBs
E. Nonsteroidal anti-inflammatory drugs
F. Cyclosporine and tacrolimus

acidosis develops along with volume depletion. Instead of an acid urine pH (as anticipated with systemic acidosis), urine pH is usually around 6 because metabolic acidosis and hypokalemia increase renal synthesis and excretion of NH_4^+, thus providing a urinary buffer that increases urine pH. Metabolic acidosis due to gastrointestinal losses with a high urine pH can be differentiated from RTA (Chap. 16) because urinary NH_4^+ excretion is typically low in RTA and high with diarrhea. Urinary NH_4^+ levels can be estimated by calculating the urine anion gap (UAG): UAG = $[Na^+ + K^+]_u − [Cl^-]_u$. When $[Cl^-]_u > [Na^+ + K^+]$, the urine gap is negative by definition. This indicates that the urine ammonium level is appropriately increased, suggesting an extrarenal cause of the acidosis. Conversely, when the urine anion gap is positive, the urine ammonium level is low, suggesting a renal cause of the acidosis.

Loss of functioning renal parenchyma by progressive renal disease leads to hyperchloremic acidosis when the glomerular filtration rate (GFR) is between 20 and 50 mL/min and to uremic acidosis with a high AG when the GFR falls to <20 mL/min. Such a progression occurs commonly with tubulointerstitial forms of renal disease, but hyperchloremic metabolic acidosis can persist with advanced glomerular disease. In advanced renal failure, ammoniagenesis is reduced in proportion to the loss of functional renal mass, and ammonium accumulation and trapping in the outer medullary collecting tubule may also be impaired. Because of adaptive increases in K^+ secretion by the collecting duct and colon, the acidosis of chronic renal insufficiency is typically normokalemic.

Proximal RTA (type 2 RTA) (Chap. 16) is most often due to generalized proximal tubular dysfunction manifested by glycosuria, generalized aminoaciduria, and phosphaturia (Fanconi syndrome). With a low plasma $[HCO_3^-]$, the urine pH is acid (pH $<$ 5.5). The fractional excretion of $[HCO_3^-]$ may exceed 10–15% when the serum HCO_3^- $>$ 20 mmol/L. Since HCO_3^- is not reabsorbed normally in the proximal tubule, therapy with $NaHCO_3$ will enhance renal potassium wasting and hypokalemia.

The typical findings in acquired or inherited forms of classic distal RTA (type 1 RTA) include hypokalemia, hyperchloremic acidosis, low urinary NH_4^+ excretion (positive UAG, low urine $[NH_4^+]$), and inappropriately high urine pH (pH $>$ 5.5). Such patients are unable to acidify the urine below a pH of 5.5. Most patients have hypocitraturia and hypercalciuria, so nephrolithiasis, nephrocalcinosis, and bone disease are common. In generalized distal nephron dysfunction (type 4 RTA), hyperkalemia is disproportionate to the reduction in GFR because of coexisting dysfunction of potassium and acid secretion. Urinary ammonium excretion is invariably depressed, and renal function may be compromised, for example, due to diabetic nephropathy, amyloidosis, or tubulointerstitial disease.

Hyporeninemic hypoaldosteronism typically causes hyperchloremic metabolic acidosis, most commonly in older adults with diabetes mellitus or tubulointerstitial disease and renal insufficiency. Patients usually have mild to moderate renal insufficiency (GFR, 20–50 mL/min) and acidosis, with elevation in serum $[K^+]$ (5.2–6.0 mmol/L), concurrent hypertension, and congestive heart failure. Both the metabolic acidosis and the hyperkalemia are out of proportion to impairment in GFR. Nonsteroidal anti-inflammatory drugs, trimethoprim, pentamidine, and angiotensin-converting enzyme (ACE) inhibitors can also cause hyperkalemia with hyperchloremic metabolic acidosis in patients with renal insufficiency (Table 5-5).

See Chap. 16 for the pathophysiology, diagnosis, and treatment of RTA.

METABOLIC ALKALOSIS

Metabolic alkalosis is manifested by an elevated arterial pH, an increase in the serum $[HCO_3^-]$, and an increase in $PaCO_2$ as a result of compensatory alveolar hypoventilation (Table 5-1). It is often accompanied by hypochloremia and hypokalemia. The arterial pH establishes the diagnosis, since it is increased in metabolic alkalosis and decreased or normal in respiratory acidosis. Metabolic alkalosis frequently occurs in association with other disorders such as respiratory acidosis or alkalosis or metabolic acidosis.

PATHOGENESIS

Metabolic alkalosis occurs as a result of net gain of $[HCO_3^-]$ or loss of nonvolatile acid (usually HCl by vomiting) from the extracellular fluid. Since it is unusual for alkali to be added to the body, the disorder involves a generative stage, in which the loss of acid usually causes alkalosis, and a maintenance stage, in which the kidneys fail to compensate by excreting HCO_3^-.

Under normal circumstances, the kidneys have an impressive capacity to excrete HCO_3^-. Continuation of metabolic alkalosis represents a failure of the kidneys to eliminate HCO_3^- in the usual manner. For HCO_3^- to be added to the extracellular fluid, it must be administered exogenously or synthesized endogenously, in part or entirely by the kidneys. The kidneys will retain, rather than excrete, the excess alkali and maintain the alkalosis if (1) volume deficiency, chloride deficiency, and K^+ deficiency exist in combination with a reduced GFR, which augments distal tubule H^+ secretion; or (2) hypokalemia exists because of autonomous hyperaldosteronism. In the first example, alkalosis is corrected by administration of NaCl and KCl, whereas in the latter it is necessary to repair the alkalosis by pharmacologic or surgical intervention, not with saline administration.

DIFFERENTIAL DIAGNOSIS

To establish the cause of metabolic alkalosis (Table 5-6), it is necessary to assess the status of the extracellular fluid volume (ECFV), the recumbent and upright blood pressure, the serum $[K^+]$, and the renin–aldosterone system. For example, the presence of chronic hypertension and chronic hypokalemia in an alkalotic patient suggests either mineralocorticoid excess or that the hypertensive patient is receiving diuretics. Low plasma renin activity and normal urine $[Na^+]$ and $[Cl^-]$ in a patient who is not taking diuretics indicate a primary mineralocorticoid excess syndrome. The combination of hypokalemia and alkalosis in a normotensive, nonedematous patient can be due to Bartter's or Gitelman's syndrome, magnesium deficiency, vomiting, exogenous alkali, or diuretic ingestion. Determination of urine electrolytes (especially the urine $[Cl^-]$) and screening of the urine for diuretics may be helpful. If the urine is alkaline, with an elevated $[Na^+]$ and $[K^+]$ but low $[Cl^-]$, the diagnosis is usually either vomiting (overt or surreptitious) or alkali ingestion. If the urine is relatively acid and has low concentrations of Na^+, K^+, and Cl^-, the most likely possibilities are prior vomiting, the posthypercapnic state, or prior diuretic ingestion. If, on

TABLE 5-6

CAUSES OF METABOLIC ALKALOSIS

I. Exogenous HCO_3^- loads
   A. Acute alkali administration
   B. Milk-alkali syndrome
II. Effective ECFV contraction, normotension, K^+ deficiency, and secondary hyperreninemic hyperaldosteronism
   A. Gastrointestinal origin
      1. Vomiting
      2. Gastric aspiration
      3. Congenital chloridorrhea
      4. Villous adenoma
   B. Renal origin
      1. Diuretics
      2. Posthypercapnic state
      3. Hypercalcemia/hypoparathyroidism
      4. Recovery from lactic acidosis or ketoacidosis
      5. Nonreabsorbable anions including penicillin, carbenicillin
      6. Mg^{2+} deficiency
      7. K^+ depletion
      8. Bartter's syndrome (loss of function mutations in TALH)
      9. Gitelman's syndrome (loss of function mutation in Na^+-Cl^- cotransporter in DCT)
III. ECFV expansion, hypertension, K^+ deficiency, and mineralocorticoid excess
   A. High renin
      1. Renal artery stenosis
      2. Accelerated hypertension
      3. Renin-secreting tumor
      4. Estrogen therapy
   B. Low renin
      1. Primary aldosteronism
         a. Adenoma
         b. Hyperplasia
         c. Carcinoma
      2. Adrenal enzyme defects
         a. 11 β-Hydroxylase deficiency
         b. 17 α-Hydroxylase deficiency
      3. Cushing's syndrome or disease
      4. Other
         a. Licorice
         b. Carbenoxolone
         c. Chewer's tobacco
IV. Gain-of-function mutation of renal sodium channel with ECFV expansion, hypertension, K^+ deficiency, and hyporeninemic-hypoaldosteronism
   A. Liddle's syndrome

Note: ECFV, extracellular fluid volume; TALH, thick ascending limb of Henle's loop; DCT, distal convoluted tubule.

disorder. The genetic and molecular basis of these two disorders has been elucidated recently (Chap. 16).

Alkali Administration

Chronic administration of alkali to individuals with normal renal function rarely, if ever, causes alkalosis. However, in patients with coexistent hemodynamic disturbances, alkalosis can develop because the normal capacity to excrete HCO_3^- may be exceeded or there may be enhanced reabsorption of HCO_3^-. Such patients include those who receive HCO_3^- (PO or IV), acetate loads (parenteral hyperalimentation solutions), citrate loads (transfusions), or antacids plus cation-exchange resins (aluminum hydroxide and sodium polystyrene sulfonate).

METABOLIC ALKALOSIS ASSOCIATED WITH ECFV CONTRACTION, K⁺ DEPLETION, AND SECONDARY HYPERRENINEMIC HYPERALDOSTERONISM

Gastrointestinal Origin

Gastrointestinal loss of H^+ from vomiting or gastric aspiration results in retention of HCO_3^-. The loss of fluid and NaCl in vomitus or nasogastric suction results in contraction of the ECFV and an increase in the secretion of renin and aldosterone. Volume contraction through a reduction in GFR results in an enhanced capacity of the renal tubule to reabsorb HCO_3^-. During active vomiting, however, the filtered load of bicarbonate is acutely increased to the point that the reabsorptive capacity of the proximal tubule for HCO_3^- is exceeded. The excess $NaHCO_3$ issuing out of the proximal tubule reaches the distal tubule, where H^+ secretion is enhanced by an aldosterone and the delivery of the poorly reabsorbed anion, HCO_3^-. Correction of the contracted ECFV with NaCl and repair of K^+ deficits corrects the acid-base disorder, and chloride deficiency.

Renal Origin

Diuretics

Drugs that induce chloruresis, such as thiazides and loop diuretics (furosemide, bumetanide, torsemide, and ethacrynic acid), acutely diminish the ECFV without altering the total body bicarbonate content. The serum $[HCO_3^-]$ increases because the reduced ECFV "contracts" the $[HCO_3^-]$ in the plasma (contraction alkalosis). The chronic administration of diuretics tends to generate an alkalosis by increasing distal salt delivery, so that K^+ and H^+ secretion are stimulated. The alkalosis is maintained by persistence of the contraction of the ECFV, secondary hyperaldosteronism, K^+ deficiency, and the direct effect of the diuretic (as long as diuretic administration continues). Repair of the alkalosis is achieved by providing isotonic saline to correct the ECFV deficit.

the other hand, neither the urine sodium, potassium, nor chloride concentrations are depressed, magnesium deficiency, Bartter's or Gitelman's syndrome, or current diuretic ingestion should be considered. Bartter's syndrome is distinguished from Gitelman's syndrome because of hypocalciuria and hypomagnesemia in the latter

Solute Losing Disorders: Bartter's Syndrome and Gitelman's Syndrome

See Chap. 16.

Nonreabsorbable Anions and Magnesium Deficiency

Administration of large quantities of nonreabsorbable anions, such as penicillin or carbenicillin, can enhance distal acidification and K^+ secretion by increasing the transepithelial potential difference (lumen negative). Mg^{2+} deficiency results in hypokalemic alkalosis by enhancing distal acidification through stimulation of renin and hence aldosterone secretion.

Potassium Depletion

Chronic K^+ depletion may cause metabolic alkalosis by increasing urinary acid excretion. Both NH_4^+ production and absorption are enhanced and HCO_3^- reabsorption is stimulated. Chronic K^+ deficiency upregulates the renal H^+, K^+-ATPase to increase K^+ absorption at the expense of enhanced H^+ secretion. Alkalosis associated with severe K^+ depletion is resistant to salt administration, but repair of the K^+ deficiency corrects the alkalosis.

After Treatment of Lactic Acidosis or Ketoacidosis

When an underlying stimulus for the generation of lactic acid or ketoacid is removed rapidly, as with repair of circulatory insufficiency or with insulin therapy, the lactate or ketones are metabolized to yield an equivalent amount of HCO_3^-. Other sources of new HCO_3^- are additive with the original amount generated by organic anion metabolism to create a surfeit of HCO_3^-. Such sources include (1) new HCO_3^- added to the blood by the kidneys as a result of enhanced acid excretion during the preexisting period of acidosis, and (2) alkali therapy during the treatment phase of the acidosis. Acidosis-induced contraction of the ECFV and K^+ deficiency act to sustain the alkalosis.

Posthypercapnia

Prolonged CO_2 retention with chronic respiratory acidosis enhances renal HCO_3^- absorption and the generation of new HCO_3^- (increased net acid excretion). If the Pa_{CO_2} is returned to normal, metabolic alkalosis results from the persistently elevated $[HCO_3^-]$. Alkalosis develops if the elevated Pa_{CO_2} is abruptly returned toward normal by a change in mechanically controlled ventilation. Associated ECFV contraction does not allow complete repair of the alkalosis by correction of the Pa_{CO_2} alone, and alkalosis persists until Cl^- supplementation is provided.

METABOLIC ALKALOSIS ASSOCIATED WITH ECFV EXPANSION, HYPERTENSION, AND HYPERALDOSTERONISM

Increased aldosterone levels may be the result of autonomous primary adrenal overproduction or of secondary aldosterone release due to renal overproduction of renin. Mineralocorticoid excess increases net acid excretion and may result in metabolic alkalosis, which may be worsened by associated K^+ deficiency. ECFV expansion from salt retention causes hypertension. The kaliuresis persists because of mineralocorticoid excess and distal Na^+ absorption causing enhanced K^+ excretion, continued K^+ depletion with polydipsia, inability to concentrate the urine, and polyuria.

Liddle's syndrome (Chap. 16) results from increased activity of the collecting duct Na^+ channel (ENaC) and is a rare inherited disorder associated with hypertension due to volume expansion manifested as hypokalemic alkalosis and normal aldosterone levels.

Symptoms

With metabolic alkalosis, changes in central and peripheral nervous system function are similar to those of hypocalcemia; symptoms include mental confusion, obtundation, and a predisposition to seizures, paresthesia, muscular cramping, tetany, aggravation of arrhythmias, and hypoxemia in chronic obstructive pulmonary disease. Related electrolyte abnormalities include hypokalemia and hypophosphatemia.

℞ Treatment: METABOLIC ALKALOSIS

This is primarily directed at correcting the underlying stimulus for HCO_3^- generation. If primary aldosteronism, renal artery stenosis, or Cushing's syndrome is present, correction of the underlying cause will reverse the alkalosis. $[H^+]$ loss by the stomach or kidneys can be mitigated by the use of proton pump inhibitors or the discontinuation of diuretics. The second aspect of treatment is to remove the factors that sustain the inappropriate increase in HCO_3^- reabsorption, such as ECFV contraction or K^+ deficiency. Although K^+ deficits should be repaired, NaCl therapy is usually sufficient to reverse the alkalosis if ECFV contraction is present, as indicated by a low urine $[Cl^-]$.

If associated conditions preclude infusion of saline, renal HCO_3^- loss can be accelerated by administration of acetazolamide, a carbonic anhydrase inhibitor, which is usually effective in patients with adequate renal function but can worsen K^+ losses. Dilute hydrochloric acid (0.1 N HCl) is also effective but can cause hemolysis, and must be delivered centrally and slowly. Hemodialysis against a dialysate low in $[HCO_3^-]$ and high in $[Cl^-]$ can be effective when renal function is impaired.

RESPIRATORY ACIDOSIS

Respiratory acidosis can be due to severe pulmonary disease, respiratory muscle fatigue, or abnormalities in ventilatory control and is recognized by an increase in

PaCO$_2$ and decrease in pH (Table 5-7). In acute respiratory acidosis, there is an immediate compensatory elevation (due to cellular buffering mechanisms) in HCO$_3^-$, which increases 1 mmol/L for every 10-mmHg increase in PaCO$_2$. In chronic respiratory acidosis (>24 h), renal adaptation increases the [HCO$_3^-$] by 4 mmol/L for every 10-mmHg increase in PaCO$_2$. The serum HCO$_3^-$ usually does not increase above 38 mmol/L.

The clinical features vary according to the severity and duration of the respiratory acidosis, the underlying disease, and whether there is accompanying hypoxemia. A rapid increase in PaCO$_2$ may cause anxiety, dyspnea, confusion, psychosis, and hallucinations and may progress to coma. Lesser degrees of dysfunction in chronic hypercapnia include sleep disturbances, loss of memory, daytime somnolence, personality changes, impairment of coordination, and motor disturbances such as tremor, myoclonic jerks, and asterixis. Headaches and other signs that mimic raised intracranial pressure, such as papilledema, abnormal reflexes, and focal muscle weakness, are due to vasoconstriction secondary to loss of the vasodilator effects of CO$_2$.

Depression of the respiratory center by a variety of drugs, injury, or disease can produce respiratory acidosis. This may occur acutely with general anesthetics, sedatives, and head trauma or chronically with sedatives, alcohol, intracranial tumors, and the syndromes of sleep-disordered breathing, including the primary alveolar and obesity-hypoventilation syndromes. Abnormalities or disease in the motor neurons, neuromuscular junction, and skeletal muscle can cause hypoventilation via respiratory muscle fatigue. Mechanical ventilation, when not properly adjusted and supervised, may result in respiratory acidosis, particularly if CO$_2$ production suddenly rises (because of fever, agitation, sepsis, or overfeeding) or alveolar ventilation falls because of worsening pulmonary function. High levels of positive end-expiratory pressure in the presence of reduced cardiac output may cause hypercapnia as a result of large increases in alveolar dead space. Permissive hypercapnia is being used with increasing frequency because of studies suggesting lower mortality rates than with conventional mechanical ventilation, especially with severe central nervous system or heart disease. The potential beneficial effects of permissive hypercapnia may be mitigated by correction of the acidemia by administration of NaHCO$_3$.

Acute hypercapnia follows sudden occlusion of the upper airway or generalized bronchospasm as in severe asthma, anaphylaxis, inhalational burn, or toxin injury. Chronic hypercapnia and respiratory acidosis occur in end-stage obstructive lung disease. Restrictive disorders involving both the chest wall and the lungs can cause respiratory acidosis because the high metabolic cost of respiration causes ventilatory muscle fatigue. Advanced stages of intrapulmonary and extrapulmonary restrictive defects present as chronic respiratory acidosis.

TABLE 5-7
RESPIRATORY ACID-BASE DISORDERS

I. Alkalosis
  A. Central nervous system stimulation
    1. Pain
    2. Anxiety, psychosis
    3. Fever
    4. Cerebrovascular accident
    5. Meningitis, encephalitis
    6. Tumor
    7. Trauma
  B. Hypoxemia or tissue hypoxia
    1. High altitude, ↓PaCO$_2$
    2. Pneumonia, pulmonary edema
    3. Aspiration
    4. Severe anemia
  C. Drugs or hormones
    1. Pregnancy, progesterone
    2. Salicylates
    3. Cardiac failure
  D. Stimulation of chest receptors
    1. Hemothorax
    2. Flail chest
    3. Cardiac failure
    4. Pulmonary embolism
  E. Miscellaneous
    1. Septicemia
    2. Hepatic failure
    3. Mechanical hyperventilation
    4. Heat exposure
    5. Recovery from metabolic acidosis
II. Acidosis
  A. Central
    1. Drugs (anesthetics, morphine, sedatives)
    2. Stroke
    3. Infection
  B. Airway
    1. Obstruction
    2. Asthma
  C. Parenchyma
    1. Emphysema
    2. Pneumoconiosis
    3. Bronchitis
    4. Adult respiratory distress syndrome
    5. Barotrauma
  D. Neuromuscular
    1. Poliomyelitis
    2. Kyphoscoliosis
    3. Myasthenia
    4. Muscular dystrophies
  E. Miscellaneous
    1. Obesity
    2. Hypoventilation
    3. Permissive hypercapnia

The diagnosis of respiratory acidosis requires, by definition, the measurement of PaCO$_2$ and arterial pH. A detailed history and physical examination often indicate the cause. Pulmonary function studies, including spirometry, diffusion capacity for carbon monoxide, lung volumes, and arterial Pa_{CO_2} and O_2 saturation, usually make it possible to determine if respiratory acidosis is secondary to lung disease. The workup for nonpulmonary causes should include a detailed drug history, measurement of hematocrit, and assessment of upper airway, chest wall, pleura, and neuromuscular function.

℞ **Treatment:**
RESPIRATORY ACIDOSIS

The management of respiratory acidosis depends on its severity and rate of onset. Acute respiratory acidosis can be life threatening, and measures to reverse the underlying cause should be undertaken simultaneously with restoration of adequate alveolar ventilation. This may necessitate tracheal intubation and assisted mechanical ventilation. Oxygen administration should be titrated carefully in patients with severe obstructive pulmonary disease and chronic CO_2 retention who are breathing spontaneously. When oxygen is used injudiciously, these patients may experience progression of the respiratory acidosis. Aggressive and rapid correction of hypercapnia should be avoided, because the falling Pa_{CO_2} may provoke the same complications noted with acute respiratory alkalosis (i.e., cardiac arrhythmias, reduced cerebral perfusion, and seizures). The Pa_{CO_2} should be lowered gradually in chronic respiratory acidosis, aiming to restore the Pa_{CO_2} to baseline levels and to provide sufficient Cl^- and K^+ to enhance the renal excretion of HCO_3^-.

Chronic respiratory acidosis is frequently difficult to correct, but measures aimed at improving lung function can help some patients and forestall further deterioration in most.

RESPIRATORY ALKALOSIS

Alveolar hyperventilation decreases Pa_{CO_2} and increases the HCO_3^-/Pa_{CO_2} ratio, thus increasing pH (Table 5-7). Nonbicarbonate cellular buffers respond by consuming HCO_3^-. Hypocapnia develops when a sufficiently strong ventilatory stimulus causes CO_2 output in the lungs to exceed its metabolic production by tissues. Plasma pH and $[HCO_3^-]$ appear to vary proportionately with Pa_{CO_2} over a range from 40–15 mmHg. The relationship between arterial $[H^+]$ concentration and Pa_{CO_2} is ~0.7 mmol/L per mmHg (or 0.01 pH unit/mmHg), and that for plasma $[HCO_3^-]$ is 0.2 mmol/L per mmHg. Hypocapnia sustained for >2–6 h is further compensated by a decrease in renal ammonium and titratable acid excretion and a reduction in filtered HCO_3^- reabsorption. Full renal adaptation to respiratory alkalosis

may take several days and requires normal volume status and renal function. The kidneys appear to respond directly to the lowered Pa_{CO_2} rather than to alkalosis per se. In chronic respiratory alkalosis a 1-mmHg fall in Pa_{CO_2} causes a 0.4- to 0.5-mmol/L drop in $[HCO_3^-]$ and a 0.3-mmol/L fall (or 0.003 rise in pH) in $[H^+]$.

The effects of respiratory alkalosis vary according to duration and severity but are primarily those of the underlying disease. Reduced cerebral blood flow as a consequence of a rapid decline in Pa_{CO_2} may cause dizziness, mental confusion, and seizures, even in the absence of hypoxemia. The cardiovascular effects of acute hypocapnia in the conscious human are generally minimal, but in the anesthetized or mechanically ventilated patient, cardiac output and blood pressure may fall because of the depressant effects of anesthesia and positive-pressure ventilation on heart rate, systemic resistance, and venous return. Cardiac arrhythmias may occur in patients with heart disease as a result of changes in oxygen unloading by blood from a left shift in the hemoglobin-oxygen dissociation curve (Bohr effect). Acute respiratory alkalosis causes intracellular shifts of Na^+, K^+, and PO_4^- and reduces free $[Ca^{2+}]$ by increasing the protein-bound fraction. Hypocapnia-induced hypokalemia is usually minor.

Chronic respiratory alkalosis is the most common acid-base disturbance in critically ill patients and, when severe, portends a poor prognosis. Many cardiopulmonary disorders manifest respiratory alkalosis in their early to intermediate stages, and the finding of normocapnia and hypoxemia in a patient with hyperventilation may herald the onset of rapid respiratory failure and should prompt an assessment to determine if the patient is becoming fatigued. Respiratory alkalosis is common during mechanical ventilation.

The hyperventilation syndrome may be disabling. Paresthesia, circumoral numbness, chest wall tightness or pain, dizziness, inability to take an adequate breath, and, rarely, tetany may themselves be sufficiently stressful to perpetuate the disorder. Arterial blood-gas analysis demonstrates an acute or chronic respiratory alkalosis, often with hypocapnia in the range of 15–30 mmHg and no hypoxemia. Central nervous system diseases or injury can produce several patterns of hyperventilation and sustained Pa_{CO_2} levels of 20–30 mmHg. Hyperthyroidism, high caloric loads, and exercise raise the basal metabolic rate, but ventilation usually rises in proportion so that arterial blood gases are unchanged and respiratory alkalosis does not develop. Salicylates are the most common cause of drug-induced respiratory alkalosis as a result of direct stimulation of the medullary chemoreceptor. The methylxanthines, theophylline, and aminophylline stimulate ventilation and increase the ventilatory response to CO_2. Progesterone increases ventilation and lowers arterial Pa_{CO_2} by as much as 5–10 mmHg. Therefore, chronic respiratory alkalosis is a common feature of pregnancy. Respiratory alkalosis is also prominent in liver failure, and the severity correlates with the degree of hepatic insufficiency. Respiratory alkalosis is often an early finding in gram-negative septicemia, before fever, hypoxemia, or hypotension develops.

The diagnosis of respiratory alkalosis depends on measurement of arterial pH and Pa_{CO_2}. The plasma $[K^+]$ is often reduced and the $[Cl^-]$ increased. In the acute phase, respiratory alkalosis is not associated with increased renal HCO_3^- excretion, but within hours net acid excretion is reduced. In general, the HCO_3^- concentration falls by 2.0 mmol/L for each 10-mmHg decrease in Pa_{CO_2}. Chronic hypocapnia reduces the serum $[HCO_3^-]$ by 4.0 mmol/L for each 10-mmHg decrease in Pa_{CO_2}. It is unusual to observe a plasma $HCO_3^- < 12$ mmol/L as a result of a pure respiratory alkalosis.

When a diagnosis of respiratory alkalosis is made, its cause should be investigated. The diagnosis of hyperventilation syndrome is made by exclusion. In difficult cases, it may be important to rule out other conditions such as pulmonary embolism, coronary artery disease, and hyperthyroidism.

℞ **Treatment:**
RESPIRATORY ALKALOSIS

The management of respiratory alkalosis is directed toward alleviation of the underlying disorder. If respiratory alkalosis complicates ventilator management, changes in dead space, tidal volume, and frequency can minimize the hypocapnia. Patients with the hyperventilation syndrome may benefit from reassurance, rebreathing from a paper bag during symptomatic attacks, and attention to underlying psychological stress. Antidepressants and sedatives are not recommended. β-Adrenergic blockers may ameliorate peripheral manifestations of the hyperadrenergic state.

FURTHER READINGS

DuBose TD Jr: Acid-base disorders, in *Brenner and Rector's The Kidney*, 8th ed, BM Brenner (ed). Philadelphia, Saunders, 2007, in press

————, Alpern RJ: Renal tubular acidosis, in *The Metabolic and Molecular Bases of Inherited Disease*, 8th ed, CR Scriver et al (eds). New York, McGraw-Hill, 2001

Galla JH: Metabolic alkalosis, in *Acid-Base and Electrolyte Disorders—A Companion to Brenner and Rector's The Kidney*, TD DuBose, LL Hamm (eds). Philadelphia, Saunders, 2002, pp 109–128

Karet FE: Mechanisms in hyperkalemic renal tubular acidosis. J Am Soc Nephrol 20:251, 2009

Laski ME, Wesson DE: Lactic acidosis, in *Acid-Base and Electrolyte Disorders—A Companion to Brenner and Rector's The Kidney*, TD DuBose, LL Hamm (eds). Philadelphia, Saunders, 2002, pp 83–107

Madias NE: Respiratory alkalosis, in *Acid-Base and Electrolyte Disorders—A Companion to Brenner and Rector's The Kidney*, TD DuBose, LL Hamm (eds). Philadelphia, Saunders, 2002, pp 147–164

Nagami GT: Role of angiotensin II in the enhancement of ammonia production and secretion by the proximal tubule in metabolic acidosis. Am J Physiol Renal Physiol 294:F874, 2008

Sabatini S et al: Bicarbonate therapy in severe metabolic acidosis. J Am Soc Nephrol 20:692, 2009

Walsh S et al: Cation transport activity of anion exchanger 1 mutations found in inherited distal renal tubular acidosis. Am J Physiol Renal Physiol 295:F343, 2008

Wesson DE et al: Clinical syndromes of metabolic alkalosis, in *The Kidney: Physiology and Pathophysiology*, 3d ed, DW Seldin, G Giebisch (eds). Philadelphia, Lippincott Williams and Wilkins, 2000, pp 2055–2072

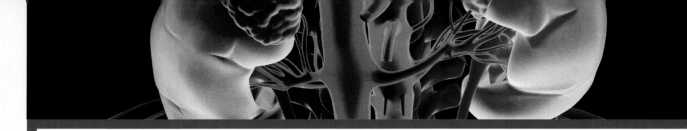

CHAPTER 6

FLUID AND ELECTROLYTE DISTURBANCES

Gary G. Singer ■ Barry M. Brenner

SODIUM AND WATER

Composition of Body Fluids

Water is the most abundant constituent in the body, comprising approximately 50% of body weight in women and 60% in men. This difference is attributable to differences in the relative proportions of adipose tissue in men and women. Total body water is distributed in two major compartments: 55–75% is intracellular [intracellular fluid (ICF)], and 25–45% is extracellular [extracellular fluid (ECF)]. The ECF is further subdivided into intravascular (plasma water) and extravascular (interstitial) spaces in a ratio of 1:3.

The solute or particle concentration of a fluid is known as its *osmolality* and is expressed as milliosmoles per kilogram of water (mosmol/kg). Water crosses cell membranes to achieve osmotic equilibrium (ECF osmolality = ICF osmolality). The extracellular and intracellular solutes or osmoles are markedly different due to disparities in permeability and the presence of transporters and active pumps. The major ECF particles are Na^+ and its accompanying anions Cl^- and HCO_3^-, whereas K^+ and organic phosphate esters [adenosine triphosphate (ATP), creatine phosphate, and phospholipids] are the predominant ICF osmoles. Solutes that are restricted to the ECF or the ICF determine the *effective osmolality* (or *tonicity*) of that compartment.

Since Na^+ is largely restricted to the extracellular compartment, total body Na^+ content is a reflection of ECF volume. Likewise, K^+ and its attendant anions are predominantly limited to the ICF and are necessary for normal cell function. Therefore, the number of intracellular particles is relatively constant, and a change in ICF osmolality is usually due to a change in ICF water content. However, in certain situations, brain cells can vary the number of intracellular solutes in order to defend against large water shifts. This process of *osmotic adaptation* is important in the defense of cell volume and occurs in chronic hyponatremia and hypernatremia. This response is mediated initially by transcellular shifts of K^+ and Na^+, followed by synthesis, import, or export of organic solutes (so-called osmolytes) such as inositol, betaine, and glutamine. During chronic hyponatremia, brain cells lose solutes, thereby defending cell volume and diminishing neurologic symptoms. The converse occurs during chronic hypernatremia. Certain solutes, such as urea, do not contribute to water shift across cell membranes and are known as *ineffective osmoles*.

Fluid movement between the intravascular and interstitial spaces occurs across the capillary wall and is determined by the Starling forces—capillary hydraulic pressure and colloid osmotic pressure. The transcapillary hydraulic pressure gradient exceeds the corresponding oncotic pressure gradient, thereby favoring the movement of plasma ultrafiltrate into the extravascular space.

The return of fluid into the intravascular compartment occurs via lymphatic flow.

Water Balance

(See also Chap. 2.) The normal plasma osmolality is 275–290 mosmol/kg and is kept within a narrow range by mechanisms capable of sensing a 1–2% change in tonicity. To maintain a steady state, water intake must equal water excretion. Disorders of water homeostasis result in hypo- or hypernatremia. Normal individuals have an obligate water loss consisting of urine, stool, and evaporation from the skin and respiratory tract. Gastrointestinal excretion is usually a minor component of total water output, except in patients with vomiting, diarrhea, or high enterostomy output states. Evaporative or insensitive water losses are important in the regulation of core body temperature. Obligatory renal water loss is mandated by the minimum solute excretion required to maintain a steady state. Normally, about 600 mosmols must be excreted per day, and since the maximal urine osmolality is 1200 mosmol/kg, a minimum urine output of 500 mL/d is required for neutral solute balance.

Water Intake

The primary stimulus for water ingestion is *thirst*, mediated either by an increase in effective osmolality or a decrease in ECF volume or blood pressure. *Osmoreceptors*, located in the anterolateral hypothalamus, are stimulated by a rise in tonicity. Ineffective osmoles, such as urea and glucose, do not play a role in stimulating thirst. The average osmotic threshold for thirst is approximately 295 mosmol/kg and varies among individuals. Under normal circumstances, daily water intake exceeds physiologic requirements.

Water Excretion

In contrast to the ingestion of water, its excretion is tightly regulated by physiologic factors. The principal determinant of renal water excretion is *arginine vasopressin* (AVP; formerly antidiuretic hormone), a polypeptide synthesized in the supraoptic and paraventricular nuclei of the hypothalamus and secreted by the posterior pituitary gland. The binding of AVP to V_2 receptors on the basolateral membrane of principal cells in the collecting duct activates adenylyl cyclase and initiates a sequence of events that leads to the insertion of water channels into the luminal membrane. These water channels that are specifically activated by AVP are encoded by the *aquaporin-2* gene. The net effect is passive water reabsorption along an osmotic gradient from the lumen of the collecting duct to the hypertonic medullary interstitium. The major stimulus for AVP secretion is hypertonicity. Since the major ECF solutes are Na^+ salts, effective osmolality is primarily determined by the plasma Na^+ concentration. An increase or decrease in tonicity is sensed by hypothalamic osmoreceptors as a decrease or increase in cell volume,

respectively, leading to enhancement or suppression of AVP secretion. The osmotic threshold for AVP release is 280–290 mosmol/kg, and the system is sufficiently sensitive that plasma osmolality varies by no more than 1–2%.

Nonosmotic factors that regulate AVP secretion include *effective circulating (arterial) volume*, nausea, pain, stress, hypoglycemia, pregnancy, and numerous drugs. The hemodynamic response is mediated by baroreceptors in the carotid sinus. The sensitivity of these receptors is significantly lower than that of the osmoreceptors. In fact, depletion of blood volume sufficient to result in a decreased mean arterial pressure is necessary to stimulate AVP release, whereas small changes in effective circulating volume have little effect.

To maintain homeostasis and a normal plasma Na^+ concentration, the ingestion of solute-free water must eventually lead to the loss of the same volume of electrolyte-free water. Three steps are required for the kidney to excrete a water load: (1) filtration and delivery of water (and electrolytes) to the diluting sites of the nephron; (2) active reabsorption of Na^+ and Cl^- without water in the thick ascending limb of the loop of Henle (TALH) and, to a lesser extent, in the distal nephron; and (3) maintenance of a dilute urine due to impermeability of the collecting duct to water in the absence of AVP. Abnormalities of any of these steps can result in impaired free water excretion, and eventual hyponatremia.

Sodium Balance

Sodium is actively pumped out of cells by the Na^+, K^+-ATPase pump. As a result, 85–90% of all Na^+ is extracellular, and the ECF volume is a reflection of total body Na^+ content. Normal volume regulatory mechanisms ensure that Na^+ loss balances Na^+ gain. If this does not occur, conditions of Na^+ excess or deficit ensue and are manifest as edematous or hypovolemic states, respectively. It is important to distinguish between disorders of osmoregulation and disorders of volume regulation since water and Na^+ balance are regulated independently. Changes in Na^+ concentration generally reflect disturbed water homeostasis, whereas alterations in Na^+ content are manifest as ECF volume contraction or expansion and imply abnormal Na^+ balance.

Sodium Intake

Individuals eating a typical Western diet consume approximately 150 mmol of NaCl daily. This normally exceeds basal requirements. As noted above, sodium is the principal extracellular cation. Therefore, dietary intake of Na^+ results in ECF volume expansion, which in turn promotes enhanced renal Na^+ excretion to maintain steady state Na^+ balance.

Sodium Excretion

(See also Chap. 2.) The regulation of Na^+ excretion is multifactorial and is the major determinant of Na^+

balance. A Na^+ deficit or excess is manifest as a decreased or increased effective circulating volume, respectively. Changes in effective circulating volume tend to lead to parallel changes in glomerular filtration rate (GFR). However, tubule Na^+ reabsorption, and not GFR, is the major regulatory mechanism controlling Na^+ excretion. Almost two-thirds of filtered Na^+ is reabsorbed in the proximal convoluted tubule; this process is electroneutral and isoosmotic. Further reabsorption (25–30%) occurs in the TALH via the apical Na^+-K^+-$2Cl^-$ co-transporter; this is an active process and is also electroneutral. Distal convoluted tubule reabsorption of Na^+ (5%) is mediated by the *thiazide-sensitive Na^+-Cl^- co-transporter*. Final Na^+ reabsorption occurs in the cortical and medullary collecting ducts, the amount excreted being reasonably equivalent to the amount ingested per day.

HYPOVOLEMIA

Etiology

True volume depletion, or hypovolemia, generally refers to a state of combined salt and water loss exceeding intake, leading to ECF volume contraction. The loss of Na^+ may be renal or extrarenal (Table 6-1).

▬ Renal
Many conditions are associated with excessive urinary NaCl and water losses, including diuretics. Pharmacologic

TABLE 6-1

CAUSES OF HYPOVOLEMIA
I. ECF volume contracted
A. Extrarenal Na^+ loss
1. Gastrointestinal (vomiting, nasogastric suction, drainage, fistula, diarrhea)
2. Skin/respiratory (insensible losses, sweat, burns)
3. Hemorrhage
B. Renal Na^+ and water loss
1. Diuretics
2. Osmotic diuresis
3. Hypoaldosteronism
4. Salt-wasting nephropathies
C. Renal water loss
1. Diabetes insipidus (central or nephrogenic)
II. ECF volume normal or expanded
A. Decreased cardiac output
1. Myocardial, valvular, or pericardial disease
B. Redistribution
1. Hypoalbuminemia (hepatic cirrhosis, nephrotic syndrome)
2. Capillary leak (acute pancreatitis, ischemic bowel, rhabdomyolysis)
C. Increased venous capacitance
1. Sepsis

Note: ECF, extracellular fluid.

diuretics inhibit specific pathways of Na^+ reabsorption along the nephron with a consequent increase in urinary Na^+ excretion. Enhanced filtration of non-reabsorbed solutes, such as glucose or urea, can also impair tubular reabsorption of Na^+ and water, leading to an osmotic or solute diuresis. This often occurs in poorly controlled diabetes mellitus and in patients receiving high-protein hyperalimentation. Mannitol is a diuretic that produces an osmotic diuresis because the renal tubule is impermeable to mannitol. Many tubule and interstitial renal disorders are associated with Na^+ wasting. Excessive renal losses of Na^+ and water may also occur during the diuretic phase of acute tubular necrosis (Chap. 10) and following the relief of bilateral urinary tract obstruction. Finally, mineralocorticoid deficiency (hypoaldosteronism) causes salt wasting in the presence of normal intrinsic renal function.

Massive renal water excretion can also lead to hypovolemia. The ECF volume contraction is usually less severe since two-thirds of the volume lost is intracellular. Conditions associated with excessive urinary water loss include *central diabetes insipidus* (CDI) and *nephrogenic diabetes insipidus* (NDI). These two disorders are due to impaired secretion of and renal unresponsiveness to AVP, respectively, and are discussed below.

▬ Extrarenal
Nonrenal causes of hypovolemia include fluid loss from the gastrointestinal tract, skin, and respiratory system and third-space accumulations (burns, pancreatitis, peritonitis). Approximately 9 L of fluid enters the gastrointestinal tract daily, 2 L by ingestion and 7 L by secretion. Almost 98% of this volume is reabsorbed so that fecal fluid loss is only 100–200 mL/d. Impaired gastrointestinal reabsorption or enhanced secretion leads to volume depletion. Since gastric secretions have a low pH (high H^+ concentration) and biliary, pancreatic, and intestinal secretions are alkaline (high HCO_3^- concentration), vomiting and diarrhea are often accompanied by metabolic alkalosis and acidosis, respectively.

Water evaporation from the skin and respiratory tract contributes to thermoregulation. These *insensible losses* amount to 500 mL/d. During febrile illnesses, prolonged heat exposure, exercise, or increased salt and water loss from skin, in the form of sweat, can be significant and lead to volume depletion. The Na^+ concentration of sweat is normally 20–50 mmol/L and decreases with profuse sweating due to the action of aldosterone. Since sweat is hypotonic, the loss of water exceeds that of Na^+. The water deficit is minimized by enhanced thirst. Nevertheless, ongoing Na^+ loss is manifest as hypovolemia. Enhanced evaporative water loss from the respiratory tract may be associated with hyperventilation, especially in mechanically ventilated febrile patients.

Certain conditions lead to fluid sequestration in a *third space*. This compartment is extracellular but is not in equilibrium with either the ECF or the ICF. The fluid is effectively lost from the ECF and can result in hypovolemia. Examples include the bowel lumen in gastrointestinal obstruction, subcutaneous tissues in severe burns, retroperitoneal space in acute pancreatitis, and peritoneal cavity in peritonitis. Finally, severe hemorrhage from any source can result in volume depletion.

Pathophysiology

ECF volume contraction is manifest as a decreased plasma volume and hypotension. Hypotension is due to decreased venous return (preload) and diminished cardiac output; it triggers baroreceptors in the carotid sinus and aortic arch and leads to activation of the sympathetic nervous system and the renin-angiotensin system. The net effect is to maintain mean arterial pressure and cerebral and coronary perfusion. In contrast to the cardiovascular response, the renal response is aimed at restoring the ECF volume by decreasing the GFR and filtered load of Na^+ and, most importantly, by promoting tubular reabsorption of Na^+. Increased sympathetic tone increases proximal tubular Na^+ reabsorption and decreases GFR by causing preferential afferent arteriolar vasoconstriction. Sodium is also reabsorbed in the proximal convoluted tubule in response to increased angiotensin II and altered peritubular capillary hemodynamics (decreased hydraulic and increased oncotic pressure). Enhanced reabsorption of Na^+ by the collecting duct is an important component of the renal adaptation to ECF volume contraction. This occurs in response to increased *aldosterone* and AVP secretion and suppressed *atrial natriuretic peptide* secretion.

Clinical Features

A careful history is often helpful in determining the etiology of ECF volume contraction (e.g., vomiting, diarrhea, polyuria, diaphoresis). Most symptoms are nonspecific and secondary to electrolyte imbalances and tissue hypoperfusion and include fatigue, weakness, muscle cramps, thirst, and postural dizziness. More severe degrees of volume contraction can lead to end-organ ischemia manifest as oliguria, cyanosis, abdominal and chest pain, and confusion or obtundation. Diminished skin turgor and dry oral mucous membranes are poor markers of decreased interstitial fluid. Signs of intravascular volume contraction include decreased jugular venous pressure, postural hypotension, and postural tachycardia. Larger and more acute fluid losses lead to hypovolemic shock, manifest as hypotension, tachycardia, peripheral vasoconstriction, and hypoperfusion—cyanosis, cold and clammy extremities, oliguria, and altered mental status.

Diagnosis

A thorough history and physical examination are generally sufficient to diagnose the etiology of hypovolemia.

Laboratory data usually confirm and support the clinical diagnosis. The blood urea nitrogen (BUN) and plasma creatinine concentrations tend to be elevated, reflecting a decreased GFR. Normally, the BUN:creatinine ratio is about 10:1. However, in *prerenal azotemia*, hypovolemia leads to increased urea reabsorption, a proportionately greater elevation in BUN than plasma creatinine, and a BUN:creatinine ratio of 20:1 or higher. An increased BUN (relative to creatinine) may also be due to increased urea production that occurs with hyperalimentation (high-protein), glucocorticoid therapy, and gastrointestinal bleeding.

The appropriate response to hypovolemia is enhanced renal Na^+ and water reabsorption, which is reflected in the urine composition. Therefore, the urine Na^+ concentration should usually be <20 mmol/L except in conditions associated with impaired Na^+ reabsorption, as in acute tubular necrosis (Chap. 10). Another exception is hypovolemia due to vomiting, since the associated metabolic alkalosis and increased filtered HCO_3^- impair proximal Na^+ reabsorption. In this case, the urine Cl^- is low (<20 mmol/L). The urine osmolality and specific gravity in hypovolemic subjects are generally >450 mosmol/kg and 1.015, respectively, reflecting the presence of enhanced AVP secretion. However, in hypovolemia due to diabetes insipidus, urine osmolality and specific gravity are indicative of inappropriately dilute urine.

R$_x$ Treatment: HYPOVOLEMIA

The therapeutic goals are to restore normovolemia with fluid similar in composition to that lost and to replace ongoing losses. Symptoms and signs, including weight loss, can help estimate the degree of volume contraction and should also be monitored to assess response to treatment. Mild volume contraction can usually be corrected via the oral route. More severe hypovolemia requires intravenous therapy. Isotonic or normal saline (0.9% NaCl or 154 mmol/L Na^+) is the solution of choice in normonatremic and most hyponatremic individuals and should be administered initially in patients with hypotension or shock. Hypernatremia reflects a proportionally greater deficit of water than Na^+, and its correction will therefore require a hypotonic solution such as half-normal saline (0.45% NaCl or 77 mmol/L Na^+) or 5% dextrose in water. Patients with significant hemorrhage, anemia, or intravascular volume depletion may require blood transfusion or colloid-containing solutions (albumin, dextran). Hypokalemia may be present initially or may ensue as a result of increased urinary K^+ excretion; it should be corrected by adding appropriate amounts of KCl to replacement solutions.

Etiology

A plasma Na^+ concentration <135 mmol/L usually reflects a hypotonic state. However, plasma osmolality may be normal or increased in some cases of hyponatremia. Isotonic or slightly hypotonic hyponatremia may complicate transurethral resection of the prostate or bladder because large volumes of isoosmotic (mannitol) or hypoosmotic (sorbitol or glycine) bladder irrigation solution can be absorbed and result in a dilutional hyponatremia. The metabolism of sorbitol and glycine to CO_2 and water may lead to hypotonicity if the accumulated fluid and solutes are not rapidly excreted. Hypertonic hyponatremia is usually due to hyperglycemia or, occasionally, intravenous administration of mannitol. Relative insulin deficiency causes myocytes to become impermeable to glucose. Therefore, during poorly controlled diabetes mellitus, glucose is an effective osmole and draws water from muscle cells, resulting in hyponatremia. Plasma Na^+ concentration falls by 1.4 mmol/L for every 100 mg/dL rise in the plasma glucose concentration.

Most causes of hyponatremia are associated with a low plasma osmolality (Table 6–2). In general, hypotonic hyponatremia is due either to a primary water gain (and secondary Na^+ loss) or a primary Na^+ loss (and secondary water gain). In the absence of water intake or hypotonic fluid replacement, hyponatremia is usually associated with hypovolemic shock due to a profound sodium deficit and transcellular water shift. Contraction of the ECF volume stimulates thirst and AVP secretion. The increased water ingestion and impaired renal excretion result in hyponatremia. It is important to note that *diuretic-induced hyponatremia* is almost always due to thiazide diuretics. Loop diuretics decrease the tonicity of the medullary interstitium and impair maximal urinary concentrating capacity. This limits the ability of AVP to promote water retention. In contrast, thiazide diuretics lead to Na^+ and K^+ depletion and AVP-mediated water retention. Hyponatremia can also occur by a process of *desalination*. This occurs when the urine tonicity (the sum of the concentrations of Na^+ and K^+) exceeds that of administered intravenous fluids (including isotonic saline). This accounts for some cases of acute postoperative hyponatremia and cerebral salt wasting after neurosurgery.

Hyponatremia in the setting of ECF volume expansion is usually associated with edematous states, such as congestive heart failure, hepatic cirrhosis, and the nephrotic syndrome. These disorders all have in common a decreased effective circulating arterial volume, leading to increased thirst and increased AVP levels. Additional factors impairing the excretion of solute-free water include a reduced GFR, decreased delivery of ultrafiltrate to the diluting site (due to increased proximal fractional reabsorption of Na^+ and water), and diuretic therapy. The degree of hyponatremia often correlates with the severity

TABLE 6-2

CAUSES OF HYPONATREMIA

I. Pseudohyponatremia
   A. Normal plasma osmolality
      1. Hyperlipidemia
      2. Hyperproteinemia
      3. Posttransurethral resection of prostate/bladder tumor
   B. Increased plasma osmolality
      1. Hyperglycemia
      2. Mannitol
II. Hypoosmolal hyponatremia
   A. Primary Na^+ loss (secondary water gain)
      1. Integumentary loss: sweating, burns
      2. Gastrointestinal loss: vomiting, tube drainage, fistula, obstruction, diarrhea
      3. Renal loss: diuretics, osmotic diuresis, hypoaldosteronism, salt-wasting nephropathy, postobstructive diuresis, nonoliguric acute tubular necrosis
   B. Primary water gain (secondary Na^+ loss)
      1. Primary polydipsia
      2. Decreased solute intake (e.g., beer potomania)
      3. AVP release due to pain, nausea, drugs
      4. Syndrome of inappropriate AVP secretion
      5. Glucocorticoid deficiency
      6. Hypothyroidism
      7. Chronic renal insufficiency
   C. Primary Na^+ gain (exceeded by secondary water gain)
      1. Heart failure
      2. Hepatic cirrhosis
      3. Nephrotic syndrome

of the underlying condition and is an important prognostic factor. Oliguric acute and chronic renal failure may be associated with hyponatremia if water intake exceeds the ability to excrete equivalent volumes.

Hyponatremia in the absence of ECF volume contraction, decreased effective circulating arterial volume, or renal insufficiency is usually due to increased AVP secretion resulting in impaired water excretion. Ingestion or administration of water is also required since high levels of AVP alone are usually insufficient to produce hyponatremia. This disorder, commonly termed the *syndrome of inappropriate antidiuretic hormone secretion* (SIADH), is the most common cause of normovolemic hyponatremia and is due to the nonphysiologic release of AVP from the posterior pituitary or an ectopic source. Renal free water excretion is impaired while the regulation of Na^+ balance is unaffected. The most common causes of SIADH include neuropsychiatric and pulmonary diseases, malignant tumors, major surgery (postoperative pain), and pharmacologic agents. Severe pain and nausea are physiologic stimuli of AVP secretion; these stimuli are inappropriate in the absence of hypovolemia or hyperosmolality.

The pattern of AVP secretion can be used to classify SIADH into four subtypes: (1) erratic autonomous AVP secretion (ectopic production); (2) normal regulation of AVP release around a lower osmolality set point or *reset osmostat* (cachexia, malnutrition); (3) normal AVP response to hypertonicity with failure to suppress completely at low osmolality (incomplete pituitary stalk section); and (4) normal AVP secretion with increased sensitivity to its actions or secretion of some other antidiuretic factor (rare). Patients with the nephrogenic syndrome of inappropriate antidiuresis have clinical and laboratory features consistent with SIADH but undetectable levels of AVP. It is hypothesized that this disorder is due to gain of function mutations in the V_2 receptor.

Hormonal excess or deficiency may cause hyponatremia. Adrenal insufficiency and hypothyroidism may present with hyponatremia and should not be confused with SIADH. Although decreased mineralocorticoids may contribute to the hyponatremia of adrenal insufficiency, it is the cortisol deficiency that leads to hypersecretion of AVP both indirectly (secondary to volume depletion) and directly (cosecreted with corticotropin-releasing factor). The mechanisms by which hypothyroidism leads to hyponatremia include decreased cardiac output and GFR and increased AVP secretion in response to hemodynamic stimuli.

Finally, hyponatremia may occur in the absence of AVP or renal failure if the kidney is unable to excrete the dietary water load. In psychogenic or primary polydipsia, compulsive water consumption may overwhelm the normally large renal excretory capacity of 12 L/d. These patients often have psychiatric illnesses and may be taking medications, such as phenothiazines, that enhance the sensation of thirst by causing a dry mouth. The maximal urine output is a function of the minimum urine osmolality achievable and the mandatory solute excretion. Metabolism of a normal diet generates about 600 mosmol/d, and the minimum urine osmolality in humans is 50 mosmol/kg. Therefore, the maximum daily urine output will be about 12 L (600 ÷ 50 = 12). A solute excretion rate of greater than ~750 mosmol/d is, by definition, an *osmotic diuresis*. A low-protein diet may yield as few as 250 mosmol/d, which translates into a maximal urine output of 5 L/d at a minimum urine tonicity of 50 mosmol/kg. Beer drinkers typically have a poor dietary intake of protein and electrolytes and consume large volumes (of beer), which may exceed the renal excretory capacity and result in hyponatremia. This phenomenon is referred to as *beer potomania*.

Clinical Features

The clinical manifestations of hyponatremia are related to osmotic water shift leading to increased ICF volume, specifically brain cell swelling or cerebral edema. Therefore, the symptoms are primarily neurologic, and their

severity is dependent on the rapidity of onset and absolute decrease in plasma Na^+ concentration. Patients may be asymptomatic or complain of nausea and malaise. As the plasma Na^+ concentration falls, the symptoms progress to include headache, lethargy, confusion, and obtundation. Stupor, seizures, and coma do not usually occur unless the plasma Na^+ concentration falls acutely below 120 mmol/L or decreases rapidly. As described above, adaptive mechanisms designed to protect cell volume occur in chronic hyponatremia. Loss of Na^+ and K^+, followed by organic osmolytes, from brain cells decreases brain swelling due to secondary transcellular water shifts (from ICF to ECF). The net effect is to minimize cerebral edema and its symptoms.

Diagnosis

(Fig. 6-1) Hyponatremia is not a disease but a manifestation of a variety of disorders. The underlying cause can often be ascertained from an accurate history and physical examination, including an assessment of ECF volume status and effective circulating arterial volume. The differential diagnosis of hyponatremia, an expanded ECF

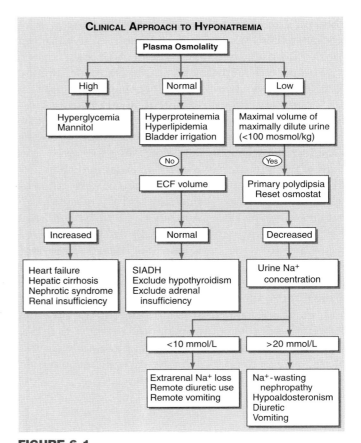

FIGURE 6-1

Algorithm depicting clinical approach to hyponatremia. ECF, extracellular fluid; SIADH, syndrome of inappropriate antidiuretic hormone secretion.

volume, and decreased effective circulating volume includes congestive heart failure, hepatic cirrhosis, and the nephrotic syndrome. Hypothyroidism and adrenal insufficiency tend to present with a near-normal ECF volume and decreased effective circulating arterial volume. All of these diseases have characteristic signs and symptoms. Patients with SIADH are usually euvolemic.

Four laboratory findings often provide useful information and can narrow the differential diagnosis of hyponatremia: (1) the plasma osmolality, (2) the urine osmolality, (3) the urine Na^+ concentration, and (4) the urine K^+ concentration. Since ECF tonicity is determined primarily by the Na^+ concentration, most patients with hyponatremia have a decreased plasma osmolality. The appropriate renal response to hypoosmolality is to excrete the maximum volume of dilute urine, i.e., urine osmolality and specific gravity of <100 mosmol/kg and 1.003, respectively. This occurs in patients with primary polydipsia. If this is not present, it suggests impaired free water excretion due to the action of AVP on the kidney. The secretion of AVP may be a physiologic response to hemodynamic stimuli or it may be inappropriate in the presence of hyponatremia and euvolemia. Since Na^+ is the major ECF cation and is largely restricted to this compartment, ECF volume contraction represents a deficit in total body Na^+ content. Therefore, volume depletion in patients with normal underlying renal function results in enhanced tubule Na^+ reabsorption and a urine Na^+ concentration <20 mmol/L. The finding of a urine Na^+ concentration >20 mmol/L in hypovolemic hyponatremia implies a salt-wasting nephropathy, diuretic therapy, hypoaldosteronism, or occasionally vomiting. Both the urine osmolality and the urine Na^+ concentration can be followed serially when assessing response to therapy.

SIADH is characterized by hypoosmotic hyponatremia in the setting of an inappropriately concentrated urine (urine osmolality >100 mosmol/kg). Patients are typically normovolemic and have normal Na^+ balance. They tend to be mildly volume-expanded secondary to water retention and have a urine Na^+ excretion rate equal to intake (urine Na^+ concentration usually >40 mmol/L). By definition, they have normal renal, adrenal, and thyroid function and usually have normal K^+ and acid–base balance. SIADH is often associated with hypouricemia due to the uricosuric state induced by volume expansion. In contrast, hypovolemic patients tend to be hyperuricemic secondary to increased proximal urate reabsorption.

℞ Treatment:
HYPONATREMIA

The goals of therapy are twofold: (1) to raise the plasma Na^+ concentration by restricting water intake and

promoting water loss and (2) to correct the underlying disorder. Mild asymptomatic hyponatremia is generally of little clinical significance and requires no treatment. The management of asymptomatic hyponatremia associated with ECF volume contraction should include Na^+ repletion, generally in the form of isotonic saline. The direct effect of the administered NaCl on the plasma Na^+ concentration is trivial. However, restoration of euvolemia removes the hemodynamic stimulus for AVP release, allowing the excess free water to be excreted. The hyponatremia associated with edematous states tends to reflect the severity of the underlying disease and is usually asymptomatic. These patients have increased total body water that exceeds the increase in total body Na^+ content. Treatment should include restriction of Na^+ and water intake, correction of hypokalemia, and promotion of water loss in excess of Na^+. The latter may require the use of loop diuretics with replacement of a proportion of the urinary Na^+ loss to ensure net free water excretion. Dietary water restriction should be less than the urine output. Correction of the K^+ deficit may raise the plasma Na^+ concentration by favoring a shift of Na^+ out of cells as K^+ moves in. Water restriction is also a component of the therapeutic approach to hyponatremia associated with primary polydipsia, renal failure, and SIADH. The recent development of nonpeptide vasopressin antagonists has introduced a new selective treatment for euvolemic and hypervolemic hyponatremia.

The rate of correction of hyponatremia depends on the absence or presence of neurologic dysfunction. This, in turn, is related to the rapidity of onset and magnitude of the fall in plasma Na^+ concentration. In asymptomatic patients, the plasma Na^+ concentration should be raised by no more than 0.5–1.0 mmol/L per hour and by less than 10–12 mmol/L over the first 24 h. Acute or severe hyponatremia (plasma Na^+ concentration <110–115 mmol/L) tends to present with altered mental status and/or seizures and requires more rapid correction. Severe symptomatic hyponatremia should be treated with hypertonic saline, and the plasma Na^+ concentration should be raised by 1–2 mmol/L per hour for the first 3–4 h or until the seizures subside. Once again, the plasma Na^+ concentration should probably be raised by no more than 12 mmol/L during the first 24 h. The quantity of Na^+ required to increase the plasma Na^+ concentration by a given amount can be estimated by multiplying the deficit in plasma Na^+ concentration by the total body water.

Under normal conditions, total body water is 50 or 60% of lean body weight in women or men, respectively. Therefore, to raise the plasma Na^+ concentration from 105 to 115 mmol/L in a 70-kg man requires 420 mmol [(115 − 105) × 70 × 0.6] of Na^+. The risk of correcting hyponatremia too rapidly is the development of the *osmotic demyelination syndrome* (ODS). This is a neurologic disorder characterized by flaccid paralysis, dysarthria, and dysphagia. The diagnosis is usually suspected clinically and can be confirmed by appropriate neuroimaging studies. There is no specific treatment for the disorder, which is associated with significant morbidity and mortality. Patients with chronic hyponatremia are most susceptible to the development of ODS, since their brain cell volume has returned to near normal as a result of the osmotic adaptive mechanisms described above. Therefore, administration of hypertonic saline to these individuals can cause sudden osmotic shrinkage of brain cells. In addition to rapid or overcorrection of hyponatremia, risk factors for ODS include prior cerebral anoxic injury, hypokalemia, and malnutrition, especially secondary to alcoholism. Water restriction in primary polydipsia and intravenous saline therapy in ECF volume–contracted patients may also lead to overly rapid correction of hyponatremia as a result of AVP suppression and a brisk water diuresis. This can be prevented by administration of water or use of an AVP analogue to slow down the rate of free water excretion.

HYPERNATREMIA

Etiology

Hypernatremia is defined as a plasma Na^+ concentration >145 mmol/L. Since Na^+ and its accompanying anions are the major effective ECF osmoles, hypernatremia is a state of hyperosmolality. As a result of the fixed number of ICF particles, maintenance of osmotic equilibrium in hypernatremia results in ICF volume contraction. Hypernatremia may be due to primary Na^+ gain or water deficit. The two components of an appropriate response to hypernatremia are increased water intake stimulated by thirst and the excretion of the minimum volume of maximally concentrated urine reflecting AVP secretion in response to an osmotic stimulus.

In practice, the majority of cases of hypernatremia result from the loss of water. Since water is distributed between the ICF and the ECF in a 2:1 ratio, a given amount of solute-free water loss will result in a twofold greater reduction in the ICF compartment than the ECF compartment. For example, consider three scenarios: the loss of 1 L of water, isotonic NaCl, or half-isotonic NaCl. If 1 L of water is lost, the ICF volume will decrease by 667 mL, whereas the ECF volume will fall by only 333 mL. Due to the fact that Na^+ is largely restricted to the ECF, this compartment will decrease by 1 L if the fluid lost is isoosmotic. One liter of half-isotonic NaCl is equivalent to 500 mL of water (one-third ECF, two-thirds ICF) plus 500 mL of isotonic saline (all ECF). Therefore, the loss of 1 L of half-isotonic saline decreases the ECF and ICF volumes by 667 mL and 333 mL, respectively.

The degree of hyperosmolality is typically mild unless the thirst mechanism is abnormal or access to water is limited. The latter occurs in infants, the physically handicapped, and patients with impaired mental status; in the postoperative state; and in intubated patients in the intensive care unit. On rare occasions, impaired thirst may be due to *primary hypodipsia*. This usually occurs as a result of damage to the hypothalamic osmoreceptors that control thirst and tends to be associated with abnormal osmotic regulation of AVP secretion. Primary hypodipsia may be due to a variety of pathologic changes, including granulomatous disease, vascular occlusion, and tumors. A subset of hypodipsic hypernatremia, referred to as *essential hypernatremia*, does not respond to forced water intake. This appears to be due to a specific osmoreceptor defect resulting in nonosmotic regulation of AVP release. Thus, the hemodynamic effects of water loading lead to AVP suppression and excretion of dilute urine.

The source of free water loss is either renal or extrarenal. Nonrenal loss of water may be due to evaporation from the skin and respiratory tract (insensible losses) or loss from the gastrointestinal tract. Insensible losses are increased with fever, exercise, heat exposure, and severe burns and in mechanically ventilated patients. Furthermore, the Na^+ concentration of sweat decreases with profuse perspiration, thereby increasing solute-free water loss. Diarrhea is the most common gastrointestinal cause of hypernatremia. Specifically, osmotic diarrheas (induced by lactulose, sorbitol, or malabsorption of carbohydrate) and viral gastroenteritides result in water loss exceeding that of Na^+ and K^+. In contrast, secretory diarrheas (e.g., cholera, carcinoid, VIPoma) have a fecal osmolality (twice the sum of the concentrations of Na^+ and K^+) similar to that of plasma and present with ECF volume contraction and a normal plasma Na^+ concentration or hyponatremia.

Renal water loss is the most common cause of hypernatremia and is due to drug-induced or osmotic diuresis or diabetes insipidus. Loop diuretics interfere with the countercurrent mechanism and produce an isoosmotic solute diuresis. This results in a decreased medullary interstitial tonicity and impaired renal concentrating ability. The presence of non-reabsorbed organic solutes in the tubule lumen impairs the osmotic reabsorption of water. This leads to water loss in excess of Na^+ and K^+, known as an osmotic diuresis. The most frequent cause of an osmotic diuresis is hyperglycemia and glucosuria in poorly controlled diabetes mellitus. Intravenous administration of mannitol and increased endogenous production of urea (high-protein diet) can also result in an osmotic diuresis.

Hypernatremia secondary to nonosmotic urinary water loss is usually due to (1) CDI characterized by impaired AVP secretion, or (2) NDI resulting from end-organ (renal) resistance to the actions of AVP. The most common cause of CDI is destruction of the neurohypophysis. This may occur as a result of trauma, neurosurgery, granulomatous

SECTION II

Alterations of Renal Function and Electrolytes

disease, neoplasms, vascular accidents, or infection. In many cases, CDI is idiopathic and may occasionally be hereditary. The familial form of the disease is inherited in an autosomal dominant fashion and has been attributed to mutations in the propressophysin (AVP precursor) gene. NDI may be either inherited or acquired. Congenital NDI is an X-linked recessive trait due to mutations in the V_2 receptor gene. Mutations in the autosomal *aquaporin-2* gene may also result in NDI. The *aquaporin-2* gene encodes the water channel protein whose membrane insertion is stimulated by AVP. The causes of sporadic NDI are numerous and include drugs (especially lithium), hypercalcemia, hypokalemia, and conditions that impair medullary hypertonicity (e.g., papillary necrosis or osmotic diuresis). Pregnant women, in the second or third trimester, may develop NDI as a result of excessive elaboration of vasopressinase by the placenta.

Finally, although infrequent, a primary Na^+ gain may cause hypernatremia. For example, inadvertent administration of hypertonic NaCl or $NaHCO_3$ or replacing sugar with salt in infant formula can produce this complication.

Clinical Features

As a consequence of hypertonicity, water shifts out of cells, leading to a contracted ICF volume. A decreased brain cell volume is associated with an increased risk of subarachnoid or intracerebral hemorrhage. Hence, the major symptoms of hypernatremia are neurologic and include altered mental status, weakness, neuromuscular irritability, focal neurologic deficits, and occasionally coma or seizures. Patients may also complain of polyuria or thirst. For unknown reasons, patients with polydipsia from CDI tend to prefer ice-cold water. The signs and symptoms of volume depletion are often present in patients with a history of excessive sweating, diarrhea, or an osmotic diuresis. As with hyponatremia, the severity of the clinical manifestations is related to the acuity and magnitude of the rise in plasma Na^+ concentration. Chronic hypernatremia is generally less symptomatic as a result of adaptive mechanisms designed to defend cell volume. Brain cells initially take up Na^+ and K^+ salts, later followed by accumulation of organic osmolytes such as inositol. This serves to restore the brain ICF volume toward normal.

Diagnosis

(Fig. 6-2) A complete history and physical examination will often provide clues as to the underlying cause of hypernatremia. Relevant symptoms and signs include the absence or presence of thirst, diaphoresis, diarrhea, polyuria, and the features of ECF volume contraction. The history should include a list of current and recent medications, and the physical examination is incomplete

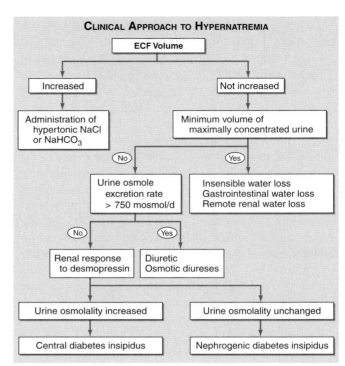

FIGURE 6-2

Algorithm depicting clinical approach to hypernatremia.

without a thorough mental status and neurologic assessment. Measurement of urine volume and osmolality are essential in the evaluation of hyperosmolality. The appropriate renal response to hypernatremia is the excretion of the minimum volume (500 mL/d) of maximally concentrated urine (urine osmolality >800 mosmol/kg). These findings suggest extrarenal or remote renal water loss or administration of hypertonic Na^+ salt solutions. The presence of a primary Na^+ excess can be confirmed by the presence of ECF volume expansion and natriuresis (urine Na^+ concentration usually >100 mmol/L).

Many causes of hypernatremia are associated with polyuria and a submaximal urine osmolality. The product of the urine volume and osmolality, i.e., the solute excretion rate, is helpful in determining the basis of the polyuria. To maintain a steady state, total solute excretion must equal solute production. As stated above, individuals eating a normal diet generate ~600 mosmol/d. Therefore, daily solute excretion in excess of 750 mosmol defines an osmotic diuresis. This can be confirmed by measuring the urine glucose and urea. In general, both CDI and NDI present with polyuria and hypotonic urine (urine osmolality <250 mosmol/kg). The degree of hypernatremia is usually mild unless there is an associated thirst abnormality. The clinical history, physical examination, and pertinent laboratory data can often rule out causes of acquired NDI. CDI and NDI can generally be distinguished by administering the AVP analogue desmopressin (10 μg intranasally) after careful water restriction. The urine osmolality should increase by at least 50% in CDI and will not change in NDI. Unfortunately, the diagnosis may sometimes be difficult due to partial defects in AVP secretion and action.

℞ Treatment: HYPERNATREMIA

The therapeutic goals are to stop ongoing water loss by treating the underlying cause and to correct the water deficit. The ECF volume should be restored in hypovolemic patients. The quantity of water required to correct the deficit can be calculated from the following equation:

$$\text{Water deficit} = \frac{\text{Plasma Na}^+ \text{ concentration} - 140}{140} \times \text{Total body water}$$

In hypernatremia due to water loss, total body water is approximately 50 and 40% of lean body weight in men and women, respectively. For example, a 50-kg woman with a plasma Na$^+$ concentration of 160 mmol/L has an estimated free water deficit of 2.9 L {[(160 − 140) ÷ 140] × (0.4 × 50)}. As in hyponatremia, rapid correction of hypernatremia is potentially dangerous. In this case, a sudden decrease in osmolality could potentially cause a rapid shift of water into cells that have undergone osmotic adaptation. This would result in swollen brain cells and increase the risk of seizures or permanent neurologic damage. Therefore, the water deficit should be corrected slowly over at least 48–72 h. When calculating the rate of water replacement, ongoing losses should be taken into account, and the plasma Na$^+$ concentration should be lowered by 0.5 mmol/L per hour and by no more than 12 mmol/L over the first 24 h.

The safest route of administration of water is by mouth or via a nasogastric tube (or other feeding tube). Alternatively, 5% dextrose in water or half-isotonic saline can be given intravenously. The appropriate treatment of CDI consists of administering desmopressin intranasally. Other options for decreasing urine output include a low-salt diet in combination with low-dose thiazide diuretic therapy. In some patients with partial CDI, drugs that either stimulate AVP secretion or enhance its action on the kidney have been useful. These include chlorpropamide, clofibrate, carbamazepine, and nonsteroidal anti-inflammatory drugs (NSAIDs). The concentrating defect in NDI may be reversible by treating the underlying disorder or eliminating the offending drug. Symptomatic polyuria

due to NDI can be treated with a low-Na$^+$ diet and thiazide diuretics, as described above. This induces mild volume depletion, which leads to enhanced proximal reabsorption of salt and water and decreased delivery to the site of action of AVP, the collecting duct. By impairing renal prostaglandin synthesis, NSAIDs potentiate AVP action and thereby increase urine osmolality and decrease urine volume. Amiloride may be useful in patients with NDI who need to be on lithium. The nephrotoxicity of lithium requires the drug to be taken up into collecting duct cells via the amiloride-sensitive Na$^+$ channel.

POTASSIUM

Potassium Balance

Potassium is the major intracellular cation. The normal plasma K$^+$ concentration is 3.5–5.0 mmol/L, whereas that inside cells is about 150 mmol/L. Therefore, the amount of K$^+$ in the ECF (30–70 mmol) constitutes <2% of the total body K$^+$ content (2500–4500 mmol). The ratio of ICF to ECF K$^+$ concentration (normally 38:1) is the principal result of the resting membrane potential and is crucial for normal neuromuscular function. The basolateral Na$^+$, K$^+$-ATPase pump actively transports K$^+$ in and Na$^+$ out of the cell in a 2:3 ratio, and the passive outward diffusion of K$^+$ is quantitatively the most important factor that generates the resting membrane potential. The activity of the electrogenic Na$^+$, K$^+$-ATPase pump may be stimulated as a result of an increased intracellular Na$^+$ concentration and inhibited in the setting of digoxin toxicity or chronic illness such as heart failure or renal failure.

The K$^+$ intake of individuals on an average Western diet is 40–120 mmol/d, or approximately 1 mmol/kg per day, 90% of which is absorbed by the gastrointestinal tract. Maintenance of the steady state necessitates matching K$^+$ ingestion with excretion. Initially, extrarenal adaptive mechanisms, followed later by urinary excretion, prevent a doubling of the plasma K$^+$ concentration that would occur if the dietary K$^+$ load remained in the ECF compartment. Immediately following a meal, most of the absorbed K$^+$ enters cells as a result of the initial elevation in the plasma K$^+$ concentration and facilitated by insulin release and basal catecholamine levels. Eventually, however, the excess K$^+$ is excreted in the urine. The regulation of gastrointestinal K$^+$ handling is not well understood. The amount of K$^+$ lost in the stool can increase from 10 to 50% or 60% (of dietary intake) in chronic renal insufficiency. In addition, colonic secretion of K$^+$ is stimulated in patients with large volumes of diarrhea, resulting in potentially severe K$^+$ depletion.

(See also Chap. 2) Renal excretion is the major route of elimination of dietary and other sources of excess K^+. The filtered load of K^+ (GFR $\times$ plasma K^+ concentration = 180 L/d $\times$ 4 mmol/L = 720 mmol/d) is ten- to twentyfold greater than the ECF K^+ content. Some 90% of filtered K^+ is reabsorbed by the proximal convoluted tubule and loop of Henle. Proximally, K^+ is reabsorbed passively with Na^+ and water, whereas the luminal Na^+-K^+-$2Cl^-$ co-transporter mediates K^+ uptake in the TALH. Therefore, K^+ delivery to the distal nephron [distal convoluted tubule and cortical collecting duct (CCD)] approximates dietary intake. Net distal K^+ secretion or reabsorption occurs in the setting of K^+ excess or depletion, respectively. The cell responsible for K^+ secretion in the late distal convoluted tubule (or connecting tubule) and CCD is the principal cell. Virtually all regulation of renal K^+ excretion and total body K^+ balance occurs in the distal nephron. Potassium secretion is regulated by two physiologic stimuli—aldosterone and hyperkalemia. Aldosterone is secreted by the zona glomerulosa cells of the adrenal cortex in response to high renin and angiotensin II or hyperkalemia. The plasma K^+ concentration, independent of aldosterone, can directly affect K^+ secretion. In addition to the K^+ concentration in the lumen of the CCD, renal K^+ loss depends on the urine flow rate, a function of daily solute excretion. Since excretion is equal to the product of concentration and volume, increased distal flow rate can significantly enhance urinary K^+ output. Finally, in severe K^+ depletion, secretion of K^+ is reduced and reabsorption in the cortical and medullary collecting ducts is upregulated.

HYPOKALEMIA

Etiology

(Table 6-3) Hypokalemia, defined as a plasma K^+ concentration <3.5 mmol/L, may result from one (or more) of the following: decreased net intake, shift into cells, increased net loss. Diminished intake is seldom the sole cause of K^+ depletion since urinary excretion can be effectively decreased to <15 mmol/d as a result of net K^+ reabsorption in the distal nephron. With the exception of the urban poor and certain cultural groups, the amount of K^+ in the diet almost always exceeds that excreted in the urine. However, dietary K^+ restriction may exacerbate the hypokalemia secondary to increased gastrointestinal or renal loss. An unusual cause of decreased K^+ intake is ingestion of clay (geophagia), which binds dietary K^+ and iron. This custom was previously common among African Americans in the American South.

Redistribution into Cells

Movement of K^+ into cells may transiently decrease the plasma K^+ concentration without altering total

TABLE 6-3

CAUSES OF HYPOKALEMIA

I. Decreased intake
   A. Starvation
   B. Clay ingestion
II. Redistribution into cells
   A. Acid-base
      1. Metabolic alkalosis
   B. Hormonal
      1. Insulin
      2. β_2-Adrenergic agonists (endogenous or exogenous)
      3. α-Adrenergic antagonists
   C. Anabolic state
      1. Vitamin B_{12} or folic acid (red blood cell production)
      2. Granulocyte-macrophage colony stimulating factor (white blood cell production)
      3. Total parenteral nutrition
   D. Other
      1. Pseudohypokalemia
      2. Hypothermia
      3. Hypokalemic periodic paralysis
      4. Barium toxicity
III. Increased loss
   A. Nonrenal
      1. Gastrointestinal loss (diarrhea)
      2. Integumentary loss (sweat)
   B. Renal
      1. Increased distal flow: diuretics, osmotic diuresis, salt-wasting nephropathies
      2. Increased secretion of potassium
         a. Mineralocorticoid excess: primary hyperaldosteronism, secondary hyperaldosteronism (malignant hypertension, renin-secreting tumors, renal artery stenosis, hypovolemia), apparent mineralocorticoid excess (licorice, chewing tobacco, carbenoxolone), congenital adrenal hyperplasia, Cushing's syndrome, Bartter's syndrome
         b. Distal delivery of non-reabsorbed anions: vomiting, nasogastric suction, proximal (type 2) renal tubular acidosis, diabetic ketoacidosis, glue-sniffing (toluene abuse), penicillin derivatives
         c. Other: amphotericin B, Liddle's syndrome, hypomagnesemia

body K^+ content. For any given cause, the magnitude of the change is relatively small, often <1 mmol/L. However, a combination of factors may lead to a significant fall in the plasma K^+ concentration and may amplify the hypokalemia due to K^+ wasting. Metabolic alkalosis is often associated with hypokalemia. This occurs as a result of K^+ redistribution as well as excessive renal K^+ loss. Treatment of diabetic ketoacidosis with insulin may lead to hypokalemia due to stimulation of the Na^+-H^+ antiporter and (secondarily) the

Na$^+$, K$^+$-ATPase pump. Furthermore, uncontrolled hyperglycemia often leads to K$^+$ depletion from an osmotic diuresis. Stress-induced catecholamine release and administration of β_2-adrenergic agonists directly induce cellular uptake of K$^+$ and promote insulin secretion by pancreatic islet β cells. *Hypokalemic periodic paralysis* is a rare condition characterized by recurrent episodic weakness or paralysis. Since K$^+$ is the major ICF cation, anabolic states can potentially result in hypokalemia due to a K$^+$ shift into cells. This may occur following rapid cell growth seen in patients with pernicious anemia treated with vitamin B$_{12}$ or with neutropenia after treatment with granulocyte-macrophage colony stimulating factor. Massive transfusion with thawed washed red blood cells (RBCs) could cause hypokalemia since frozen RBCs lose up to half of their K$^+$ during storage.

Nonrenal Loss of Potassium

Excessive sweating may result in K$^+$ depletion from increased integumentary and renal K$^+$ loss. Hyperaldosteronism, secondary to ECF volume contraction, enhances K$^+$ excretion in the urine. Normally, K$^+$ lost in the stool amounts to 5–10 mmol/d in a volume of 100–200 mL. Hypokalemia subsequent to increased gastrointestinal loss can occur in patients with profuse diarrhea (usually secretory), villous adenomas, VIPomas, or laxative abuse. However, the loss of gastric secretions does not account for the moderate to severe K$^+$ depletion often associated with vomiting or nasogastric suction. Since the K$^+$ concentration of gastric fluid is 5–10 mmol/L, it would take 30–80 L of vomitus to achieve a K$^+$ deficit of 300–400 mmol typically seen in these patients. In fact, the hypokalemia is primarily due to increased renal K$^+$ excretion. Loss of gastric contents results in volume depletion and metabolic alkalosis, both of which promote kaliuresis. Hypovolemia stimulates aldosterone release, which augments K$^+$ secretion by the principal cells. In addition, the filtered load of HCO$_3^-$ exceeds the reabsorptive capacity of the proximal convoluted tubule, thereby increasing distal delivery of NaHCO$_3$, which enhances the electrochemical gradient favoring K$^+$ loss in the urine.

Renal Loss of Potassium

In general, most cases of chronic hypokalemia are due to renal K$^+$ wasting. This may be due to factors that increase the K$^+$ concentration in the lumen of the CCD or augment distal flow rate. Mineralocorticoid excess commonly results in hypokalemia. *Primary hyperaldosteronism* is due to dysregulated aldosterone secretion by an adrenal adenoma (Conn's syndrome) or carcinoma or to adrenocortical hyperplasia. In a rare subset of patients, the disorder is familial (autosomal dominant) and aldosterone levels can be suppressed by administering low doses of exogenous glucocorticoid. The molecular defect responsible for *glucocorticoid-remediable hyperaldosteronism* is a rearranged gene (due to a chromosomal crossover), containing the 5′-regulatory region of the 11β-hydroxylase gene and the coding sequence of the aldosterone synthase gene. Consequently, mineralocorticoid is synthesized in the zona fasciculata and regulated by corticotropin. A number of conditions associated with hyperreninemia result in secondary hyperaldosteronism and renal K$^+$ wasting. High renin levels are commonly seen in both renovascular and malignant hypertension. Renin-secreting tumors of the juxtaglomerular apparatus are a rare cause of hypokalemia. Other tumors that have been reported to produce renin include renal cell carcinoma, ovarian carcinoma, and Wilms' tumor. Hyperreninemia may also occur secondary to decreased effective circulating arterial volume.

In the absence of elevated renin or aldosterone levels, enhanced distal nephron secretion of K$^+$ may result from increased production of non-aldosterone mineralocorticoids in *congenital adrenal hyperplasia*. Glucocorticoid-stimulated kaliuresis does not normally occur due to the conversion of cortisol to cortisone by 11β-hydroxysteroid dehydrogenase (11β-HSDH). Therefore, 11β-HSDH deficiency or suppression allows cortisol to bind to the aldosterone receptor and leads to the *syndrome of apparent mineralocorticoid excess*. Drugs that inhibit the activity of 11β-HSDH include glycyrrhetinic acid, present in licorice, chewing tobacco, and carbenoxolone. The presentation of Cushing's syndrome may include hypokalemia if the capacity of 11β-HSDH to inactivate cortisol is overwhelmed by persistently elevated glucocorticoid levels.

Liddle's syndrome is a rare familial (autosomal dominant) disease characterized by hypertension, hypokalemic metabolic alkalosis, renal K$^+$ wasting, and suppressed renin and aldosterone secretion. Increased distal delivery of Na$^+$ with a nonreabsorbable anion (not Cl$^-$) enhances K$^+$ secretion. Classically, this is seen with *proximal (type 2) renal tubular acidosis* (RTA) and vomiting, associated with bicarbonaturia. Diabetic ketoacidosis and toluene abuse (glue sniffing) can lead to increased delivery of β-hydroxybutyrate and hippurate, respectively, to the CCD and to renal K$^+$ loss. High doses of penicillin derivatives administered to volume-depleted patients may likewise promote renal K$^+$ secretion as well as an osmotic diuresis. *Classic distal (type 1) RTA* is associated with hypokalemia due to increased renal K$^+$ loss, the mechanism of which is uncertain. Amphotericin B causes hypokalemia due to increased distal nephron permeability to Na$^+$ and K$^+$ and to renal K$^+$ wasting.

Bartter's syndrome is a disorder characterized by hypokalemia, metabolic alkalosis, hyperreninemic hyperaldosteronism secondary to ECF volume contraction, and juxtaglomerular apparatus hyperplasia. Finally, diuretic use and abuse are common causes of K$^+$ depletion. Carbonic anhydrase inhibitors, loop diuretics, and thiazides are all kaliuretic. The degree of hypokalemia tends to be greater with long-acting agents and is dose dependent.

Increased renal K⁺ excretion is primarily due to increased distal solute delivery and secondary hyperaldosteronism (due to volume depletion).

See also Chap. 16.

Clinical Features

The clinical manifestations of K⁺ depletion vary greatly between individual patients, and their severity depends on the degree of hypokalemia. Symptoms seldom occur unless the plasma K⁺ concentration is <3 mmol/L. Fatigue, myalgia, and muscular weakness of the lower extremities are common complaints and are due to a lower (more negative) resting membrane potential. More severe hypokalemia may lead to progressive weakness, hypoventilation (due to respiratory muscle involvement), and eventually complete paralysis. Impaired muscle metabolism and the blunted hyperemic response to exercise associated with profound K⁺ depletion increase the risk of rhabdomyolysis. Smooth-muscle function may also be affected and manifest as paralytic ileus.

The electrocardiographic changes of hypokalemia are due to delayed ventricular repolarization and do not correlate well with the plasma K⁺ concentration. Early changes include flattening or inversion of the T wave, a prominent U wave, ST-segment depression, and a prolonged QU interval. Severe K⁺ depletion may result in a prolonged PR interval, decreased voltage and widening of the QRS complex, and an increased risk of ventricular arrhythmias, especially in patients with myocardial ischemia or left ventricular hypertrophy. Hypokalemia may also predispose to digitalis toxicity. Hypokalemia is often associated with acid-base disturbances related to the underlying disorder. In addition, K⁺ depletion results in intracellular acidification and an increase in net acid excretion or new HCO₃⁻ production. This is a consequence of enhanced proximal HCO₃⁻ reabsorption, increased renal ammoniagenesis, and increased distal H⁺ secretion. This contributes to the generation of metabolic alkalosis frequently present in hypokalemic patients. NDI is not uncommonly seen in K⁺ depletion and is manifest as polydipsia and polyuria. Glucose intolerance may also occur with hypokalemia and has been attributed to either impaired insulin secretion or peripheral insulin resistance.

Diagnosis

(**Fig. 6-3**) In most cases, the etiology of K⁺ depletion can be determined by a careful history. Diuretic and laxative abuse as well as surreptitious vomiting may be difficult to identify but should be excluded. Rarely, patients with a marked leukocytosis (e.g., acute myeloid leukemia) and normokalemia may have a low measured plasma K⁺ concentration due to white blood cell uptake of K⁺ at room temperature. This *pseudohypokalemia* can be avoided by storing the blood sample on ice or rapidly separating the plasma (or serum) from the cells.

After eliminating decreased intake and intracellular shift as potential causes of hypokalemia, examination of the renal response can help to clarify the source of K⁺ loss. The appropriate response to K⁺ depletion is to excrete <15 mmol/d of K⁺ in the urine, due to increased reabsorption and decreased distal secretion. Hypokalemia with minimal renal K⁺ excretion suggests that K⁺ was lost via the skin or gastrointestinal tract or that there is a remote history of vomiting or diuretic use. As described above, renal K⁺ wasting may be due to factors that either increase the K⁺ concentration in the CCD or increase the distal flow rate (or both). The ECF volume status, blood pressure, and associated acid-base disorder may help to differentiate the causes of excessive renal K⁺ loss. A rapid and simple test designed to evaluate the driving force for net K⁺ secretion is the *transtubular K⁺ concentration gradient* (TTKG). The TTKG is the ratio of the K⁺ concentration in the lumen of the CCD ($[K^+]_{CCD}$) to that in peritubular capillaries or plasma ($[K^+]_p$). The validity of this measurement depends on three assumptions: (1) few solutes are reabsorbed in the medullary collecting

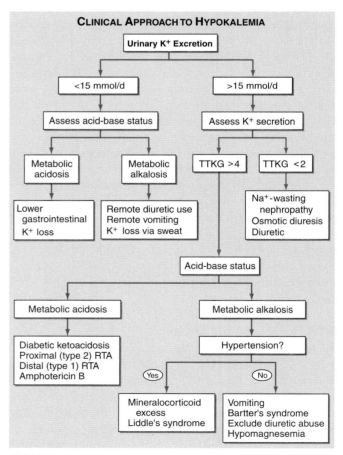

FIGURE 6-3

Algorithm depicting clinical approach to hypokalemia. TTKG, transtubular K⁺ concentration gradient; RTA, renal tubular acidosis.

duct (MCD), (2) K^+ is neither secreted nor reabsorbed in the MCD, and (3) the osmolality of the fluid in the terminal CCD is known. Significant reabsorption or secretion of K^+ in the MCD seldom occurs, except in profound K^+ depletion or excess, respectively. When AVP is acting ($OSM_U \geq OSM_P$), the osmolality in the terminal CCD is the same as that of plasma, and the K^+ concentration in the lumen of the distal nephron can be estimated by dividing the urine K^+ concentration ($[K^+]_U$) by the ratio of the urine to plasma osmolality (OSM_U/OSM_P):

$$[K^+]_{CCD} = [K^+]_U \div (OSM_U/OSM_P) \, TTKG$$

$$= [K^+]_{CCD}/[K^+]_P$$

$$= [K^+]_U \div (OSM_U/OSM_P)/[K^+]_P$$

Hypokalemia with a TTKG greater than 4 suggests renal K^+ loss due to increased distal K^+ secretion. Plasma renin and aldosterone levels are often helpful in differentiating the various causes of hyperaldosteronism. Bicarbonaturia and the presence of other non-reabsorbed anions also increase the TTKG and lead to renal K^+-wasting.

℞ Treatment:
HYPOKALEMIA

The therapeutic goals are to correct the K^+ deficit and to minimize ongoing losses. With the exception of periodic paralysis, hypokalemia resulting from transcellular shifts rarely requires intravenous K^+ supplementation, which can lead to rebound hyperkalemia. It is generally safer to correct hypokalemia via the oral route. The degree of K^+ depletion does not correlate well with the plasma K^+ concentration. A decrement of 1 mmol/L in the plasma K^+ concentration (from 4.0 to 3.0 mmol/L) may represent a total body K^+ deficit of 200–400 mmol, and patients with plasma levels under 3.0 mmol/L often require in excess of 600 mmol of K^+ to correct the deficit. Furthermore, factors promoting K^+ shift out of cells (e.g., insulin deficiency in diabetic ketoacidosis) may result in underestimation of the K^+ deficit. Therefore, the plasma K^+ concentration should be monitored frequently when assessing the response to treatment. Potassium chloride is usually the preparation of choice and will promote more rapid correction of hypokalemia and metabolic alkalosis. Potassium bicarbonate and citrate (metabolized to HCO_3^-) tend to alkalinize the patient and would be more appropriate for hypokalemia associated with chronic diarrhea or RTA.

Patients with severe hypokalemia or those unable to take anything by mouth require intravenous replacement therapy with KCl. The maximum concentration of administered K^+ should be no more than 40 mmol/L via a peripheral vein or 60 mmol/L via a central vein. The rate of infusion should not exceed 20 mmol/h unless paralysis or malignant ventricular arrhythmias are present. Ideally, KCl should be mixed in normal saline since dextrose solutions may initially exacerbate hypokalemia due to insulin-mediated movement of K^+ into cells. Rapid intravenous administration of K^+ should be used judiciously and requires close observation of the clinical manifestations of hypokalemia (electrocardiogram and neuromuscular examination).

HYPERKALEMIA
Etiology

Hyperkalemia, defined as a plasma K^+ concentration >5.0 mmol/L, occurs as a result of either K^+ release from cells or decreased renal loss. Increased K^+ intake is rarely the sole cause of hyperkalemia since the phenomenon of *potassium adaptation* ensures rapid K^+ excretion in response to increases in dietary consumption. Iatrogenic hyperkalemia may result from overzealous parenteral K^+ replacement or in patients with renal insufficiency. *Pseudohyperkalemia* represents an artificially elevated plasma K^+ concentration due to K^+ movement out of cells immediately prior to or following venipuncture. Contributing factors include prolonged use of a tourniquet with or without repeated fist clenching, hemolysis, and marked leukocytosis or thrombocytosis. The latter two result in an elevated serum K^+ concentration due to release of intracellular K^+ following clot formation. Pseudohyperkalemia should be suspected in an otherwise asymptomatic patient with no obvious underlying cause. If proper venipuncture technique is used and a plasma (not serum) K^+ concentration is measured, it should be normal. Intravascular hemolysis, tumor lysis syndrome, and rhabdomyolysis all lead to K^+ release from cells as a result of tissue breakdown.

Metabolic acidoses, with the exception of those due to the accumulation of organic anions, can be associated with mild hyperkalemia resulting from intracellular buffering of H^+. Insulin deficiency and hypertonicity (e.g., hyperglycemia) promote K^+ shift from the ICF to the ECF. The severity of exercise-induced hyperkalemia is related to the degree of exertion. It is due to release of K^+ from muscles and is usually rapidly reversible, often associated with rebound hypokalemia. Treatment with beta blockers rarely causes hyperkalemia but may contribute to the elevation in plasma K^+ concentration seen with other conditions. *Hyperkalemic periodic paralysis* is a rare autosomal dominant disorder characterized by episodic weakness or paralysis, precipitated by stimuli that normally lead to mild hyperkalemia (e.g., exercise). The genetic defect appears to be a single amino acid substitution due to a mutation in the gene for the skeletal muscle Na^+ channel. Hyperkalemia may occur with severe digitalis toxicity due to inhibition of the Na^+,K^+-ATPase pump. Depolarizing muscle relaxants such as succinylcholine can increase the plasma K^+ concentration, especially in patients with massive trauma, burns, or neuromuscular disease.

Chronic hyperkalemia is virtually always associated with decreased renal K^+ excretion due to either impaired secretion or diminished distal solute delivery (Table 6-4). The latter is seldom the only cause of impaired K^+ excretion but may significantly contribute to hyperkalemia in protein-malnourished (low urea excretion) and ECF volume–contracted (decreased distal NaCl delivery) patients. Decreased K^+ secretion by the principal cells results from either impaired Na^+ reabsorption or increased Cl^- reabsorption.

Hyporeninemic hypoaldosteronism is a syndrome characterized by euvolemia or ECF volume expansion and suppressed renin and aldosterone levels. This disorder is commonly seen in mild renal insufficiency, diabetic nephropathy, or chronic tubulointerstitial disease. Patients frequently have an impaired kaliuretic response to exogenous mineralocorticoid administration, suggesting that enhanced distal Cl^- reabsorption (electroneutral Na^+ reabsorption) may account for many of the findings of hyporeninemic hypoaldosteronism. NSAIDs inhibit renin secretion and the synthesis of vasodilatory renal prostaglandins. The resultant decrease in GFR and K^+ secretion is often manifest as hyperkalemia. As a rule, the degree of hyperkalemia due to hypoaldosteronism is mild in the absence of increased K^+ intake or renal dysfunction.

Angiotensin-converting enzyme (ACE) inhibitors block the conversion of angiotensin I to angiotensin II. Angiotensin receptor antagonists directly inhibit the actions of angiotensin II on AT1 angiotensin II receptors. The actions of both of these classes of drugs result in impaired aldosterone release. Patients at increased risk of ACE inhibitor or angiotensin receptor antagonist–induced hyperkalemia include those with diabetes mellitus, renal insufficiency, decreased effective circulating arterial volume, bilateral renal artery stenosis, or concurrent use of K^+-sparing diuretics or NSAIDs.

Decreased aldosterone synthesis may be due to *primary adrenal insufficiency* (Addison's disease) or congenital adrenal enzyme deficiency. Heparin (including low-molecular-weight heparin) inhibits production of aldosterone by the cells of the zona glomerulosa and can lead to severe hyperkalemia in a subset of patients with underlying renal disease, diabetes mellitus, or those receiving K^+-sparing diuretics, ACE inhibitors, or NSAIDs. *Pseudohypoaldosteronism* is a rare familial disorder characterized by hyperkalemia, metabolic acidosis, renal Na^+ wasting, hypotension, high renin and aldosterone levels, and end-organ resistance to aldosterone. The gene encoding the mineralocorticoid receptor is normal in these patients, and the electrolyte abnormalities can be reversed with suprapharmacologic doses of an exogenous mineralocorticoid (e.g., 9α-fludrocortisone) or an inhibitor of 11β-HSDH (e.g., carbenoxolone). The kaliuretic response to aldosterone is impaired by K^+-sparing diuretics. Spironolactone is a competitive mineralocorticoid antagonist, whereas amiloride and triamterene block the apical Na^+ channel of the principal cell. Two other drugs that impair K^+ secretion by blocking distal nephron Na^+ reabsorption are trimethoprim and pentamidine. These antimicrobial agents may contribute to the hyperkalemia often seen in patients infected with HIV who are being treated for *Pneumocystis carinii* pneumonia.

Hyperkalemia frequently complicates acute oliguric renal failure due to increased K^+ release from cells (acidosis, catabolism) and decreased excretion. Increased distal flow rate and K^+ secretion per nephron compensate for decreased renal mass in chronic renal insufficiency. However, these adaptive mechanisms eventually fail to maintain K^+ balance when the GFR falls below 10–15 mL/min or oliguria ensues. Otherwise asymptomatic urinary tract obstruction is an often overlooked cause of hyperkalemia. Other nephropathies associated with impaired K^+ excretion include drug-induced interstitial nephritis, lupus nephritis, sickle cell disease, and diabetic nephropathy.

Gordon's syndrome is a rare condition characterized by hyperkalemia, metabolic acidosis, and a normal GFR. These patients are usually volume-expanded with suppressed renin and aldosterone levels as well as refractory to the kaliuretic effect of exogenous mineralocorticoids. It has been suggested that these findings could all be accounted for by increased distal Cl^- reabsorption (electroneutral Na^+ reabsorption), also referred to as a

TABLE 6-4

CAUSES OF HYPERKALEMIA

I. Renal failure
II. Decreased distal flow (i.e., decreased effective circulating arterial volume)
III. Decreased K^+ secretion
   A. Impaired Na^+ reabsorption
     1. Primary hypoaldosteronism: adrenal insufficiency, adrenal enzyme deficiency (21-hydroxylase, 3β-hydroxysteroid dehydrogenase, corticosterone methyl oxidase)
     2. Secondary hypoaldosteronism: hyporeninemia, drugs (ACE inhibitors, NSAIDs, heparin)
     3. Resistance to aldosterone: pseudohypoaldosteronism, tubulointerstitial disease, drugs (K^+-sparing diuretics, trimethoprim, pentamidine)
   B. Enhanced Cl^- reabsorption (chloride shunt)
     1. Gordon's syndrome
     2. Cyclosporine

Note: ACE, angiotensin-converting enzyme; NSAIDs, nonsteroidal anti-inflammatory drugs.

Cl⁻ shunt. A similar mechanism may be partially responsible for the hyperkalemia associated with cyclosporine nephrotoxicity. *Hyperkalemic distal (type 4) RTA* may be due to either hypoaldosteronism or a Cl⁻ shunt (aldosterone–resistant).

Clinical Features

Since the resting membrane potential is related to the ratio of the ICF to ECF K⁺ concentration, hyperkalemia partially depolarizes the cell membrane. Prolonged depolarization impairs membrane excitability and is manifest as weakness, which may progress to flaccid paralysis and hypoventilation if the respiratory muscles are involved. Hyperkalemia also inhibits renal ammonia-genesis and reabsorption of NH_4^+ in the TALH. Thus, net acid excretion is impaired and results in metabolic acidosis, which may further exacerbate the hyperkalemia due to K⁺ movement out of cells.

The most serious effect of hyperkalemia is cardiac toxicity, which does not correlate well with the plasma K⁺ concentration. The earliest electrocardiographic changes include increased T-wave amplitude, or peaked T waves. More severe degrees of hyperkalemia result in a prolonged PR interval and QRS duration, atrioventricular conduction delay, and loss of P waves. Progressive widening of the QRS complex and merging with the T wave produces a sine wave pattern. The terminal event is usually ventricular fibrillation or asystole.

Diagnosis

(**Fig. 6-4**) With rare exceptions, chronic hyperkalemia is always due to impaired K⁺ excretion. If the etiology is not readily apparent and the patient is asymptomatic, pseudohyperkalemia should be excluded, as described above. Oliguric acute renal failure and severe chronic renal insufficiency should also be ruled out. The history should focus on medications that impair K⁺ handling and potential sources of K⁺ intake. Evaluation of the ECF compartment, effective circulating volume, and urine output are essential components of the physical examination. The severity of hyperkalemia is determined by the symptoms, plasma K⁺ concentration, and electrocardiographic abnormalities.

The appropriate renal response to hyperkalemia is to excrete at least 200 mmol of K⁺ daily. In most cases, diminished renal K⁺ loss is due to impaired K⁺ secretion, which can be assessed by measuring the TTKG. A TTKG <10 implies a decreased driving force for K⁺ secretion due to either hypoaldosteronism or resistance to the renal effects of mineralocorticoid. This can be determined by evaluating the kaliuretic response to administration of mineralocorticoid (e.g., 9α–fludrocortisone). Primary adrenal insufficiency can be differentiated from hyporeninemic hypoaldosteronism by examining the

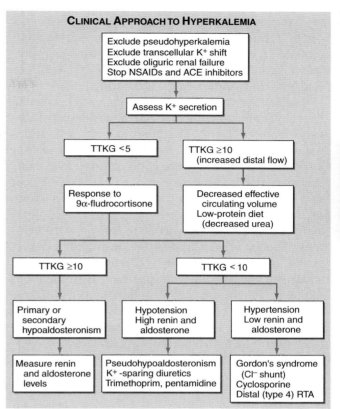

FIGURE 6-4

Algorithm depicting clinical approach to hyperkalemia. NSAID, nonsteroidal anti-inflammatory drug; ACE, angiotensin-converting enzyme; RTA, renal tubular acidosis; TTKG, transtubular K⁺ concentration gradient.

renin–aldosterone axis. Renin and aldosterone levels should be measured in the supine and upright positions following 3 days of Na⁺ restriction (Na⁺ intake <10 mmol/d) in combination with a loop diuretic to induce mild volume contraction. Aldosterone-resistant hyperkalemia can result from the various causes of impaired distal Na⁺ reabsorption or from a Cl⁻ shunt. The former leads to salt wasting, ECF volume contraction, and high renin and aldosterone levels. In contrast, enhanced distal Cl⁻ reabsorption is associated with volume expansion and suppressed renin and aldosterone secretion. As mentioned above, hypoaldosteronism seldom causes severe hyperkalemia in the absence of increased dietary K⁺ intake, renal insufficiency, transcellular K⁺ shifts, or antikaliuretic drugs.

℞ **Treatment:**
HYPERKALEMIA

The approach to therapy depends on the degree of hyperkalemia as determined by the plasma K⁺ concentration, associated muscular weakness, and changes on the electrocardiogram. Potentially fatal hyperkalemia rarely occurs unless the plasma K+ concentration exceeds 7.5 mmol/L and is usually associated with profound weakness and absent P waves, QRS widening, or ventricular arrhythmias on the electrocardiogram.

Severe hyperkalemia requires emergent treatment directed at minimizing membrane depolarization, shifting K+ into cells, and promoting K+ loss. In addition, exogenous K+ intake and antikaliuretic drugs should be discontinued. Administration of calcium gluconate decreases membrane excitability. The usual dose is 10 mL of a 10% solution infused over 2–3 min. The effect begins within minutes but is short-lived (30–60 min), and the dose can be repeated if no change in the electrocardiogram is seen after 5–10 min. Insulin causes K+ to shift into cells by mechanisms described previously and will temporarily lower the plasma K+ concentration. Although glucose alone will stimulate insulin release from normal pancreatic β cells, a more rapid response generally occurs when exogenous insulin is administered (with glucose to prevent hypoglycemia). A commonly recommended combination is 10–20 units of regular insulin and 25–50 g of glucose. Obviously, hyperglycemic patients should not be given glucose. If effective, the plasma K+ concentration will fall by 0.5–1.5 mmol/L in 15–30 min, and the effect will last for several hours. Alkali therapy with intravenous NaHCO$_3$ can also shift K+ into cells. This is safest when administered as an isotonic solution of three ampules per liter (134 mmol/L NaHCO$_3$) and ideally should be reserved for severe hyperkalemia associated with metabolic acidosis. Patients with end-stage renal disease seldom respond to this intervention and may not tolerate the Na+ load and resultant volume expansion. When administered parenterally or in nebulized form, β$_2$-adrenergic agonists promote cellular uptake of K+. The onset of action is 30 min, lowering the plasma K+ concentration by 0.5 to 1.5 mmol/L, and the effect lasts 2–4 h.

Removal of K+ can be achieved using diuretics, cation-exchange resin, or dialysis. Loop and thiazide diuretics, often in combination, may enhance K+ excretion if renal function is adequate. Sodium polystyrene sulfonate is a cation-exchange resin that promotes the exchange of Na+ for K+ in the gastrointestinal tract. Each gram binds 1 mmol of K+ and releases 2–3 mmol of Na+. When given by mouth, the usual dose is 25–50 g mixed with 100 mL of 20% sorbitol to prevent constipation. This will generally lower the plasma K+ concentration by 0.5–1.0 mmol/L within 1–2 h and last for 4–6 h. Sodium polystyrene sulfonate can also be administered as a retention enema consisting of 50 g of resin and 50 mL of 70% sorbitol mixed in 150 mL of tap water. The sorbitol should be omitted from the enema in postoperative patients due to the increased incidence of sorbitol-induced colonic necrosis, especially following renal transplantation. The most rapid and effective way of lowering the plasma K+ concentration is hemodialysis. This should be reserved for patients with renal failure and those with severe life-threatening hyperkalemia unresponsive to more conservative measures. Peritoneal dialysis also removes K+ but is only 15–20% as effective as hemodialysis. Finally, the underlying cause of the hyperkalemia should be treated. This may involve dietary modification, correction of metabolic acidosis, cautious volume expansion, and administration of exogenous mineralocorticoid.

FURTHER READINGS

ADROGUE HJ, MADIAS NE: Hypernatremia. N Engl J Med 342:1493, 2000

———: Hyponatremia. N Engl J Med 342:1581, 2000

BERL T, VERBALIS J: Pathophysiology of water metabolism, in Brenner & Rector's The Kidney, 7th ed, BM Brenner (ed). Philadelphia, Saunders, 2004

COHN JN et al: New guidelines for potassium replacement in clinical practice: A contemporary review by the National Council on Potassium in Clinical Practice. Arch Intern Med 160:2429, 2000

GOLDSZMIDT MA, ILIESCU EA: DDAVP to prevent rapid correction in hyponatremia. Clin Nephrol 53:226, 2000

GREENBERG A, VERBALIS JG: Vasopressin receptor antagonists. Kidney Int 69:2124, 2006

GREENLEE M et al: Narrative review: Evolving concepts in potassium homeostasis and hypokalemia. Ann Intern Med 150:619, 2009

GROSS P: Treatment of severe hyponatremia. Kidney Int 60:2417, 2001

JAITLY M et al: Hypokalemia during sickle cell crises apparently due to intermittent mineralocorticoid excess. Am J Kidney Dis 51:319, 2008

KIM WR et al: Hyponatremia and mortality among patients on the liver-transplant waiting list. N Engl J Med 359:1018, 2008

LIAMIS G et al: A review of drug-induced hyponatremia. Am J Kidney Dis 52:144, 2008

MOUNT DB: Disorders of potassium balance, in Brenner & Rector's The Kidney, 7th ed, BM Brenner (ed). Philadelphia, Saunders, 2004

NIELSEN S et al: Aquaporins in the kidney: From molecules to medicine. Physiol Rev 82:205, 2002

WARNOCK DG: Genetic forms of renal potassium and magnesium wasting. Am J Med 112:235, 2002

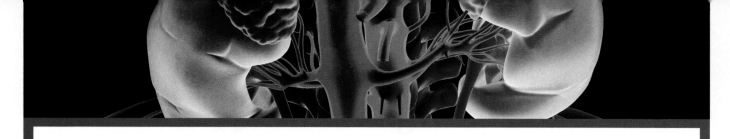

CHAPTER 7
HYPERCALCEMIA AND HYPOCALCEMIA

Sundeep Khosla

The calcium ion plays a critical role in normal cellular function and signaling, regulating diverse physiologic processes such as neuromuscular signaling, cardiac contractility, hormone secretion, and blood coagulation. Thus, extracellular calcium concentrations are maintained within an exquisitely narrow range through a series of feedback mechanisms that involve parathyroid hormone (PTH) and the active vitamin D metabolite 1,25-dihydroxyvitamin D $[1,25(OH)_2D]$. These feedback mechanisms are orchestrated by integrating signals between the parathyroid glands, kidney, intestine, and bone (Fig. 7-1).

Disorders of serum calcium concentration are relatively common and often serve as a harbinger of underlying disease. This chapter provides a brief summary of the approach to patients with altered serum calcium levels.

HYPERCALCEMIA

ETIOLOGY

The causes of hypercalcemia can be understood and classified based on derangements in the normal feedback mechanisms that regulate serum calcium (Table 7-1). Excess PTH production, which is not appropriately suppressed by increased serum calcium concentrations, occurs in primary neoplastic disorders of the parathyroid glands (parathyroid adenomas, hyperplasia, or, rarely, carcinoma) that are associated with increased parathyroid cell mass and impaired feedback inhibition by calcium. Inappropriate PTH secretion for the ambient level of serum calcium also occurs with heterozygous inactivating calcium sensor receptor (CaSR) mutations, which impair extracellular calcium sensing by the parathyroid glands and the kidneys, resulting in familial hypocalciuric hypercalcemia (FHH). Although PTH secretion by tumors is extremely rare, many solid tumors produce PTH-related peptide (PTHrP), which shares homology with PTH in the first 13 amino acids and binds the PTH receptor, thus mimicking effects of PTH on bone and the kidney. In PTHrP-mediated hypercalcemia of malignancy, PTH levels are suppressed by the high serum calcium levels. Hypercalcemia associated with granulomatous disease (e.g., sarcoidosis) or lymphomas is caused by enhanced conversion of 25(OH)D to the potent $1,25(OH)_2D$. In these disorders, $1,25(OH)_2D$ enhances intestinal calcium absorption, resulting in hypercalcemia and suppressed PTH. Disorders that directly increase calcium mobilization from bone, such as hyperthyroidism or osteolytic metastases, also lead to hypercalcemia with suppressed PTH secretion, as does exogenous calcium overload, as in milk-alkali syndrome, or total parenteral nutrition with excessive calcium supplementation.

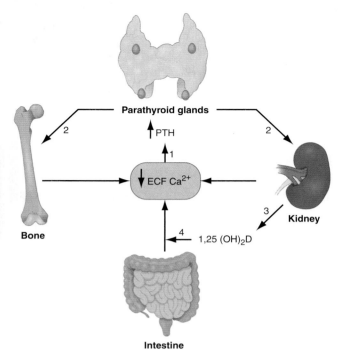

FIGURE 7-1

Feedback mechanisms maintaining extracellular calcium concentrations within a narrow, physiologic range [8.9–10.1 mg/dL (2.2–2.5 mM)]. A decrease in extracellular (ECF) calcium (Ca^{2+}) triggers an increase in parathyroid hormone (PTH) secretion (1) via activation of the calcium sensor receptor on parathyroid cells. PTH, in turn, results in increased tubular reabsorption of calcium by the kidney (2) and resorption of calcium from bone (2) and also stimulates renal 1,25(OH)$_2$D production (3) 1,25(OH)$_2$D, in turn, acts principally on the intestine to increase calcium absorption (4) Collectively, these homeostatic mechanisms serve to restore serum calcium levels to normal.

CLINICAL MANIFESTATIONS

Mild hypercalcemia (up to 11–11.5 mg/dL) is usually asymptomatic and recognized only on routine calcium measurements. Some patients may complain of vague neuropsychiatric symptoms, including trouble concentrating, personality changes, or depression. Other presenting symptoms may include peptic ulcer disease or nephrolithiasis, and fracture risk may be increased. More severe hypercalcemia (>12–13 mg/dL), particularly if it develops acutely, may result in lethargy, stupor, or coma, as well as gastrointestinal symptoms (nausea, anorexia, constipation, or pancreatitis). Hypercalcemia decreases renal concentrating ability, which may cause polyuria and polydipsia. With long-standing hyperparathyroidism, patients may present with bone pain or pathologic fractures. Finally, hypercalcemia can result in significant electrocardiographic changes, including bradycardia, AV block, and short QT interval; changes in serum calcium can be monitored by following the QT interval.

TABLE 7-1

CAUSES OF HYPERCALCEMIA
Excessive PTH production
Primary hyperparathyroidism (adenoma, hyperplasia, rarely carcinoma)
Tertiary hyperparathyroidism (long-term stimulation of PTH secretion in renal insufficiency)
Ectopic PTH secretion (very rare)
Inactivating mutations in the CaSR (FHH)
Alterations in CaSR function (lithium therapy)
Hypercalcemia of malignancy
Overproduction of PTHrP (many solid tumors)
Lytic skeletal metastases (breast, myeloma)
Excessive 1,25(OH)$_2$D production
Granulomatous diseases (sarcoidosis, tuberculosis, silicosis)
Lymphomas
Vitamin D intoxication
Primary increase in bone resorption
Hyperthyroidism
Immobilization
Excessive calcium intake
Milk-alkali syndrome
Total parenteral nutrition
Other causes
Endocrine disorders (adrenal insufficiency, pheochromocytoma, VIPoma)
Medications (thiazides, vitamin A, antiestrogens)

Note: CaSR, calcium sensor receptor; FHH, familial hypocalciuric hypercalcemia; PTH, parathyroid hormone; PTHrP, PTH-related peptide.

DIAGNOSTIC APPROACH

The first step in the diagnostic evaluation of hyper- or hypocalcemia is to ensure that the alteration in serum calcium levels is not due to abnormal albumin concentrations. About 50% of total calcium is ionized, and the rest is bound principally to albumin. Although direct measurements of ionized calcium are possible, they are easily influenced by collection methods and other artifacts; thus, it is generally preferable to measure total calcium and albumin to "correct" the serum calcium. When serum albumin concentrations are reduced, a corrected calcium concentration is calculated by adding 0.2 mM (0.8 mg/dL) to the total calcium level for every decrement in serum albumin of 1.0 g/dL below the reference value of 4.1 g/dL for albumin, and conversely for elevations in serum albumin.

A detailed history may provide important clues regarding the etiology of the hypercalcemia (Table 7-1). Chronic hypercalcemia is most commonly caused by primary hyperparathyroidism, as opposed to the second most common etiology of hypercalcemia, an underlying malignancy. The history should include medication use, previous neck surgery, and systemic symptoms suggestive of sarcoidosis or lymphoma.

Once true hypercalcemia is established, the second most important laboratory test in the diagnostic evaluation is a PTH level using a two-site assay for the intact hormone. Increases in PTH are often accompanied by hypophosphatemia. In addition, serum creatinine should be measured to assess renal function; hypercalcemia may impair renal function, and renal clearance of PTH may be altered depending on the fragments detected by the assay. If the PTH level is increased (or "inappropriately normal") in the setting of an elevated calcium and low phosphorus, the diagnosis is almost always primary hyperparathyroidism. Since individuals with FHH may also present with mildly elevated PTH levels and hypercalcemia, this diagnosis should be considered and excluded because parathyroid surgery is ineffective in this condition. A calcium/creatinine clearance ratio (calculated as urine calcium/serum calcium divided by urine creatinine/serum creatinine) of <0.01 is suggestive of FHH, particularly when there is a family history of mild, asymptomatic hypercalcemia. Ectopic PTH secretion is extremely rare.

A suppressed PTH level in the face of hypercalcemia is consistent with non-parathyroid-mediated hypercalcemia, most often due to underlying malignancy. Although a tumor that causes hypercalcemia is generally overt, a PTHrP level may be needed to establish the diagnosis of hypercalcemia of malignancy. Serum $1,25(OH)_2D$ levels are increased in granulomatous disorders, and clinical evaluation in combination with laboratory testing will generally provide a diagnosis for the various disorders listed in Table 7-1.

℞ Treatment:
HYPERCALCEMIA

Mild, asymptomatic hypercalcemia does not require immediate therapy, and management should be dictated by the underlying diagnosis. By contrast, significant, symptomatic hypercalcemia usually requires therapeutic intervention independent of the etiology of hypercalcemia. Initial therapy of significant hypercalcemia begins with volume expansion since hypercalcemia invariably leads to dehydration; 4–6 L of intravenous saline may be required over the first 24 h, keeping in mind that underlying comorbidities (e.g., congestive heart failure) may require the use of loop diuretics to enhance sodium and calcium excretion. However, loop diuretics should not be initiated until the volume status has been restored to normal. If there is increased calcium mobilization from bone (as in malignancy or severe hyperparathyroidism), drugs that inhibit bone resorption should be considered. Zoledronic acid (e.g., 4 mg intravenously over ~30 min), pamidronate (e.g., 60–90 mg intravenously over 2–4 h), and etidronate

(e.g., 7.5 mg/kg per day for 3–7 consecutive days) are approved by the U.S. Food and Drug Administration for the treatment of hypercalcemia of malignancy in adults. Onset of action is within 1–3 days, with normalization of serum calcium levels occurring in 60–90% of patients. Bisphosphonate infusions may need to be repeated if hypercalcemia relapses. Because of their effectiveness, bisphosphonates have replaced calcitonin or plicamycin, which are rarely used in current practice for the management of hypercalcemia. In rare instances, dialysis may be necessary. Finally, while intravenous phosphate chelates calcium and decreases serum calcium levels, this therapy can be toxic because calcium-phosphate complexes may deposit in tissues and cause extensive organ damage.

In patients with $1,25(OH)_2D$-mediated hypercalcemia, glucocorticoids are the preferred therapy, as they decrease $1,25(OH)_2D$ production. Intravenous hydrocortisone (100–300 mg daily) or oral prednisone (40–60 mg daily) for 3–7 days are used most often. Other drugs, such as ketoconazole, chloroquine, and hydroxychloroquine, may also decrease $1,25(OH)_2D$ production and are used occasionally.

HYPOCALCEMIA
ETIOLOGY

The causes of hypocalcemia can be differentiated according to whether serum PTH levels are low (hypoparathyroidism) or high (secondary hyperparathyroidism). Although there are many potential causes of hypocalcemia, impaired PTH or vitamin D production are the most common etiologies (Table 7-2). Because PTH is the main defense against hypocalcemia, disorders associated with deficient PTH production or secretion may be associated with profound, life-threatening hypocalcemia. In adults, hypoparathyroidism most commonly results from inadvertent damage to all four glands during thyroid or parathyroid gland surgery. Hypoparathyroidism is a cardinal feature of autoimmune endocrinopathies; rarely, it may be associated with infiltrative diseases such as sarcoidosis. Impaired PTH secretion may be secondary to magnesium deficiency or to activating mutations in the CaSR, which suppress PTH, leading to effects that are opposite to those that occur in FHH.

Vitamin D deficiency, impaired $1,25(OH)_2D$ production (primarily secondary to renal insufficiency), or, rarely, vitamin D resistance also cause hypocalcemia. However, the degree of hypocalcemia in these disorders is generally not as severe as that seen with hypoparathyroidism because the parathyroids are capable of mounting a compensatory increase in PTH secretion.

TABLE 7-2

CAUSES OF HYPOCALCEMIA

Low Parathyroid Hormone Levels (Hypoparathyroidism)

Parathyroid agenesis
  Isolated
  DiGeorge syndrome
Parathyroid destruction
  Surgical
  Radiation
  Infiltration by metastases or systemic diseases
  Autoimmune
Reduced parathyroid function
  Hypomagnesemia
  Activating CaSR mutations

High Parathyroid Hormone Levels (Secondary Hyperparathyroidism)

Vitamin D deficiency or impaired $1,25(OH)_2D$
  production/action
    Nutritional vitamin D deficiency (poor intake or absorption)
    Renal insufficiency with impaired $1,25(OH)_2D$ production
    Vitamin D resistance, including receptor defects
Parathyroid hormone resistance syndromes
  PTH receptor mutations
  Pseudohypoparathyroidism (G protein mutations)
Drugs
  Calcium chelators
  Inhibitors of bone resorption (bisphosphonates, plicamycin)
  Altered vitamin D metabolism (phenytoin, ketoconazole)
Miscellaneous causes
  Acute pancreatitis
  Acute rhabdomyolysis
  Hungry bone syndrome after parathyroidectomy
  Osteoblastic metastases with marked stimulation of bone formation (prostate cancer)

Note: CaSR, calcium sensor receptor; PTH, parathyroid hormone.

Hypocalcemia may also occur in conditions associated with severe tissue injury such as burns, rhabdomyolysis, tumor lysis, or pancreatitis. The cause of hypocalcemia in these settings may include a combination of low albumin, hyperphosphatemia, tissue deposition of calcium, and impaired PTH secretion.

CLINICAL MANIFESTATIONS

Patients with hypocalcemia may be asymptomatic if the decreases in serum calcium are relatively mild and chronic, or they may present with life-threatening complications. Moderate to severe hypocalcemia is associated with paresthesias, usually of the fingers, toes, and circumoral regions, and is caused by increased neuromuscular irritability. On physical examination, a Chvostek's sign

(twitching of the circumoral muscles in response to gentle tapping of the facial nerve just anterior to the ear) may be elicited, although it is also present in ~10% of normal individuals. Carpal spasm may be induced by inflation of a blood pressure cuff to 20 mmHg above the patient's systolic blood pressure for 3 min (Trousseau's sign). Severe hypocalcemia can induce seizures, carpopedal spasm, bronchospasm, laryngospasm, and prolongation of the QT interval.

DIAGNOSTIC APPROACH

In addition to measuring serum calcium, it is useful to determine albumin, phosphorus, and magnesium levels. As for the evaluation of hypercalcemia, determining the PTH level is central to the evaluation of hypocalcemia. A suppressed (or "inappropriately low") PTH level in the setting of hypocalcemia establishes absent or reduced PTH secretion (hypoparathyroidism) as the cause of the hypocalcemia. Further history will often elicit the underlying cause (i.e., parathyroid agenesis vs. destruction). By contrast, an elevated PTH level (secondary hyperparathyroidism) should direct attention to the vitamin D axis as the cause of the hypocalcemia. Nutritional vitamin D deficiency is best assessed by obtaining serum 25-hydroxyvitamin D levels, which reflect vitamin D stores. In the setting of renal insufficiency or suspected vitamin D resistance, serum $1,25(OH)_2D$ levels are informative.

℞ Treatment: HYPOCALCEMIA

The approach to treatment depends on the severity of the hypocalcemia, the rapidity with which it develops, and the accompanying complications (e.g., seizures, laryngospasm). Acute, symptomatic hypocalcemia is initially managed with calcium gluconate, 10 mL of 10% wt/vol (90 mg or 2.2 mmol) intravenously, diluted in 50 mL of 5% dextrose or 0.9% sodium chloride, given intravenously over 5 min. Continuing hypocalcemia often requires a constant intravenous infusion (typically 10 ampules of calcium gluconate or 900 mg of calcium in 1 L of 5% dextrose or 0.9% sodium chloride administered over 24 h). Accompanying hypomagnesemia, if present, should be treated with appropriate magnesium supplementation.

Chronic hypocalcemia due to hypoparathyroidism is treated with calcium supplements (1000–1500 mg/d elemental calcium in divided doses) and either vitamin D_2 or D_3 (25,000–100,000 U daily) or calcitriol [$1,25(OH)_2D$, 0.25–2 µg/d]. Other vitamin D metabolites (dihydrotachysterol, alfacalcidiol) are now used less frequently. Vitamin D deficiency, however, is best treated using vitamin D supplementation, with the dose depending on the severity of the deficit and the underlying cause. Thus, nutritional vitamin D deficiency generally responds to relatively low doses of vitamin D (50,000 U, two to three times per week for several months), while vitamin D deficiency due to malabsorption may require much higher doses (100,000 U/d or more). The treatment goal is to bring serum calcium into the low normal range and to avoid hypercalciuria, which may lead to nephrolithiasis.

FURTHER READINGS

BILEZIKIAN JP, SILVERBERG SJ: Asymptomatic primary hyperparathyroidism. N Engl J Med 350:1746, 2004

FARFORD B et al: Nonsurgical management of primary hyperparathyroidism. Mayo Clin Proc 82(3):351, 2007

FINKELSTEIN JS, POTTS JT JR: Medical management of hypercalcemia, in *Endocrinology*, 5th ed, LJ DeGroot, JL Jameson (eds). Philadelphia, Elsevier, 2006

KIFOR O et al: Activating antibodies to the calcium-sensing receptor in two patients with autoimmune hypoparathyroidism. J Clin Endocrinol Metab 89:548, 2004

LEGRAND SB et al: Narrative review: Furosemide for hypercalcemia: An unproven yet common practice. Ann Intern Med 149:259, 2008

MUNDY GR et al: PTH-related peptide (PTHrP) in hypercalcemia. J Am Soc Nephrol 19:672, 2008

STEWART AF: Hypercalcemia associated with cancer. N Engl J Med 352:373, 2005

THAKKER RV: Genetics of endocrine and metabolic disorders: Parathyroid. Rev Endocr Metab Disord 5:37, 2004

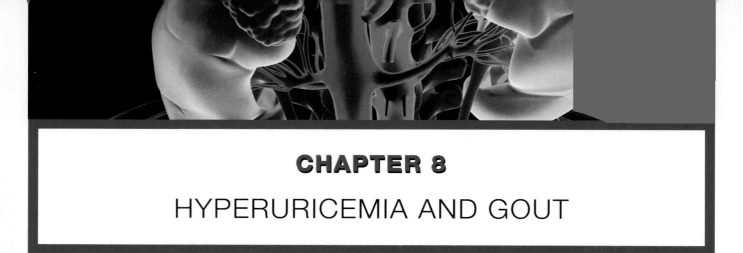

CHAPTER 8

HYPERURICEMIA AND GOUT

Robert L. Wortmann ■ H. Ralph Schumacher ■ Lan X. Chen

Purines (adenine and guanine) and pyrimidines (cytosine, thymine, uracil) serve fundamental roles in the replication of genetic material, gene transcription, protein synthesis, and cellular metabolism. Disorders that involve abnormalities of nucleotide metabolism range from relatively common diseases such as hyperuricemia and gout, in which there is increased production or impaired excretion of a metabolic end product of purine metabolism (uric acid), to rare enzyme deficiencies that affect purine and pyrimidine synthesis or degradation. Understanding these biochemical pathways has led, in some instances, to the development of specific forms of treatment, such as the use of allopurinol to reduce uric acid production.

URIC ACID METABOLISM

Uric acid is the final breakdown product of purine degradation in humans. It is a weak acid with pK_as of 5.75 and 10.3. Urates, the ionized forms of uric acid, predominate in plasma extracellular fluid and synovial fluid, with ~98% existing as monosodium urate at pH 7.4.

Plasma is saturated with monosodium urate at a concentration of 415 μmol/L (6.8 mg/dL) at 37°C. At higher concentrations, plasma is therefore supersaturated, creating the potential for urate crystal precipitation. However,

plasma urate concentrations can reach 4800 μmol/L (80 mg/dL) without precipitation, perhaps because of the presence of solubilizing substances.

The pH of urine greatly influences the solubility of uric acid. At pH 5.0, urine is saturated with uric acid at concentrations ranging from 360–900 μmol/L (6–15 mg/dL). At pH 7.0, saturation is reached at concentrations between 9480 and 12,000 μmol/L (158 and 200 mg/dL). Ionized forms of uric acid in urine include mono- and disodium, potassium, ammonium, and calcium urates.

Although purine nucleotides are synthesized and degraded in all tissues, urate is produced only in tissues that contain xanthine oxidase, primarily the liver and small intestine. Urate production varies with the purine content of the diet and the rates of purine biosynthesis, degradation, and salvage (Fig. 8-1). Normally, two-thirds to three-fourths of urate is excreted by the kidneys, and most of the remainder is eliminated through the intestines.

The kidneys clear urate from the plasma and maintain physiologic balance by utilizing specific organic anion transporters (OATs) including urate transporter 1 (URAT1) and human uric acid transporter (hUAT) (Fig. 8-2). URAT1 and other OATs carry urate into the tubular cells from the apical side of the lumen. Once inside the cell, urate must pass to the basolateral side of the lumen

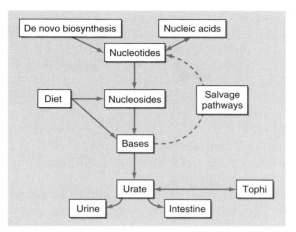

FIGURE 8-1

The total-body urate pool is the net result between urate production and excretion. Urate production is influenced by dietary intake of purines and the rates of de novo biosynthesis of purines from nonpurine precursors, nucleic acid turnover, and salvage by phosphoribosyltransferase activities. The formed urate is normally excreted by urinary and intestinal routes. Hyperuricemia can result from increased production, decreased excretion, or a combination of both mechanisms. When hyperuricemia exists, urate can precipitate and deposit in tissues as tophi.

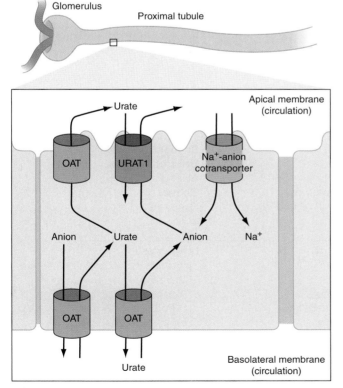

FIGURE 8-2

Schematic for handling of uric acid by the kidney. Organic anion transporters (OATs) including urate transporter 1 (URAT1) carry uric acid into the tubular cell. Uricosuric compounds inhibit URAT1 on the apical side of the tubular cell.

TABLE 8-1

MEDICATIONS WITH URICOSURIC ACTIVITY	
Acetohexamide	Glyceryl guaiacolate
ACTH	Glycopyrrolate
Ascorbic acid	Halofenate
Azauridine	Losartan
Benzbromarone	Meclofenamate
Calcitonin	Phenolsulfonphthalein
Chlorprothixene	Phenylbutazone
Citrate	Probenecid
Dicumarol	Radiographic contrast agents
Diflunisal	Salicylates (>2 g/2d)
Estrogens	Sulfinpyrazone
Fenofibrate	Tetracycline that is outdated
Glucocorticoids	Zoxazolamine

in a process controlled by the voltage-dependent carrier hUAT. Until recently, a four-component model has been used to describe the renal handling of urate/uric acid: (1) glomerular filtration, (2) tubular reabsorption, (3) secretion, and (4) postsecretory reabsorption. Although these processes have been considered sequential, it is now apparent that they are carried out in parallel by these transporters. URAT1 is a novel transporter expressed at the apical brush border of the proximal nephron. Uricosuric compounds (Table 8-1) directly inhibit URAT1 on the apical side of the tubular cell (so-called *cis*-inhibition). In contrast, antiuricosuric compounds (those that promote hyperuricemia), such as nicotinate, pyrazinoate, lactate, and other aromatic organic acids, serve as the exchange anion inside the cell, thereby stimulating anion exchange and urate reabsorption (*trans*-stimulation). The activities of URAT1, other OATs, and sodium anion transporter result in 8–12% of the filtered urate being executed as uric acid.

Most children have serum urate concentrations of 180–240 μmol/L (3.0–4.0 mg/dL). Levels begin to rise in males during puberty but remain low in females until menopause. Mean serum urate values of adult men and premenopausal women are 415 and 360 μmol/L (6.8 and 6.0 mg/dL), respectively. After menopause, values for women increase to approximate those of men. In adulthood, concentrations rise steadily over time and vary with height, body weight, blood pressure, renal function, and alcohol intake.

HYPERURICEMIA

Hyperuricemia can result from increased production or decreased excretion of uric acid or from a combination of the two processes. Sustained hyperuricemia predisposes some individuals to develop clinical manifestations including gouty arthritis, urolithiasis, and renal dysfunction.

Hyperuricemia is defined as a plasma (or serum) urate concentration >408 µmol/L (6.8 mg/dL). The risk of developing gouty arthritis or urolithiasis increases with higher urate levels and escalates in proportion to the degree of elevation. Hyperuricemia is present in between 2.0 and 13.2% of ambulatory adults and is even more frequent in hospitalized individuals.

CAUSES OF HYPERURICEMIA

Hyperuricemia may be classified as primary or secondary depending on whether the cause is innate or is the result of an acquired disorder. However, it is more useful to classify hyperuricemia in relation to the underlying pathophysiology, i.e., whether it results from increased production, decreased excretion, or a combination of the two (Fig. 8-1, Table 8-2).

Increased Urate Production

Diet contributes to the serum urate in proportion to its purine content. Strict restriction of purine intake reduces the mean serum urate level by about 60 µmol/L (1.0 mg/dL) and urinary uric acid excretion by ~1.2 mmol/d (200 mg/d). Foods high in nucleic acid content include liver, "sweetbreads" (i.e., thymus and pancreas), kidney, and anchovy.

Endogenous sources of purine production also influence the serum urate level (Fig. 8-3). De novo purine biosynthesis is an 11-step process that forms inosine monophosphate (IMP). The rates of purine biosynthesis and urate production are determined, for the most part, by amidophosphoribosyltransferase (amidoPRT), which combines phosphoribosylpyrophosphate (PRPP) and glutamine. A secondary regulatory pathway is the salvage of purine bases by hypoxanthine phosphoribosyltransferase (HPRT). HPRT catalyzes the combination of the purine bases hypoxanthine and guanine with PRPP to form the respective ribonucleotides IMP and guanosine monophosphate (GMP).

Serum urate levels are closely coupled to the rates of de novo purine biosynthesis, which is driven in part by the level of PRPP, as evidenced by two X-linked inborn errors of purine metabolism. Both increased PRPP synthetase activity and HPRT deficiency are associated with overproduction of purines, hyperuricemia, and hyperuricaciduria (see below for clinical descriptions).

Accelerated purine nucleotide degradation can also cause hyperuricemia, i.e., with conditions of rapid cell turnover, proliferation, or cell death, as in leukemic blast crises, cytotoxic therapy for malignancy, hemolysis, or rhabdomyolysis. Hyperuricemia can result from excessive degradation of skeletal muscle ATP after strenuous physical exercise or status epilepticus and in glycogen storage diseases types III, V, and VII. The hyperuricemia of myocardial infarction, smoke inhalation, and acute respiratory failure may also be related to accelerated breakdown of adenosine triphosphate (ATP).

TABLE 8-2

CLASSIFICATION OF HYPERURICEMIA BY PATHOPHYSIOLOGY

Urate Overproduction

Primary idiopathic	Myeloproliferative diseases	Rhabdomyolysis
HPRT deficiency	Polycythemia vera	Exercise
PRPP synthetase overactivity	Psoriasis	Alcohol
Hemolytic processes	Paget's disease	Obesity
Lymphoproliferative diseases	Glycogenosis III, V, and VII	Purine-rich diet

Decreased Uric Acid Excretion

Primary idiopathic	Starvation ketosis	Drug ingestion
Renal insufficiency	Berylliosis	Salicylates (>2 g/d)
Polycystic kidney disease	Sarcoidosis	Diuretics
Diabetes insipidus	Lead intoxication	Alcohol
Hypertension	Hyperparathyroidism	Levodopa
Acidosis	Hypothyroidism	Ethambutol
Lactic acidosis	Toxemia of pregnancy	Pyrazinamide
Diabetic ketoacidosis	Bartter's syndrome	Nicotinic acid
	Down syndrome	Cyclosporine

Combined Mechanism

Glucose-6-phosphatase deficiency	Fructose-1-phosphate aldolase deficiency	Alcohol
		Shock

Note: HPRT, hypoxanthine phosphoribosyltransferase; PRPP, phosphoribosylpyrophosphate.

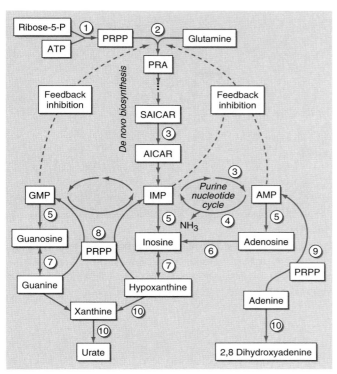

FIGURE 8-3

Abbreviated scheme of purine metabolism. (1) Phosphoribosylpyrophosphate (PRPP) synthetase, (2) amidophosphoribosyltransferase (amidoPRT), (3) adenylosuccinate lyase, (4) (myo-)adenylate (AMP) deaminase, (5) 5′-nucleotidase, (6) adenosine deaminase, (7) purine nucleoside phosphorylase, (8) hypoxanthine phosphoribosyltransferase (HPRT), (9) adenine phosphoribosyltransferase (APRT), and (10) xanthine oxidase. PRA, phosphoribosylamine; SAICAR, succinylaminoimidazole carboxamide ribotide; AICAR, aminoimidazole carboxamide ribotide; GMP, guanylate; IMP, inosine monophosphate.

Decreased Uric Acid Excretion

Over 90% of individuals with sustained hyperuricemia have a defect in the renal handling of uric acid. Gouty individuals excrete ~40% less uric acid than nongouty individuals for any given plasma urate concentration. Uric acid excretion increases in gouty and nongouty individuals when plasma urate levels are raised by purine ingestion or infusion, but in those with gout, plasma urate concentrations must be 60–120 μmol/L (1–2 mg/dL) higher than normal to achieve equivalent uric acid excretion rates.

Altered uric acid excretion could theoretically result from decreased glomerular filtration, decreased tubular secretion, or enhanced tubular reabsorption. Decreased urate filtration does not appear to cause primary hyperuricemia but does contribute to the hyperuricemia of renal insufficiency. Although hyperuricemia is invariably present in chronic renal disease, the correlation between serum creatinine, urea nitrogen, and urate concentration

is poor. Uric acid excretion per unit of glomerular filtration rate increases progressively with chronic renal insufficiency, but tubular secretory capacity tends to be preserved, tubular reabsorptive capacity is reduced, and extrarenal clearance of uric acid increases as renal damage becomes more severe.

Many agents that cause hyperuricemia exert their effects by stimulating reabsorption rather than inhibiting secretion. This appears to occur through a process of "priming" renal urate reabsorption through the sodium-dependent loading of proximal tubular epithelial cells with anions capable of *trans*-stimulating urate reabsorption. A transporter in the brush border of the proximal tubular cells mediates sodium-dependent resorption of components recognized to cause hyperuricemia by renal mechanisms. These include pyrazinoate (from pyrazinamide treatment), nicotinate (from niacin therapy), and the organic acids lactate, β-hydroxybutyrate, and acetoacetate. These monovalent anions are also substrates for URAT1. Thus, increased blood levels of these substances result in their increased glomerular filtration and greater reabsorption by proximal tubular cells. The increased intraepithelial cell concentrations lead to increased reabsorption of urate by promoting URAT1-dependent anion exchange. Low doses of salicylates also promote hyperuricemia by this mechanism. In addition, sodium loading of proximal tubular cells stimulates brush border urate exchange, explaining urate retention provoked by reduced extracellular fluid volume and states of angiotensin II, insulin, and parathyroid hormone excess.

Alcohol promotes hyperuricemia because of increased urate production and decreased uric acid excretion. Excessive alcohol consumption accelerates hepatic breakdown of ATP to increase urate production. Alcohol consumption can also induce hyperlacticacidemia, which blocks uric acid secretion. The higher purine content in some alcoholic beverages such as beer may also be a factor.

EVALUATION

Hyperuricemia does not necessarily represent a disease, nor is it a specific indication for therapy. The decision to treat depends on the cause and the potential consequences of the hyperuricemia in each individual.

Quantification of uric acid excretion can be used to determine whether hyperuricemia is caused by overproduction or decreased excretion. On a purine-free diet, men with normal renal function excrete <3.6 mmol/d (600 mg/d). Thus, the hyperuricemia of individuals who excrete uric acid above this level while on a purine-free diet is due to purine overproduction; for those who excrete lower amounts on the purine-free diet, it is due to decreased excretion. If the assessment is performed while the patient is on a regular diet, the level of 4.2 mmol/d (800 mg/d) can be used as the discriminating value.

GOUT

COMPLICATIONS

Gout is a metabolic disease most often affecting middle-aged to elderly men and postmenopausal women. It is the result of an increased body pool of urate with hyperuricemia. It is typically characterized by episodic acute and chronic arthritis, due to deposition of monosodium urate (MSU) crystals in joints and connective tissue tophi, and the risk for deposition in kidney interstitium or uric acid nephrolithiasis.

Acute and Chronic Arthritis

Acute arthritis is the most frequent early clinical manifestation of gout. Usually, only one joint is affected initially, but polyarticular acute gout can occur in subsequent episodes. The metatarsophalangeal joint of the first toe is often involved, but tarsal joints, ankles, and knees are also commonly affected. Especially in elderly patients or in advanced disease, finger joints may be involved. Inflamed Heberden's or Bouchard's nodes may be a first manifestation of gouty arthritis. The first episode of acute gouty arthritis frequently begins at night with dramatic joint pain and swelling. Joints rapidly become warm, red, and tender, with a clinical appearance that often mimics cellulitis. Early attacks tend to subside spontaneously within 3–10 days, and most patients have intervals of varying length with no residual symptoms until the next episode. Several events may precipitate acute gouty arthritis: dietary excess, trauma, surgery, excessive ethanol ingestion, hypouricemic therapy, and serious medical illnesses such as myocardial infarction and stroke.

After many acute mono- or oligoarticular attacks, a proportion of gouty patients may present with a chronic nonsymmetric synovitis, causing potential confusion with rheumatoid arthritis. Less commonly, chronic gouty arthritis will be the only manifestation and, more rarely, the disease will manifest only as periarticular tophaceous deposits in the absence of synovitis. Women represent only 5–20% of all patients with gout. Premenopausal gout is rare; it is seen mostly in individuals with a strong family history of gout. Kindreds of precocious gout in young females caused by decreased renal urate clearance and renal insufficiency have been described. Most women with gouty arthritis are postmenopausal and elderly, have osteoarthritis and arterial hypertension causing mild renal insufficiency, and are usually receiving diuretics.

Laboratory Diagnosis

Even if the clinical appearance strongly suggests gout, the diagnosis should be confirmed by needle aspiration

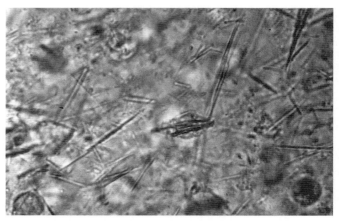

FIGURE 8-4

Extracellular and intracellular monosodium urate crystals, as seen in a fresh preparation of synovial fluid, illustrate needle- and rod-shaped strongly negative birefringent crystals (compensated polarized light microscopy; 400×).

of acutely or chronically involved joints or tophaceous deposits. Acute septic arthritis, several of the other crystalline-associated arthropathies, palindromic rheumatism, and psoriatic arthritis may present with similar clinical features. During acute gouty attacks, strongly birefringent needle-shaped MSU crystals with negative elongation are typically seen both intracellularly and extracellularly (Fig. 8-4). Synovial fluid cell counts are elevated from 2000 to 60,000/μL. Effusions appear cloudy due to the increased numbers of leukocytes. Large amounts of crystals occasionally produce a thick pasty or chalky joint fluid. Bacterial infection can coexist with urate crystals in synovial fluid; if there is any suspicion of septic arthritis, joint fluid must also be cultured.

MSU crystals can also often be demonstrated in the first metatarsophalangeal joint and in knees not acutely involved with gout. Arthrocentesis of these joints is a useful technique to establish the diagnosis of gout between attacks.

Serum uric acid levels can be normal or low at the time of the acute attack, as inflammatory cytokines can be uricosuric and effective initiation of hypouricemic therapy can precipitate attacks. This limits the value of serum uric acid determinations for the diagnosis of gout. Nevertheless, serum urate levels are almost always elevated at some time and are important to use to follow the course of hypouricemic therapy. A 24-h urine collection for uric acid can, in some cases, be useful in assessing the risk of stones, in elucidating overproduction or underexcretion of uric acid, and in deciding if it might be appropriate to use a uricosuric therapy. Excretion of >800 mg of uric acid per 24 h on a regular diet suggests that causes of overproduction of purine should be considered. Urinalysis, serum creatinine, hemoglobin, white blood cell (WBC) count, liver function tests, and serum lipids should be obtained because of possible pathologic sequelae of gout and other associated diseases requiring treatment, and as baselines because of possible adverse effects of gout treatment.

Radiographic Features

Early in the disease, radiographic studies may only confirm clinically evident swelling. Cystic changes, well-defined erosions with sclerotic margins (often with overhanging bony edges), and soft tissue masses are characteristic radiographic features of advanced chronic tophaceous gout.

Rx Treatment: GOUT

ACUTE GOUTY ARTHRITIS The mainstay of treatment during an acute attack is the administration of anti-inflammatory drugs such as nonsteroidal anti-inflammatory drugs (NSAIDs), colchicine, or glucocorticoids. NSAIDs are most often used in individuals without complicating comorbid conditions. Both colchicine and NSAIDs may be poorly tolerated and dangerous in the elderly and in the presence of renal insufficiency and gastrointestinal disorders. In attacks involving one or two joints, intraarticular glucocorticoid injections may be preferable and effective. Ice pack applications and rest of the involved joints can be helpful. Colchicine given orally is a traditional and effective treatment, if used early in the attack. One to two 0.6-mg tablets can be given every 6–8 h over several days with subsequent tapering. This is generally better tolerated than the formerly advised hourly regimen. The drug must be stopped promptly at the first sign of loose stools, and symptomatic treatment must be given for the diarrhea. Intravenous colchicine is occasionally used, e.g., as pre- or postoperative prophylaxis in 1- to 2-mg doses when patients cannot take medications orally. Life-threatening colchicine toxicity and sudden death have been described with the administration of >4 mg/d IV. The IV colchicine should be given slowly through an established venous line over 10 min in a soluset. The total dose should never exceed 4 mg.

NSAIDs given in full anti-inflammatory doses are effective in ~90% of patients, and the resolution of signs and symptoms usually occurs in 5–8 days. The most effective drugs are any of those with a short half-life and include indomethacin, 25–50 mg tid; ibuprofen, 800 mg tid; or diclofenac, 50 mg tid. Oral glucocorticoids such as prednisone, 30–50 mg/d as the initial dose and gradually tapered with the resolution of the attack, can be effective in polyarticular gout. For single or few involved joints intraarticular triamcinolone acetonide, 20–40 mg, or methylprednisolone, 25–50 mg, have been effective

and well tolerated. Adrenocorticotropic hormone (ACTH) as an intramuscular injection of 40–80 IU in a single dose or every 12 h for 1–2 days can be effective in patients with acute polyarticular refractory gout or in those with a contraindication for using colchicine or NSAIDs.

HYPOURICEMIC THERAPY Ultimate control of gout requires correction of the basic underlying defect, the hyperuricemia. Attempts to normalize serum uric acid to <300–360 μmol/L (5.0–6.0 mg/dL) to prevent recurrent gouty attacks and eliminate tophaceous deposits entail a commitment to long-term hypouricemic regimens and medications that generally are required for life. Hypouricemic therapy should be considered when, as in most patients, the hyperuricemia cannot be corrected by simple means (control of body weight, low-purine diet, increase in liquid intake, limitation of ethanol use, and avoidance of diuretics). The decision to initiate hypouricemic therapy is usually made taking into consideration the number of acute attacks (urate lowering may be cost effective after two attacks), serum uric acid levels [progression is more rapid in patients with serum uric acid >535 μmol/L (>9.0 mg/dL)], patient's willingness to commit to lifelong therapy, or presence of uric acid stones. Urate-lowering therapy should be initiated in any patient who already has tophi or chronic gouty arthritis. Uricosuric agents, such as probenecid, can be used in patients with good renal function who underexcrete uric acid, with <600 mg in a 24-h urine sample. Urine volume must be maintained by ingestion of 1500 mL of water every day. Probenecid can be started at a dosage of 250 mg twice daily and increased gradually as needed up to 3 g in order to maintain a serum uric acid level <300 μmol/L (5 mg/dL). Probenecid is generally not effective in patients with serum creatinine levels of >177 μmol/L (2.0 mg/dL). These patients may require allopurinol or benzbromarone (not available in the United States). The latter is another uricosuric drug that is more effective in patients with renal failure. Recent reports have identified that losartan, fenofibrate, and amlodipine have some mild uricosuric effects.

The xanthine oxidase inhibitor allopurinol is by far the most commonly used hypouricemic agent and is the best drug to lower serum urate in overproducers, urate stone formers, and patients with renal disease. It can be given in a single morning dose, 100–300 mg initially and increasing up to 800 mg if needed. In patients with chronic renal disease, the initial allopurinol dosage should be lower and adjusted depending on the serum creatinine concentration; for example, with a creatinine clearance of 10 mL/min, one would generally use 100 mg every other day. Doses can gradually be increased to reach the target urate level; however, more studies are needed to provide exact guidance. Patients with frequent, acute attacks may also require lower initial doses to prevent exacerbations. Toxicity of allopurinol has been recognized increasingly in patients with renal failure who use thiazide diuretics and in those patients allergic to penicillin and ampicillin. The most serious side effects include skin rash with progression to life-threatening toxic epidermal necrolysis, systemic vasculitis, bone marrow suppression, granulomatous hepatitis, and renal failure. Patients with mild cutaneous reactions to allopurinol can reconsider the use of a uricosuric agent or undergo an attempt at desensitization to allopurinol. They can also pay increased attention to diet and should be aware of new alternative agents under investigation. Urate-lowering drugs are generally not initiated during acute attacks but after the patient is stable and low-dose colchicine has been initiated to decrease the risk of flares that often occur with urate lowering. Colchicine prophylaxis in doses of 0.6 mg one to two times daily is usually continued, along with the hypouricemic therapy, until the patient is normouricemic and without gouty attacks for 6 months or as long as tophi are present. New urate-lowering drugs undergoing investigation include a PEGylated uricase and a new specific xanthine oxidase inhibitor, febuxostat.

The most recognized complication of hyperuricemia is *gouty arthritis*. In the general population the prevalence of hyperuricemia ranges between 2.0 and 13.2%, and the prevalence of gout is between 1.3 and 3.7%. The higher the serum urate level, the more likely an individual is to develop gout. In one study, the incidence of gout was 4.9% for individuals with serum urate concentrations >540 μmol/L (9.0 mg/dL) compared with 0.5% for those with values between 415 and 535 μmol/L (7.0 and 8.9 mg/dL). The complications of gout correlate with both the duration and severity of hyperuricemia.

Hyperuricemia also causes several renal problems: (1) nephrolithiasis; (2) urate nephropathy, a rare cause of renal insufficiency attributed to MSU crystal deposition in the renal interstitium; and (3) uric acid nephropathy, a reversible cause of acute renal failure resulting from deposition of large amounts of uric acid crystals in the renal collecting ducts, pelvis, and ureters.

Nephrolithiasis

Uric acid nephrolithiasis occurs most commonly, but not exclusively, in individuals with gout. In gout, the prevalence of nephrolithiasis correlates with the serum and urinary uric acid levels, reaching ~50% with serum urate levels of 770 μmol/L (13 mg/dL) or urinary uric acid excretion >6.5 mmol/d (1100 mg/d).

Uric acid stones can develop in individuals with no evidence of arthritis, only 20% of whom are hyperuricemic. Uric acid can also play a role in other types of kidney stones. Some nongouty individuals with calcium oxalate or calcium phosphate stones have hyperuricemia or hyperuricaciduria. Uric acid may act as a nidus on which calcium oxalate can precipitate or lower the formation product for calcium oxalate crystallization.

Urate Nephropathy

Urate nephropathy, sometimes referred to as *urate nephrosis*, is a late manifestation of severe gout and is characterized histologically by deposits of monosodium urate crystals surrounded by a giant cell inflammatory reaction in the medullary interstitium and pyramids. The disorder is now rare and cannot be diagnosed in the absence of gouty arthritis. The lesions may be clinically silent or cause proteinuria, hypertension, and renal insufficiency.

Uric Acid Nephropathy

This reversible cause of acute renal failure is due to precipitation of uric acid in renal tubules and collecting ducts that causes obstruction to urine flow. Uric acid nephropathy develops following sudden urate overproduction and marked hyperuricaciduria. Factors that favor uric acid crystal formation include dehydration and acidosis. This form of acute renal failure occurs most often during an aggressive "blastic" phase of leukemia or lymphoma prior to or coincident with cytolytic therapy, but has also been observed in individuals with other neoplasms, following epileptic seizures, and after vigorous exercise with heat stress. Autopsy studies have demonstrated intraluminal precipitates of uric acid, dilated proximal tubules, and normal glomeruli. The initial pathogenic events are believed to include obstruction of collecting ducts with uric acid and obstruction of distal renal vasculature.

If recognized, uric acid nephropathy is potentially reversible. Appropriate therapy has reduced the mortality from about 50% to practically nil. Serum levels cannot be relied on for diagnosis because this condition has developed in the presence of urate concentrations varying from 720 to 4800 μmol/L (12 to 80 mg/dL). The distinctive feature is the urinary uric acid concentration. In most forms of acute renal failure with decreased urine output, urinary uric acid content is either normal or reduced, and the ratio of uric acid to creatinine is <1. In acute uric acid nephropathy the ratio of uric acid to creatinine in a random urine sample or 24-h specimen is >1, and a value that high is essentially diagnostic.

HYPERURICEMIA AND METABOLIC SYNDROME

Metabolic syndrome is characterized by abdominal obesity with visceral adiposity, impaired glucose tolerance due to insulin resistance with hyperinsulinemia, hypertriglyceridemia, increased low-density lipoprotein cholesterol, decreased high-density lipoprotein cholesterol, and hyperuricemia. Hyperinsulinemia reduces the renal excretion of uric acid and sodium. Not surprisingly, hyperuricemia resulting from euglycemic hyperinsulinemia may precede the onset of Type 2 diabetes, hypertension, coronary artery disease, and gout in individuals with metabolic syndrome.

℞ Treatment:
   HYPERURICEMIA

ASYMPTOMATIC HYPERURICEMIA Hyperuricemia is present in ~5% of the population and in up to 25% of hospitalized individuals. The vast majority are at no clinical risk. In the past, the association of hyperuricemia with cardiovascular disease and renal failure led to the use of urate-lowering agents for patients with asymptomatic hyperuricemia. This practice is no longer recommended except for individuals receiving cytolytic therapy for neoplastic disease, in which treatment is given in an effort to prevent uric acid nephropathy. Because hyperuricemia can be a component of the metabolic syndrome, its presence is an indication to screen for and aggressively treat any accompanying obesity, hyperlipidemia, diabetes mellitus, or hypertension.

Hyperuricemic individuals are at risk to develop gouty arthritis, especially those with higher serum urate levels. However, most hyperuricemic persons never develop gout and prophylactic treatment is not indicated. Furthermore, neither structural kidney damage nor tophi are identifiable before the first attack. Reduced renal function cannot be attributed to asymptomatic hyperuricemia, and treatment of asymptomatic hyperuricemia does not alter the progression of renal dysfunction in patients with renal disease. Increased risk of stone formation in those with asymptomatic hyperuricemia is not established.

Thus, because treatment with specific antihyperuricemic agents entails inconvenience, cost, and potential toxicity, routine treatment of asymptomatic hyperuricemia cannot be justified other than for prevention of acute uric acid nephropathy. In addition, routine screening for asymptomatic hyperuricemia is not recommended. If hyperuricemia is diagnosed, however, the cause should be determined. Causal factors should be corrected if the condition is secondary, and associated problems such as hypertension, hypercholesterolemia, diabetes mellitus, and obesity should be treated.

SYMPTOMATIC HYPERURICEMIA
Nephrolithiasis Antihyperuricemic therapy is recommended for the individual who has both gouty arthritis and either uric acid– or calcium-containing stones, both of which may occur in association with hyperuricaciduria. Regardless of the nature of the calculi, fluid

ingestion should be sufficient to produce a daily urine volume >2 L. Alkalinization of the urine with sodium bicarbonate or acetazolamide may be justified to increase the solubility of uric acid. Specific treatment of uric acid calculi requires reducing the urine uric acid concentration with a xanthine oxidase inhibitor, such as allopurinol or febuxostat. These agents decrease the serum urate concentration and the urinary excretion of uric acid in the first 24 h, with a maximum reduction occurring within 2 weeks. The average effective dose of allopurinol is 300–400 mg/d. Allopurinol can be given once a day because of the long half-life (18 h) of its active metabolite oxypurinol. The drug is effective in patients with renal insufficiency, but the dose should be reduced. Allopurinol is also useful in reducing the recurrence of calcium oxalate stones in gouty patients and in nongouty individuals with hyperuricemia or hyperuricaciduria. Febuxostat (80–240 mg/d) is also taken once daily, and doses do not need to be adjusted in the presence of mild to moderate renal dysfunction. Potassium citrate (30–80 mmol/d orally in divided doses) is an alternative therapy for patients with uric acid stones alone or mixed calcium/uric acid stones. A xanthine oxidase inhibitor is also indicated for the treatment of 2,8-dihydroxyadenine kidney stones.

Uric Acid Nephropathy Uric acid nephropathy is often preventable, and immediate, appropriate therapy has greatly reduced the mortality rate. Vigorous IV hydration and diuresis with furosemide dilute the uric acid in the tubules and promote urine flow to ≥100 mL/h. The administration of acetazolamide, 240–500 mg every 6–8 h, and sodium bicarbonate, 89 mmol/L, IV enhances urine alkalinity and thereby solubilizes more uric acid. It is important to ensure that the urine pH remains >7.0 and to watch for circulatory overload. In addition, antihyperuricemic therapy in the form of allopurinol in a single dose of 8 mg/kg is administered to reduce the amount of urate that reaches the kidney. If renal insufficiency persists, subsequent daily doses should be reduced to 100–200 mg because oxypurinol, the active metabolite of allopurinol, accumulates in renal failure. Despite these measures, hemodialysis may be required. Urate oxidase (Rasburicase) can also be administered IV to prevent or to treat tumor lysis syndrome.

HYPOURICEMIA

Hypouricemia, defined as a serum urate concentration <120 μmol/L (2.0 mg/dL) can result from decreased production of urate, increased excretion of uric acid, or a combination of both mechanisms. It occurs in <0.2% of the general population and <0.8% of hospitalized individuals. Hypouricemia causes no symptoms or pathology and therefore requires no therapy.

Most hypouricemia results from increased renal uric acid excretion. The finding of normal amounts of uric acid in a 24-h urine collection in an individual with hypouricemia is evidence for a renal cause. Medications with uricosuric properties (Table 8-1) include aspirin (at doses >2.0 g/d), losartan, fenofibrate, x-ray contrast materials, and glycerylguaiacholate. Total parenteral hyperalimentation can also cause hypouricemia, possibly a result of the high glycine content of the infusion formula. Other causes of increased urate clearance include conditions such as neoplastic disease, hepatic cirrhosis, diabetes mellitus, and inappropriate secretion of vasopressin; defects in renal tubular transport such as primary Fanconi syndrome and Fanconi syndromes caused by Wilson's disease, cystinosis, multiple myeloma, and heavy metal toxicity; and isolated congenital defects in the bidirectional transport of uric acid. Hypouricemia can be familial. Some of these cases result from a loss-of-function mutation in *SLC22A12*, the gene that encodes for URAT1.

SELECTED INBORN ERRORS OF PURINE METABOLISM

(See also Table 8-3, Fig. 8-3.)

HPRT DEFICIENCY

The HPRT gene is located on the X chromosome. Affected males are hemizygous for the mutant gene; carrier females are asymptomatic. A complete deficiency of HPRT, the Lesch-Nyhan syndrome, is characterized by hyperuricemia, self-mutilative behavior, choreoathetosis, spasticity, and mental retardation. A partial deficiency of HPRT, the Kelley-Seegmiller syndrome, is associated with hyperuricemia but no central nervous system manifestations. In both disorders, the hyperuricemia results from urate overproduction and can cause uric acid crystalluria, nephrolithiasis, obstructive uropathy, and gouty arthritis. Early diagnosis and appropriate therapy with allopurinol can prevent or eliminate all the problems attributable to hyperuricemia but have no effect on the behavioral or neurologic abnormalities.

INCREASED PRPP SYNTHETASE ACTIVITY

Like the HPRT deficiency states, PRPP synthetase overactivity is X-linked and results in gouty arthritis and uric acid nephrolithiasis. Nerve deafness occurs in some families.

TABLE 8-3

INBORN ERRORS OF PURINE METABOLISM

ENZYME	ACTIVITY	INHERITANCE	CLINICAL FEATURES	LABORATORY FEATURES
Hypoxanthine phosphoribosyltransferase	Complete deficiency	X-linked	Self-mutilation, choreoathetosis, gout, and uric acid lithiasis	Hyperuricemia, hyperuricosuria
	Partial deficiency	X-linked	Gout, and uric acid lithiasis	Hyperuricemia, hyperuricosuria
Phosphoribosylpyrophosphate synthetase	Overactivity	X-linked	Gout, uric acid lithiasis, and deafness	Hyperuricemia, hyperuricosuria
Adenine phosphoribosyltransferase	Deficiency	Autosomal recessive	2,8-Dihydroxyadenine lithiasis	—
Xanthine oxidase	Deficiency	Autosomal recessive	Xanthinuria and xanthine lithiasis	Hypouricemia, hypouricosuria
Adenylosuccinate lyase	Deficiency	Autosomal recessive	Autism and psychomotor retardation	—
Myoadenylate deaminase	Deficiency	Autosomal recessive	Myopathy with exercise intolerance or asymptomatic	—
Adenosine deaminase	Deficiency	Autosomal recessive	Severe combined immunodeficiency disease and chrondro-osseous dysplasia	—
Purine nucleoside phosphorylase	Deficiency	Autosomal recessive	T cell–mediated immunodeficiency	—

ADENINE PHOSPHORIBOSYLTRANSFERASE (APRT) DEFICIENCY

APRT deficiency is inherited as an autosomal recessive trait. Affected individuals develop kidney stones composed of 2,8-dihydroxyadenine. Caucasians with the disorder have a complete deficiency (type I), whereas Japanese subjects have some measurable enzyme activity (type II). Expression of the defect is similar in the two populations, as is the frequency of the heterozygous state (0.4–1.1 per 100). Allopurinol treatment prevents stone formation.

HEREDITARY XANTHINURIA

A deficiency of xanthine oxidase causes all purine in the urine to occur in the form of hypoxanthine and xanthine. About two-thirds of deficient individuals are asymptomatic. The remainder develop kidney stones composed of xanthine.

MYOADENYLATE DEAMINASE DEFICIENCY

Primary (inherited) and secondary (acquired) forms of myoadenylate deaminase deficiency have been described. The primary form is inherited as an autosomal recessive trait. Clinically, some may have relatively mild myopathic symptoms with exercise or other triggers, but most individuals with this defect are asymptomatic. Therefore, another explanation for the myopathy should be sought in symptomatic patients with this deficiency. The acquired deficiency occurs in association with a wide variety of neuromuscular disease, including muscular dystrophies, neuropathies, inflammatory myopathies, and collagen vascular diseases.

ADENYLOSUCCINATE LYASE DEFICIENCY

Deficiency of this enzyme is due to an autosomal recessive trait and causes profound psychomotor retardation, seizures, and other movement disorders. All individuals with this deficiency are mentally retarded, and most are autistic.

FURTHER READINGS

BECKER MA et al: Febuxostat compared to allopurinol in patients with hyperuricemia and gout. N Engl J Med 353:2450, 2005

CHOI HK et al: Pathogenesis of gout. Ann Intern Med 143:499, 2005

COHEN SD et al: Association of incident gout and mortality in dialysis patients. J Am Soc Nephrol 19:2204, 2008

DEHGHAN A et al: Association of three genetic loci with uric acid concentration and risk of gout: A genome-wide association study. Lancet 372:1953, 2008

GAFFO AL et al: Management of hyperuricemia and gout in CKD. Am J Kidney Dis 52:994, 2008

LEE SJ, TERKELTAUB RA: New developments in clinically relevant mechanisms and treatment of gout. Curr Rheum Rep 8:224, 2006

SCHUMACHER HR, Chen LX: Newer therapeutic approaches: Gout. Rheum Dis Clin North Am 32:235, 2006

SCRIVER CR et al (eds): Part 11. Purines and Pyrimidines, in *The Metabolic and Molecular Bases of Inherited Disease,* 8th ed. New York, McGraw-Hill, 2001, pp 2513–2702; OMMBID, 2006

WORTMANN RL, KELLEY WN: Gout and hyperuricemia, in *Kelly's Textbook of Rheumatology,* 7th ed, ED Harris, Jr et al (eds). Philadelphia, Saunders, 2005, pp 1402–1429

———— et al (eds): *Crystal-Induced Arthropathies.* New York, Informa Healthcare, 2006, pp 189–212, 255–276, 369–400

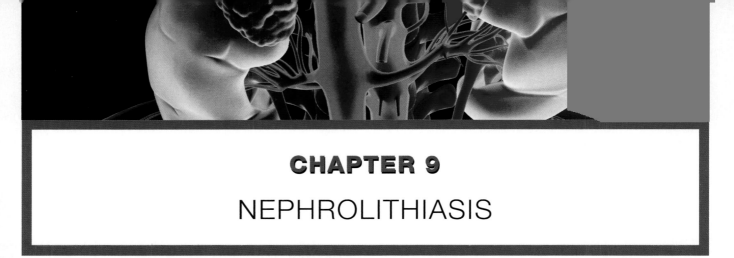

CHAPTER 9

NEPHROLITHIASIS

John R. Asplin ■ Fredric L. Coe ■ Murray J. Favus

Kidney stones are one of the most common urological problems. In the United States, ~13% of men and 7% of women will develop a kidney stone during their lifetime, and the prevalence is increasing throughout the industrialized world.

TYPES OF STONES

Calcium salts, uric acid, cystine, and struvite ($MgNH_4PO_4$) are the basic constituents of most kidney stones in the western hemisphere. Calcium oxalate and calcium phosphate stones make up 75–85% of the total (Table 9–1) and may be admixed in the same stone. Calcium phosphate in stones is usually hydroxyapatite [$Ca_5(PO_4)_3OH$] or, less commonly, brushite ($CaHPO_4H_2O$).

Calcium stones are more common in men; the average age of onset is the third to fourth decade. Approximately 50% of people who form a single calcium stone eventually form another within the next 10 years. The average rate of new stone formation in recurrent stone formers is about one stone every 2 or 3 years. *Uric acid stones* account for 5–10% of kidney stones and are also more common in men. Half of patients with uric acid stones have gout; uric acid lithiasis is usually familial whether or not gout is present. *Cystine stones* are uncommon, comprising ~1% of cases in most series of nephrolithiasis. *Struvite stones* are common and potentially dangerous. These stones occur mainly in women or patients who require chronic bladder catheterization and result from urinary tract infection with urease-producing bacteria, usually *Proteus* species. The stones can grow to a large size and fill the renal pelvis and calyces to produce a "staghorn" appearance.

MANIFESTATIONS OF STONES

As stones grow on the surfaces of the renal papillae or within the collecting system, they need not produce symptoms. Asymptomatic stones may be discovered during the course of radiographic studies undertaken for unrelated reasons. Stones rank, along with benign and malignant neoplasms and renal cysts, among the common causes of isolated hematuria. Stones become symptomatic when they enter the ureter or occlude the ureteropelvic junction, causing pain and obstruction.

Stone Passage

A stone can traverse the ureter without symptoms, but passage usually produces pain and bleeding. The pain begins gradually, usually in the flank, but increases over the next 20–60 min to become so severe that narcotic drugs may be needed for its control. The pain may remain in the flank or spread downward and anteriorly toward the ipsilateral loin, testis, or vulva. A stone in the portion of the ureter within the bladder wall causes frequency, urgency, and dysuria that may be confused with urinary tract infection. The vast majority of ureteral stones <0.5 cm in diameter will pass spontaneously.

TABLE 9-1

MAJOR CAUSES OF RENAL STONES

STONE TYPE AND CAUSES	PERCENT OF ALL STONES[a]	PERCENT OCCURRENCE OF SPECIFIC CAUSES[a]	RATIO OF MALES TO FEMALES	ETIOLOGY	DIAGNOSIS	TREATMENT
Calcium stones	75–85		2:1 to 3:1			
Idiopathic hypercalciuria		50–55	2:1	Hereditary (?)	Normocalcemia, unexplained hypercalciuria[b]	Low-sodium, low-protein diet; thiazide diuretics
Hyperuricosuria		20	4:1	Diet	Urine uric acid >750 mg per 24 h (women), >800 mg per 24 h (men)	Allopurinol or diet
Primary hyperparathyroidism		3–5	3:10	Neoplasia	Unexplained hypercalcemia	Surgery
Distal renal tubular acidosis		Rare	1:1	Hereditary	Hyperchloremic acidosis, minimum urine pH >5.5	Alkali replacement
Dietary hyperoxaluria		10–30	1:1	High oxalate diet or low calcium diet	Urine oxalate >50 mg per 24 h	Low oxalate diet
Enteric hyperoxaluria		~1–2	1:1	Bowel surgery	Urine oxalate >75 mg per 24 h	Cholestyramine or oral calcium loading
Primary hyperoxaluria		Rare	1:1	Hereditary	Urine oxalate and glycolic or l-glyceric acid increased	Fluids and pyridoxine
Hypocitraturia		20–40	1:1 to 2:1	Hereditary (?), diet	Urine citrate <320 mg per 24 h	Alkali supplements
Idiopathic stone disease		20	2:1	Unknown	None of the above present	Oral phosphate, fluids
Uric acid stones	5–10					
Gout		~50	3:1 to 4:1	Hereditary	Clinical diagnosis	Alkali and allopurinol
Idiopathic		~50	1:1	Hereditary (?)	Uric acid stones, no gout	Alkali and allopurinol if daily urine uric acid above 1000 mg
Dehydration		?	1:1	Intestinal, habit	History, intestinal fluid loss	Alkali, fluids, reversal of cause
Lesch-Nyhan syndrome		Rare	Males only	Hereditary	Reduced hypoxanthine-guanine phosphoribosyl-transferase level	Allopurinol
Malignant tumors		Rare	1:1	Neoplasia	Clinical diagnosis	Allopurinol
Cystine stones	1		1:1	Hereditary	Stone type; elevated cystine excretion	Massive fluids, alkali, D-penicillamine if needed
Struvite stones	5–10		1:3	Infection	Stone type	Antimicrobial agents and judicious surgery

[a]Values are percent of patients who form a particular type of stone and who display each specific cause of stones.

[b]Urine calcium above 300 mg/24 h (men), 250 mg/24 h (women), or 4 mg/kd per 24 h either sex. Hyperthyroidism, Cushing's syndrome, sarcoidosis, malignant tumors, immobilization, vitamin D intoxication, rapidly progressive bone disease, and Paget's disease all cause hypercalciuria and must be excluded in diagnosis of idiopathic hypercalciuria.

It has been standard practice to diagnose acute renal colic by intravenous pyelography; however, helical CT scan without radiocontrast enhancement is now the preferred procedure. The advantages of CT include detection of uric acid stones in addition to the traditional radiopaque stones, no exposure to the risk of radiocontrast agents, and possible diagnosis of other causes of abdominal pain in a patient suspected of having renal colic from stones. Ultrasound is not as sensitive as CT in detecting renal or ureteral stones. Standard abdominal x-rays may be used to monitor patients for formation and growth of kidney stones, as they are less expensive and provide less radiation exposure than CT scans. Calcium, cystine, and struvite stones are all radiopaque on standard x-rays, whereas uric acid stones are radiolucent.

Other Syndromes

Staghorn Calculi

Struvite, cystine, and uric acid stones often grow too large to enter the ureter. They gradually fill the renal pelvis and may extend outward through the infundibula to the calyces themselves. Very large staghorn stones can have surprisingly few symptoms and may lead to the eventual loss of kidney function.

Nephrocalcinosis

Calcium stones grow on the papillae. Most break loose and cause colic, but they may remain in place so that multiple papillary calcifications are found by x-ray, a condition termed *nephrocalcinosis*. Papillary nephrocalcinosis is common in hereditary distal renal tubular acidosis (RTA) and in other types of severe hypercalciuria. In medullary sponge kidney disease (Chap. 16), calcification may occur in dilated distal collecting ducts.

Infection

Although urinary tract infection is not a direct consequence of stone disease, it can occur after instrumentation and surgery of the urinary tract, which are frequent in the treatment of stone disease. Stone disease and urinary tract infection can enhance their respective seriousness and interfere with treatment. Obstruction of an infected kidney by a stone may lead to sepsis and extensive damage of renal tissue, since it converts the urinary tract proximal to the obstruction into a closed, or partially closed, space that can become an abscess. Stones may harbor bacteria in the stone matrix, leading to recurrent urinary tract infection. On the other hand, infection due to bacteria that possess the enzyme urease can cause stones composed of struvite.

Activity of Stone Disease

Active disease means that new stones are forming or that preformed stones are growing. Sequential radiographs are needed to document the growth or appearance of new stones and to ensure that passed stones are actually newly formed, not preexistent.

PATHOGENESIS OF STONES

Urinary stones usually arise because of the breakdown of a delicate balance between solubility and precipitation of salts. The kidneys must conserve water, but they must excrete materials that have a low solubility. These two opposing requirements must be balanced during adaptation to diet, climate, and activity. The problem is mitigated to some extent by the fact that urine contains substances that inhibit crystallization. These protective mechanisms are less than perfect. When the urine becomes supersaturated with insoluble materials, because excretion rates are excessive and/or because water conservation is extreme, crystals form and may grow and aggregate to form a stone.

Supersaturation

A solution in equilibrium with crystals of calcium oxalate is said to be saturated with respect to calcium oxalate. If crystals are removed, and if either calcium or oxalate ions are added to the solution, the chemical activities increase, but no new crystals form. Such a solution is *metastably supersaturated*. If calcium oxalate crystals are now added, they will grow in size. Ultimately, as calcium or oxalate is added to the solution, supersaturation reaches a critical value at which a solid phase begins to develop spontaneously. This value is called the *upper limit of metastability*. Kidney stone growth requires a urine that, on average, is supersaturated. Excessive supersaturation is common in stone formation.

Calcium, oxalate, and phosphate form many soluble complexes among themselves and with other substances in urine, such as citrate. As a result, their free ion activities are below their chemical concentrations. Reduction in ligands such as citrate can increase ion activity and, therefore, supersaturation. Urine supersaturation can be increased by dehydration or by overexcretion of calcium, oxalate, phosphate, cystine, or uric acid. Urine pH is also important; phosphate and uric acid are acids that dissociate readily over the physiologic range of urine pH. Alkaline urine contains more dibasic phosphate, favoring deposits of brushite and apatite. Below a urine pH of 5.5, uric acid crystals (pK 5.47) predominate, whereas phosphate crystals are rare. The solubility of calcium oxalate is not influenced by changes in urine pH. Measurements of supersaturation in a 24-h urine sample probably underestimate the risk of precipitation. Transient dehydration, variation of urine pH, and postprandial bursts of overexcretion may cause values considerably above average.

SECTION II

Alterations of Renal Function and Electrolytes

Crystallization

When urine supersaturation exceeds the upper limit of metastability, crystals begin to nucleate. Cell debris and other crystals present in the urinary tract can serve as templates for crystal formation, a process known as *heterogeneous nucleation*. Heterogeneous nucleation lowers the level of supersaturation required for crystal formation. Once formed, crystal nuclei will grow in size if urine is supersaturated with respect to that crystal phase. Multiple crystals can then aggregate to form a kidney stone.

In order for a kidney stone to form, crystals must be retained in the renal pelvis long enough to grow and aggregate to a clinically significant size. The mechanism of crystal retention has been a matter of much debate. Recent studies have shown that common calcium oxalate kidney stones form as overgrowths on apatite plaques in the renal papillae. These plaques, called Randall's plaques, provide an excellent surface for heterogeneous nucleation of calcium oxalate salts. The Randall's plaques begin in the deep medulla in the basement membrane of the thin limb of the loop of Henle and then spread through the interstitium to the basement membrane of the papillary urothelium. If the urothelium becomes damaged, the plaque is exposed to the urine, and calcium oxalate crystallization and stone formation begins.

Inhibitors of Crystal Formation

Urine contains potent inhibitors of nucleation, growth, and aggregation for calcium salts. Inorganic pyrophosphate is a potent inhibitor that appears to affect formation of calcium phosphate more than calcium oxalate crystals. Citrate inhibits crystal growth and nucleation, although most of the stone inhibitory activity of citrate is due to lowering urine supersaturation via complexation of calcium. Other urine components such as glycoproteins inhibit calcium oxalate crystallization.

EVALUATION AND TREATMENT OF PATIENTS WITH NEPHROLITHIASIS

Most patients with nephrolithiasis have remediable metabolic disorders that cause stones and can be detected by chemical analyses of serum and urine. Adults with recurrent kidney stones and children with even a single kidney stone should be evaluated. A practical outpatient evaluation consists of two 24-h urine collections, with a corresponding blood sample; measurements of serum and urine calcium, uric acid, electrolytes, and creatinine, and urine pH, volume, oxalate, and citrate should be made. Since stone risks vary with diet, activity, and environment, at least one urine collection should be made on a weekend when the patient is at home and another on a work day. When possible, the composition of kidney stones should be determined because treatment depends on stone type (Table 9-1). No matter what disorders are

found, every patient should be counseled to avoid dehydration and to drink copious amounts of water. The efficacy of high fluid intake was confirmed in a prospective study of first-time stone formers. Increasing urine volume to 2.5 L per day resulted in a 50% reduction of stone recurrence compared to the control group.

℞ Treatment: NEPHROLITHIASIS

The management of stones already present in the kidneys or urinary tract requires a combined medical and surgical approach. The specific treatment depends on the location of the stone, the extent of obstruction, the nature of the stone, the function of the affected and unaffected kidney, the presence or absence of urinary tract infection, the progress of stone passage, and the risks of operation or anesthesia given the clinical state of the patient. Medical therapy can enhance passage of ureteral stones. Oral α_1-adrenergic blockers relax ureteral muscle and have been shown to reduce time to stone passage and the need for surgical removal of small stones. In general, severe obstruction, infection, intractable pain, and serious bleeding are indications for removal of a stone.

Advances in urologic technology have rendered open surgery for stones a rare event. There are now three alternatives for stone removal. *Extracorporeal lithotripsy* causes the in situ fragmentation of stones in the kidney, renal pelvis, or ureter by exposing them to shock waves. The kidney stone is centered at a focal point of high-intensity shock waves. The waves are transmitted to the patient using water as a conduction medium, either by placing the patient in a water tank or by placing water-filled cushions between the patient and the shock wave generators. After multiple shock waves, most stones are reduced to powder that moves through the ureter into the bladder. *Percutaneous nephrolithotomy* requires the passage of a cystoscope-like instrument into the renal pelvis through a small incision in the flank. Stones are then disrupted by a small ultrasound transducer or holmium laser. The last method is *ureteroscopy* with stone disruption using a holmium laser. Ureteroscopy is generally used for stones in the ureter but some surgeons are now using ureteroscopy for stones in the renal pelvis as well.

Calcium Stones

Idiopathic Hypercalciuria

This condition is the most common metabolic abnormality found in patients with nephrolithiasis (Table 9-1). It is familial and is likely a polygenic trait, although there are some rare monogenic causes of hypercalciuria and kidney stones such as Dent's disease, which is an X-linked disorder characterized by hypercalciuria, nephrocalcinosis, and progressive kidney failure. Idiopathic hypercalciuria is diagnosed by the presence of hypercalciuria without hypercalcemia and the absence of other systemic disorders known to affect mineral metabolism. In the past, the separation of "absorptive" and "renal" forms of hypercalciuria was used to guide treatment. However, these may not be distinct entities but the extremes of a continuum of behavior. Vitamin D overactivity, either through high calcitriol levels or excess vitamin D receptor, is a likely explanation for the hypercalciuria in many of these patients. Hypercalciuria contributes to stone formation by raising urine saturation with respect to calcium oxalate and calcium phosphate.

℞ **Treatment:**
HYPERCALCIURIA

For many years the standard therapy for hypercalciuria was dietary calcium restriction. However, recent studies have shown that low-calcium diets increase the risk of incident stone formation. Low-calcium diets may lead to stone formation by reducing the amount of calcium to bind oxalate in the intestine, thereby increasing urine oxalate levels. However, the mechanism by which a low-calcium diet increases stone risk has not been clearly defined. In addition, hypercalciuric stone formers have reduced bone mineral density and an increased risk of fracture compared to the non-stone-forming population. Low calcium intake likely contributes to the low bone mineral density. A 5-year prospective trial compared the efficacy of a low-calcium diet to a low-protein, low-sodium, normal-calcium diet in preventing stone recurrence in male calcium stone formers. The group on the low-calcium diet had a significantly greater rate of stone relapse. Low-calcium diets are of unknown efficacy in preventing stone formation and carry a long-term risk of bone disease in the stone-forming population. Low-sodium and low-protein diets are a superior option in stone formers. If diet therapy is not sufficient to prevent stones, then thiazide diuretics may be used. Thiazide diuretics lower urine calcium and are effective in preventing the formation of stones. Three 3-year randomized trials have shown a 50% decrease in stone formation in the thiazide-treated groups as compared to the placebo-treated controls. The drug effect requires slight contraction of the extracellular fluid volume, and high dietary NaCl intake reduces its therapeutic effect. Thiazide-induced hypokalemia should be aggressively treated since hypokalemia will reduce urine citrate, an important inhibitor of calcium crystallization.

Hyperuricosuria

About 20% of calcium oxalate stone formers are hyperuricosuric, primarily because of an excessive intake of

purine from meat, fish, and poultry. The mechanism of stone formation is probably due to salting out calcium oxalate by urate. A low-purine diet is desirable but difficult for many patients to achieve. The alternative is allopurinol, which has been shown to be effective in a randomized, controlled trial. A dose of 100 mg bid is usually sufficient.

Primary Hyperparathyroidism

The diagnosis of this condition is established by documenting that hypercalcemia that cannot be otherwise explained is accompanied by inappropriately elevated serum concentrations of parathyroid hormone. Hypercalciuria, usually present, raises the urine supersaturation of calcium phosphate and/or calcium oxalate (Table 9-1). Prompt diagnosis is important because parathyroidectomy should be carried out before renal damage or bone disease occurs.

Distal Renal Tubular Acidosis

(See also Chap. 16.) The defect in this condition seems to reside in the distal nephron, which cannot establish a normal pH gradient between urine and blood, leading to hyperchloremic acidosis. The diagnosis is suggested by a minimum urine pH > 5.5 in the presence of systemic acidosis. If the diagnosis is in doubt because metabolic abnormalities are mild, an ammonium chloride loading test can be performed. Patients with distal RTA will not lower urine pH below 5.5. Hypercalciuria, an alkaline urine, and a low urine citrate level increase urine saturation with respect to calcium phosphate. Calcium phosphate stones form, nephrocalcinosis is common, and osteomalacia or rickets may occur. Renal damage is frequent, and glomerular filtration rate falls gradually.

Treatment with supplemental alkali reduces hypercalciuria and limits the production of new stones. The usual dose of sodium bicarbonate is 0.5–2.0 mmol/kg of body weight per day in four to six divided doses. An alternative is potassium citrate supplementation, given at the same dose per day but needing to be given only two to three times per day. In incomplete distal RTA, systemic acidosis is absent, but urine pH cannot be lowered below 5.5 after an exogenous acid load such as ammonium chloride. Incomplete RTA may develop in some patients who form calcium oxalate stones because of idiopathic hypercalciuria; the importance of RTA in producing stones in this situation is uncertain, and thiazide treatment is a reasonable alternative. Alkali can also be used in incomplete RTA. When treating patients with alkali, it is prudent to monitor changes in urine citrate and pH. If urine pH increases without an increase in citrate, then calcium phosphate supersaturation will increase and stone disease may worsen.

Hyperoxaluria

Oxalate is a metabolic end product in humans. Urine oxalate comes from diet and endogenous metabolic production, with ~40–50% originating from dietary sources. The upper limit of normal for oxalate excretion is generally considered to be 40–50 mg/d. Mild hyperoxaluria (50–80 mg/d) is usually caused by excessive intake of high-oxalate foods such as spinach, nuts, and chocolate. In addition, low-calcium diets may promote hyperoxaluria as there is less calcium available to bind oxalate in the intestine. Enteric hyperoxaluria is a consequence of small-bowel disease resulting in fat malabsorption. Oxalate excretion is often >100 mg/d. Enteric hyperoxaluria may be caused by jejunoileal bypass for obesity, pancreatic insufficiency, or extensive small-intestine involvement from Crohn's disease. With fat malabsorption, calcium in the bowel lumen is bound by fatty acids instead of oxalate, which is left free for absorption in the colon. Delivery of unabsorbed fatty acids and bile salts to the colon may injure the colonic mucosa and enhance oxalate absorption. Primary hyperoxaluria is a rare autosomal recessive disease that causes severe hyperoxaluria. Patients usually present with recurrent calcium oxalate stones during childhood. Primary hyperoxaluria type 1 is due to a deficiency in the peroxisomal enzyme alanine:glyoxylate aminotransferase. Type 2 is due to a deficiency of D-glyceric dehydrogenase. Severe hyperoxaluria from any cause can produce tubulointerstitial nephropathy (Chap. 17) and lead to stone formation.

℞ Treatment:
HYPEROXALURIA

Patients with mild to moderate hyperoxaluria should be treated with a diet low in oxalate and with a normal intake of calcium and magnesium to reduce oxalate absorption. Enteric hyperoxaluria can be treated with a low-fat, low-oxalate diet and calcium supplements, given with meals, to bind oxalate in the gut lumen. The oxalate-binding resin cholestyramine at a dose of 8–16 g/d provides an additional form of therapy. Treatment for primary hyperoxaluria includes a high fluid intake, neutral phosphate, and pyridoxine (25–200 mg/d). Citrate supplementation may also have some benefit. Even with aggressive therapy, irreversible renal failure may occur. Liver transplantation, to correct the enzyme defect, combined with a kidney transplantation has been successfully utilized in patients with primary hyperoxaluria.

▮ Hypocitraturia

Urine citrate prevents calcium stone formation by creating a soluble complex with calcium, effectively reducing free urine calcium. Hypocitraturia is found in 20–40% of stone formers, either as a single disorder or in combination with other metabolic abnormalities. It can be secondary to systemic disorders, such as RTA, chronic diarrheal illness, or hypokalemia, or it may be a primary disorder, in which case it is called *idiopathic hypocitraturia*.

℞ Treatment:
HYPOCITRATURIA

Treatment is with alkali, which increases urine citrate excretion; generally bicarbonate or citrate salts are used. Potassium salts are preferred as sodium loading increases urinary excretion of calcium, reducing the effectiveness of treatment. Two randomized, placebo-controlled trials have demonstrated the effectiveness of citrate supplements in calcium oxalate stone formers.

▮ Idiopathic Calcium Lithiasis

Some patients have no metabolic cause for stones despite a thorough metabolic evaluation (Table 9-1). The best treatment appears to be high fluid intake so that the urine specific gravity remains at ≤1.005 throughout the day and night. Thiazide diuretics, allopurinol, and citrate therapy may help reduce crystallization of calcium salts, but there are no prospective trials in this patient population. Oral phosphate at a dose of 2 g phosphorus daily may lower urine calcium and increase urine pyrophosphate and thereby reduce the rate of recurrence. Orthophosphate causes mild nausea and diarrhea, but tolerance may improve with continued intake.

Uric Acid Stones

In gout, idiopathic uric acid lithiasis, and dehydration, the average urine pH is usually <5.4 and often below 5.0. Metabolic syndrome has also been found to be a cause of acidic urine as insulin resistance leads to a decrease in renal ammoniagenesis. When urine pH is low, the protonated form of uric acid predominates and is soluble in urine only in concentrations of 100 mg/L. Concentrations above this level represent supersaturation that causes crystals and stones to form. Hyperuricosuria, when present, increases supersaturation, but urine of low pH can be supersaturated with undissociated uric acid even though the daily excretion rate is normal. Myeloproliferative syndromes, chemotherapy of malignant tumors, and Lesch–Nyhan syndrome cause such massive production of uric acid and consequent hyperuricosuria that stones and uric acid sludge form even at a normal urine pH. Plugging of the renal collecting tubules by uric acid crystals can cause acute renal failure.

℞ Treatment:
URIC ACID LITHIASIS

The two goals of treatment are to raise urine pH and to lower excessive urine uric acid excretion to <1 g/d. Supplemental alkali, 1–3 mmol/kg of body weight per day, should be given in three or four divided doses, one of which should be given at bedtime. The goal of treatment should be a urine pH between 6.0 and 6.5 in a 24-h urine collection. Increasing urine pH above 6.5 will not provide additional benefit in preventing uric acid crystallization but does increase the risk of calcium phosphate stone formation. The form of the alkali may be important. Potassium citrate may reduce the risk of calcium salts crystallizing when urine pH is increased, whereas sodium citrate or sodium bicarbonate may increase the risk. A low-purine diet should be instituted in uric acid stone formers with hyperuricosuria. Patients who continue to form uric acid stones despite treatment with fluids, alkali, and a low-purine diet should have allopurinol added to their regimen.

Cystinuria and Cystine Stones

In this inherited disorder, proximal tubular and jejunal transport of the dibasic amino acids cysteine (cysteine disulfide), lysine, arginine, and ornithine are defective, and excessive amounts are lost in the urine. Clinical disease is due solely to the insolubility of cystine, which forms stones.

■ Pathogenesis

Cystinuria occurs because of defective transport of dibasic amino acids by the brush borders of renal tubule and intestinal epithelial cells. Disease-causing mutations have been identified in both the heavy and light chain of a heteromeric amino acid transporter found in the proximal tubule of the kidney. Cystinuria is classified into two main types, based on the urinary excretion of cystine in obligate heterozygotes. In type I cystinuria, heterozygotes have normal urine cystine excretion; thus type I has an autosomal recessive pattern of inheritance. A gene located on chromosome 2 and designated *SLC3A1* encodes the heavy chain of the transporter and has been found to be abnormal in type I. In non-type-I cystinuria, heterozygotes have moderately elevated urine cystine excretion, with homozygotes having a much higher urine cystine excretion. Non-type-I is inherited as a dominant trait with incomplete penetrance. Non-type-I is due to mutations in the *SLC7A9* gene on chromosome 19, which encodes the light chain of the heteromeric transporter. In rare cases, mutations of the *SLC7A9* gene can lead to a type I phenotype.

■ Diagnosis

Cystine stones are formed only by patients with cystinuria, but 10% of stones in cystinuric patients do not contain cystine; therefore, every stone former should be screened for the disease. The sediment from a first morning urine specimen in many patients with homozygous cystinuria reveals typical hexagonal, platelike cystine crystals. Cystinuria can also be detected using the urine sodium nitroprusside test. Because the test is sensitive, it is positive in many asymptomatic heterozygotes for cystinuria. A positive nitroprusside test or the finding of cystine crystals in

the urine sediment should be evaluated by measurement of daily cystine excretion. Cystine stones seldom form in adults unless urine excretion is at least 300 mg/d.

℞ Treatment:
CYSTINURIA AND CYSTINE STONES

High fluid intake, even at night, is the cornerstone of therapy. Daily urine volume should exceed 3 L. Raising urine pH with alkali is helpful, provided the urine pH exceeds 7.5. A low-salt diet (100 mmol/d) can reduce cystine excretion up to 40%. Because side effects are frequent, drugs such as penicillamine and tiopronin, which form the mixed soluble disulfide cysteine-drug complexes, should be used only when fluid loading, salt reduction, and alkali therapy are ineffective. Low-methionine diets have not proved to be practical for clinical use, but patients should avoid protein gluttony.

Struvite Stones

These stones are a result of urinary infection with bacteria, usually *Proteus* species, which possess urease, an enzyme that degrades urea to NH_3 and CO_2. The NH_3 hydrolyzes to NH_4^+ and raises urine pH to 8 or 9. The CO_2 hydrates to H_2CO_3 and then dissociates to CO_3^{2-} that precipitates with calcium as $CaCO_3$. The NH_4^+ precipitates PO_4^{3-} and Mg^{2+} to form $MgNH_4PO_4$ (struvite). The result is a stone of calcium carbonate admixed with struvite. Struvite does not form in urine in the absence of infection, because NH_4^+ concentration is low in urine that is alkaline in response to physiologic stimuli. Chronic *Proteus* infection can occur because of impaired urinary drainage, urologic instrumentation or surgery, and especially with chronic antibiotic treatment, which can favor the dominance of *Proteus* in the urinary tract. The presence of struvite crystals in urine, rectangular prisms said to resemble coffin lids, indicates infection with urease-producing organisms.

℞ Treatment:
STRUVITE STONES

Complete removal of the stone with subsequent sterilization of the urinary tract is the treatment of choice for patients who can tolerate the procedures. Percutaneous nephrolithotomy is the preferred surgical approach for most patients. At times, extracorporeal lithotripsy may be used in combination with a percutaneous approach. Open surgery is rarely required. Irrigation of the renal pelvis and calyces with hemiacidrin, a solution that dissolves struvite, can reduce recurrence after surgery. Stone-free rates of 50–90% have been reported after surgical intervention. Antimicrobial treatment is best reserved for dealing with acute infection and for maintenance of a sterile urine after surgery. Urine cultures and culture of stone fragments removed at surgery should guide the choice of antibiotic. For patients who are not candidates for surgical removal of stone, acetohydroxamic acid, an inhibitor of urease, can be used. Unfortunately, acetohydroxamic acid has many side effects, such as headache, tremor, and thrombophlebitis, that limit its use.

FURTHER READINGS

ABATE N et al: The metabolic syndrome and uric acid nephrolithiasis: Novel features of renal manifestation of insulin resistance. Kidney Int 65:386, 2004

COE FL et al: Kidney stone disease. J Clin Invest 115:2598, 2005

CURHAN GC et al: 24-h uric acid excretion and the risk of kidney stones. Kidney Int 73:489, 2008

EVAN AP et al: Randall's plaque of patients with nephrolithiasis begins in basement membranes of thin loops of Henle. J Clin Invest 111:607, 2003

GAMBARO G et al: Genetics of hypercalciuria and calcium nephrolithiasis: From the rare monogenic to the common polygenic forms. Am J Kidney Dis 44:963, 2004

MILLER NL, LINGEMAN JE: Management of kidney stones. Br Med J 334:468, 2007

PREMINGER GM et al: AUA guideline on management of staghorn calculi: Diagnosis and treatment recommendations. J Urol 173: 1991, 2005

RENKEMA KY et al: The calcium-sensing receptor promotes urinary acidification to prevent nephrolithiasis. J Am Soc Nephrol 20: 1705, 2009

SAKHAEE K: Recent advances in the pathophysiology of nephrolithiasis. Kidney Int 75:585, 2009

STAMATELOU K et al: Time trends in reported prevalence of kidney stones in the United States: 1976–1994. Kidney Int 63:1817, 2003

TAYLOR EN et al: Fructose consumption and the risk of kidney stones. Kidney Int 73:207, 2008

WEST B et al: Metabolic syndrome and self-reported history of kidney stones: The National Health and Nutrition Examination Survey (NHANES III) 1988–1994. Am J Kidney Dis 51:741, 2008

Nephrolithiasis

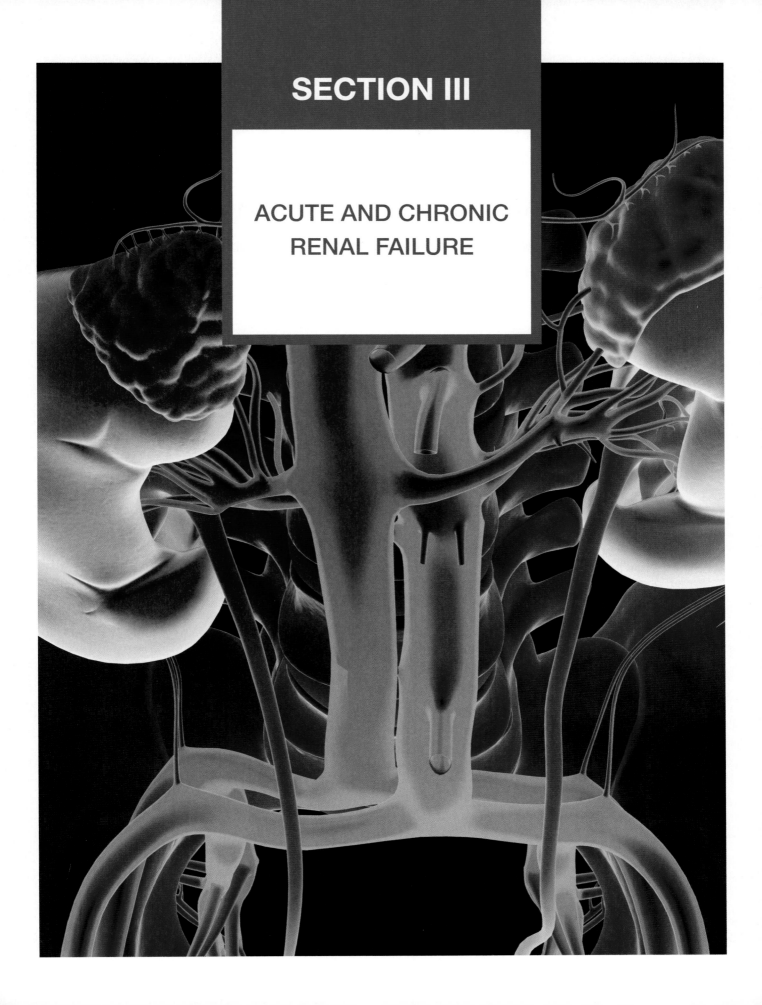

SECTION III

ACUTE AND CHRONIC RENAL FAILURE

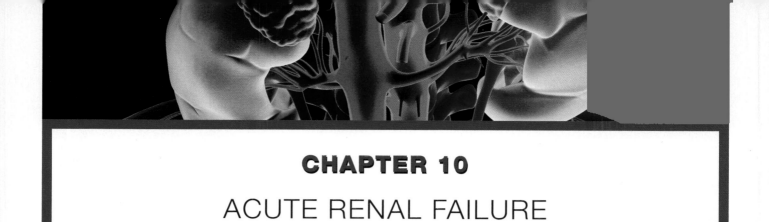

CHAPTER 10

ACUTE RENAL FAILURE

Kathleen D. Liu ■ Glenn M. Chertow

Acute renal failure (ARF) is characterized by a rapid decline in glomerular filtration rate (GFR) over hours to days. Depending on the exact definition used, ARF complicates approximately 5–7% of hospital admissions and up to 30% of admissions to intensive care units. Retention of nitrogenous waste products, oliguria (urine output <400 mL/d contributing to extracellular fluid overload), and electrolyte and acid-base abnormalities are frequent clinical features. ARF is usually asymptomatic and diagnosed when biochemical monitoring of hospitalized patients reveals a new increase in blood urea and serum creatinine concentrations. For purposes of diagnosis and management, causes of ARF are generally divided into three major categories: (1) diseases that cause renal hypoperfusion, resulting in decreased function without frank parenchymal damage (*prerenal ARF*, or azotemia) (~55%); (2) diseases that directly involve the renal parenchyma (*intrinsic ARF*) (~40%); and (3) diseases associated with urinary tract obstruction (*postrenal ARF*) (~5%). ARF is often considered to be reversible, although a return to baseline serum creatinine concentrations postinjury might not be sufficiently sensitive to detect clinically significant irreversible damage that may ultimately contribute to chronic kidney disease. ARF is associated with significant in-hospital morbidity and mortality, the latter in the range of 30–60%, depending on the clinical setting and presence or absence of nonrenal organ system failure.

ETIOLOGY AND PATHOPHYSIOLOGY

PRERENAL ARF (PRERENAL AZOTEMIA)

The most common form of ARF is prerenal ARF, which occurs in the setting of renal hypoperfusion. Prerenal ARF is generally reversible when renal perfusion pressure is restored. By definition, renal parenchymal tissue is not damaged. More severe or prolonged hypoperfusion may lead to ischemic injury, often termed *acute tubular necrosis*, or ATN. Thus, prerenal ARF and ischemic ATN fall along a spectrum of manifestations of renal hypoperfusion. As shown in **Table 10-1**, prerenal ARF can complicate any disease that induces hypovolemia, low cardiac output, systemic vasodilatation, or selective intrarenal vasoconstriction.

Hypovolemia leads to a fall in mean systemic arterial pressure, which is detected as reduced stretch by arterial (e.g., carotid sinus) and cardiac baroreceptors. In turn, this triggers a coordinated series of neurohormonal responses that aim to restore blood volume and arterial pressure. These include activation of the sympathetic nervous system and renin-angiotensin-aldosterone system, as well as release of arginine vasopressin. Relatively "nonessential" vascular beds (such as the musculocutaneous and splanchnic circulations) undergo vasoconstriction in an attempt to preserve cardiac and cerebral perfusion pressure. In addition, salt loss through sweat

TABLE 10-1

CLASSIFICATION AND MAJOR CAUSES OF ACUTE RENAL FAILURE

Prerenal ARF

I. Hypovolemia
  A. Increased extracellular fluid losses: hemorrhage
  B. Gastrointestinal fluid loss: vomiting, diarrhea, enterocutaneous fistula
  C. Renal fluid loss: diuretics, osmotic diuresis, hypoadrenalism, nephrogenic diabetes insipidus
  D. Extravascular sequestration: burns, pancreatitis, severe hypoalbuminemia (hypoproteinemia)
  E. Decreased intake: dehydration, altered mental status
II. Altered renal hemodynamics resulting in hypoperfusion
  A. Low cardiac output state: diseases of the myocardium, valves, and pericardium (including tamponade); pulmonary hypertension or massive pulmonary embolism leading to right and left heart failure; impaired venous return (e.g., abdominal compartment syndrome or positive pressure ventilation)
  B. Systemic vasodilation: sepsis, antihypertensives, afterload reducers, anaphylaxis
  C. Renal vasoconstriction: hypercalcemia, catecholamines, calcineurin inhibitors, amphotericin B
  D. Impairment of renal autoregulatory responses: cyclooxygenase inhibitors (e.g., nonsteroidal anti-inflammatory drugs), angiotensin-converting enzyme inhibitors, or angiotensin II receptor blockers
  E. Hepatorenal syndrome

Intrinsic ARF

I. Renovascular obstruction (bilateral, or unilateral in the setting of one kidney)
  A. Renal artery obstruction: atherosclerotic plaque, thrombosis, embolism, dissection aneurysm, large vessel vasculitis
  B. Renal vein obstruction: thrombosis or compression
II. Diseases of the glomeruli or vasculature
  A. Glomerulonephritis or vasculitis
  B. Other: thrombotic microangiopathy, malignant hypertension, collagen vascular diseases (systemic lupus erythematosus, scleroderma), disseminated intravascular coagulation, preeclampsia
III. Acute tubular necrosis
  A. Ischemia: causes are the same as for prerenal ARF, but generally the insult is more severe and/or more prolonged
  B. Infection, with or without sepsis syndrome
  C. Toxins:
    1. Exogenous: radiocontrast, calcineurin inhibitors, antibiotics (e.g., aminoglycosides), chemotherapy (e.g., cisplatin), antifungals (e.g., amphotericin B), ethylene glycol
    2. Endogenous: rhabdomyolysis, hemolysis
IV. Interstitial nephritis
  A. Allergic: antibiotics (β-lactams, sulfonamides, quinolones, rifampin), nonsteroidal anti-inflammatory drugs, diuretics, other drugs
  B. Infection: pyelonephritis (if bilateral)
  C. Infiltration: lymphoma, leukemia, sarcoidosis
  D. Inflammatory, nonvascular: Sjögren's syndrome, tubulointerstitial nephritis with uveitis
V. Intratubular obstruction
  A. Endogenous: myeloma proteins, uric acid (tumor lysis syndrome), systemic oxalosis
  B. Exogenous: acyclovir, ganciclovir, methotrexate, indinavir

Postrenal ARF (Obstruction)

I. Ureteric (bilateral, or unilateral in the case of one kidney): calculi, blood clots, sloughed papillae, cancer, external compression (e.g., retroperitoneal fibrosis)
II. Bladder neck: neurogenic bladder, prostatic hypertrophy, calculi, blood clots, cancer
III. Urethra: stricture or congenital valves

CHAPTER 10

Acute Renal Failure

glands is inhibited, and thirst and salt appetite are stimulated. Renal salt and water retention also occur.

In states of mild hypoperfusion, glomerular perfusion and the filtration fraction are preserved through several compensatory mechanisms. In response to the reduction in perfusion pressure, stretch receptors in afferent arterioles trigger afferent arteriolar vasodilatation through a local myogenic reflex (autoregulation). Angiotensin II increases biosynthesis of vasodilator prostaglandins (e.g., prostaglandin E_2 and prostacyclin), also resulting in afferent arteriolar vasodilation. In addition, angiotensin II induces preferential constriction of efferent arterioles. As a result, the fraction of plasma flowing through glomerular capillaries that is filtered is increased (filtration fraction), intraglomerular pressure is maintained, and GFR is preserved. With more severe hypoperfusion, these compensatory responses are overwhelmed and GFR falls, leading to prerenal ARF.

Autoregulatory dilatation of afferent arterioles allows for maintenance of GFR despite systemic hypotension; however, when hypotension is severe or prolonged, these autoregulatory mechanisms fail, resulting in a precipitous decline in GFR. Lesser degrees of hypotension may provoke prerenal ARF in those at risk: the elderly and patients with diseases that affect the integrity of afferent arterioles [e.g., hypertensive nephrosclerosis, diabetic vasculopathy, and other forms of occlusive (including atherosclerotic) renovascular disease]. In addition, drugs that interfere with adaptive responses to hypoperfusion may convert compensated renal hypoperfusion into overt prerenal ARF or ATN. Pharmacologic inhibitors of renal prostaglandin biosynthesis [nonsteroidal anti-inflammatory drugs (NSAIDs)] or angiotensin-converting enzyme (ACE) activity (ACE inhibitors) and angiotensin II receptor blockers (ARBs) are major culprits. While NSAIDs do not compromise GFR in healthy individuals, these medications may precipitate prerenal ARF in patients with volume depletion or in those with chronic kidney disease (in whom GFR is maintained, in part, through prostaglandin-mediated hyperfiltration by the remaining functional nephrons). ACE inhibitors should be used with special care in patients with bilateral renal artery stenosis or unilateral stenosis in a solitary functioning kidney. In these settings, glomerular perfusion and filtration may be exquisitely dependent on the actions of angiotensin II. Angiotensin II preserves GFR in these circumstances by raising systemic arterial pressure and by triggering selective constriction of efferent arterioles. ACE inhibitors and ARBs blunt these responses and can precipitate ARF.

Hepatorenal Syndrome

Hepatorenal syndrome (HRS) is a unique form of prerenal ARF that frequently complicates advanced cirrhosis as well as acute liver failure. In HRS the kidneys are structurally normal but fail due to splanchnic vasodilation and arteriovenous shunting, resulting in profound renal vasoconstriction. Correction of the underlying liver disease (e.g., by liver transplantation) results in resolution of the acute renal failure. There are two forms of HRS, type I and type II, that differ in their clinical course. In type I HRS, the more aggressive form of the disease, ARF progresses even after optimization of systemic hemodynamics and carries a mortality rate of >90%.

INTRINSIC ARF

Intrinsic causes of ARF can be conceptually divided based on the predominant compartment of the kidney that is affected: (1) ischemic or nephrotoxic tubular injury, (2) tubulointerstitial diseases, (3) diseases of the renal microcirculation and glomeruli, and (4) diseases of larger renal vessels (Table 10-1). Ischemia and nephrotoxins

classically induce acute tubular injury. Although many patients with ischemic or nephrotoxic ARF do not have morphologic evidence of cellular necrosis, this disease is often referred to as *acute tubular necrosis*, or ATN. More recently, because of the important role of sublethal injury to tubular epithelial and other renal cells (e.g., endothelial cells) in the pathogenesis of this syndrome, the term *acute kidney injury* (AKI) has been proposed.

Etiology and Pathophysiology of Ischemic ATN

Prerenal ARF and ischemic ATN are part of a spectrum of manifestations of renal hypoperfusion. In its most extreme form, ischemia leads to bilateral renal cortical necrosis and irreversible renal failure. ATN differs from prerenal ARF in that the renal tubular epithelial cells are injured in the latter. ATN occurs most frequently in patients undergoing major cardiovascular surgery or suffering severe trauma, hemorrhage, sepsis, and/or volume depletion (Table 10-1). Patients with other risk factors for ARF (e.g., exposure to nephrotoxins or preexisting chronic kidney disease) are at increased risk for ATN. Recovery typically takes 1–2 weeks after normalization of renal perfusion, as it requires repair and regeneration of renal cells.

The course of ischemic ATN is typically characterized by four phases: initiation, extension, maintenance, and recovery (Fig. 10-1). These phases are often preceded by a period of prerenal azotemia. During the *initiation phase* (lasting hours to days), GFR declines because (1) glomerular ultrafiltration pressure is reduced as renal blood flow falls, (2) the flow of filtrate within tubules is obstructed by casts comprised of shed epithelial cells and necrotic debris, and (3) there is backleak of glomerular filtrate through injured tubular epithelium. Ischemic injury is most prominent in the S_3 segment of the proximal tubule and the medullary portion of the thick ascending limb of the loop of Henle. These segments of the tubule are particularly sensitive to ischemia because of high rates of active [adenosine triphosphate (ATP)-dependent] solute transport and location in the outer medulla, where the partial pressure of oxygen is low, even under basal conditions. Cellular ischemia results in ATP depletion, inhibition of active sodium transport, cytoskeletal disruption, loss of cell polarity, cell-cell and cell-matrix attachment, and oxygen free-radical formation. Renal injury may be limited by restoration of renal blood flow during this period. If severe, cell injury results in apoptosis or necrosis.

The *extension phase* follows the initiation phase and is characterized by continued ischemic injury and inflammation. It has been proposed that endothelial damage (resulting in vascular congestion) contributes to both of these processes. During the *maintenance phase* (typically 1–2 weeks), GFR stabilizes at its nadir (typically 5–10 mL/min), urine output is lowest, and uremic complications may arise. It is not clear why the GFR remains

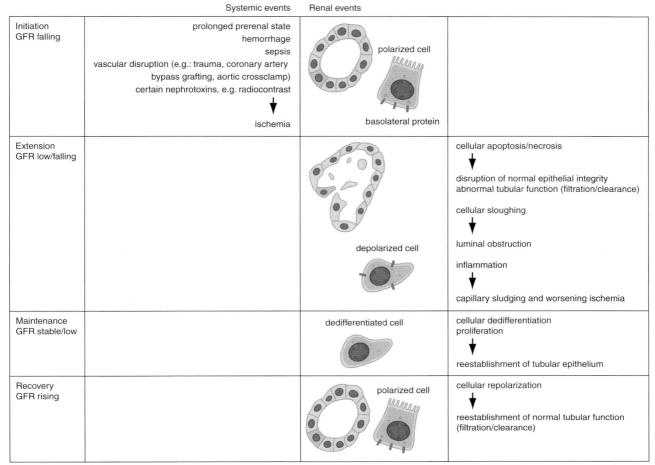

Systemic events	Renal events

Initiation
GFR falling

prolonged prerenal state
hemorrhage
sepsis
vascular disruption (e.g.: trauma, coronary artery
bypass grafting, aortic crossclamp)
certain nephrotoxins, e.g. radiocontrast

ischemia

polarized cell

basolateral protein

Extension
GFR low/falling

depolarized cell

cellular apoptosis/necrosis

disruption of normal epithelial integrity
abnormal tubular function (filtration/clearance)

cellular sloughing

luminal obstruction

inflammation

capillary sludging and worsening ischemia

Maintenance
GFR stable/low

dedifferentiated cell

cellular dedifferentiation
proliferation

reestablishment of tubular epithelium

Recovery
GFR rising

polarized cell

cellular repolarization

reestablishment of normal tubular function
(filtration/clearance)

FIGURE 10-1
Four phases of acute tubular necrosis.

low during this phase, despite correction of systemic hemodynamics. Proposed mechanisms include persistent intrarenal vasoconstriction and medullary ischemia triggered by dysregulated release of vasoactive mediators from injured endothelial cells, congestion of medullary blood vessels, and reperfusion injury induced by reactive oxygen species and inflammatory mediators released by leukocytes or renal parenchymal cells. In addition, epithelial cell injury may contribute to persistent intrarenal vasoconstriction through *tubuloglomerular feedback*. Specialized epithelial cells in the macula densa region of distal tubules detect increases in distal salt delivery that occur as a consequence of impaired reabsorption by more proximal nephron segments. Macula densa cells, in turn, stimulate constriction of adjacent afferent arterioles by a poorly defined mechanism and further compromise glomerular perfusion and filtration, thereby contributing to a vicious circle.

The *recovery phase* is characterized by tubular epithelial cell repair and regeneration as well as a gradual return of GFR toward premorbid levels. The recovery phase may be complicated by a marked diuretic phase due to delayed recovery of epithelial cell function (solute and water reabsorption) relative to glomerular filtration.

Etiology and Pathophysiology of Nephrotoxic ARF

Nephrotoxic ATN may complicate exposure to many structurally diverse pharmacologic agents (Table 10-1). With most nephrotoxins, the incidence of ARF is increased in the elderly and in patients with preexisting chronic kidney disease, true or "effective" hypovolemia, or concomitant exposure to other toxins.

Radiocontrast agents, cyclosporine, and tacrolimus (FK506) cause kidney injury through intrarenal vasoconstriction. Consequently, ATN in association with these medications is characterized by an acute fall in renal blood flow and GFR, a relatively benign urine sediment, and a low fractional excretion of sodium. Severe cases may show clinical or pathologic evidence of tubular cell necrosis. Contrast nephropathy is also thought to result from the generation of reactive oxygen species that are directly toxic to renal tubular epithelial cells. Contrast nephropathy classically presents as an acute (onset within 24–48 h) but reversible (peak 3-5 days, resolution within 1 week) rise in blood urea nitrogen and serum creatinine. Contrast nephropathy is most common in individuals with preexisting chronic kidney disease, diabetes mellitus, congestive heart failure, hypovolemia, or multiple myeloma. The type (low vs. isoosmolar contrast) and dose of contrast also influence the likelihood of injury associated with its administration.

Antibiotics and anticancer drugs typically cause ATN through direct toxicity to the tubular epithelial cells and/or intratubular obstruction. ARF complicates 10–30% of courses of *aminoglycoside antibiotics*. Aminoglycosides accumulate in renal tubular epithelial cells, where they cause oxidative stress and cell injury; thus, ARF usually occurs after several days of aminoglycoside therapy. Damage may occur in both the proximal and distal tubules; defects in the distal tubule may result in decreased concentrating ability. *Amphotericin B* causes dose-related ARF through intrarenal vasoconstriction and direct toxicity to proximal tubule epithelium. Newer (liposomal) formulations of amphotericin B may be associated with less nephrotoxicity. Acyclovir may precipitate in the renal tubules and cause acute renal failure. Foscarnet and pentamidine are less commonly prescribed antimicrobials also frequently associated with acute renal failure. Cisplatin and carboplatin, like the aminoglycosides, are accumulated by proximal tubule cells and typically provoke ARF after 7–10 days of exposure, typically in association with potassium and magnesium wasting. Ifosfamide administration may lead to hemorrhagic cystitis, manifested by hematuria, as well as acute and chronic renal failure. Type II renal tubular acidosis (Fanconi syndrome) often accompanies ifosfamide-associated ARF.

Endogenous nephrotoxins include calcium, myoglobin, hemoglobin, urate, oxalate, and myeloma light chains. Hypercalcemia can compromise GFR, predominantly by inducing intrarenal vasoconstriction as well as volume depletion from obligate water loss. Both *rhabdomyolysis* and *hemolysis* can induce ARF. Common causes of rhabdomyolysis include traumatic crush injury, acute muscle ischemia, prolonged seizure activity, excessive exercise, heat stroke or malignant hyperthermia, and infectious or metabolic disorders (e.g., hypophosphatemia, severe hypothyroidism). ARF due to hemolysis is relatively rare and is observed following blood transfusion reactions. It has been postulated that myoglobin and hemoglobin promote intrarenal oxidative stress, resulting in injury to tubular epithelial cells and inducing intratubular cast formation. In addition, cell-free hemoglobin and myoglobin are potent inhibitors of nitric oxide bioactivity and may trigger intrarenal vasoconstriction and ischemia. Hypovolemia or acidosis may further promote intratubular cast formation. Intratubular casts containing filtered immunoglobulin light chains and other proteins (including Tamm-Horsfall protein produced by thick ascending limb cells) cause ARF in patients with *multiple myeloma* (myeloma cast nephropathy). Light chains are also directly toxic to tubule epithelial cells. Intratubular obstruction is an important cause of ARF in patients with severe *hyperuricosuria* or *hyperoxaluria*. Acute uric acid nephropathy can complicate the treatment of selected lymphoproliferative or myeloproliferative disorders (e.g., Burkitt's lymphoma, acute myelogenous leukemia), especially after the administration of chemotherapy, resulting in increased cell lysis ("tumor lysis syndrome").

Pathology of Ischemic and Nephrotoxic ATN

The classic pathologic features of ischemic ATN are patchy and focal necrosis of the tubular epithelium, with detachment of cells from the basement membrane, and occlusion of tubule lumens with casts composed of intact or degenerating epithelial cells, Tamm-Horsfall protein, and pigments. Leukocyte accumulation is frequently observed in vasa recta; however, the morphology of the glomeruli and renal vasculature is characteristically normal. Necrosis is most severe in the S_3 segment of proximal tubules but may also affect the medullary thick ascending limb of the loop of Henle.

With exposure to nephrotoxins, morphologic changes tend to be most prominent in both the convoluted and straight portions of proximal tubules. Cellular necrosis is less pronounced than in ischemic ATN.

Other Causes of Intrinsic ARF

Virtually any pharmacologic agent may trigger allergic interstitial nephritis, which is characterized by infiltration of the tubulointerstitium by granulocytes (typically but not invariably eosinophils), macrophages, and/or lymphocytes and by interstitial edema. The most common offenders are antibiotics (e.g., penicillins, cephalosporins, quinolones, sulfonamides, rifampin) and NSAIDs (Table 10-1).

Patients with advanced atherosclerosis can develop ARF after manipulation of the aorta or renal arteries during surgery or angiography, following trauma, or, rarely, spontaneously (atheroembolic ARF). Cholesterol crystals embolize to the renal vasculature, lodge in small- and medium-sized arteries, and incite a giant cell and fibrotic reaction in the vessel wall with narrowing or obstruction of the vessel lumen. Atheroembolic ARF is often associated with hypocomplementemia and eosinophiluria, and it is frequently irreversible. The acute glomerulonephritides are immune-mediated diseases characterized by proliferative or crescentic glomerular inflammation (glomerulonephritis). These diseases are discussed in detail in Chap. 15.

POSTRENAL ARF

(See also Chap. 21.) Urinary tract obstruction accounts for fewer than 5% of cases of hospital-acquired ARF. Because one kidney has sufficient reserve to handle generated nitrogenous waste products, ARF from obstruction requires obstruction to urine flow between the external urethral meatus and bladder neck, bilateral ureteric obstruction, or unilateral ureteric obstruction in a patient with one functioning kidney or with significant preexisting chronic kidney disease. Bladder neck obstruction is the most common cause of postrenal ARF and is usually due to prostatic disease (e.g., hypertrophy, neoplasia, or infection), neurogenic bladder, or therapy with anticholinergic drugs. Less common causes of acute lower urinary tract obstruction include blood clots, calculi, and urethritis with spasm. Ureteric obstruction may result from intraluminal obstruction (e.g., calculi, blood clots, sloughed renal papillae), infiltration of the ureteric wall (e.g., neoplasia), or external compression (e.g., retroperitoneal fibrosis, neoplasia or abscess, inadvertent surgical ligature). During the early stages of obstruction (hours to days), continued glomerular filtration leads to increased intraluminal pressure upstream to the site of obstruction. As a result, there is gradual distention of the proximal ureter, renal pelvis, and calyces and a fall in GFR.

CLINICAL FEATURES AND DIFFERENTIAL DIAGNOSIS

The first step in evaluating a patient with renal failure is to determine if the disease is acute or chronic. If review of laboratory records demonstrates that the rise in blood urea nitrogen and creatinine is recent, this suggests that the process is acute. However, previous measurements are not always available. Findings that suggest chronic kidney disease (Chap. 11) include anemia, evidence of renal osteodystrophy (radiologic or laboratory), and small scarred kidneys. However, anemia may also complicate ARF, and renal size may be normal or increased in several chronic renal diseases (e.g., diabetic nephropathy, amyloidosis, polycystic kidney disease, HIV associated nephropathy). Once a diagnosis of ARF has been established, the etiology of ARF needs to be determined. Depending on the cause, specific therapies may need to be instituted. If the etiology is felt to be an exogenous nephrotoxin (often a medication), the nephrotoxin should be eliminated or discontinued. Lastly, the prevention and management of complications should be instituted.

CLINICAL ASSESSMENT

Symptoms of *prerenal* ARF include thirst and orthostatic dizziness. Physical signs of orthostatic hypotension, tachycardia, reduced jugular venous pressure, decreased skin turgor, and dry mucous membranes suggest prerenal ARF. Careful clinical examination may reveal stigmata of chronic liver disease and portal hypertension, advanced cardiac failure, sepsis, or other causes of reduced "effective" arterial blood volume (Table 10-1). Case records should be reviewed for documentation of a progressive fall in urine output and body weight and recent initiation of treatment with diuretics, NSAIDs, ACE inhibitors, or ARBs.

Hypovolemia, septic shock, and major surgery are important risk factors for ischemic ATN. The risk of ischemic ATN is increased further if ARF persists despite normalization of systemic hemodynamics. Diagnosis of nephrotoxic ATN requires careful review of the clinical data and records for evidence of recent exposure to nephrotoxic medications, radiocontrast agents, or endogenous toxins.

Although ischemic and nephrotoxic ATN account for >90% of cases of intrinsic ARF, other renal parenchymal diseases must be considered (Table 10-2). Fever, arthralgias, and a pruritic erythematous rash following exposure to a new drug suggest allergic interstitial nephritis, although systemic features of hypersensitivity are frequently absent. Flank pain may be a prominent symptom following occlusion of a renal artery or vein and with other parenchymal diseases distending the renal capsule (e.g., severe glomerulonephritis or pyelonephritis). Subcutaneous nodules, livedo reticularis, bright orange retinal arteriolar plaques, and digital ischemia ("purple toes"), despite palpable pedal pulses, suggest atheroembolization. ARF in association with oliguria, edema, and hypertension, with an "active" urine sediment (nephritic syndrome), suggests acute glomerulonephritis or vasculitis. Malignant hypertension may result in ARF, often in association with hypertensive injury to other organs (e.g., papilledema, neurologic dysfunction, left ventricular hypertrophy) and may mimic glomerulonephritis in its other clinical manifestations.

Postrenal ARF may present with suprapubic and flank pain due to distention of the bladder and of the renal collecting system and capsule, respectively. Colicky flank pain radiating to the groin suggests acute ureteric obstruction. Prostatic disease is likely if there is a history of nocturia, frequency, and hesitancy and enlargement of the prostate on rectal examination. Neurogenic bladder should be suspected in patients receiving anticholinergic medications or with physical evidence of autonomic dysfunction. Definitive diagnosis of postrenal ARF hinges on judicious use of radiologic investigations and rapid improvement in renal function following relief of obstruction.

URINALYSIS

(See also Chap. 4.) Anuria suggests complete urinary tract obstruction but may complicate severe cases of prerenal or intrinsic renal ARF. Wide fluctuations in urine output raise the possibility of intermittent obstruction, whereas patients with partial urinary tract obstruction may present with polyuria due to impairment of urine concentrating mechanisms.

In prerenal ARF, the sediment is characteristically acellular and contains transparent hyaline casts ("bland," "benign," "inactive" urine sediment). Hyaline casts are formed in concentrated urine from normal constituents of urine—principally Tamm-Horsfall protein, which is

TABLE 10-2

EPIDEMIOLOGY, CLINICAL FEATURES, AND DIAGNOSTIC STUDIES FOR MAJOR CAUSES OF ACUTE RENAL FAILURE

ETIOLOGY	EPIDEMIOLOGY	CLINICAL FEATURES	SERUM STUDIES	URINE STUDIES	OTHER TESTING
Prerenal ARF	Most common cause of community-acquired ARF; history of poor fluid intake, treatment with NSAIDs/ACE inhibitors/ARBs, worsening heart failure	Volume depletion (absolute/postural hypotension, low jugular venous pressure, dry mucous membranes) or decreased effective circulatory volume (e.g., heart failure or liver disease)	High BUN/CR ratio (≥20) is suggestive but not diagnostic	Hyaline casts FE_{Na} <1% U_{Na} <10 mmol/L SG >1.018	
Intrinsic ARF					
Diseases of large renal vessels					
Renal artery thrombosis	More common in those with atrial fibrillation or arterial thrombosis	Flank or abdominal pain	Elevated LDH	Mild proteinuria Occasional hematuria	Renal angiogram or MR angiogram are diagnostic
Atheroembolic disease	Vascular disease; classically occurs within days–weeks of manipulation of the aorta or other large vessels, often in the setting of anticoagulation	Retinal plaques, palpable purpura, livedo reticularis	Eosinophilia Hypocomplementemia	Eosinophiluria	Skin or renal biopsy
Renal vein thrombosis	History of nephrotic syndrome or pulmonary embolism	Flank pain		Mild proteinuria Occasional hematuria	Renal venogram or MR venogram are diagnostic
Diseases of small vessels and glomeruli					
Glomerulonephritis/ vasculitis	Associated with recent infection (postinfectious or endocarditis), systemic lupus erythematosus, liver disease (hepatitis B or C) Anti-GBM disease: Typically men in their 20s–40s ANCA disease: Two peaks: 20s–30s and 50s–60s	New cardiac murmur (postinfectious) Skin rash/ulcers, arthralgias (lupus) Sinusitis (anti-GBM disease) Lung hemorrhage (anti-GBM, ANCA, lupus)	ANA, ANCA, anti-GBM antibody, hepatitis serologies, cryoglobulins, blood cultures, ASO, complements (positive tests depend on etiology)	Hematuria with red cell casts/ dysmorphic red blood cells Granular casts Proteinuria (usually <1 g/d)	Renal biopsy
Hemolytic-uremic syndrome/ thrombotic thrombo-cytopenic	Recent GI infection (*E. coli*) or use of calcineurin inhibitors (FK506 and cyclosporine)	Fever, neurologic abnormalities	Schistocytes on peripheral blood smear, elevated LDH, anemia, thrombocytopenia	Hematuria Mild proteinuria Red cell casts (rare)	Renal biopsy

(Continued)

TABLE 10-2 (CONTINUED)

EPIDEMIOLOGY, CLINICAL FEATURES, AND DIAGNOSTIC STUDIES FOR MAJOR CAUSES OF ACUTE RENAL FAILURE

ETIOLOGY	EPIDEMIOLOGY	CLINICAL FEATURES	SERUM STUDIES	URINE STUDIES	OTHER TESTING
Malignant hypertension	Severe/uncontrolled hypertension	Evidence of damage to other organs: headache, papilledema, heart failure with LVH by echocardiography/ ECG Typically resolves with blood pressure control		Hematuria with red cell casts/ proteinuria	
Acute tubular necrosis					
Ischemia	Recent hemorrhage or severe hypotension			Muddy brown granular or tubular epithelial cell casts $FE_{Na} >1\%$ $U_{Na} >20$ mmol/L SG <1.015	
Exogenous toxins	Recent exposure to nephrotoxic antibiotics or chemotherapy, often in association with sepsis, or volume depletion			Muddy brown granular or tubular epithelial cell casts $FE_{Na} >1\%$ $U_{Na} >20$ mmol/L SG <1.015	
	Recent exposure to radiocontrast, often in association with volume depletion, diabetes or CKD			Muddy brown granular or tubular epithelial cell casts Urinalysis may be normal FE_{Na} often <1% U_{Na} often <20 mmol/L	
Endogenous toxins	Rhabdomyolysis	Post ictal state (seizures), evidence of trauma or prolonged immobilization	Increased myoglobin, creatine kinase	U/A positive for heme but no hematuria	
	Hemolysis: recent blood transfusion	Fever, other evidence of transfusion reaction	Pink plasma, increased LDH	Pink, heme-positive urine without hematuria	Transfusion reaction workup
	Tumor lysis: recent chemotherapy		Hyperuricemia, increased LDH	Urate crystals	
	Multiple myeloma	Individuals >60 years of age, ongoing constitutional symptoms (fatigue, malaise)	Circulating monoclonal spike, anemia	Dipstick-negative proteinuria, monoclonal spike on electrophoresis	Bone marrow or renal biopsy
	Ethylene glycol ingestion	History of alcohol abuse, altered mental status	Metabolic gap acidosis with osmolal gap, positive toxicology	Oxalate crystals	

(Continued)

TABLE 10-2 (CONTINUED)

EPIDEMIOLOGY, CLINICAL FEATURES, AND DIAGNOSTIC STUDIES FOR MAJOR CAUSES OF ACUTE RENAL FAILURE

ETIOLOGY	EPIDEMIOLOGY	CLINICAL FEATURES	SERUM STUDIES	URINE STUDIES	OTHER TESTING
Diseases of the tubulointerstitium					
Allergic interstitial nephritis	Recent medication exposure	Fever, rash, arthralgias	Eosinophilia	White cell casts, eosinophiluria	Renal biopsy
Acute bilateral pyelonephritis		Fever, flank pain and tenderness	Positive blood cultures	Leukocytes, proteinuria, positive urine culture	
Postrenal ARF	History of renal stones or prostatic disease	Palpable bladder, flank or abdominal pain		Usually normal; hematuria if due to stones	Imaging to assess obstruction: CT scan and/or ultrasound

Note: ACE, angiotensin-converting enzyme; ANA, antinuclear antibody; ANCA, antineutrophil cytoplasmic antibody; ARBs, angiotensin II receptor blockers; ARF, acute renal failure; ASO, antistreptolysin O; BUN, blood urea nitrogen; CKD, chronic kidney disease; CR, creatinine; CT, computed tomography; ECG, electrocardiogram; FE_{Na}, fractional excretion of sodium; GBM, glomerular basement membrane; GI, gastrointestinal; LDH, lactate dehydrogenase; LVH, left ventricular hypertrophy; MR, magnetic resonance; NSAIDs, nonsteroidal anti-inflammatory drugs; SG, specific gravity; U/A, urinalysis; U_{Na}, urine sodium concentration.

secreted by epithelial cells of the loop of Henle. Postrenal ARF may also present with an inactive sediment, although hematuria and pyuria are common in patients with intraluminal obstruction or prostatic disease. Pigmented "muddy brown" granular casts and casts containing tubule epithelial cells are characteristic of ATN and suggest an ischemic or nephrotoxic etiology. These casts are usually found in association with mild "tubular" proteinuria (<1 g/d), reflecting impaired reabsorption and processing of filtered proteins by injured proximal tubules. Casts may be absent in 20–30% of patients with ATN and are not required for diagnosis. In general, red blood cell casts indicate glomerular injury or, less often, acute tubulointerstitial nephritis. White cell casts and nonpigmented granular casts suggest interstitial nephritis, whereas broad granular casts are characteristic of chronic kidney disease and probably reflect interstitial fibrosis and dilatation of tubules. Eosinophiluria (>5% of urine leukocytes) is a common finding (~90%) in antibiotic-induced allergic interstitial nephritis and can be detected with Hansel's stain; however, lymphocytes may predominate in allergic interstitial nephritis induced by NSAIDs and some other drugs (i.e., ampicillin, rifampicin, and interferon α). Occasional uric acid crystals (pleomorphic in shape) are common in the concentrated urine of prerenal ARF but suggest acute urate nephropathy if seen in abundance. Oxalate (envelope-shaped) and hippurate (needle-shaped) crystals raise the possibility of ethylene glycol ingestion and toxicity.

Proteinuria of >1 g/d suggests injury to the glomerular ultrafiltration barrier ("glomerular proteinuria") or excretion of myeloma light chains. The latter may not be detected by conventional dipstick analysis, and other tests may be needed (e.g., sulfosalicylic acid precipitation, immunoelectrophoresis). Hemoglobinuria or myoglobinuria should be suspected if urine is strongly positive for heme by dipstick but contains few red cells, and if the supernatant of centrifuged urine is positive for free heme. Bilirubinuria may provide a clue to the presence of HRS.

RENAL FAILURE INDICES

Analysis of urine and blood biochemistry may be useful for distinguishing prerenal ARF from ischemic or nephrotoxic intrinsic renal ARF. The fractional excretion of sodium (FE_{Na}) is most useful in this regard. The FE_{Na} relates sodium clearance to creatinine clearance. Sodium is reabsorbed avidly from glomerular filtrate in patients with prerenal ARF, in an attempt to restore intravascular volume. The FE_{Na} tends to be high in ischemic ATN but is often low in patients with sepsis-induced, pigment-induced, and some forms of nephrotoxic ATN (e.g., contrast-associated). In contrast, creatinine is not reabsorbed in either setting. Consequently, patients with prerenal ARF typically have a FE_{Na} of <1.0% (frequently <0.1%). In patients with metabolic alkalosis, where there may be obligate losses of sodium in the urine to maintain electroneutrality, the fractional excretion of chloride (FE_{Cl})

may be more sensitive than the FE_{Na} in detecting prerenal azotemia. The *urine sodium concentration* is a less-sensitive index for distinguishing prerenal ARF from ischemic and nephrotoxic ARF as values overlap between groups. Similarly, indices of urinary concentrating ability such as urine specific gravity, urine osmolality, urine-to-plasma urea ratio, and blood urea-to-creatinine ratio are of limited value in differential diagnosis.

Many caveats apply when interpreting biochemical renal failure indices. The FE_{Na} may be >1.0% in prerenal ARF if patients are receiving diuretics or with preexisting chronic kidney disease, certain salt-wasting syndromes, or adrenal insufficiency.

LABORATORY FINDINGS

Serial serum creatinine measurements can provide useful insights to the cause of ARF. Prerenal ARF is typified by fluctuating serum creatinine levels that parallel changes in hemodynamic status. Creatinine rises rapidly (within 24–48 h) in patients with ARF following renal ischemia, atheroembolization, and radiocontrast exposure. Peak serum creatinine concentrations are observed after 3–5 days with contrast nephropathy and return to baseline after 5–7 days. In contrast, serum creatinine concentrations typically peak later (7–10 days) in ATN and atheroembolic disease. The initial rise in serum creatinine is characteristically delayed until the second week of therapy with many tubular epithelial cell toxins (e.g., aminoglycosides, cisplatin) and is thought to reflect the need for accumulation of these agents within tubular epithelial cells to cause injury.

Hyperkalemia, hyperphosphatemia, hypocalcemia, and elevations in serum uric acid and creatine kinase (MM isoenzyme) levels at presentation suggest a diagnosis of rhabdomyolysis. Hyperuricemia [>890 µmol/L (>15 mg/dL)] in association with hyperkalemia, hyperphosphatemia, and increased circulating levels of intracellular enzymes such as lactate dehydrogenase may indicate acute urate nephropathy and tumor lysis syndrome following cancer chemotherapy. A wide anion and osmolal gap [the latter calculated as the difference between the observed (measured) serum osmolality minus the expected osmolality calculated from serum sodium, glucose, and urea concentrations] indicate the presence of an unusual anion or osmole in the circulation (e.g., ingestion of ethylene glycol or methanol). Severe anemia in the absence of hemorrhage raises the possibility of hemolysis, multiple myeloma, or thrombotic microangiopathy. Systemic eosinophilia suggests allergic interstitial nephritis but is also a feature of atheroembolic disease and polyarteritis nodosa.

RADIOLOGIC FINDINGS

Imaging of the urinary tract by ultrasonography is useful to exclude postrenal ARF. CT and MRI are alternative imaging modalities. Whereas pelvicalyceal dilatation is usual with urinary tract obstruction (98% sensitivity), dilatation may be absent immediately following obstruction or in patients with ureteric encasement (e.g., retroperitoneal fibrosis, neoplasia). Retrograde or anterograde pyelography is a more definitive investigation in complex cases and provides precise localization of the site of obstruction. A plain film of the abdomen or unenhanced helical CT scan is a valuable initial screening technique in patients with suspected nephrolithiasis. Magnetic resonance angiography (MRA) is often used to assess patency of renal arteries and veins in patients with suspected vascular obstruction. Alternative methods include Doppler ultrasound (which is much more operator dependent than MRA) and CT-based angiography. Catheter-based angiography may be required for definitive diagnosis and treatment.

RENAL BIOPSY

Biopsy is reserved for patients in whom prerenal and postrenal ARF have been excluded and the cause of intrinsic ARF is unclear. Renal biopsy is particularly useful when clinical assessment and laboratory investigations suggest diagnoses other than ischemic or nephrotoxic injury that may respond to disease-specific therapy. Examples include glomerulonephritis, vasculitis, and allergic interstitial nephritis.

COMPLICATIONS

ARF impairs renal excretion of sodium, potassium, and water and perturbs divalent cation homeostasis and urinary acidification mechanisms. As a result, ARF is frequently complicated by intravascular volume overload, hyponatremia, hyperkalemia, hyperphosphatemia, hypocalcemia, hypermagnesemia, and metabolic acidosis. In addition, patients are unable to excrete nitrogenous waste products and are prone to develop the uremic syndrome (Chap. 3). The speed of development and the severity of these complications reflect the degree of renal impairment and catabolic state of the patient.

Expansion of extracellular fluid volume is an inevitable consequence of diminished salt and water excretion in oliguric or anuric individuals. Whereas milder forms are characterized by weight gain, bibasilar lung rales, raised jugular venous pressure, and dependent edema, continued volume expansion may precipitate life-threatening pulmonary edema. Excessive administration of free water, either through ingestion and nasogastric administration or as hypotonic saline or isotonic dextrose solutions, can induce *hypoosmolality* and *hyponatremia*, which, if severe, lead to neurologic abnormalities, including seizures.

Hyperkalemia is a frequent complication of ARF. Coexistent metabolic acidosis may exacerbate hyperkalemia by promoting potassium efflux from cells. Hyperkalemia may be particularly severe, even at the time of diagnosis, in patients with rhabdomyolysis, hemolysis, and tumor lysis syndrome. Mild hyperkalemia (<6.0 mmol/L) is usually asymptomatic. Higher levels may trigger electrocardiographic abnormalities and/or arrhythmias.

ARF is typically complicated by *metabolic acidosis,* often with an increased anion gap (Chap. 5). Acidosis can be particularly severe when endogenous production of hydrogen ions is increased by other mechanisms (e.g., diabetic or fasting ketoacidosis; lactic acidosis complicating generalized tissue hypoperfusion, liver disease, or sepsis; metabolism of ethylene glycol or methanol).

Hyperphosphatemia is an almost invariable complication of ARF. Severe hyperphosphatemia may develop in highly catabolic patients or following rhabdomyolysis, hemolysis, or tissue ischemia. Metastatic deposition of calcium phosphate can lead to *hypocalcemia,* particularly with elevation of serum calcium (mg/dL) and phosphate (mg/dL) concentrations. Other factors that contribute to hypocalcemia include tissue resistance to the actions of parathyroid hormone and reduced levels of 1,25-dihydroxyvitamin D. Hypocalcemia is often asymptomatic but can cause perioral paresthesia, muscle cramps, seizures, altered mental status, prolongation of the QT interval, and other nonspecific T-wave changes on electrocardiography.

Anemia develops rapidly in ARF and is usually multifactorial in origin. Contributing factors include impaired erythropoiesis, hemolysis, bleeding, hemodilution, and reduced red cell survival time. Prolongation of the *bleeding time* is also common. Common contributors to the bleeding diathesis include mild thrombocytopenia, platelet dysfunction, and/or clotting factor abnormalities (e.g., factor VIII dysfunction). *Infection* is a common and serious complication of ARF. It is unclear whether patients with ARF have a clinically significant defect in host immune responses or whether the high incidence of infection reflects repeated breaches of mucocutaneous barriers (e.g., intravenous cannulae, mechanical ventilation, bladder catheterization). *Cardiopulmonary complications* of ARF include arrhythmias, pericarditis and pericardial effusion, and pulmonary edema.

Protracted periods of severe ARF are invariably associated with the development of the *uremic syndrome* (Chap. 3).

A *vigorous diuresis* can occur during the recovery phase of ARF, which may be inappropriate on occasion and lead to intravascular volume depletion. *Hypernatremia* can also complicate recovery if water losses via hypotonic urine are not replaced or if losses are inappropriately replaced by relatively hypertonic saline solutions. *Hypokalemia, hypomagnesemia, hypophosphatemia,* and *hypocalcemia* are less common metabolic complications during this period but may develop in response to injury associated with selected drugs (e.g., ifosfamide may lead to Fanconi syndrome or type II renal tubular acidosis associated with hypokalemia, acidosis, hypophosphatemia, and glycosuria).

℞ **Treatment:**
ACUTE RENAL FAILURE

PREVENTION Because there are no specific therapies for ischemic or nephrotoxic ARF, prevention is of paramount importance. Many cases of ischemic ARF can be avoided by close attention to cardiovascular function and intravascular volume in high-risk patients, such as the elderly and those with preexisting chronic kidney disease. Indeed, aggressive restoration of intravascular volume has been shown to dramatically reduce the incidence of ischemic ARF after major surgery or trauma, burns, or cholera. The incidence of nephrotoxic ARF can be reduced by tailoring the administration (dose and frequency) of nephrotoxic drugs to body size and GFR. In this regard, it should be noted that serum creatinine is a relatively insensitive index of GFR and may overestimate GFR considerably in small or elderly patients. For purposes of drug dosing, it is advisable to estimate the GFR using the Cockcroft-Gault formula (which factors in age, sex, and weight) or the simplified Modification of Diet in Renal Disease (MDRD) equation (which factors in age, sex, weight, and race) (Chap. 15). Of note, these equations cannot be used to estimate GFR when creatinine is not at steady state (e.g., during evolving ARF). Adjusting drug dosage according to circulating drug levels also appears to limit renal injury in patients receiving aminoglycoside antibiotics, cyclosporine, or tacrolimus. Diuretics, NSAIDs, ACE inhibitors, ARBs, and vasodilators should be used with caution in patients with suspected true or "effective" hypovolemia or renovascular disease as they may precipitate prerenal ARF or convert the latter to ischemic ARF. Allopurinol and forced alkaline diuresis are useful prophylactic measures in patients at high risk for acute urate nephropathy (e.g., cancer chemotherapy in hematologic malignancies) to limit uric acid generation and prevent precipitation of urate crystals in renal tubules. Rasburicase, a recombinant urate-oxidase enzyme, catalyzes enzymatic oxidation of uric acid into a soluble metabolite, allantoin. Forced alkaline diuresis may also prevent or attenuate ARF in patients receiving high-dose methotrexate or suffering from rhabdomyolysis. N-acetylcysteine limits acetaminophen-induced renal injury if given within 24 h of ingestion.

A number of preventive measures have been proposed for contrast nephropathy. It is clear that hydration is an effective preventive measure. Other measures that have been proposed include loop diuretics and mannitol, dopamine, fenoldopam, N-acetylcysteine, theophylline, and sodium bicarbonate. Despite favorable experimental data, there is insufficient evidence to support the use of loop diuretics or mannitol to prevent radiocontrast nephropathy or any other cause of ARF. Likewise, despite its widespread use, dopamine has proved ineffective as a prophylactic agent. Fenoldopam, a dopamine a-1 specific agonist approved for use as a parenteral antihypertensive agent, has been tested in several clinical trials and does not appear to reduce the incidence of contrast nephropathy. Moreover, fenoldopam is associated with significant side effects, including systemic hypotension, and its use as an agent to prevent radiocontrast nephropathy should be discouraged. In contrast, several (relatively small) randomized clinical trials (RCTs) have suggested a clinical benefit to the use of *N*-acetylcysteine, although meta-analyses have been inconclusive. However, aside from the potential hazards associated with a delay in radiographic imaging, *N*-acetylcysteine appears to be safe, and its use in patients at high risk for radiocontrast nephropathy is reasonable, based on its low side effect profile. Larger RCTs will be required to show definitive benefit. Theophylline and aminophylline (adenosine antagonists) offer the potential advantage of use immediately preceding radiocontrast administration, although the benefit, if present, appears marginal in most studies. Lastly, volume expansion with bicarbonate-containing intravenous fluids has been suggested to be superior to sodium chloride (saline) administration and showed a significant benefit in a single center RCT. Unlike *N*-acetylcysteine, the use of sodium bicarbonate does not obligate a delay in imaging (the published protocol began IV fluids 1 h before the imaging study was begun). Whether a combination of strategies (e.g., *N*-acetylcysteine + sodium bicarbonate) offers additive benefit and that patients require treatment remain unclear and warrant further study.

SPECIFIC THERAPIES By definition, prerenal ARF is rapidly reversible upon correction of the primary hemodynamic abnormality, and postrenal ARF resolves upon relief of obstruction. To date there are no specific therapies for established AKI. Management of these disorders should focus on elimination of the causative hemodynamic abnormality or toxin, avoidance of additional insults, and prevention and treatment of complications. Specific treatment of other causes of intrinsic renal ARF depends on the underlying pathology.

Prerenal ARF The composition of replacement fluids for treatment of prerenal ARF due to hypovolemia should be tailored according to the composition of the lost fluid. Severe hypovolemia due to hemorrhage should be corrected with packed red cells, whereas isotonic saline is usually appropriate replacement for mild to moderate hemorrhage or plasma loss (e.g., burns, pancreatitis). Urinary and gastrointestinal fluids can vary greatly in composition but are usually hypotonic. Hypotonic solutions (e.g., 0.45% saline) are usually recommended as initial replacement in patients with prerenal ARF due to increased urinary or gastrointestinal fluid losses, although isotonic saline may be more appropriate in severe cases. Subsequent therapy should be based on measurements of the volume and ionic content

of excreted or drained fluids. Serum potassium and acid-base status should be monitored carefully, and potassium and bicarbonate supplemented as appropriate. Cardiac failure may require aggressive management with inotropic agents, preload and afterload reducing agents, antiarrhythmic drugs, and mechanical aids such as intraaortic balloon pumps. Invasive hemodynamic monitoring may be required in selected cases to guide therapy for complications in patients in whom clinical assessment of cardiovascular function and intravascular volume is difficult.

Fluid management may be particularly challenging in patients with cirrhosis complicated by ascites. In this setting, it is important to distinguish between full-blown HRS, which carries a grave prognosis, and reversible ARF due to true or "effective" hypovolemia induced by overzealous use of diuretics or sepsis (e.g., spontaneous bacterial peritonitis). The contribution of hypovolemia to ARF can be definitively assessed only by administration of a fluid challenge. Fluids should be administered slowly and titrated to jugular venous pressure and, if necessary, central venous and pulmonary capillary wedge pressure. Patients with a reversible prerenal component typically have an increase in urine output and fall in serum creatinine with fluid challenge, whereas patients with HRS do not. Patients with HRS may suffer increased ascites formation and pulmonary compromise if not monitored closely during fluid challenge. Large volumes of ascitic fluid can usually be drained by paracentesis without deterioration in renal function if intravenous albumin is administered simultaneously. Indeed, "large-volume paracentesis" may afford an increase in GFR, likely by lowering intraabdominal pressure and improving flow in renal veins. Alternatively, for patients with refractory ascites, transjugular intrahepatic portosystemic shunting is an alternative. Older peritoneal-venous shunts (LaVeen or Denver shunt) have largely fallen out of favor. Transjugular intrahepatic portosystemic shunts may improve renal function through increased central blood volume and suppression of aldosterone and norepinephrine secretion.

Intrinsic ARF Many different approaches to attenuate injury or hasten recovery have been tested in ischemic and nephrotoxic AKI. These include atrial natriuretic peptide, low-dose dopamine, endothelin antagonists, loop-blocking diuretics, calcium channel blockers, α-adrenoreceptor blockers, prostaglandin analogues, antioxidants, antibodies against leukocyte adhesion molecules, and insulin-like growth factor type I. Whereas many of these are beneficial in experimental models of ischemic or nephrotoxic ATN, they have either failed to confer consistent benefit or proved ineffective in humans.

ARF due to other intrinsic renal diseases such as acute glomerulonephritis or vasculitis may respond to immunosuppressive agents (glucocorticoids, alkylating agents, and/or plasmapheresis, depending on the primary pathology). Glucocorticoids also may hasten remission in allergic interstitial nephritis, although data are limited to small-case series. Aggressive control of systemic arterial pressure is of paramount importance in limiting renal injury in malignant hypertensive nephrosclerosis. Hypertension and ARF due to scleroderma may be exquisitely sensitive to treatment with ACE inhibitors.

Postrenal ARF Management of postrenal ARF requires close collaboration between nephrologist, urologist, and radiologist. Obstruction of the urethra or bladder neck is usually managed initially by transurethral or suprapubic placement of a bladder catheter, which provides

temporary relief while the obstructing lesion is identified and treated definitively. Similarly, ureteric obstruction may be treated initially by percutaneous catheterization of the dilated renal pelvis or ureter. Indeed, obstructing lesions can often be removed percutaneously (e.g., calculus, sloughed papilla) or bypassed by insertion of a ureteric stent (e.g., carcinoma). Most patients experience an appropriate diuresis for several days following relief of obstruction. Approximately 5% of patients develop a transient salt-wasting syndrome that may require administration of intravenous saline to maintain blood pressure.

SUPPORTIVE MEASURES (Table 10-3) Following correction of hypovolemia, salt and water

TABLE 10-3

MANAGEMENT OF ISCHEMIC AND NEPHROTOXIC ACUTE RENAL FAILURE[a]

MANAGEMENT ISSUE	THERAPY
Reversal of Renal Insult	
Ischemic ATN	Restore systemic hemodynamics and renal perfusion through volume resuscitation and use of vasopressors
Nephrotoxic ATN	Eliminate nephrotoxic agents
	Consider toxin-specific measures: e.g., forced alkaline diuresis for rhabdomyolysis, allopurinol/rasburicase for tumor lysis syndrome
Prevention and Treatment of Complications	
Intravascular volume overload	Salt and water restriction
	Diuretics
	Ultrafiltration
Hyponatremia	Restriction of enteral free water intake
	Avoidance of hypotonic intravenous solutions, including dextrose-containing solutions
Hyperkalemia	Restriction of dietary K^+ intake
	Eliminate K^+ supplements and K^+-sparing diuretics
	Loop diuretics to promote K^+ excretion
	Potassium binding ion-exchange resins (e.g., sodium polystyrene sulfonate or Kayexalate)
	Insulin (10 units regular) and glucose (50 mL of 50% dextrose) to promote intracellular mobilization
	Inhaled β-agonist therapy to promote intracellular mobilization
	Calcium gluconate or calcium chloride (1 g) to stabilize the myocardium
	Dialysis
Metabolic acidosis	Sodium bicarbonate (maintain serum bicarbonate >15 mmol/L or arterial pH > 7.2)
	Administration of other bases, e.g., THAM
	Dialysis
Hyperphosphatemia	Restriction of dietary phosphate intake
	Phosphate binding agents (calcium carbonate, calcium acetate, sevelamer hydrochloride, aluminum hydroxide)
Hypocalcemia	Calcium carbonate or gluconate (if symptomatic)
Hypermagnesemia	Discontinue Mg^{++} containing antacids
Hyperuricemia	Treatment usually not necessary if <890 μmol/L or <15 mg/dL
	Allopurinol, forced alkaline diuresis, rasburicase
Nutrition	Protein and calorie intake to avoid net negative nitrogen balance
Dialysis	To prevent complications of acute renal failure
Choice of agents	Avoid other nephrotoxins: ACE inhibitors/ARBs, aminoglycosides, NSAIDs, radiocontrast unless absolutely necessary and no alternative
Drug dosing	Adjust doses and frequency of administration for degree of renal impairment

[a]Note that these are general recommendations and need to be tailored to the individual patient.
Note: ATN, acute tubular necrosis; THAM, tris(hydroxymethyl)aminomethane; ACE, angiotensin-converting enzyme; ARBs, angiotensin II receptor blockers; NSAIDs, nonsteroidal anti-inflammatory drugs.

intake are tailored to match losses. Hypervolemia can usually be managed by restriction of salt and water intake and diuretics. Indeed, there is, as yet, no proven rationale for administration of diuretics in ARF except to treat this complication. Despite the fact that subpressor doses of dopamine may transiently promote salt and water excretion by increasing renal blood flow and GFR and by inhibiting tubule sodium reabsorption, subpressor ("low-dose," "renal-dose") dopamine has proved ineffective in clinical trials, may trigger arrhythmias, and should not be used as a renoprotective agent in this setting. Ultrafiltration or dialysis is used to treat severe hypervolemia when conservative measures fail. Hyponatremia and hypoosmolality can usually be controlled by restriction of free water intake. Conversely, hypernatremia is treated by administration of water or intravenous hypotonic saline or isotonic dextrose-containing solutions. The management of hyperkalemia is described in Chap. 6.

Metabolic acidosis is not usually treated unless serum bicarbonate concentration falls below 15 mmol/L or arterial pH falls below 7.2. More severe acidosis is corrected by oral or intravenous sodium bicarbonate. Initial rates of replacement are guided by estimates of bicarbonate deficit and adjusted thereafter according to serum levels (Chap. 5). Patients should be monitored for complications of sodium bicarbonate administration such as hypervolemia, metabolic alkalosis, hypocalcemia, and hypokalemia. From a practical point of view, most patients who require supplemental sodium bicarbonate administration will need emergency dialysis within days. Hyperphosphatemia is usually controlled by restriction of dietary phosphate and by oral phosphate binders (calcium carbonate, calcium acetate, sevelamer, and aluminum hydroxide) to reduce gastrointestinal absorption of phosphate. Hypocalcemia does not usually require treatment unless severe, as may occur with rhabdomyolysis or pancreatitis or following administration of bicarbonate. Hyperuricemia is typically mild [<890 μmol/L (<15 mg/dL)] and does not require intervention.

The objective of *nutritional management* during the maintenance phase of ARF is to provide sufficient calories and protein to minimize catabolism. Nutritional requirements will vary based on the underlying disease process; for example, those with sepsis-associated AKI are likely to be hypercatabolic. The presence of oliguria complicates nutritional management, and if the patient is not on dialysis, minimizing production of nitrogenous waste is a consideration. Often, the institution of dialysis facilitates the provision of adequate nutritional support. There is no clear benefit of parenteral nutrition compared with enteral nutrition; indeed, those supported with parenteral nutrition are at increased risk of complications, including infection.

Anemia may necessitate blood transfusion if severe. Recombinant human erythropoietin is rarely used in ARF because bone marrow resistance to erythropoietin is common, and more immediate treatment of anemia (if any) is required. Uremic bleeding may respond to administration of desmopressin or estrogens. Often dialysis is instituted to control bleeding that appears to be related to uremia. Gastrointestinal prophylaxis with histamine receptor (H2) antagonists or proton pump inhibitors should be prescribed, especially in the setting of critical illness. Meticulous care of intravenous and bladder catheters, and other invasive devices is mandatory to avoid infections.

Indications and Modalities of Dialysis (See also Chap. 12.) During ARF, dialysis is often used to support renal function until renal repair/recovery occur. Absolute indications for dialysis include symptoms or signs of the uremic syndrome and management of refractory hypervolemia, hyperkalemia, or acidosis. Many nephrologists also initiate dialysis empirically for blood urea levels of >100 mg/dL; however, this approach has yet to be validated in controlled clinical trials. Although direct clinical comparisons are limited, hemodialysis appears to be somewhat more effective than peritoneal dialysis for management of ARF. Peritoneal dialysis may be useful when hemodialysis is unavailable or if it is impossible to obtain vascular access. However, peritoneal dialysis is associated with increased protein losses and is contraindicated in those patients who have undergone recent abdominal surgery or those with ongoing infection. Peritoneal dialysis access requires insertion of a cuffed catheter into the peritoneal cavity.

Vascular access for hemodialysis requires insertion of a temporary double-lumen hemodialysis catheter into the internal jugular or femoral vein. Insertion into the subclavian vein is generally avoided owing to the risk of subclavian stenosis. Hemodialysis may be provided in the form of intermittent hemodialysis (typically performed for 3–4 hours per day, three to four times per week), slow low-efficiency dialysis (performed for 6–12 hours per day, three to six times per week), or continuous renal replacement therapy (CRRT). CRRTs are particularly valuable techniques in patients in whom intermittent therapy fails to control hypervolemia, uremia, or acidosis or in those who do not tolerate intermittent hemodialysis due to hemodynamic instability. In those patients where hemodynamic instability is a primary consideration, slow low-efficiency hemodialysis (SLED), a relatively new hybrid mode of dialysis, is an excellent alternative to CRRT.

Continuous arteriovenous modalities [continuous arteriovenous hemofiltration, hemodialysis, and hemodiafiltration (CAVH, CAVHD, and CAVHDF, respectively)] require both arterial and venous access. The patient's own blood pressure generates an ultrafiltrate of plasma across a porous biocompatible dialysis membrane. With the advent of peristaltic pumps, the arteriovenous modalities have fallen out of favor, in part because of the complications associated with cannulation of a large artery with a large-bore catheter. In continuous venovenous hemodialysis (CVVHD), a blood pump generates ultrafiltration pressure across the dialysis membrane. In continuous venovenous hemofiltration (CVVH), the hemodialysis (diffusive clearance) component is eliminated, and an ultrafiltrate of plasma is removed across the dialysis membrane and replaced by a physiologic crystalloid solution (convective clearance). In continuous venovenous hemodiafiltration (CVVHDF), these two methods of clearance are combined. The bulk of evidence to date suggests that intermittent and continuous dialytic therapies are equally effective for the treatment of ARF. The choice of technique is currently tailored to the specific needs of the patient, the resources of the institution, and the expertise of the physician. Potential disadvantages of continuous techniques include the need for prolonged immobilization, systemic anticoagulation, and prolonged exposure of blood to synthetic (albeit biocompatible) dialysis membranes.

The optimal dose of dialysis for ARF remains unclear at present. Recent evidence (from a single center, non-randomized trial) suggests that more intensive hemodialysis (e.g., daily rather than alternate-day intermittent dialysis) may be clinically superior and confers improved survival in ARF once dialysis is required. This conclusion may not be as intuitive as it first appears since dialysis itself has been postulated to prolong ARF by inducing hypotension and other adverse effects related to the blood-dialyzer contact (e.g., complement activation and inflammation). Similarly, data suggest that increased doses of CRRT may be of benefit for ARF, although these results need to be confirmed in a larger, multicenter study.

Outcome and Long-Term Prognosis The in-hospital mortality rate among patients with ARF ranges from 20–50% or more, depending on underlying conditions, and has declined only marginally over the past 15 years. Most patients who survive an episode of ARF recover sufficient renal function to remain dialysis independent, although a fraction (roughly 10–20%) go on to require maintenance dialysis.

Common etiologies for acute renal failure will vary, depending on the availability of health care in a given country. In general, the most common cause of community-acquired ARF is prerenal azotemia. However, in countries with less well-developed health care systems, infective etiologies for ARF predominate. In developed countries, postoperative and ischemic/nephrotoxic causes of ARF are more common.

ACKNOWLEDGMENT

We are grateful to Dr. Hugh Brady and Dr. Barry Brenner, authors of this chapter in the 16th edition of Harrison's Principles of Internal Medicine, for contributions to this edition.

FURTHER READINGS

Ho KM et al: Meta-analysis of N-acetylcysteine to prevent acute renal failure after major surgery. Am J Kidney Dis 53:33, 2009

Lameire N: The pathophysiology of acute renal failure. Crit Care Clin 21:197, 2005

——— et al: Acute renal failure. Lancet 365:417, 2005

Pannu N et al: Prophylaxis strategies for contrast-induced nephropathy. JAMA 295:2765, 2006

——— et al: Renal replacement therapy in patients with acute renal failure: A systematic review. JAMA 299:793, 2008

Tumlin J et al: Efficacy and safety of renal tubule cell therapy for acute renal failure. J Am Soc Nephrol 19:1034, 2008

Weisbord SD, Palevsky P: Radiocontrast-induced acute renal failure. J Intensive Care Med 20:63, 2005

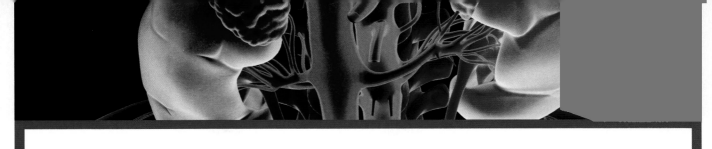

CHAPTER 11

CHRONIC KIDNEY DISEASE

Joanne M. Bargman   ■   Karl Skorecki

Chronic kidney disease (CKD) encompasses a spectrum of different pathophysiologic processes associated with abnormal kidney function, and a progressive decline in glomerular filtration rate (GFR). **Table 11-1** provides a widely accepted classification, based on recent guidelines of the National Kidney Foundation [Kidney Dialysis Outcomes Quality Initiative (KDOQI)], in which stages of CKD are defined according to the estimated GFR.

The term *chronic renal failure* applies to the process of continuing significant, irreversible reduction in nephron number, and typically corresponds to CKD stages 3–5. The pathophysiologic processes and adaptations associated with chronic renal failure is the focus of this chapter. The dispiriting term *end-stage renal disease* represents a stage of CKD where the accumulation of toxins, fluid, and electrolytes normally excreted by the kidneys results in the *uremic syndrome*. This syndrome leads to death unless the toxins are removed by renal replacement therapy, using dialysis or kidney transplantation. These latter interventions are discussed in Chaps. 12 and 13. *End-stage renal disease* is supplanted in this chapter by the term *stage 5 CKD*.

PATHOPHYSIOLOGY OF CHRONIC KIDNEY DISEASE

The pathophysiology of CKD involves two broad sets of mechanisms of damage: (1) initiating mechanisms specific to the underlying etiology (e.g., immune complexes and mediators of inflammation in certain types of glomerulonephritis, or toxin exposure in certain diseases of the renal tubules and interstitium); and (2) a set of progressive mechanisms, involving hyperfiltration and hypertrophy of the remaining viable nephrons, that are a common consequence following long-term reduction of renal mass, irrespective of underlying etiology (Chap. 2). The responses to reduction in nephron number are mediated by vasoactive hormones, cytokines, and growth factors. Eventually, these short-term adaptations of hypertrophy and hyperfiltration become maladaptive as the increased pressure and flow predisposes to sclerosis and dropout of the remaining nephrons. Increased intrarenal activity of the renin-angiotensin axis appears to contribute both to the initial adaptive hyperfiltration and to the subsequent maladaptive hypertrophy and sclerosis, the latter, in part, owing to the stimulation of transforming growth factor β (TGF-β). This process explains why a reduction in renal mass from an isolated insult may lead to a progressive decline in renal function over many years.

THE STAGES OF CKD AND IDENTIFICATION OF AT-RISK POPULATIONS

It is important to identify factors that increase the risk for CKD, even in individuals with normal GFR. Risk

TABLE 11-1

CLASSIFICATION OF CHRONIC KIDNEY DISEASE (CKD)	
STAGE	GFR, mL/min per 1.73 m²
0	>90[a]
1	≥90[b]
2	60–89
3	30–59
4	15–29
5	<15

[a]With risk factors for CKD (see text).
[b]With demonstrated kidney damage (e.g., persistent proteinuria, abnormal urine sediment, abnormal blood and urine chemistry, abnormal imaging studies).
Note: GFR, glomerular filtration rate.
Source: Modified from National Kidney Foundation. K/DOQI Clinical Practice Guidelines for Chronic Kidney Disease: Evaluation, classification and stratification. Am J Kidney Dis 39:suppl 1, 2002.

factors include hypertension, diabetes mellitus, autoimmune disease, older age, African ancestry, a family history of renal disease, a previous episode of acute renal failure, and the presence of proteinuria, abnormal urinary sediment, or structural abnormalities of the urinary tract.

In order to stage CKD, it is necessary to estimate the GFR. Two equations commonly used to estimate GFR are shown in Table 11-2, and incorporate the measured plasma creatinine concentration, age, sex, and ethnic origin. Many laboratories now report an estimated GFR, or "e-GFR," using one of these equations.

The normal annual mean decline in GFR with age from the peak GFR (~120 mL/min per 1.73 m²) attained during the third decade of life is ~1 mL/min per year per 1.73 m², reaching a mean value of 70 mL/min per 1.73 m² at age 70. The mean GFR is lower in women than in men. For example, a woman in her 80s

with a normal serum creatinine may have a GFR of just 50 mL/min per 1.73 m². Thus, even a mild elevation in serum creatinine concentration [e.g., 130 μmol/L (1.5 mg/dL)], often signifies a substantial reduction in GFR in most individuals.

Measurement of albuminuria is also helpful for monitoring nephron injury and the response to therapy in many forms of CKD, especially chronic glomerular diseases. While an accurate 24-h urine collection is the "gold standard" for measurement of albuminuria, the measurement of albumin-to-creatinine ratio in a spot first-morning urine sample is often more practical to obtain and correlates well, but not perfectly, with 24-h urine collections. Persistence in the urine of >17 mg of albumin per gram of creatinine in adult males and 25 mg albumin per gram of creatinine in adult females usually signifies chronic renal damage. *Microalbuminuria* refers to the excretion of amounts of albumin too small to detect by urinary dipstick or conventional measures of urine protein. It is a good screening test for early detection of renal disease, in particular, and may be a marker for the presence of microvascular disease in general. If a patient has a large amount of excreted albumin, there is no reason to perform an assay for microalbuminuria.

Stages 1 and 2 CKD are usually not associated with any symptoms arising from the decrement in GFR. However, there may be symptoms from the underlying renal disease itself, such as edema in patients with nephrotic syndrome or signs of hypertension secondary to the renal parenchymal disease in patients with polycystic kidney disease, some forms of glomerulonephritis, and many other parenchymal and vascular renal diseases, even with well-preserved GFR. If the decline in GFR progresses to stages 3 and 4, clinical and laboratory complications of CKD become more prominent. Virtually all organ systems are affected, but the most evident complications include anemia and associated easy fatigability; decreasing appetite with progressive malnutrition, abnormalities in

TABLE 11-2

RECOMMENDED EQUATIONS FOR ESTIMATION OF GLOMERULAR FILTRATION RATE (GFR) USING SERUM CREATININE CONCENTRATION (P_{Cr}), AGE, SEX, RACE, AND BODY WEIGHT

1. Equation from the Modification of Diet in Renal Disease study[a]
   Estimated GFR (mL/min per 1.73 m²) $= 1.86 \times (P_{Cr})^{-1.154} \times (age)^{-0.203}$
   Multiply by 0.742 for women
   Multiply by 1.21 for African Americans
2. Cockcroft-Gault equation
   Estimated creatinine clearance (mL/min)

$$= \frac{(140 - age \times body\ weight,\ kg)}{72 \times P_{Cr}\ (mg/dL)}$$

   Multiply by 0.85 for women

[a]Equation is *available* in hand-held calculators and in tabular form.
Source: Adapted from AS Levey et al: Am J Kidney Dis 39 (Suppl 1): S1, 2002, with permission.

calcium, phosphorus, and mineral-regulating hormones, such as $1,25(OH)_2D_3$ (calcitriol) and parathyroid hormone (PTH); and abnormalities in sodium, potassium, water, and acid-base homeostasis. If the patient progresses to stage 5 CKD, toxins accumulate such that patients usually experience a marked disturbance in their activities of daily living, well-being, nutritional status, and water and electrolyte homeostasis, eventuating in the *uremic syndrome*. As discussed above, this state will culminate in death unless renal replacement therapy (dialysis or transplantation) is instituted.

ETIOLOGY AND EPIDEMIOLOGY

It has been estimated from population survey data that at least 6% of the adult population in the United States has chronic kidney disease at stages 1 and 2. An unknown subset of this group will progress to more advanced stages of CKD. An additional 4.5% of the U.S. population is estimated to have stages 3 and 4 CKD. The most frequent cause of CKD is diabetic nephropathy, most often secondary to Type 2 diabetes mellitus. Hypertensive nephropathy is a common cause of CKD in the elderly, in whom chronic renal ischemia as a result of small and large vessel renovascular disease may be underrecognized. Progressive nephrosclerosis from vascular disease is the renal correlate of the same processes that lead to coronary heart disease and cerebrovascular disease. The increasing incidence of CKD in the elderly has been ascribed, in part, to decreased mortality from the cardiac and cerebral complications of atherosclerotic vascular disease in these individuals, enabling a greater segment of the population to manifest the renal component of generalized vascular disease. Nevertheless, it should be appreciated that overwhelmingly the vast majority of those with early stages of renal disease, especially of vascular origin, will succumb to the cardiovascular and cerebrovascular consequences of the vascular disease before they can progress to the most advanced stages of CKD. The early stage of CKD, manifesting as albuminuria and even a minor decrement in GFR, is now recognized as a major risk factor for cardiovascular disease.

The striking interindividual variability in the rate of progression to CKD has an important heritable component, and a number of genetic loci that contribute to the progression of CKD have been identified. Similarly, it has been noted that women of reproductive age are relatively protected against progression of many renal diseases, and sex-specific responses to angiotensin II and its blockade have been identified.

PATHOPHYSIOLOGY AND BIOCHEMISTRY OF UREMIA

Although serum urea and creatinine concentrations are used to measure the excretory capacity of the kidneys,

accumulation of these two molecules themselves do not account for the many symptoms and signs that characterize the uremic syndrome in advanced renal failure. Hundreds of toxins that accumulate in renal failure have been implicated in the uremic syndrome. These include water-soluble, hydrophobic, protein-bound, charged, and uncharged compounds. Additional categories of nitrogenous excretory products include guanido compounds, urates and hippurates, products of nucleic acid metabolism, polyamines, myoinositol, phenols, benzoates, and indoles. Compounds with a molecular mass between 500 and 1500 Da, the so-called middle molecules, are also retained and contribute to morbidity and mortality. It is thus evident that the plasma concentrations of urea and creatinine should be viewed as being readily measured, but incomplete, surrogate markers for these compounds, and monitoring the levels of urea and creatinine in the patient with impaired kidney function represents a vast oversimplification of the uremic state.

The uremic syndrome and the disease state associated with advanced renal impairment involve more than renal excretory failure. A host of metabolic and endocrine functions normally undertaken by the kidneys are also impaired, and this results in anemia, malnutrition, and abnormal metabolism of carbohydrates, fats, and proteins. Furthermore, plasma levels of many hormones, including PTH, insulin, glucagon, sex hormones, and prolactin, change with renal failure as a result of urinary retention, decreased degradation, or abnormal regulation. Finally, progressive renal impairment is associated with worsening systemic inflammation. Elevated levels of C-reactive protein are detected along with other acute-phase reactants, while levels of so-called negative acute-phase reactants, such as albumin and fetuin, decline with progressive renal impairment. Thus, renal impairment is important in the malnutrition-inflammation-atherosclerosis/calcification syndrome, which contributes in turn to the acceleration of vascular disease and comorbidity associated with advanced renal disease.

In summary, the pathophysiology of the uremic syndrome can be divided into manifestations in three spheres of dysfunction: (1) those consequent to the accumulation of toxins normally undergoing renal excretion, including products of protein metabolism; (2) those consequent to the loss of other renal functions, such as fluid and electrolyte homeostasis and hormone regulation; and (3) progressive systemic inflammation and its vascular and nutritional consequences.

CLINICAL AND LABORATORY MANIFESTATIONS OF CHRONIC KIDNEY DISEASE AND UREMIA

Uremia leads to disturbances in the function of virtually every organ system. Chronic dialysis can reduce the incidence and severity of many of these disturbances, so that the overt and florid manifestations of uremia have largely disappeared in the modern health setting. However, as indicated in Table 11-3, even optimal dialysis therapy is not completely effective as renal replacement therapy, because some disturbances resulting from impaired renal function fail to respond to dialysis.

FLUID, ELECTROLYTE, AND ACID-BASE DISORDERS

Sodium and Water Homeostasis

In most patients with stable CKD, the total-body content of sodium and water is modestly increased, although this may not be apparent on clinical examination. Normal renal function guarantees that the tubular reabsorption of filtered sodium and water is adjusted so that urinary excretion matches net intake. Many forms of renal disease (e.g., glomerulonephritis) disrupt this glomerulotubular balance such that dietary intake of sodium exceeds its urinary excretion, leading to sodium retention and attendant extracellular fluid volume (ECFV) expansion. This expansion may contribute to hypertension, which itself can accelerate the nephron injury. As long as water intake does not exceed the capacity for water clearance, the ECFV expansion will be isotonic and the patient will have a normal plasma sodium concentration and effective osmolality (Chap. 2). Hyponatremia is not commonly seen in CKD patients but, when present, can respond to water restriction. If the patient has evidence of ECFV expansion (peripheral edema, sometimes hypertension poorly responsive to therapy) he or she should be counseled regarding salt restriction. Thiazide diuretics have limited utility in stages 3–5 CKD, such that administration of loop diuretics, including furosemide, bumetanide, or torsemide, may also be needed. Resistance to loop diuretics in renal failure often mandates use of higher doses than those used in patients with near-normal kidney function. The combination of loop diuretics with metolazone, which inhibits the

TABLE 11-3

CLINICAL ABNORMALITIES IN UREMIA[a]

Fluid and electrolyte disturbances	Neuromuscular disturbances	Dermatologic disturbances
Volume expansion (I)	Fatigue (I)[b]	Pallor (I)[b]
Hyponatremia (I)	Sleep disorders (P)	Hyperpigmentation (I, P, or D)
Hyperkalemia (I)	Headache (P)	Pruritus (P)
Hyperphosphatemia (I)	Impaired mentation (I)[b]	Ecchymoses (I)
Endocrine-metabolic disturbances	Lethargy (I)[b]	Nephrogenic fibrosing dermopathy (D)
Secondary hyperparathyroidism (I or P)	Asterixis (I)	Uremic frost (I)
Adynamic bone (D)	Muscular irritability	**Gastrointestinal disturbances**
Vitamin D–deficient osteomalacia (I)	Peripheral neuropathy (I or P)	Anorexia (I)
Carbohydrate resistance (I)	Restless legs syndrome (I or P)	Nausea and vomiting (I)
Hyperuricemia (I or P)	Myoclonus (I)	Gastroenteritis (I)
Hypertriglyceridemia (I or P)	Seizures (I or P)	Peptic ulcer (I or P)
Increased Lp(a) level (P)	Coma (I)	Gastrointestinal bleeding (I, P, or D)
Decreased high-density lipoprotein level (P)	Muscle cramps (P or D)	Idiopathic ascites (D)
Protein-energy malnutrition (I or P)	Dialysis disequilibrium syndrome (D)	Peritonitis (D)
Impaired growth and development (P)	Myopathy (P or D)	**Hematologic and immunologic disturbances**
Infertility and sexual dysfunction (P)	**Cardiovascular and pulmonary disturbances**	Anemia (I)[b]
Amenorrhea (I/P)	Arterial hypertension (I or P)	Lymphocytopenia (P)
β₂-Microglobulin associated amyloidosis (P or D)	Congestive heart failure or pulmonary edema (I)	Bleeding diathesis (I or D)[b]
	Pericarditis (I)	Increased susceptibility to infection (I or P)
	Hypertrophic or dilated cardiomyopathy (I, P, or D)	Leukopenia (D)
	Uremic lung (I)	Thrombocytopenia (D)
	Accelerated atherosclerosis (P or D)	
	Hypotension and arrhythmias (D)	
	Vascular calcification (P or D)	

[a]Virtually all abnormalities in this table are completely reversed in time by successful renal transplantation. The response of these abnormalities to hemodialysis or peritoneal dialysis therapy is more variable. (I) denotes an abnormality that usually improves with an optimal program of dialysis and related therapy; (P) denotes an abnormality that tends to persist or even progress, despite an optimal program; (D) denotes an abnormality that develops only after initiation of dialysis therapy.
[b]Improves with dialysis and erythropoietin therapy.
Note: Lp(a), lipoprotein A.

sodium-chloride co-transporter of the distal convoluted tubule, can help effect renal salt excretion. Ongoing diuretic resistance with intractable edema and hypertension in advanced CKD may serve as an indication to initiate dialysis.

In addition to problems with salt and water excretion, some patients with CKD may also have impaired renal conservation of sodium and water. When an extrarenal cause for fluid loss, such as gastrointestinal (GI) loss, is present, these patients may be prone to ECFV depletion because of the inability of the failing kidney to reclaim filtered sodium adequately. Furthermore, depletion of ECFV, whether due to GI losses or overzealous diuretic therapy, can further compromise kidney function on a "pre-renal" basis, lead to acute-on-chronic kidney failure, and result in overt uremia. In this setting, cautious volume repletion with normal saline may return the ECFV to normal and restore renal function to baseline without having to intervene with dialysis.

Potassium Homeostasis

In CKD, the decline in GFR is not necessarily accompanied by a parallel decline in urinary potassium excretion, which is predominantly mediated by aldosterone-dependent secretory events in the distal nephron segments. Another defense against potassium retention in these patients is augmented potassium excretion in the GI tract. Notwithstanding these two homeostatic responses, hyperkalemia may be precipitated in certain settings. These include increased dietary potassium intake, protein catabolism, hemolysis, hemorrhage, transfusion of stored red blood cells, and metabolic acidosis. In addition, a host of medications can inhibit potassium entry into cells and renal potassium excretion. The most important medications in this respect include the angiotensin-converting enzyme (ACE) inhibitors, angiotensin receptor blockers (ARBs), and spironolactone and other potassium-sparing diuretics such as amiloride, eplerenone, and triamterene.

Certain causes of CKD can be associated with earlier and more severe disruption of potassium-secretory mechanisms in the distal nephron, out of proportion to the decline in GFR. These include conditions associated with hyporeninemic hypoaldosteronism, such as diabetes, and renal diseases that preferentially affect the distal nephron, such as obstructive uropathy and sickle cell nephropathy.

Hypokalemia is not common in CKD and usually reflects markedly reduced dietary potassium intake, especially in association with excessive diuretic therapy or concurrent GI losses. Hypokalemia can also occur as a result of primary renal potassium wasting in association with other solute transport abnormalities, such as Fanconi's syndrome, renal tubular acidosis, or other forms of hereditary or acquired tubulointerstitial disease. However, even with these conditions, as the GFR declines,

the tendency to hypokalemia diminishes and hyperkalemia may supervene. Therefore, the use of potassium supplements and potassium-sparing diuretics should be constantly reevaluated as GFR declines.

Metabolic Acidosis

Metabolic acidosis is a common disturbance in advanced CKD. The majority of patients can still acidify the urine, but they produce less ammonia and, therefore, cannot excrete the normal quantity of protons in combination with this urinary buffer. Hyperkalemia, if present, further depresses ammonia production. The combination of hyperkalemia and hyperchloremic metabolic acidosis (known as type IV renal tubular acidosis, or hyporeninemic hypoaldosteronism) is often seen in patients with diabetic nephropathy or in those with predominant tubulointerstitial disease or obstructive uropathy; this is a non–anion-gap metabolic acidosis. Treatment of hyperkalemia may increase renal ammonia production, improve renal generation of bicarbonate, and improve the metabolic acidosis.

With worsening renal function, the total urinary net daily acid excretion is usually limited to 30–40 mmol, and the anions of retained organic acids can then lead to an anion-gap metabolic acidosis. Thus, the non–anion-gap metabolic acidosis that can be seen in earlier stages of CKD may be complicated by the addition of an anion-gap metabolic acidosis as CKD progresses. In most patients, the metabolic acidosis is mild; the pH is rarely <7.35 and can usually be corrected with oral sodium bicarbonate supplementation. Animal and human studies have suggested that even modest degrees of metabolic acidosis may be associated with the development of net protein catabolism, and it has been suggested that alkali supplementation be considered when the serum bicarbonate concentration falls below 20–23 mmol/L. The concomitant sodium load mandates careful attention to volume status and the potential need for diuretic agents.

Rx Treatment: FLUID, ELECTROLYTE, AND ACID-BASE DISORDERS

Adjustments in the dietary intake of salt and use of loop diuretics, occasionally in combination with metolazone, may be needed to maintain euvolemia. In contrast, overzealous salt restriction or diuretic use can lead to ECFV depletion and precipitate a further decline in GFR. The rare patient with salt-losing nephropathy may require a sodium-rich diet or salt supplementation. Water restriction is indicated only if there is a problem with hyponatremia. Otherwise, patients with CKD and an intact thirst mechanism may be instructed to drink fluids in a quantity that keeps them just ahead of their thirst. Intractable ECFV expansion, despite dietary salt restriction and diuretic therapy, may be an indication to start renal replacement therapy. Hyperkalemia often responds to dietary restriction of potassium, avoidance of potassium supplements (including occult sources, such as dietary salt substitutes) or potassium-retaining medications (especially ACE inhibitors or ARBs), or the use of kaliuretic diuretics. Potassium-binding resins, such as calcium resonium or sodium polystyrene, can promote potassium loss through the GI tract and may reduce the incidence of hyperkalemia in CKD patients. Intractable hyperkalemia is an indication (although uncommon) to consider institution of dialysis in a CKD patient. The renal tubular acidosis and subsequent anion-gap metabolic acidosis in progressive CKD will respond to alkali supplementation, typically with sodium bicarbonate. Recent studies suggest that this replacement should be considered when the serum bicarbonate concentration falls to 20 mmol/L to avoid the protein catabolic state seen with even mild degrees of metabolic acidosis.

DISORDERS OF CALCIUM AND PHOSPHATE METABOLISM

The principal complications of abnormalities of calcium and phosphate metabolism in CKD occur in the skeleton and the vascular bed, with occasional severe involvement of extraosseous soft tissues. It is likely that disorders of bone turnover and disorders of vascular and soft tissue calcification are related to each other (Fig. 11-1).

Bone Manifestations of CKD

The major disorders of bone disease can be classified into those associated with high bone turnover with increased PTH levels (including osteitis fibrosa cystica, the classic lesion of secondary hyperparathyroidism) and low bone turnover with low or normal PTH levels (adynamic bone disease and osteomalacia).

The pathophysiology of secondary hyperparathyroidism and the consequent high-turnover bone disease is related to abnormal mineral metabolism through the following events: (1) declining GFR leads to reduced excretion of phosphate, and thus phosphate retention; (2) the retained phosphate stimulates increased synthesis of PTH and growth of parathyroid gland mass; and (3) decreased levels of ionized calcium, resulting from diminished calcitriol production by the failing kidney as well as phosphate retention, also stimulate PTH production. Low calcitriol levels contribute to hyperparathyroidism, both by leading to hypocalcemia and by a direct effect on PTH gene transcription.

In addition to increased production of PTH from the parathyroid cells, the mass of the parathyroid glands increases progressively with CKD. The cell mass may assume one of the following growth patterns: (1) diffuse hyperplasia (polyclonal), (2) nodular growth (monoclonal) within diffuse hyperplasia, or (3) diffuse monoclonal hyperplasia ("adenoma" or tertiary autonomous hyperparathyroidism).

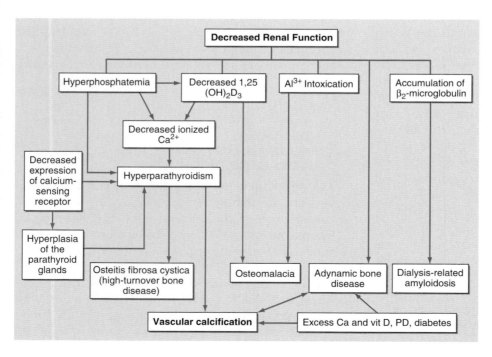

FIGURE 11-1

Flowchart for the development of bone, phosphate, and calcium abnormalities in chronic renal disease. PD, peritoneal dialysis.

Patients with the monoclonal ("autonomous") hyperplasia are especially prone to develop resistant hypercalcemia and may require surgical parathyroidectomy.

The hyperparathyroidism stimulates bone turnover and leads to osteitis fibrosa cystica. Bone histology shows abnormal osteoid, bone and bone marrow fibrosis, and formation of bone cysts, sometimes with hemorrhagic elements so that they appear brown in color, hence the term *brown tumor*. Clinical manifestations of severe hyperparathyroidism include bone pain and fragility, the brown tumors, rare compression syndromes caused by brown tumors, and erythropoietin resistance in part related to the bone marrow fibrosis. Furthermore, PTH is a uremic toxin, and high levels are associated with muscle weakness, fibrosis of cardiac muscle, and nonspecific constitutional symptoms.

Low-turnover bone disease can be grouped into two categories—adynamic bone disease and osteomalacia. In the latter condition, there is accumulation of unmineralized bone matrix that may be caused by vitamin D deficiency, excess aluminum deposition, or even metabolic acidosis. Adynamic bone disease is increasing in prevalence, especially among diabetics and the elderly. It is characterized by reduced bone volume and mineralization and may result from excessive suppression of PTH production. The latter can result from the use of vitamin D preparations or from excessive calcium exposure in the form of calcium-containing phosphate binders or high-calcium dialysis solutions. Complications of adynamic bone disease include an increased incidence of fracture and an association with increased vascular and cardiac calcification.

Calcium, Phosphorus, and the Cardiovascular System

Recent epidemiologic evidence has shown a strong association between hyperphosphatemia and increased cardiovascular mortality in patients with stage 5 CKD and even in patients with earlier stages of CKD. Hyperphosphatemia and hypercalcemia are associated with increased vascular calcification, but it is unclear whether the excessive mortality is mediated by this mechanism. Studies using CT and electron-beam CT scanning show that CKD patients have calcification of coronary arteries and even heart valves that appear to be orders of magnitude greater than that in patients without renal disease. The magnitude of the calcification is proportional to age and hyperphosphatemia and is also associated with low PTH levels and low bone turnover. It is possible that in patients with advanced kidney disease, ingested calcium intake cannot be deposited in bones with low turnover, and therefore is deposited at extraosseous sites, such as the vascular bed and soft tissues. It is interesting in this regard that there is also an association between osteoporosis and vascular calcification in the general population. Finally, there is recent evidence indicating that hyperphosphatemia can induce a change in gene expression in vascular cells to an osteoblast-like profile.

Other Complications of Abnormal Mineral Metabolism

Calciphylaxis is a devastating condition seen almost exclusively in patients with advanced CKD. It is heralded by livedo reticularis and advances to patches of ischemic necrosis, especially on the legs, thighs, abdomen, and breasts (Fig. 11-2). Pathologically, there is evidence of vascular occlusion in association with extensive vascular calcification. It appears that this condition is increasing in incidence. Originally it was ascribed to severe abnormalities in calcium and phosphorus control in dialysis patients, usually associated with advanced hyperparathyroidism. However, more recently, calciphylaxis has been seen with increasing frequency in the absence of severe hyperparathyroidism. Other etiologies have been suggested, including the increased use of oral calcium as a phosphate binder. Warfarin is commonly used in hemodialysis patients, and one of the effects of warfarin therapy is to decrease the vitamin K–dependent regeneration of matrix GLA protein. This latter protein is important in preventing vascular calcification. Thus, warfarin treatment is considered a risk factor for calciphylaxis, and if a patient develops this syndrome, this medication should be discontinued and replaced with alternative forms of anticoagulation.

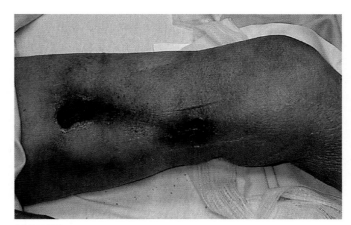

FIGURE 11-2

Calciphylaxis. This peritoneal dialysis patient was on chronic warfarin therapy for prophylactic anticoagulation for a mechanical heart valve. She slept with the dialysis catheter pressed between her legs. A small abrasion was followed by progressive skin necrosis along the catheter tract on her inner thighs. Despite treatment with hyperbaric oxygen, intravenous thiosulfate, and discontinuation of warfarin, she succumbed to systemic complications of the necrotic process.

Treatment:
℞ **DISORDERS OF CALCIUM AND PHOSPHATE METABOLISM**

The optimal management of secondary hyperparathyroidism and osteitis fibrosa is prevention. Once the parathyroid gland mass is very large, it is difficult to control the disease. Careful attention should be paid to the plasma phosphate concentration in CKD patients, who should be counseled on a low-phosphate diet as well as the appropriate use of phosphate-binding agents. These are agents that are taken with meals and complex the dietary phosphate to limit its GI absorption. Examples of phosphate binders are calcium acetate and calcium carbonate. A major side effect of calcium-based phosphate binders is total-body calcium accumulation and hypercalcemia, especially in patients with low-turnover bone disease. Sevelamer, a non-calcium-containing polymer, also functions as a phosphate binder; it does not predispose CKD patients to hypercalcemia, and may attenuate calcium deposition in the vascular bed.

Calcitriol exerts a direct suppressive effect on PTH secretion and also indirectly suppresses PTH secretion by raising the concentration of ionized calcium. However, calcitriol therapy may result in hypercalcemia and/or hyperphosphatemia through increased GI absorption of these minerals. Certain analogues of calcitriol are available (e.g., paricalcitol) that suppress PTH secretion with less attendant hypercalcemia.

Recognition of the role of the extracellular calcium-sensing receptor has led to the development of calcimimetic agents that enhance the sensitivity of the parathyroid cell to the suppressive effect of calcium. This class of drug produces a dose-dependent reduction in PTH and plasma calcium concentration in some patients.

Current KDOQI recommendations call for a target PTH level between 150 and 300 pg/mL, recognizing that very low PTH levels are associated with adynamic bone disease and possible consequences of fracture and ectopic calcification.

CARDIOVASCULAR ABNORMALITIES

Cardiovascular disease is the leading cause of morbidity and mortality in patients at every stage of CKD. The incremental risk of cardiovascular disease in those with CKD compared to the age- and sex-matched general population ranges from 10- to 200-fold, depending on the stage of CKD (Fig. 11-3). Between 30 and 45% of patients reaching stage 5 CKD already have advanced cardiovascular complications. As a result, most patients with CKD succumb to cardiovascular disease (Fig. 11-4) before ever reaching stage 5 CKD. Thus, the focus of patient care in earlier CKD stages should be directed to prevention of cardiovascular complications.

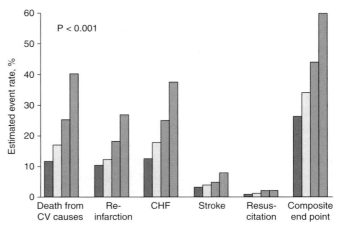

FIGURE 11-3

An analysis of the correlation between the decline in kidney function, as estimated by glomerular filtration rate (GFR), and the increasing incidence of cardiovascular (CV) complications and death from CV disease. Studies such as these suggest that a GFR that is less than normal should be considered a risk factor for CV events and mortality. CHF, congestive heart failure. Volume of GFR in mL/min per 1.73 m^2: 1, ≥75.0; 2, 60.0–74.9; 3, 45.0–59.9; 4, <45. *(From NS Anavekar et al: N Engl J Med 351:1285, 2004.)*

Ischemic Vascular Disease

The presence of any stage of CKD is a major risk factor for ischemic cardiovascular disease, including occlusive coronary, cerebrovascular, and peripheral vascular disease. The increased prevalence of vascular disease in CKD patients derives from both traditional ("classic") and nontraditional (CKD-related) risk factors. Traditional risk factors include hypertension, hypervolemia, dyslipidemia, sympathetic overactivity, and hyperhomocysteinemia. The CKD-related risk factors comprise anemia, hyperphosphatemia,

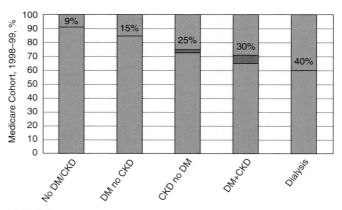

FIGURE 11-4

U.S. Renal Data System showing increased likelihood of dying rather than starting dialysis or reaching stage 5 chronic kidney disease (CKD). 1, Death; 2, ESRD/D; 3, event-free. DM; diabetes mellitus. *(Adapted from Collins, Adv Studies in Med (3c) 2003, Medicare Cohort, 1998–1999.)*

hyperparathyroidism, sleep apnea, and generalized inflammation. The inflammatory state associated with a reduction in kidney function is reflected in increased circulating acute-phase reactants, such as inflammatory cytokines and C-reactive protein, with a corresponding fall in the "negative acute-phase reactants," such as serum albumin and fetuin. The inflammatory state appears to accelerate vascular occlusive disease, and low levels of fetuin may permit more rapid vascular calcification, especially in the face of hyperphosphatemia. Other abnormalities seen in CKD may augment myocardial ischemia, including left ventricular hypertrophy and microvascular disease. Coronary reserve, defined as the increase in coronary blood flow in response to greater demand, is also attenuated. There is diminished availability of nitric oxide because of increased concentration of asymmetric dimethyl-1-arginine and increased scavenging by reactive oxygen species. In addition, hemodialysis, with its attendant episodes of hypotension and hypovolemia, may further aggravate coronary ischemia.

Heart Failure

Abnormal cardiac function secondary to myocardial ischemia, left ventricular hypertrophy, and frank cardiomyopathy, in combination with the salt and water retention that can be seen with CKD, often results in heart failure or even episodes of pulmonary edema. Heart failure can be a consequence of diastolic or systolic dysfunction, or both. A form of "low-pressure" pulmonary edema can also occur in advanced CKD, manifesting as shortness of breath and a "bat wing" distribution of alveolar edema fluid on the chest x-ray. This finding can occur even in the absence of ECFV overload and is associated with normal or mildly elevated pulmonary capillary wedge pressure. This process has been ascribed to increased permeability of alveolar capillary membranes as a manifestation of the uremic state, and it responds to dialysis. Other CKD-related risk factors, including anemia and sleep apnea, may contribute to the risk of heart failure.

Hypertension and Left Ventricular Hypertrophy

Hypertension is one of the most common complications of CKD. It usually develops early during the course of CKD and is associated with adverse outcomes, including the development of ventricular hypertrophy and a more rapid loss of renal function. Many studies have shown a relationship between the level of blood pressure and the rate of progression of diabetic and non–diabetic kidney disease. Left ventricular hypertrophy and dilated cardiomyopathy are among the strongest risk factors for cardiovascular morbidity and mortality in patients with CKD and are thought to be related primarily, but not exclusively, to prolonged hypertension and ECFV overload. In addition, anemia and the placement of an arteriovenous fistula for

hemodialysis can generate a high cardiac output state and consequent heart failure.

The absence of hypertension may signify the presence of a salt-wasting form of renal disease, the effect of antihypertensive therapy, or volume depletion, or may signify poor left ventricular function. Indeed, in epidemiologic studies of dialysis patients, low blood pressure actually carries a worse prognosis than high blood pressure. This mechanism, in part, accounts for the "reverse causation" seen in dialysis patients, wherein the presence of traditional risk factors, such as hypertension, hyperlipidemia, and obesity, appear to portend a better prognosis. Importantly, these observations derive from cross-sectional studies of late-stage CKD patients and should not be interpreted to discourage appropriate management of these risk factors in CKD patients, especially at early stages. In contrast to the general population, it is possible that in late-stage CKD, low blood pressure, reduced body mass index, and hypolipidemia indicate the presence of a malnutrition-inflammation state, with poor prognosis.

The use of exogenous erythropoietic products can increase blood pressure and the requirement for antihypertensive drugs. Chronic ECFV overload is also a contributor to hypertension, and improvement in blood pressure can often be seen with the use of oral sodium restriction, diuretics, and fluid removal with dialysis. Nevertheless, because of activation of the renin–angiotensin–aldosterone axis and other disturbances in the balance of vasoconstrictors and vasodilators, some patients remain hypertensive despite careful attention to ECFV status.

℞ **Treatment:**
CARDIOVASCULAR ABNORMALITIES

MANAGEMENT OF HYPERTENSION There are two overall goals of therapy for hypertension in these patients: to slow the progression of the kidney disease itself, and to prevent the extrarenal complications of high blood pressure, such as cardiovascular disease and stroke. In all patients with CKD, blood pressure should be controlled to levels recommended by national guideline panels. In CKD patients with diabetes or proteinuria >1 g per 24 h, blood pressure should be reduced to 125/75 mmHg, if achievable without prohibitive adverse effects. Salt restriction and diuretics should be the first line of therapy. When volume management alone is not sufficient, the choice of antihypertensive agent is similar to that in the general population. The ACE inhibitors and ARBs slow the rate of decline of kidney function, even in dialysis patients, but their use may be complicated by the development of hyperkalemia. Often the concomitant use of a kaliuretic diuretic, such as metolazone, can improve potassium excretion in addition to improving blood pressure control. Potassium-sparing diuretics should be used with caution or avoided altogether in most patients.

MANAGEMENT OF CARDIOVASCULAR DISEASE There are many strategies available to treat the traditional and nontraditional risk factors in CKD patients. While these have been proven effective in the general population, there is little evidence for their benefit in patients with advanced CKD, especially those on dialysis. Certainly hypertension, elevated serum levels of homocysteine, and dyslipidemia promote atherosclerotic disease and are treatable complications of CKD. Renal disease complicated by nephrotic syndrome is associated with a very atherogenic lipid profile and hypercoagulability, which increases the risk of occlusive vascular disease. Since diabetes mellitus and hypertension are the two most frequent causes of advanced CKD, it is not surprising that cardiovascular disease is the most frequent cause of death in dialysis patients. The role of "inflammation" may be quantitatively more important in patients with kidney disease, and the treatment of more traditional risk factors may result in only modest success. However, modulation of traditional risk factors may be the only weapon in the therapeutic armamentarium for these patients until the nature of inflammation in CKD and its treatment are better understood.

Lifestyle changes, including regular exercise, should be advocated but are not often implemented. Hyperhomocysteinemia may respond to vitamin therapy, including oral folate supplementation, but this therapy is of unproven benefit. Hyperlipidemia in patients with CKD should be managed according to national guidelines. If dietary measures are not sufficient, preferred lipid-lowering medications, such as statins, should be used. Again, the use of these agents has not been of proven benefit for patients with advanced CKD.

Pericardial Disease

Pericardial pain with respiratory accentuation, accompanied by a friction rub, is diagnostic of uremic pericarditis. Classic electrocardiographic abnormalities include PR–interval depression and diffuse ST-segment elevation. Pericarditis can be accompanied by pericardial effusion that is seen on echocardiography and can rarely lead to tamponade. However, the pericardial effusion can be asymptomatic, and pericarditis can be seen without significant effusion.

Pericarditis is observed in advanced uremia, and with the advent of timely initiation of dialysis, is not as common as it once was. It is now more often observed in underdialyzed, nonadherent patients than in those starting dialysis.

℞ **Treatment:**
PERICARDIAL DISEASE

Uremic pericarditis is an absolute indication for the urgent initiation of dialysis or for intensification of the dialysis prescription in those already receiving dialysis. Because of the propensity to hemorrhage in pericardial fluid, hemodialysis should be performed without heparin. A pericardial drainage procedure should be considered in patients with recurrent pericardial effusion. Nonuremic causes of pericarditis and effusion include viral, malignant, tuberculous, and autoimmune etiologies. It may also be seen after myocardial infarction and as a complication of treatment with minoxidil.

HEMATOLOGIC ABNORMALITIES

Anemia

A normocytic, normochromic anemia is observed as early as stage 3 CKD and is almost universal by stage 4. The primary cause in patients with CKD is insufficient production of erythropoietin (EPO) by the diseased kidneys. Additional factors include iron deficiency, acute and chronic inflammation with impaired iron utilization ("anemia of chronic disease"), severe hyperparathyroidism with consequent bone marrow fibrosis, and shortened red cell survival in the uremic environment. Less common causes include folate and vitamin B_{12} deficiency and aluminum toxicity. In addition, comorbid conditions such as hemoglobinopathy can worsen the anemia (Table 11-4).

The anemia of CKD is associated with a number of adverse pathophysiologic consequences, including decreased tissue oxygen delivery and utilization, increased cardiac output, ventricular dilatation, and ventricular hypertrophy. Clinical manifestations include angina, heart failure, decreased cognition and mental acuity, and impaired host defense against infection. In addition, anemia may play a role in growth retardation in children with CKD.

TABLE 11-4

CAUSES OF ANEMIA IN CKD
Relative deficiency of erythropoietin
Diminished red blood cell survival
Bleeding diathesis
Iron deficiency
Hyperparathyroidism/bone marrow fibrosis
"Chronic inflammation"
Folate or vitamin B_{12} deficiency
Hemoglobinopathy
Comorbid conditions: hypo/hyperthyroidism, pregnancy, HIV-associated disease, autoimmune disease, immunosuppressive drugs

While many studies in CKD patients have found that anemia and resistance to exogenous EPO are associated with a poor prognosis, it is unclear as to how much the low hematocrit itself versus inflammation leads to a poor outcome.

℞ Treatment: ANEMIA

The availability of recombinant human EPO and modified EPO products, such as darbepoetin-alpha, has been one of the most significant advances in the care of renal patients since the introduction of dialysis and renal transplantation. The routine use of these products has obviated the need for regular blood transfusions in severely anemic CKD patients, thus dramatically reducing the incidence of transfusion-associated infections and iron overload. Frequent blood transfusions in dialysis patients also led to the development of alloantibodies that could sensitize the patient to donor kidney antigens and make renal transplantation more problematic.

Adequate bone marrow iron stores should be available before treatment with EPO is initiated. Iron supplementation is usually essential to ensure an adequate response to EPO in patients with CKD because the demand for iron by the marrow frequently exceeds the amount of iron that is immediately available for erythropoiesis (measured by percent transferrin saturation), as well as the amount in iron stores (measured by serum ferritin). For the CKD patient not yet on dialysis or the patient treated with peritoneal dialysis, oral iron supplementation should be attempted. If there is GI intolerance, the patient may have to undergo IV iron infusion, often during the dialysis session. In addition to iron, an adequate supply of other major substrates and cofactors for red cell production must be assured, including vitamin B_{12} and folate. Anemia resistant to recommended doses of EPO in the face of adequate iron stores may be due to some combination of the following: acute or chronic inflammation, inadequate dialysis, severe hyperparathyroidism, chronic blood loss or hemolysis, chronic infection, or malignancy. Patients with a hemoglobinopathy, such as sickle cell disease or thalassemia, will usually not respond normally to exogenous EPO; however, an increase in hemoglobin concentration is still seen in many of these patients. Blood transfusions may contribute to suppression of erythropoiesis in CKD; because they increase the risk of hepatitis, iron overload, and transplant sensitization, they should be avoided unless the anemia fails to respond to EPO and the patient is symptomatic.

Normalization of the hemoglobin concentration has not been demonstrated to be of incremental benefit to

dialysis patients. Current practice is to target a hemoglobin concentration of 110 to 120 g/L.

Abnormal Hemostasis

Patients with later stages of CKD may have a prolonged bleeding time, decreased activity of platelet factor III, abnormal platelet aggregation and adhesiveness, and impaired prothrombin consumption. Clinical manifestations include an increased tendency to bleeding and bruising, prolonged bleeding from surgical incisions, menorrhagia, and spontaneous GI bleeding. Interestingly, CKD patients also have a greater susceptibility to thromboembolism, especially if they have renal disease that includes nephrotic-range proteinuria. The latter condition results in hypoalbuminemia and renal loss of anticoagulant factors, which can lead to a thrombophilic state.

℞ Treatment: ABNORMAL HEMOSTASIS

Abnormal bleeding time and coagulopathy in patients with renal failure may be reversed temporarily with desmopressin (DDAVP), cryoprecipitate, IV conjugated estrogens, blood transfusions, and EPO therapy. Optimal dialysis will often correct a prolonged bleeding time.

Given the coexistence of bleeding disorders and a propensity to thrombosis that is unique in the CKD patient, decisions about anticoagulation that have a favorable risk-benefit profile in the general population may not be applicable to the patient with advanced CKD. One example is warfarin anticoagulation for atrial fibrillation: the decision to anticoagulate should be made on an individual basis in the CKD patient.

Certain anticoagulants, such as fractionated low-molecular-weight heparin, may need to be avoided or dose-adjusted in these patients, with monitoring of factor Xa activity where available. It is often more prudent to use conventional high-molecular-weight heparin, titrated to the measured partial thromboplastin time, in hospitalized patients requiring an alternative to warfarin anticoagulation.

NEUROMUSCULAR ABNORMALITIES

Central nervous system (CNS), peripheral, and autonomic neuropathy as well as abnormalities in muscle structure and function are all well-recognized complications of CKD. Retained nitrogenous metabolites and middle molecules, including PTH, contribute to the pathophysiology of neuromuscular abnormalities. Subtle clinical manifestations of uremic neuromuscular disease usually become evident at stage 3 CKD. Early manifestations of CNS complications include mild disturbances in memory and concentration and sleep disturbance. Neuromuscular irritability, including hiccups, cramps, and fasciculations or twitching of muscles, becomes evident at later stages. In advanced untreated kidney failure, asterixis, myoclonus, seizures, and coma can be seen.

Peripheral neuropathy usually becomes clinically evident after the patient reaches stage 4 CKD, although electrophysiologic and histologic evidence occurs earlier. Initially, sensory nerves are involved more than motor, lower extremities more than upper, and distal parts of the extremities more than proximal. The "restless leg syndrome" is characterized by ill-defined sensations of sometimes debilitating discomfort in the legs and feet relieved by frequent leg movement. If dialysis is not instituted soon after onset of sensory abnormalities, motor involvement follows, including muscle weakness. Evidence of peripheral neuropathy without another cause (e.g., diabetes mellitus) is a firm indication for starting renal replacement therapy. Many of the complications described above will resolve with dialysis, although subtle nonspecific abnormalities may persist. Successful renal transplantation may reverse residual neurologic changes.

GASTROINTESTINAL AND NUTRITIONAL ABNORMALITIES

Uremic fetor, a urine-like odor on the breath, derives from the breakdown of urea to ammonia in saliva and is often associated with an unpleasant metallic taste (dysgeusia). Gastritis, peptic disease, and mucosal ulcerations at any level of the GI tract occur in uremic patients and can lead to abdominal pain, nausea, vomiting, and GI bleeding. These patients are also prone to constipation, which can be worsened by the administration of calcium and iron supplements. The retention of uremic toxins also leads to anorexia, nausea, and vomiting.

Protein restriction may be useful to decrease nausea and vomiting; however, it may put the patient at risk for malnutrition and should be carried out, if possible, in consultation with a registered dietitian. Protein-energy malnutrition, a consequence of low protein and caloric intake, is common in advanced CKD and is often an indication for initiation of renal replacement therapy. In addition to diminished intake, these patients are resistant to the anabolic actions of insulin and other hormones and growth factors. Metabolic acidosis and the activation of inflammatory cytokines can promote protein catabolism. Assessment for protein-energy malnutrition should begin at stage 3 CKD. A number of indices are useful in this assessment and include dietary history, including diary and subjective global assessment; edema-free body weight; serum albumin concentration; and measurement of urinary protein nitrogen appearance. Dual-energy x-ray absorptiometry is now widely used to estimate lean body mass versus ECFV. Adjunctive tools include clinical signs, such as skinfold thickness, mid-arm muscle circumference, and additional laboratory tests such as serum pre-albumin and cholesterol levels. Nutritional guidelines for patients with CKD are summarized in the section on "Treatment of Chronic Kidney Disease."

ENDOCRINE-METABOLIC DISTURBANCES

Glucose metabolism is impaired in CKD, as evidenced by slowing of the rate at which blood glucose levels decline after a glucose load. However, fasting blood glucose is usually normal or only slightly elevated, and the mild glucose intolerance does not require specific therapy. Because the kidney contributes to insulin removal from the circulation, plasma levels of insulin are slightly to moderately elevated in most uremic patients, both in the fasting and postprandial states. Because of this diminished renal degradation of insulin, patients on insulin therapy may need progressive reduction in dose as their renal function worsens. Many hypoglycemic agents require dose reduction in renal failure, and some, such as metformin, are contraindicated when the GFR is less than half of normal.

In women with CKD, estrogen levels are low, and menstrual abnormalities and inability to carry pregnancies to term are common. When the GFR has declined to ~40 mL/min, pregnancy is associated with a high rate of spontaneous abortion, with only ~20% of pregnancies leading to live births, and pregnancy may hasten the progression of the kidney disease itself. Men with CKD have reduced plasma testosterone levels, and sexual dysfunction and oligospermia may supervene. Sexual maturation may be delayed or impaired in adolescent children with CKD, even among those treated with dialysis. Many of these abnormalities improve or reverse with intensive dialysis or successful renal transplantation.

DERMATOLOGIC ABNORMALITIES

Abnormalities of the skin are prevalent in progressive CKD. Anemic patients may be pale, and those with defective hemostasis may show multiple ecchymoses. Pruritus is quite common. In advanced CKD, even on dialysis, patients may become more pigmented, and this is felt to reflect the deposition of retained pigmented metabolites, or *urochromes*. Although many of the cutaneous abnormalities improve with dialysis, pruritus is often tenacious. The first lines of management are to rule out unrelated skin disorders, such as scabies, and to control phosphate concentration. EPO therapy was initially reported to improve uremic pruritus, although that is not always the case. Local moisturizers, mild topical glucocorticoids, oral antihistamines, and ultraviolet radiation have been reported to be helpful.

A skin condition called *nephrogenic fibrosing dermopathy* has recently been reported in which progressive subcutaneous induration, especially on the arms and legs, is described. The condition is similar to scleromyxedema and is seen in patients with CKD, most commonly on dialysis. Recent reports suggest that exposure to the magnetic resonance contrast agent, gadolinium, may precipitate this syndrome.

EVALUATION AND MANAGEMENT OF PATIENTS WITH CKD

INITIAL APPROACH

History and Physical Examination

Symptoms and overt signs of kidney disease are often absent until renal failure supervenes. Thus, the diagnosis of kidney disease often surprises patients and may be a cause of skepticism and denial. Particular aspects of the history that are germane to renal disease include a history of hypertension (which can cause CKD or be a reflection of CKD), diabetes mellitus, abnormal urinalyses, and problems with pregnancy such as preeclampsia or early pregnancy loss. A careful drug history should be elicited: patients may not volunteer use of analgesics, for example. Other drugs to consider include nonsteroidal anti-inflammatory agents, gold, penicillamine, antimicrobials, antiretroviral agents, proton pump inhibitors, and lithium. In evaluating the uremic syndrome, questions about appetite, weight loss, nausea, hiccups, peripheral edema, muscle cramps, pruritus, and restless legs are especially helpful.

The physical examination should focus on blood pressure and target organ damage from hypertension. Thus, funduscopy and precordial examination (left ventricular heave, a fourth heart sound) should be carried out. Funduscopy is important in the diabetic patient, seeking evidence of diabetic retinopathy, which is associated with nephropathy. Other physical examination manifestations of CKD include edema and sensory polyneuropathy. The finding of asterixis or a pericardial friction rub not attributable to other causes usually signifies the presence of the uremic syndrome.

Laboratory Investigation

Laboratory studies should focus on a search for clues to an underlying causative or aggravating disease process and on the degree of renal damage and its consequences. If appropriate, tests for systemic lupus erythematosus and vasculitis should be performed. Serum and urine protein electrophoresis should be obtained in all patients >35 years with unexplained CKD, especially if there is associated anemia and elevated, or even inappropriately normal, serum calcium concentration in the face of renal insufficiency. In the presence of glomerulonephritis, underlying infectious etiologies such as hepatitis B and C and HIV should be assessed. Serial measurements of renal function should be obtained to determine the pace of renal deterioration and ensure that the disease is truly chronic rather than subacute and hence potentially reversible. Serum concentrations of calcium, phosphorus, and PTH should be measured to evaluate metabolic bone disease. Hemoglobin concentration, iron, B_{12}, and folate should also be evaluated. A 24-h urine collection may be helpful, as protein excretion >300 mg may be an indication for therapy with ACE inhibitors or ARBs.

Imaging Studies

The most useful imaging study is a renal ultrasound, which can verify the presence of two kidneys, determine if they are symmetric, provide an estimate of kidney size, and rule out renal masses and evidence of obstruction. Since it takes time for kidneys to shrink as a result of chronic disease, the finding of bilaterally small kidneys supports the diagnosis of CKD of long-standing duration, with an irreversible component of scarring. If the kidney size is normal, it is possible that the renal disease is acute or subacute. The exceptions are diabetic nephropathy (where kidney size is increased at the outset of diabetic nephropathy before CKD with loss of GFR supervenes), amyloidosis, and HIV nephropathy, where kidney size may be normal in the face of CKD. Polycystic kidney disease that has reached some degree of renal failure will almost always present with enlarged kidneys with multiple cysts (Chap. 16). A discrepancy >1 cm in kidney length suggests either a unilateral developmental abnormality or disease process or renovascular disease with arterial insufficiency affecting one kidney more than the other. The diagnosis of renovascular disease can be undertaken with different techniques, including Doppler sonography, nuclear medicine studies, or CT or MRI studies. If there is a suspicion of reflux nephropathy (recurrent childhood urinary tract infection, asymmetric renal size with scars on the renal poles), a voiding cystogram may be indicated. However, in most cases by the time the patient has CKD, the reflux has resolved, and even if still present, repair does not improve renal function. Radiographic contrast imaging studies are not particularly helpful in the investigation of CKD. Intravenous or intraarterial dye should be avoided where possible in the CKD patient, especially with diabetic nephropathy, because of the risk of radiographic contrast dye–induced renal failure. When unavoidable, appropriate precautionary measures include avoidance of hypovolemia at the time of contrast exposure, minimization of the dye load, and choice of radiographic contrast preparations with the least nephrotoxic potential.

Renal Biopsy

In the patient with bilaterally small kidneys, renal biopsy is not advised because (1) it is technically difficult and has a greater likelihood of causing bleeding and other adverse consequences, (2) there is usually so much scarring that the underlying disease may not be apparent, and (3) the window of opportunity to render disease-specific therapy has passed. Other contraindications to renal biopsy include uncontrolled hypertension, active urinary tract infection, bleeding diathesis, and morbid obesity. Ultrasound-guided percutaneous biopsy is the favored approach, but a surgical or laparoscopic approach can be considered, especially in the patient with a single kidney where direct visualization and control of bleeding are crucial. In the CKD patient in whom a kidney biopsy is indicated (e.g., suspicion of a concomitant or superimposed active process, such as interstitial nephritis or accelerated loss of GFR), the bleeding time should be measured, and, if increased, desmopressin should be administered immediately prior to the procedure. A brief run of hemodialysis (without heparin) may also be considered prior to renal biopsy to normalize the bleeding time.

ESTABLISHING THE DIAGNOSIS AND ETIOLOGY OF CKD

The most important initial diagnostic step in the evaluation of a patient presenting with elevated serum creatinine is to distinguish newly diagnosed CKD from acute or subacute renal failure because the latter two conditions may respond to therapy specific to the disease. Previous measurements of plasma creatinine concentration are particularly helpful in this regard. Normal values from recent months or even years suggest that the current extent of renal dysfunction could be more acute, and hence reversible, than might otherwise be appreciated. In contrast, elevated plasma creatinine concentration in the past suggests that the renal disease represents the progression of a chronic process. Even if there is evidence of chronicity, there is the possibility of a superimposed acute process, such as ECFV depletion, supervening on the chronic condition. If the history suggests multiple systemic manifestations of recent onset (e.g., fever, polyarthritis, and rash) it should be assumed that renal insufficiency is part of the acute process.

Some of the laboratory tests and imaging studies outlined above can be helpful. Evidence of metabolic bone disease with hyperphosphatemia, hypocalcemia, and elevated PTH and bone alkaline phosphatase levels suggests chronicity. Normochromic, normocytic anemia suggests that the process has been ongoing for some time. The finding of bilaterally reduced kidney size (<8.5 cm in all but the smallest adults) favors CKD.

While renal biopsy can usually be performed in early CKD (stages 1–3), it is not always indicated. For example,

in a patient with a history of Type 1 diabetes mellitus for 15–20 years with retinopathy, nephrotic-range proteinuria, and absence of hematuria, the diagnosis of diabetic nephropathy is very likely and biopsy is not necessary. However, if there were some other finding not typical of diabetic nephropathy, such as hematuria or white blood cell casts, some other disease may be present and a biopsy may be indicated. Hypertensive nephrosclerosis and progressive ischemic nephropathy are usually diagnosed clinically by the presence of long-standing hypertension, evidence of ischemic disease elsewhere (e.g., cardiac or peripheral vascular disease), and the finding of only mild (<3 g/d) proteinuria in the absence of urinary blood or red cell casts. It is important to consider progressive ischemic nephropathy because a small subset of these patients may respond to revascularization procedures, although this remains controversial.

In the absence of a clinical diagnosis, renal biopsy may be the only recourse to establish an etiology in early-stage CKD. However, as noted above, once the CKD is advanced and the kidneys are small and scarred, there is little utility and significant risk in attempting to arrive at a specific diagnosis.

℞ **Treatment:**
CHRONIC KIDNEY DISEASE

Treatments aimed at specific causes of CKD are discussed elsewhere. The optimal timing of therapy is usually well before there has been a measurable decline in GFR and certainly before CKD is established (Table 11-5). It is helpful to sequentially measure and plot the rate of decline of GFR in all patients. Any acceleration in the rate of decline should prompt a search for superimposed acute or subacute processes that may be reversible. These include ECFV depletion, uncontrolled hypertension, urinary tract infection, new obstructive uropathy, exposure to nephrotoxic agents [such as nonsteroidal anti-inflammatory drugs (NSAIDs) or radiographic dye], and reactivation or flare of the original disease, such as lupus or vasculitis.

SLOWING THE PROGRESSION OF CKD There is variation in the rate of decline of GFR among patients with CKD. However, the following interventions should be considered in an effort to stabilize or slow the decline of renal function.

Protein Restriction While protein restriction has been advocated to reduce symptoms associated with uremia, it may also slow the rate of renal decline at earlier stages of renal disease. This concept is based on clinical and experimental evidence that protein-mediated hyperfiltration contributes to ongoing decline in renal function in many different forms of renal disease.

TABLE 11-5

CLINICAL ACTION PLAN

STAGE	DESCRIPTION	GFR, mL/min PER 1.73 m²	ACTION[a]
1	Kidney damage with normal or ↑ GFR	≥90	Diagnosis and treatment, treatment of comorbid conditions, slowing progression, CVD risk reduction
2	Kidney damage with mild ↓ GFR	60–89	Estimating progression
3	Moderate ↓ GFR	30–59	Evaluating and treating complications
4	Severe ↓ GFR	15–29	Preparation for kidney replacement therapy
5	Kidney failure	<15 (or dialysis)	Kidney replacement (if uremia present)

[a]Includes actions from preceding stages.
Note: CVD, cardiovascular disease.
Source: National Kidney Foundation: Am J Kidney Dis 39 (2 Suppl 1): S1, 2002.

A number of studies have shown that protein restriction may be effective in slowing the progression of CKD, especially proteinuric and diabetic renal diseases. However, the Modification of Diet in Renal Disease study was unable to demonstrate a robust benefit in delaying progression to advanced stages of CKD with dietary restriction of protein intake. Nonetheless, restriction of dietary protein intake has been recommended for CKD patients. KDOQI clinical practice guidelines include a daily protein intake of between 0.60 and 0.75 g/kg/d, depending upon patient adherence, comorbid disease, presence of proteinuria, and nutritional status. It is further advised that at least 50% of the protein intake be of high biologic value. As patients approach stage 5 CKD, spontaneous protein intake tends to decrease, and patients may enter a state of protein-energy malnutrition. In these circumstances, a protein intake of up to 0.90 g/kg/d might be recommended, again, with an emphasis on proteins of high biologic value.

Sufficient energy intake is important to prevent protein-calorie malnutrition, and 35 kcal/kg is recommended. Monitoring of parameters of nutritional status must accompany the dietary intervention, using the parameters outlined above in the section on GI and nutritional abnormalities.

Reducing Intraglomerular Hypertension and Proteinuria Increased intraglomerular filtration pressures and glomerular hypertrophy develop as a response to loss of nephron number from different kidney diseases. This response is maladaptive, as it promotes the ongoing decline of kidney function even if the inciting process has been treated or spontaneously resolved. Control of systemic and glomerular hypertension is at least as important as dietary protein restriction in slowing the progression of CKD. Therefore, in addition to reduction of cardiovascular disease risk, antihypertensive therapy in patients with CKD also aims to slow the progression of nephron injury by reducing intraglomerular hypertension. Elevated blood pressure increases proteinuria through its transmission to the glomerulus. Conversely, the renoprotective effect of antihypertensive medications is gauged through the consequent reduction of proteinuria. Thus, the more effective a given treatment is in lowering protein excretion, the greater the subsequent impact on protection from decline in GFR. This observation is the basis for the treatment guideline establishing 125/75 mmHg as the target blood pressure in proteinuric CKD patients.

ACE inhibitors and ARBs inhibit the angiotensin-induced vasoconstriction of the efferent arterioles of the glomerular microcirculation. This inhibition leads to a reduction in both intraglomerular filtration pressure and proteinuria. Several controlled studies have shown that these drugs are effective in slowing the progression of renal failure in patients with both diabetic and nondiabetic renal failure. This slowing in progression of CKD is strongly associated with their proteinuria-lowering effect. In the absence of an anti-proteinuric response with either agent alone, combined treatment with both ACE inhibitors and ARBs can be tried. Adverse effects from these agents include cough and angioedema with ACE inhibitors, anaphylaxis, and hyperkalemia with either class. A progressive increase in plasma creatinine concentration may suggest the presence of renovascular disease within the large or small arteries. Development of these side effects may mandate the use of second-line antihypertensive agents instead of the ACE inhibitors or ARBs. Among the calcium channel blockers, diltiazem and verapamil may exhibit superior anti-proteinuric and renoprotective effects compared to the dihydropyridines. At least two different categories of response can be considered: one in which progression is strongly associated with systemic and intraglomerular hypertension and proteinuria (e.g., diabetic nephropathy,

CHAPTER 11 Chronic Kidney Disease

SECTION III

Acute and Chronic Renal Failure

glomerular diseases) and in which ACE inhibitors and ARBs are likely to be the first choice; and another in which proteinuria is mild or absent initially (e.g., adult polycystic kidney disease and other tubulointerstitial diseases) and hence the contribution of intraglomerular hypertension less prominent, for which reason other antihypertensive agents can be useful for control of systemic hypertension.

SLOWING PROGRESSION OF DIABETIC RENAL DISEASE

Diabetic nephropathy is now the leading cause of CKD requiring renal replacement therapy in many parts of the world, and its prevalence is increasing disproportionately in the developing world. Furthermore, the prognosis of diabetic patients on dialysis is poor, with survival comparable to many forms of cancer. Accordingly, it is mandatory to develop strategies whose aim is to prevent or slow the progression of diabetic nephropathy in these patients.

Control of Blood Glucose Excellent glycemic control reduces the risk of kidney disease and its progression in both Type 1 and Type 2 diabetes mellitus. It is recommended that plasma values for preprandial glucose be kept in the 5.0–7.2 mmol/L (90–130 mg/dL) range and hemoglobin A_{1C} should be <7%. As the GFR decreases with progressive nephropathy, the use and dose of oral hypoglycemics needs to be reevaluated. For example, chlorpropamide may be associated with prolonged hypoglycemia in patients with decreased renal function; metformin has been reported to cause lactic acidosis in the patient with renal impairment and should be discontinued when the GFR is reduced; and the thiazolidinediones (e.g., rosiglitazone, pioglitazone, and others) may increase renal salt and water absorption and aggravate volume-overloaded states. Finally, as renal function declines, renal degradation of administered insulin will also decline, so that less insulin may be required for glycemic control.

Control of Blood Pressure and Proteinuria Hypertension is found in the majority of Type 2 diabetic patients at diagnosis. This finding correlates with the presence of albuminuria and is a strong predictor of cardiovascular events and nephropathy. Microalbuminuria, the finding of albumin in the urine not detectable by the urine dipstick, precedes the decline in GFR and heralds renal and cardiovascular complications. Testing for microalbumin is recommended in all diabetic patients, at least annually. If the patient already has established proteinuria, then testing for microalbumin is not necessary. Antihypertensive treatment reduces albuminuria and diminishes its progression even in normotensive diabetic patients. In addition to treatment of hypertension in general, the use of ACE inhibitors and ARBs in particular is associated with additional renoprotection. These salutary effects are mediated by reducing intraglomerular pressure and inhibition of angiotensin-driven sclerosing pathways, in part through inhibition of TGF-β-mediated pathways.

MANAGING OTHER COMPLICATIONS OF CHRONIC KIDNEY DISEASE

Medication Dose Adjustment Although the loading dose of most drugs is not affected by CKD because no renal elimination is used in the calculation, the maintenance doses of many drugs will need to be adjusted. For those agents in which >70% excretion is by a nonrenal route, such as hepatic elimination, dose adjustment may not be needed. Some drugs that should be avoided include metformin, meperidine, and oral hypoglycemics that are eliminated by the kidney. NSAIDs should be avoided because of the risk of further worsening of kidney function. Many antibiotics, antihypertensives, and antiarrhythmics may require a reduction in dosage or change in the dose interval. For a comprehensive, detailed listing of the dose adjustments for most of the commonly used medications, see "Drug Prescribing in Renal Failure" published by the American College of Physicians (see *www.acponline.org*).

Preparation for Renal Replacement Therapy (See also Chap. 13.) Temporary relief of symptoms and signs of impending uremia, such as anorexia, nausea, vomiting, lassitude, and pruritus, may sometimes be achieved with protein restriction. However, this carries a significant risk of protein-energy malnutrition, and thus plans for more long-term management should be in place.

The institution of maintenance dialysis and kidney transplantation has extended the lives of hundreds of thousands of patients with CKD worldwide. Clear indications for initiation of renal replacement therapy for patients with CKD include pericarditis, encephalopathy, intractable muscle cramping, anorexia, and nausea not attributable to reversible causes such as peptic ulcer disease, evidence of malnutrition, and fluid and electrolyte abnormalities, principally hyperkalemia, that are refractory to other measures.

Recommendations for the optimal time for initiation of renal replacement therapy have been established by the National Kidney Foundation in their KDOQI guidelines and are based on recent evidence demonstrating that delaying initiation of renal replacement therapy until patients are malnourished or have severe uremic complications leads to a worse prognosis on dialysis or with transplantation. Because of the interindividual variability in the severity of uremic symptoms and renal function, it is ill-advised to assign an arbitrary urea nitrogen or creatinine level to the need to start dialysis. Moreover, patients may become accustomed to chronic uremia and deny symptoms, only to find that they feel better with dialysis and realize in retrospect how poorly they were feeling before its initiation.

Previous studies suggested that starting dialysis before the onset of severe symptoms and signs of uremia was associated with prolongation of survival. This led to the concept of a "healthy" start and is congruent with the philosophy that it is better to keep patients feeling well all along, rather than allowing them to become ill with uremia before trying to return them to better health with dialysis. Although recent studies have not confirmed a clear association of early-start dialysis with improved patient survival, there is still merit in this approach. On a practical level, advanced preparation may help to avoid problems with the dialysis process itself (e.g., a poorly functioning fistula for hemodialysis or malfunctioning peritoneal dialysis catheter) and thus preempt the morbidity associated with resorting to the insertion of temporary hemodialysis access with its attendant risks of sepsis, bleeding, and thrombosis.

Patient Education Social, psychological, and physical preparation for the transition to renal replacement therapy and the choice of the optimal initial modality are best accomplished with a gradual approach involving a multidisciplinary team. Along with conservative measures discussed in the sections above, it is important to prepare patients with an intensive educational program, explaining the likelihood and timing of initiation of renal replacement therapy and the various forms of therapy available. The more knowledgeable that patients are about hemodialysis (both in-center and home based), peritoneal dialysis, and kidney transplantation, the easier and more appropriate will be their decisions. Patients who are provided with educational programs are more likely to choose home-based dialysis therapy. This approach is of societal benefit because home-based therapy is less expensive and is associated with improved quality of life. The educational programs should be commenced no later than stage 4 CKD so that the patient has sufficient cognitive function to learn the important concepts.

Exploration of social service support is also important. In those who may perform home dialysis or undergo preemptive renal transplantation, early education of family members for selection and preparation of a home dialysis helper or a related (or unrelated) kidney donor should occur long before the onset of symptomatic renal failure.

Kidney transplantation (Chap. 13) offers the best potential for complete rehabilitation, because dialysis replaces only a small fraction of the kidneys' filtration function and none of the other renal functions, including endocrine and anti-inflammatory effects. Generally, kidney transplantation follows a period of dialysis treatment, although preemptive kidney transplantation (usually from a living donor) can be carried out if it is certain that the renal failure is irreversible.

IMPLICATIONS FOR GLOBAL HEALTH

In distinction to the natural decline and successful eradication of many devastating infectious diseases, there is rapid growth in the prevalence of hypertension and vascular disease in developing countries. Diabetes mellitus is becoming increasingly prevalent in these countries, perhaps due in part to change in dietary habits, diminished physical activity, and weight gain. Therefore, it follows that there will be a proportionate increase in vascular and renal disease. Health care agencies must plan for improved screening for early detection, prevention, and treatment plans in these nations and must start considering options for improved availability of renal replacement therapies.

FURTHER READINGS

BANSAL N et al: Long-term outcomes of patients with chronic kidney disease. Nat Clin Pract Nephrol 4:532, 2008

BAUER C et al: Staging of chronic kidney disease: Time for a course correction. J Am Soc Nephrol 19:844, 2008

CHOUDHURY D et al: Preventive health care in chronic kidney disease and end-stage renal disease. Nat Clin Pract Nephrol 4:194, 2008

DELANAYE P et al: Determining prevalence of chronic kidney disease using estimated glomerular filtration rate. JAMA 299:631, 2008

GO A et al: Chronic kidney disease and the risks of death, cardiovascular events, and hospitalization. N Engl J Med 351:1296, 2004

KETTELER M et al: Calcification and cardiovascular health: New insights into an old phenomenon. Hypertension 47:1027, 2006

LEVEY AS et al: CKD: Common, harmful and treatable—World Kidney Day 2007. Am J Kidney Dis 49(2), 2007

NATIONAL KIDNEY FOUNDATION: Kidney Disease Outcomes Quality Initiative *Clinical Practice Guidelines for Nutrition in Chronic Renal Failure.* Am J Kidney Dis 35 (suppl 2): S1, 2000

————: K/DOQI Clinical Practice Guidelines for Chronic Kidney Disease: Evaluation, classification and stratification. Am J Kidney Dis 39 (suppl 1), 2000

O'HARE AM et al: Current guidelines for using angiotensin-converting enzyme inhibitors and angiotensin II-receptor antagonists in chronic kidney disease: Is the evidence base relevant to older adults? Ann Intern Med 150:717, 2009

SARNAK M et al: Kidney disease as a risk factor for development of cardiovascular disease: A statement from the American Heart Association Councils on Kidney in Cardiovascular Disease, High Blood Pressure Research, Clinical Cardiology, and Epidemiology and Prevention. Circulation 108:2154, 2003

STRONG K et al: Preventing chronic disease: How many lives can we save? Lancet 366:1578, 2005

WATTANAKIT K et al: Chronic kidney disease increases risk for venous thromboembolism. J Am Soc Nephrol 19:135, 2008

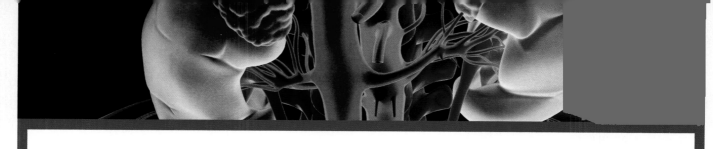

CHAPTER 12

DIALYSIS IN THE TREATMENT OF RENAL FAILURE

Kathleen D. Liu ■ Glenn M. Chertow

Dialysis may be required for the treatment of either acute or chronic kidney disease. The use of continuous renal replacement therapies (CRRT) and slow, low-efficiency dialysis (SLED) is specific to the management of acute renal failure and is discussed in Chap. 10. These modalities are performed continuously (CRRT) or over 6–12 hours per session (SLED), in contrast to the 3–4 hours of an intermittent hemodialysis session. Advantages and disadvantages of CRRT and SLED are discussed in Chap. 10.

Peritoneal dialysis is rarely used in developed countries for the treatment of acute renal failure because of the increased risk of infection and less efficient clearance per unit of time. The focus of the majority of this chapter is on the use of dialysis for end-stage renal disease (ESRD).

With the widespread availability of dialysis, the lives of hundreds of thousands of patients with ESRD have been prolonged. In the United States alone, there are now approximately 450,000 patients with ESRD, the vast majority of whom require dialysis. The incidence rate for ESRD is 330 cases per million people per year. The incidence of ESRD is disproportionately higher in African Americans (approximately 1000 per million people per year) as compared with white Americans (259 per million people per year). In the United States, the leading cause of ESRD is diabetes mellitus, currently accounting for nearly 45% of newly diagnosed cases of ESRD. Over one-quarter (27%) of patients have ESRD that has been attributed to hypertension, although it is unclear in these cases whether hypertension is the cause or a consequence of vascular disease or other unknown causes of kidney failure. Other important causes of ESRD include glomerulonephritis, polycystic kidney disease, and obstructive uropathy.

Globally, mortality rates for patients with ESRD are lowest in Europe and Japan but very high in the developing world because of the limited availability of dialysis. In the United States, the mortality rate of patients on dialysis is approximately 18–20% per year, with a 5-year survival rate of approximately 30–35%. Deaths are due mainly to cardiovascular diseases and infections (approximately 50 and 15% of deaths, respectively). Older age, male sex, nonblack race, diabetes mellitus, malnutrition, and underlying heart disease are important predictors of death.

TREATMENT OPTIONS FOR ESRD PATIENTS

Commonly accepted criteria for initiating patients on maintenance dialysis include the presence of uremic symptoms, the presence of hyperkalemia unresponsive to conservative measures, persistent extracellular volume expansion despite diuretic therapy, acidosis refractory to medical therapy, a bleeding diathesis, and a creatinine clearance or estimated glomerular filtration rate (GFR) below 10 mL/min per 1.73 m^2 (see Chap. 11 for estimating equations). Timely referral to a nephrologist for advanced planning and creation of a dialysis access, education about ESRD treatment options, and management of the complications of advanced chronic kidney disease, including hypertension, anemia, acidosis, and secondary hyperparathyroidism, is advisable.

In ESRD, treatment options include hemodialysis (in center or at home); peritoneal dialysis, as either continuous ambulatory peritoneal dialysis (CAPD) or continuous cyclic peritoneal dialysis (CCPD); or transplantation (Chap. 13). Although there are geographic variations, hemodialysis remains the most common therapeutic modality for ESRD (>90% of patients) in the United States. In contrast to hemodialysis, peritoneal dialysis is continuous, but much less efficient, in terms of solute clearance. While no large-scale clinical trials have been completed comparing outcomes among patients randomized to either hemodialysis or peritoneal dialysis, outcomes associated with both therapies are similar in most reports, and the decision of which modality to select is often based on personal preferences and quality-of-life considerations.

Hemodialysis relies on the principles of solute diffusion across a semipermeable membrane. Movement of metabolic waste products takes place down a concentration gradient from the circulation into the dialysate. The rate of diffusive transport increases in response to several factors, including the magnitude of the concentration gradient, the membrane surface area, and the mass transfer coefficient of the membrane. The latter is a function of the porosity and thickness of the membrane, the size of the solute molecule, and the conditions of flow on the two sides of the membrane. According to the laws of diffusion, the larger the molecule, the slower its rate of transfer across the membrane. A small molecule, such as urea (60 Da), undergoes substantial clearance, whereas a larger molecule, such as creatinine (113 Da), is cleared less efficiently. In addition to diffusive clearance, movement of waste products from the circulation into the dialysate may occur as a result of ultrafiltration. Convective clearance occurs because of solvent drag, with solutes being swept along with water across the semipermeable dialysis membrane.

THE DIALYZER

There are three essential components to hemodialysis: the dialyzer, the composition and delivery of the dialysate, and the blood delivery system (**Fig. 12-1**). The dialyzer

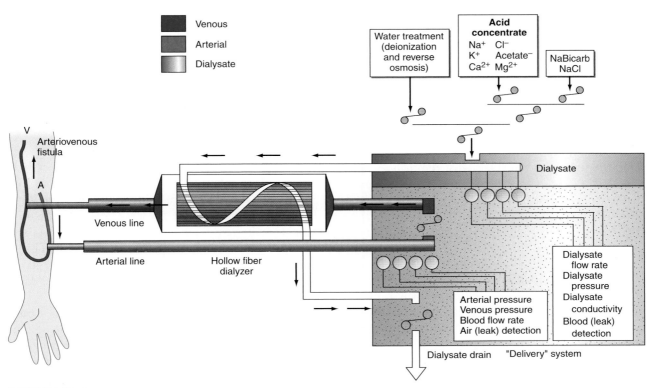

FIGURE 12-1
Schema for hemodialysis.

consists of a plastic device with the facility to perfuse blood and dialysate compartments at very high flow rates. The surface area of modern dialysis membranes in adult patients is usually in the range of 1.5–2.0 m². The hollow-fiber dialyzer is the most common in use in the United States. These dialyzers are composed of bundles of capillary tubes through which blood circulates while dialysate travels on the outside of the fiber bundle.

Recent advances have led to the development of many different types of membrane material. Broadly, there are four categories of dialysis membranes: cellulose, substituted cellulose, cellulosynthetic, and synthetic. Over the past three decades, there has been a gradual switch from cellulose-derived to synthetic membranes, because the latter are more "biocompatible." *Bioincompatibility* is generally defined as the ability of the membrane to activate the complement cascade. Cellulosic membranes are bioincompatible because of the presence of free hydroxyl groups on the membrane surface. In contrast, with the substituted cellulose membranes (e.g., cellulose acetate) or the cellulosynthetic membranes, the hydroxyl groups are chemically bound to either acetate or tertiary amino groups, resulting in limited complement activation. Synthetic membranes, such as polysulfone, polymethylmethacrylate, and polyacrylonitrile membranes, are even more biocompatible because of the absence of these hydroxyl groups. Polysulfone membranes are now used in >60% of the dialysis treatments in the United States.

Reprocessing and reuse of hemodialyzers are often employed for patients on maintenance hemodialysis in the United States. However, as the manufacturing costs for disposable dialyzers have declined, more and more outpatient dialysis facilities are no longer reprocessing dialyzers. In most centers employing reuse, only the dialyzer unit is reprocessed and reused, whereas in the developing world blood lines are also frequently reused. The reprocessing procedure can be either manual or automated. It consists of the sequential rinsing of the blood and dialysate compartments with water, a chemical cleansing step with reverse ultrafiltration from the dialysate to the blood compartment, the testing of the patency of the dialyzer, and, finally, disinfection of the dialyzer. Formaldehyde, peracetic acid–hydrogen peroxide, glutaraldehyde, and bleach have all been used as reprocessing agents.

DIALYSATE

The potassium concentration of dialysate may be varied from 0 to 4 mmol/L depending on the predialysis plasma potassium concentration. The usual dialysate calcium concentration in U.S. hemodialysis centers is 1.25 mmol/L (2.5 meq/L), although modification may be required in selected settings (e.g., higher dialysate calcium concentrations may be used in patients with hypocalcemia associated with secondary hyperparathyroidism or following parathyroidectomy). The usual dialysate sodium concentration is 140 mmol/L. Lower dialysate sodium concentrations are associated with a higher frequency of hypotension, cramping, nausea, vomiting, fatigue, and dizziness. In patients who frequently develop hypotension during their dialysis run, "sodium modeling" to counterbalance urea-related osmolar gradients is often used. When sodium modeling, the dialysate sodium concentration is gradually lowered from the range of 145–155 meq/L to isotonic concentrations (140 meq/L) near the end of the dialysis treatment, typically declining either in steps or in a linear or exponential fashion. Because patients are exposed to approximately 120 L of water during each dialysis treatment, water used for the dialysate is subjected to filtration, softening, deionization, and, ultimately, reverse osmosis. During the reverse osmosis process, water is forced through a semipermeable membrane at very high pressure to remove microbiologic contaminants and >90% of dissolved ions.

BLOOD DELIVERY SYSTEM

The blood delivery system is composed of the extracorporeal circuit in the dialysis machine and the dialysis access. The dialysis machine consists of a blood pump, dialysis solution delivery system, and various safety monitors. The blood pump moves blood from the access site, through the dialyzer, and back to the patient. The blood flow rate may range from 250–500 mL/min, depending largely on the type and integrity of the vascular access. Negative hydrostatic pressure on the dialysate side can be manipulated to achieve desirable fluid removal or *ultrafiltration*. Dialysis membranes have different ultrafiltration coefficients (i.e., mL removed/min per mmHg) so that along with hydrostatic changes, fluid removal can be varied. The dialysis solution delivery system dilutes the concentrated dialysate with water and monitors the temperature, conductivity, and flow of dialysate.

Dialysis Access

The fistula, graft, or catheter through which blood is obtained for hemodialysis is often referred to as a *dialysis access*. A native fistula created by the anastomosis of an artery to a vein (e.g., the Brescia-Cimino fistula, in which the cephalic vein is anastomosed end-to-side to the radial artery) results in arterialization of the vein. This facilitates its subsequent use in the placement of large needles (typically 15 gauge) to access the circulation. Although fistulas have the highest long-term patency rate of all dialysis access options, fistulas are created in a minority of patients in the United States. Many patients undergo placement of an arteriovenous graft (i.e., the interposition of prosthetic material, usually polytetrafluoroethylene, between an artery and a vein) or a tunneled dialysis catheter. In recent years, nephrologists, vascular surgeons, and health care policy makers in the United States have encouraged creation of arteriovenous fistulas in a larger fraction of patients (the "fistula first" initiative). Unfortunately, even when created, arteriovenous fistulas may not mature sufficiently to provide reliable access to the circulation, or they may thrombose early in their development. Novel surgical approaches (e.g., brachiobasilic fistula creation with transposition of the basilic vein fistula to the arm surface) have increased options for "native" vascular access.

Grafts and catheters tend to be used among persons with smaller-caliber veins or persons whose veins have been damaged by repeated venipuncture, or after prolonged hospitalization. The most important complication of arteriovenous grafts is thrombosis of the graft and graft failure, due principally to intimal hyperplasia at the anastomosis between the graft and recipient vein. When grafts (or fistulas) fail, catheter-guided angioplasty can be used to dilate stenoses; monitoring of venous pressures on dialysis and of access flow, though not routinely performed, may assist in the early recognition of impending vascular access failure. In addition to an increased rate of access failure, grafts and (in particular) catheters are associated with much higher rates of infection than fistulas.

Intravenous large-bore catheters are often used in patients with acute and chronic kidney disease. For persons on maintenance hemodialysis, tunneled catheters (either two separate catheters or a single catheter with two lumens) are often used when arteriovenous fistulas and grafts have failed or are not feasible due to anatomical considerations. These catheters are tunneled under the skin; the tunnel reduces bacterial translocation from the skin, resulting in a lower infection rate than with nontunneled temporary catheters. Most tunneled catheters are placed in the internal jugular veins; the external jugular, femoral, and subclavian veins may also be used. Nephrologists, interventional radiologists, and vascular surgeons generally prefer to avoid placement of catheters into the subclavian veins; while flow rates are usually excellent, subclavian stenosis is a frequent complication and, if present, will likely prohibit permanent vascular access (i.e., a fistula or graft) in the ipsilateral extremity. Infection rates may be higher with femoral catheters. For patients with multiple vascular access complications and no other options for permanent vascular access, tunneled catheters may be the last "lifeline" for hemodialysis. Translumbar or transhepatic approaches into the inferior vena cava may be required if the superior vena cava or other central veins draining the upper extremities are stenosed or thrombosed.

GOALS OF DIALYSIS

The hemodialysis procedure is targeted at removing both low- and high-molecular-weight solutes. The procedure consists of pumping heparinized blood through the dialyzer at a flow rate of 300–500 mL/min, while dialysate flows in an opposite *counter-current* direction at 500–800 mL/min. The efficiency of dialysis is determined by blood and dialysate flow through the dialyzer as well as dialyzer characteristics (i.e., its efficiency in removing solute). The *dose* of dialysis, which is currently defined as a derivation of the fractional urea clearance during a single dialysis treatment, is further governed by patient size, residual kidney function, dietary protein intake, the degree of anabolism or catabolism, and the presence of comorbid conditions.

Since the landmark studies of Sargent and Gotch relating the measurement of the dose of dialysis using urea concentrations with morbidity in the National Cooperative Dialysis Study, the *delivered* dose of dialysis has been measured and considered as a quality assurance and improvement tool. While the fractional removal of urea nitrogen and derivations thereof are considered to be the standard methods by which "adequacy of dialysis" is measured, a large multicenter randomized clinical trial (the HEMO Study) failed to show a difference in mortality associated with a large difference in urea clearance. Still, multiple observational studies and widespread expert opinion have suggested that higher dialysis dose is warranted; current targets include a urea reduction ratio (the fractional reduction in blood urea nitrogen per hemodialysis session) of >65–70% and a body water–indexed clearance × time product (KT/V) above 1.3 or 1.05, depending on whether urea concentrations are "equilibrated."

For the majority of patients with ESRD, between 9 and 12 h of dialysis are required each week, usually divided into three equal sessions. Several studies have suggested that longer hemodialysis session lengths may be beneficial, although these studies are confounded by a variety of patient characteristics, including body size and nutritional status. Hemodialysis "dose" should be individualized, and factors other than the urea nitrogen should be considered, including the adequacy of ultrafiltration or fluid removal. Several authors have highlighted improved intermediate outcomes associated with more frequent hemodialysis (i.e., more than three times a week), although these studies are also confounded by multiple factors. A randomized clinical trial is currently under way to test whether more frequent dialysis results in differences in a variety of physiologic and functional markers.

COMPLICATIONS DURING HEMODIALYSIS

Hypotension is the most common acute complication of hemodialysis, particularly among diabetics. Numerous factors appear to increase the risk of hypotension, including excessive ultrafiltration with inadequate compensatory vascular filling, impaired vasoactive or autonomic responses, osmolar shifts, overzealous use of antihypertensive agents, and reduced cardiac reserve.

Patients with arteriovenous fistulas and grafts may develop high output cardiac failure due to shunting of blood through the dialysis access; on rare occasions, this may necessitate ligation of the fistula or graft. Because of the vasodilatory and cardiodepressive effects of acetate, its use as the buffer in dialysate was once a common cause of hypotension. Since the introduction of bicarbonate-containing dialysate, dialysis-associated hypotension has become less common. The management of hypotension during dialysis consists of discontinuing ultrafiltration, the administration of 100–250 mL of isotonic saline or 10 mL of 23% saturated hypertonic saline, and administration of salt-poor albumin. Hypotension during dialysis can frequently be prevented by careful evaluation of the dry weight and by ultrafiltration modeling, such that more fluid is removed at the beginning rather than the end of the dialysis procedure. Additional maneuvers include the performance of sequential ultrafiltration followed by dialysis; the use of midodrine, a selective α_1-adrenergic pressor agent; cooling of the dialysate during dialysis treatment; and avoiding heavy meals during dialysis.

Muscle cramps during dialysis are also a common complication of the procedure. The etiology of dialysis-associated cramps remains obscure. Changes in muscle perfusion because of excessively aggressive volume removal, particularly below the estimated dry weight, and the use of low-sodium-containing dialysate, have been proposed as precipitants of dialysis-associated cramps. Strategies that may be used to prevent cramps include reducing volume removal during dialysis, ultrafiltration profiling, and the use of higher concentrations of sodium in the dialysate or sodium modeling.

Anaphylactoid reactions to the dialyzer, particularly on its first use, have been reported most frequently with the bioincompatible cellulosic-containing membranes. With the gradual phasing out of cuprophane membranes in the United States, dialyzer reactions have become relatively uncommon. Dialyzer reactions can be divided into two types, A and B. Type A reactions are attributed to an IgE-mediated intermediate hypersensitivity reaction to ethylene oxide used in the sterilization of new dialyzers. This reaction typically occurs soon after the initiation of a treatment (within the first few minutes) and can progress to full-blown anaphylaxis if the therapy is not promptly discontinued. Treatment with steroids or epinephrine may be needed if symptoms are severe. The type B reaction consists of a symptom complex of nonspecific chest and back pain, which appears to result from complement activation and cytokine release. These symptoms typically occur several minutes into the dialysis run and typically resolve over time with continued dialysis.

Cardiovascular diseases constitute the major causes of death in patients with ESRD. Cardiovascular mortality and event rates are higher in dialysis patients than in patients posttransplantation, although rates are extraordinarily high in both populations. The underlying cause of cardiovascular disease is unclear but may be related to shared risk factors (e.g., diabetes mellitus), chronic inflammation, massive changes in extracellular volume (especially with high interdialytic weight gains), inadequate treatment of hypertension, dyslipidemia, anemia, dystrophic vascular calcification, hyperhomocysteinemia, and, perhaps, alterations in cardiovascular dynamics during the dialysis treatment. Few studies have targeted cardiovascular risk reduction in ESRD patients; none have demonstrated consistent benefit. Nevertheless, most experts recommend conventional cardioprotective strategies (e.g., lipid-lowering agents, aspirin, β-adrenergic antagonists) in dialysis patients based on the patients' cardiovascular risk profile, which appears to be increased by more than an order of magnitude relative to persons unaffected by kidney disease.

PERITONEAL DIALYSIS

In peritoneal dialysis, 1.5–3 L of a dextrose-containing solution is infused into the peritoneal cavity and allowed to dwell for a set period of time, usually 2–4 h. As with hemodialysis, toxic materials are removed through a combination of convective clearance generated through ultrafiltration and diffusive clearance down a concentration gradient. The clearance of solutes and water during a peritoneal dialysis exchange depends on the balance between the movement of solute and water into the peritoneal cavity versus absorption from the peritoneal cavity. The rate of diffusion diminishes with time and eventually stops when equilibration between plasma and dialysate is reached. Absorption of solutes and water from the peritoneal cavity occurs across the peritoneal membrane into the peritoneal capillary circulation and via peritoneal lymphatics into the lymphatic circulation. The rate of peritoneal solute transport varies from patient to patient and may be altered by the presence of infection (peritonitis), drugs, and physical factors such as position and exercise.

FORMS OF PERITONEAL DIALYSIS

Peritoneal dialysis may be carried out as continuous ambulatory peritoneal dialysis (CAPD), continuous cyclic peritoneal dialysis (CCPD), or a combination of both. In CAPD, dialysis solution is manually infused into the peritoneal cavity during the day and exchanged three to five times daily. A nighttime dwell is frequently instilled at bedtime and remains in the peritoneal cavity through the night. The drainage of spent dialysate is performed manually with the assistance of gravity to move fluid out of the abdomen. In CCPD, exchanges are performed in an automated fashion, usually at night; the patient is connected to an automated cycler that performs a series of exchange cycles while the patient sleeps. The number of exchange cycles required to optimize peritoneal solute clearance varies by the peritoneal membrane characteristics; as with hemodialysis, experts suggest careful tracking of solute clearances to ensure dialysis "adequacy."

Peritoneal dialysis solutions are available in volumes typically ranging from 1.5 to 3.0 L. Lactate is the preferred buffer in peritoneal dialysis solutions. The most common additives to peritoneal dialysis solutions are heparin to prevent obstruction of the dialysis catheter lumen with fibrin and antibiotics during an episode of acute peritonitis. Insulin may also be added in patients with diabetes mellitus.

ACCESS TO THE PERITONEAL CAVITY

Access to the peritoneal cavity is obtained through a peritoneal catheter. Catheters used for maintenance peritoneal dialysis are flexible, being made of silicon rubber with numerous side holes at the distal end. These catheters usually have two Dacron cuffs to promote fibroblast proliferation, granulation, and invasion of the cuff. The scarring that occurs around the cuffs anchors the catheter and seals it from bacteria tracking from the skin surface into the peritoneal cavity; it also prevents the external leakage of fluid from the peritoneal cavity. The cuffs are placed in the preperitoneal plane and ~2 cm from the skin surface.

The *peritoneal equilibrium test* is a formal evaluation of peritoneal membrane characteristics that measures the transfer rates of creatinine and glucose across the peritoneal membrane. Patients are classified as low, low–average, high–average, and high "transporters." Patients with rapid equilibration (i.e., high transporters) tend to absorb more glucose and lose efficiency of ultrafiltration with long daytime dwells. High transporters also tend to lose larger quantities of albumin and other proteins across the peritoneal membrane. In general, patients with rapid transporting characteristics require more frequent, shorter dwell time exchanges, nearly always obligating use of a cycler for feasibility. Slower (low and low–average) transporters tend to do well with fewer exchanges. The efficiency of solute clearance also depends on the volume of dialysate infused. Larger volumes allow for greater solute clearance, particularly with CAPD in patients with low and low–average transport characteristics. Interestingly, solute clearance also increases with physical activity, presumably related to more efficient flow dynamics within the peritoneal cavity.

As with hemodialysis, the optimal dose of peritoneal dialysis is unknown. Several observational studies have suggested that higher rates of urea and creatinine clearance (the latter generally measured in L/week) are associated with lower mortality rates and fewer uremic complications. However, a randomized clinical trial (ADEMEX) failed to show a significant reduction in mortality or complications with a relatively large increment in urea

clearance. In general, patients on peritoneal dialysis do well when they retain residual kidney function. The rates of technique failure increase with years on dialysis and have been correlated with loss of residual function to a greater extent than loss of peritoneal membrane capacity. Recently, a nonabsorbable carbohydrate (icodextrin) has been introduced as an alternative osmotic agent. Studies have demonstrated more efficient ultrafiltration with icodextrin than with dextrose-containing solutions. Icodextrin is typically used as the "last fill" for patients on CCPD or for the longest dwell in patients on CAPD. For some patients in whom CCPD does not provide sufficient solute clearance, a hybrid approach can be adopted where one or more daytime exchanges are added to the CCPD regimen. While this approach can enhance solute clearance and prolong a patient's capacity to remain on peritoneal dialysis, the burden of the hybrid approach can be overwhelming to some.

COMPLICATIONS DURING PERITONEAL DIALYSIS

The major complications of peritoneal dialysis are peritonitis, catheter-associated nonperitonitis infections, weight gain and other metabolic disturbances, and residual uremia (especially among patients with no residual kidney function).

Peritonitis typically develops when there has been a break in sterile technique during one or more of the exchange procedures. Peritonitis is usually defined by an elevated peritoneal fluid leukocyte count ($100/mm^3$, of which at least 50% are polymorphonuclear neutrophils). The clinical presentation typically consists of pain and cloudy dialysate, often with fever and other constitutional symptoms. The most common culprit organisms are gram-positive cocci, including *Staphylococcus*, reflecting the origin from the skin. Gram-negative rod infections are less common; fungal and mycobacterial infections can be seen in selected patients, particularly after antibacterial therapy. Most cases of peritonitis can be managed either with intraperitoneal or oral antibiotics, depending on the organism; many patients with peritonitis do not require hospitalization. In cases where peritonitis is due to hydrophilic gram-negative rods (e.g., *Pseudomonas* sp.) or yeast, antimicrobial therapy is usually not sufficient, and catheter removal is required to ensure complete eradication of infection. Nonperitonitis catheter-associated infections (often termed *tunnel infections*) vary widely in severity. Some cases can be managed with local antibiotic or silver nitrate administration, while others are severe enough to require parenteral antibiotic therapy and catheter removal.

Peritoneal dialysis is associated with a variety of metabolic complications. As noted above, albumin and other proteins can be lost across the peritoneal membrane in concert with the loss of metabolic wastes. The hypoproteinemia induced by peritoneal dialysis obligates a higher dietary protein intake in order to maintain nitrogen balance. Hyperglycemia and weight gain are also common complications of peritoneal dialysis. Several hundred calories in the form of dextrose are absorbed each day, depending on the concentration employed. Peritoneal dialysis patients, particularly those with Type II diabetes mellitus, are then prone to other complications of insulin resistance, including hypertriglyceridemia. On the positive side, the continuous nature of peritoneal dialysis usually allows for a more liberal diet, due to continuous removal of potassium and phosphorus—two major dietary components whose accumulation can be hazardous in ESRD.

GLOBAL PERSPECTIVE

The incidence of ESRD is increasing worldwide with longer life expectancies and improved care of infectious and cardiovascular diseases. The management of ESRD varies widely by country and within country by region, and it is influenced by economic and other major factors. In general, peritoneal dialysis is more commonly performed in poorer countries owing to its lower expense and the high cost of establishing in-center hemodialysis units.

ACKNOWLEDGMENT

We are grateful to Dr. Ajay Singh and Dr. Barry Brenner, authors of "Dialysis in the Treatment of Renal Failure" in the 16th edition of Harrison's Principles of Internal Medicine, for contributions to this chapter.

FURTHER READINGS

BURKART JM et al: Peritoneal dialysis, in *Brenner and Rector's The Kidney*, 7th ed, BM Brenner (ed). Philadelphia, Saunders, 2004

EKNOYAN G et al: Effect of dialysis dose and membrane flux in maintenance hemodialysis. N Engl J Med 346:2010, 2002

GOLPER TA: Learning about the practice of peritoneal dialysis. Kidney Int 76:12, 2009

HIMMELFARB J, KLIGER AS: End-stage renal disease measures of quality. Annu Rev Med 58:387, 2007

KUMAR VA et al: Hospitalization rates in daily home hemodialysis versus peritoneal dialysis patients in the United States. Am J Kidney Dis 52:737, 2008

MCINTYRE CW: Effects of hemodialysis on cardiac function. Kidney Int 76:371, 2009

NATIONAL KIDNEY FOUNDATION: Kidney Disease Quality Initiative Clinical Practice Guidelines: Hemodialysis and peritoneal dialysis adequacy, 2001. Available online at *http://www.kidney.org/professionals/ kdoqi/guidelines.cfm*

PANIAGUA R et al: Effects of increased peritoneal clearances on mortality rates in peritoneal dialysis: ADEMEX, a prospective, randomized, controlled trial. J Am Soc Nephrol 13:1307, 2002

POLKINGHORNE KR: Vascular access practice in hemodialysis: Instrumental in determining patient mortality. Am J Kidney Dis 53:359, 2009

RAYNER HC et al: Vascular access results from the Dialysis Outcomes and Practice Patterns Study (DOPPS): Performance against Kidney Disease Outcomes Quality Initiative (K/DOQI) Clinical Practice Guidelines. Am J Kidney Dis 44:S22, 2004

US RENAL DATA SYSTEM: USRDS 2005 Annual Data Report: Atlas of End-Stage Renal Disease in the United States. Bethesda, National Institutes of Health, National Institute of Diabetes and Digestive and Kidney Disease, 2005

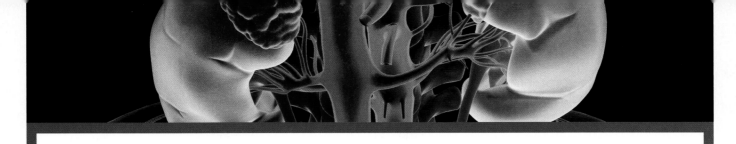

CHAPTER 13

TRANSPLANTATION IN THE TREATMENT OF RENAL FAILURE

Charles B. Carpenter ■ Edgar L. Milford ■ Mohamed H. Sayegh

Transplantation of the human kidney is the treatment of choice for advanced chronic renal failure. Worldwide, tens of thousands of such procedures have been performed. When azathioprine and prednisone were initially used as immunosuppressive drugs in the 1960s, the results with properly matched familial donors were superior to those with organs from deceased donors—ñamely, 75–90% compared with 50–60% graft survival rates at 1 year. During the 1970s and 1980s, the success rate at the 1-year mark for deceased-donor transplants rose progressively. By the time cyclosporine was introduced in the early 1980s, deceased-donor grafts had a 70% 1-year survival and reached the 82% level in the mid-1990s. After the first year, graft survival curves show an exponential decline in numbers of functioning grafts from which a half-life ($t_{1/2}$) in years is calculated; this has increased by only 2 years since the 1980s.

Mortality rates after transplantation are highest in the first year and are age related: 2% for ages 18–34 years, 3% for ages 35–49 years, and 6.8% for ages ≥50–60 years. These rates compare favorably with those in the chronic dialysis population, even after risk adjustments for age, diabetes, and cardiovascular status. Occasionally, acute irreversible rejection may occur after many months of good function, especially if the patient neglects to take the prescribed immunosuppressive drugs. Most grafts, however, succumb at varying rates to a chronic vascular obliterative process termed *chronic allograft nephropathy*, the pathogenesis of which is incompletely understood. Overall, transplantation returns most patients to an improved lifestyle and an improved life expectancy compared with patients on dialysis. There are at least 100,000 patients with functioning kidney transplants in the United States, and when one adds in the numbers of kidney transplants in centers around the world, the total activity is doubled.

RECENT ACTIVITY AND RESULTS

In 1994 there were more than 7000 deceased donor kidney transplants and 3000 living donor transplants in the United States. Table 13-1 shows an increase in numbers of transplants for deceased and living donors over the decade ending in 2003. Whereas deceased donor availability rose by 11%, the living donor rate more than doubled. The backlog of patients with end-stage renal disease (ESRD) has been increasing every year, and it always lags behind the number of available donors. In this decade, the size of the waiting list more than doubled, and the percentage of those on the waiting list

TABLE 13-1

GROWTH IN KIDNEY TRANSPLANTATION FROM 1994 TO 2003 IN THE UNITED STATES					
	1994			**2003**		
	NUMBER OF TRANSPLANTS	**SIZE OF WAIT LIST**	**PATIENTS RECEIVING GRAFTS, %**	**NUMBER OF TRANSPLANTS**	**SIZE OF WAIT LIST**	**PATIENTS RECEIVING GRAFTS, %**
Deceased donor	7533	27,196	28	8389	57,211	14
Living donor	3007			6464		
Total	10,540			14,853		

Source: Data from Summary Tables, 2004 and 2005 Annual Reports, Scientific Registry of Transplant Recipients.

receiving deceased donor transplants dropped from 28 to 14%. The increase in the living donor rate is in response to the demand; it continues to rise to exceed the number of deceased donor grafts. As there were 16,534 new registrants added to the waiting list in 1994 and 24,493 in 2003, demand will continue to exceed supply. Waiting lists continue to grow, and the average wait time for a cadaver kidney is now >4 years in many locations.

The overall results of transplantation are presented in Table 13-2 as the survival of grafts and of patients. At the 1-year mark, graft survival is higher for living donor recipients, most likely because those grafts are not subject to as much ischemic injury. The more powerful drugs now in use for immunosuppression have almost equalized the risk of graft rejection in all patients for the first year. At 5 and 10 years, however, there has been a steeper decline in survival of those with deceased–donor kidneys.

RECIPIENT SELECTION

There are few absolute contraindications to renal transplantation. The transplant procedure is relatively noninvasive, as the organ is placed in the inguinal fossa without entering the peritoneal cavity. Recipients without perioperative complications can often be discharged from the hospital in excellent condition within 5 days of the operation.

Virtually all patients with ESRD who receive a transplant have a higher life expectancy than risk-matched patients who remain on dialysis. Even though diabetics and older candidates have a higher mortality rate than other transplant recipients, their survival is improved with transplantation compared with remaining on dialysis. This global benefit of transplantation as a treatment modality poses substantial ethical issues for policy makers, as the number of deceased kidneys available is far from sufficient to meet the current needs of the candidates. The current standard of care is that the candidate should have a life expectancy of >5 years to be put on a deceased organ wait list. Even for living donation, the candidate should have >5 years of life expectancy. This standard has been established because the benefits of kidney transplantation over dialysis are realized only after a perioperative period in which the mortality is higher in transplanted patients than in dialysis patients with comparable risk profiles.

All candidates must have a thorough risk–versus–benefit evaluation prior to being approved for transplantation. In particular, an aggressive approach to diagnosis of correctable coronary artery disease, presence of latent or indolent infection (HIV, hepatitis B or C, tuberculosis), and neoplasm should be a routine part of the candidate workup. Most transplant centers consider overt AIDS and active hepatitis to be absolute contraindications to transplantation because of the high risk of opportunistic infection. Some centers

TABLE 13-2

MEAN RATES OF GRAFT AND PATIENT SURVIVALS FOR KIDNEYS TRANSPLANTED IN THE UNITED STATES FROM 1992 TO 2002[a]					
	1-YEAR FOLLOW-UP		**5-YEAR FOLLOW-UP**		**10-YEAR FOLLOW-UP**	
	GRAFTS, %	**PATIENTS, %**	**GRAFTS, %**	**PATIENTS, %**	**GRAFTS, %**	**PATIENTS, %**
Deceased donor	89	95	67	81	41	61
Living donor	95	98	80	90	56	76

[a]All patients transplanted are included, and the follow-up unadjusted survival data from the 1-, 5-, and 10-year periods are presented to show the attrition rates over time within the two types of organ donors.
Source: Data from Summary Tables, 2004 and 2005 Annual Reports, Scientific Registry of Transplant Recipients.

are now transplanting individuals with hepatitis and even HIV infection under strict protocols to determine whether the risks and benefits favor transplantation over dialysis.

Among the few absolute "immunologic" contraindications to transplantation is the presence of a potentially harmful antibody against the donor kidney at the time of the anticipated transplant. Harmful antibodies that can cause very early graft loss include natural antibodies against the ABO blood group antigens and antibodies against human leukocyte antigen (HLA) class I (A, B, C) or class II (DR) antigens. These antibodies are routinely excluded by proper screening of the candidate's ABO compatibility, HLA typing of donor and recipient, and direct cross-matching of candidate serum with lymphocytes of the donor.

DONOR SELECTION

Donors can be deceased or volunteer living donors. The latter are usually family members selected to have at least partial compatibility for HLA antigens. Living volunteer donors should be normal on physical examination and of the same major ABO blood group, because crossing major blood group barriers prejudices survival of the allograft. It is possible, however, to transplant a kidney of a type O donor into an A, B, or AB recipient. Selective renal arteriography should be performed on donors to rule out the presence of multiple or abnormal renal arteries because the surgical procedure is difficult and the ischemic time of the transplanted kidney long when vascular abnormalities exist. Transplant surgeons are now using a laparoscopic method to isolate and remove the living donor kidney. This operation has the advantage of less evident surgical scars, and, because there is less tissue trauma, the laparoscopic donors have a substantially shorter hospital stay and less discomfort than those who have the traditional surgery. Deceased donors should be free of malignant neoplastic disease, hepatitis, and HIV because of possible transmission to the recipient. Increased risk of graft failure exists when the donor is elderly or has renal failure and when the kidney has a prolonged period of ischemia and storage.

In the United States, there is a coordinated national system of regulations, allocation support, and outcomes analysis for kidney transplantation called the Organ Procurement Transplant Network. It is now possible to remove deceased donor kidneys and to maintain them for up to 48 h on cold pulsatile perfusion or simple flushing and cooling. This approach permits adequate time for typing, cross-matching, transportation, and selection problems to be solved.

TISSUE TYPING AND CLINICAL IMMUNOGENETICS

Matching for antigens of the HLA major histocompatibility gene complex is an important criterion for selection of donors for renal allografts. Each mammalian

species has a single chromosomal region that encodes the strong, or major, transplantation antigens, and this region on the human sixth chromosome is called *HLA*. HLA antigens have been classically defined by serologic techniques, but methods to define specific nucleotide sequences in genomic DNA are increasingly being used. Other "minor" antigens may play crucial roles, in addition to the ABH(O) blood groups and endothelial antigens that are not shared with lymphocytes. The Rh system is not expressed on graft tissue. Evidence for designation of HLA as the genetic region encoding major transplantation antigens comes from the success rate in living related donor renal and bone marrow transplantation, with superior results in HLA-identical sibling pairs. Nevertheless, 5% of HLA-identical renal allografts are rejected, often within the first weeks after transplantation. These failures represent states of prior sensitization to non-HLA antigens. Non-HLA minor antigens are relatively weak when initially encountered, and are therefore suppressible by conventional immunosuppressive therapy. Once priming has occurred, however, secondary responses are much more refractory to treatment.

LIVING DONORS

When first-degree relatives are donors, graft survival rates at 1 year are 5–7% greater than those for deceased-donor grafts. The 5-year survival rates still favor the partially matched (3/6 HLA mismatched) family donor over a randomly selected cadaver donor (Table 13–3). In addition, living donors provide the advantage of immediate availability. For both living and deceased donors, the 5-year outcomes are poor if there is a complete (6/6) HLA mismatch.

TABLE 13-3

EFFECT OF HLA-A, -B, -DR MISMATCHING ON KIDNEY GRAFT SURVIVAL

DEGREE OF DONOR MISMATCH	1-YEAR SURVIVAL, %	5-YEAR SURVIVAL, %
Cadaver donor (all)	89.2	61.3
0/6-HLA mismatch	91.3	68.2
3/6-HLA mismatch	90.1	60.8
6/6-HLA mismatch	85.2	55.3
Living related donor (all)	94.7	76.0
0/6-HLA mismatch	96.7	87.0
3/6-HLA mismatch	94.3	73.2
6/6-HLA mismatch	92.7	57.7
Living unrelated donor	95.3	77.4

Note: 0-mismatched related donor transplants are virtually all from HLA-identical siblings, while 3/6-mismatched transplants can be one haplotype mismatched (1-A, 1-B, and 1-DR antigen) from parent, child or sibling; 6/6-HLA-mismatched living related kidneys are derived from siblings or relatives outside of the nuclear family.

The survival rate of living unrelated renal allografts is as high as that of perfectly HLA-matched cadaver renal transplants and comparable to that of kidneys from living relatives. This outcome is likely a consequence of both short cold ischemia time and the extra care taken to document that the condition and renal function of the donor are optimal before proceeding with a living unrelated donation. It is illegal in the United States to purchase organs for transplantation.

Concern has been expressed regarding the potential risk to a volunteer kidney donor of premature renal failure after several years of increased blood flow and hyperfiltration per nephron in the remaining kidney. There are a few reports of the development of hypertension, proteinuria, and even lesions of focal segmental sclerosis in donors over long-term follow-up. Difficulties in donors followed for ≥20 years are unusual, however, and it may be that having a single kidney becomes significant only when another condition, such as hypertension, is superimposed. It is also desirable to consider the risk of development of Type 1 diabetes mellitus in a family member who is a potential donor to a diabetic renal failure patient. Anti-insulin and anti-islet cell antibodies should be measured, and glucose tolerance tests should be performed in such donors to exclude a prediabetic state.

PRESENSITIZATION

A positive cross-match of recipient serum with donor T lymphocytes representing anti-HLA class I is usually predictive of an acute vasculitic event termed *hyperacute rejection*. Patients with anti-HLA antibodies can be safely transplanted if careful cross-matching of donor blood lymphocytes with recipient serum is performed. The known sources of such sensitization are blood transfusion, prior transplant, and pregnancy. Patients sustained by dialysis often show fluctuating antibody titers and specificity patterns. At the time of assignment of a cadaveric kidney, cross-matches are performed with at least a current serum. Previously analyzed antibody specificities and additional cross-matches are performed accordingly. Techniques for cross-matching are not universally standardized; however, at least two techniques are employed in most laboratories. The minimal purpose for the cross-match is avoidance of hyperacute rejection mediated by recipient antibodies to donor HLA class I antigens. Sensitive tests, such as the use of flow cytometry, can be useful for avoidance of accelerated, and often untreatable, early graft rejection in patients receiving second or third transplants. Donor T lymphocytes, which express only class I antigens, are used as targets for detection of anti–class I (HLA-A and -B) antibodies. Preformed anti–class II (HLA-DR) antibodies against the donor carry a higher risk of graft loss as well, particularly in recipients who have suffered early loss of a prior kidney transplant. B lymphocytes expressing both class I and class II antigens are used in these assays. Non-HLA antigens restricted in expression to endothelium and sometimes monocytes have been described, but clinical relevance is not well established. A series of minor histocompatibility antigens do not elicit antibodies, and sensitization to these is detectable only by cytotoxic T cells, an assay too cumbersome for routine use. Desensitization prior to transplantation by reducing the level of antidonor antibodies via plasmapheresis of blood, administration of large doses of immunoglobulin, or both has been useful in reducing the hazard of hyperacute rejection.

IMMUNOLOGY OF REJECTION

Both cellular and humoral (antibody-mediated) effector mechanisms can play roles in kidney transplant rejection. Antibodies can also initiate a form of antibody–dependent but cell-mediated cytotoxicity by recipient cells that bear receptors for the Fc portion of immunoglobulin.

Cellular rejection is mediated by lymphocytes that respond to HLA antigens expressed within the organ. The CD4+ lymphocyte responds to class II (HLA-DR) incompatibility by proliferating and releasing proinflammatory cytokines that augment the proliferative response of both CD4+ and CD8+ cells. CD8+ cytotoxic lymphocyte precursors respond primarily to class I (HLA-A, -B) antigens and mature into cytotoxic effector cells. The cytotoxic effector ("killer") T cells cause organ damage through direct contact and lysis of donor target cells. The natural role of HLA antigen molecules is to present processed peptide fragments of antigen to T lymphocytes, the fragments residing in a "groove" of the HLA molecule distal to the cell surface. T cells can be directly stimulated by intact non-self HLA molecules expressed on donor parenchymal cells and residual donor leukocytes residing in the kidney interstitium. In addition, donor HLA molecules can be processed by a variety of donor or recipient cells capable of antigen presentation of peptides and then presented to T cells in the same manner as most other antigens. The former mode of stimulation is sometimes called *direct presentation* and the latter mode is called *indirect presentation* (**Fig. 13-1**). There is evidence that non-HLA antigens can also play a role in renal transplant rejection episodes. Recipients who receive a kidney from an HLA-identical sibling can have rejection episodes and require maintenance immunosuppression, while identical twin transplants require no immunosuppression. There are documented non-HLA antigens, such as an endothelial-specific antigen system with limited polymorphism and a tubular antigen, which can be targets of humoral or cellular rejection responses, respectively.

IMMUNOSUPPRESSIVE TREATMENT

Immunosuppressive therapy, as presently available, generally suppresses all immune responses, including those to

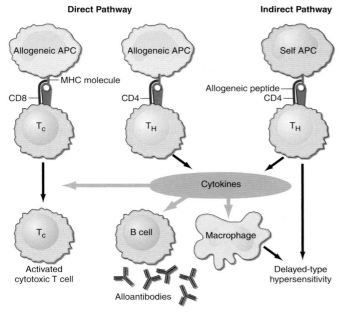

FIGURE 13-1

Recognition pathways for major histocompatibility complex (MHC) antigens. Graft rejection is initiated by CD4 helper T lymphocytes (T$_H$) having antigen receptors that bind to specific complexes of peptides and MHC class II molecules on antigen-presenting cells (APC). In transplantation, in contrast to other immunologic responses, there are two sets of T cell clones involved in rejection. In the direct pathway the class II MHC of donor allogeneic APCs is recognized by CD4 T$_H$ cells that bind to the intact MHC molecule, and class I MHC allogeneic cells are recognized by CD8 T cells. The latter generally proliferate into cytotoxic cells (T$_C$). In the indirect pathway, the incompatible MHC molecules are processed into peptides that are presented by the self-APCs of the recipient. The indirect, but not the direct, pathway is the normal physiologic process in T cell recognition of foreign antigens. Once T$_H$ cells are activated, they proliferate, and by secretion of cytokines and direct contact exert strong helper effects on macrophages, T$_C$, and B cells. *(From Sayegh and Turka, Copyright 1998, Massachusetts Medical Society. All rights reserved.)*

bacteria, fungi, and even malignant tumors. In the 1950s when clinical renal transplantation began, sublethal total-body irradiation was employed. We have now reached the point where sophisticated pharmacologic immunosuppression is available, but it still has the hazard of promoting infection and malignancy. In general, all clinically useful drugs are more selective to primary than to memory immune responses. Agents to suppress the immune response are discussed in the following paragraphs, and those currently in clinical use are listed in Table 13-4.

DRUGS

Azathioprine, an analogue of mercaptopurine, was for two decades the keystone to immunosuppressive therapy

in humans but has now given way to more effective agents. This agent can inhibit synthesis of DNA, RNA, or both. Because cell division and proliferation are a necessary part of the immune response to antigenic stimulation, suppression by this agent may be mediated by the inhibition of mitosis of immunologically competent lymphoid cells, interfering with synthesis of DNA. Alternatively, immunosuppression may be brought about by blocking the synthesis of RNA (possibly messenger RNA), inhibiting processing of antigens prior to lymphocyte stimulation. Therapy with azathioprine in doses of 1.5–2.0 mg/kg per day is generally added to cyclosporine as a means of decreasing the requirements for the latter. Because azathioprine is rapidly metabolized by the liver, its dosage need not be varied directly in relation to renal function, even though renal failure results in retention of the metabolites of azathioprine. Reduction in dosage is required because of leukopenia and occasionally thrombocytopenia. Excessive amounts of azathioprine may also cause jaundice, anemia, and alopecia. If it is essential to administer allopurinol concurrently, the azathioprine dose must be reduced. As inhibition of xanthine oxidase delays degradation, this combination is best avoided.

Mycophenolate mofetil (MMF) is now used in place of azathioprine in most centers. It has a similar mode of action and a mild degree of gastrointestinal toxicity but produces minimal bone marrow suppression. Its advantage is its increased potency in preventing or reversing rejection. Patients with hyperuricemia can be given allopurinol without adjustment of the MMF dose. The usual dose is 2–3 g/d in divided doses.

Glucocorticoids are important adjuncts to immunosuppressive therapy. Of all the agents employed, prednisone has effects that are easiest to assess, and in large doses it is usually effective for the reversal of rejection. In general, 200–300 mg prednisone is given immediately prior to or at the time of transplantation, and the dosage is reduced to 30 mg within a week. The side effects of the glucocorticoids, particularly impairment of wound healing and predisposition to infection, make it desirable to taper the dose as rapidly as possible in the immediate postoperative period. Many centers have protocols for early discontinuance or avoidance of steroids because of long-term adverse effects on bone, skin, and glucose metabolism. For treatment of acute rejection, methylprednisolone, 0.5–1.0 g IV, is administered immediately upon diagnosis of beginning rejection and continued once daily for 3 days. When the drug is effective, the results are usually apparent within 96 h. Such "pulse" doses are not effective in chronic rejection. Most patients whose renal function is stable after 6 months or a year do not require large doses of prednisone; maintenance doses of 10–15 mg/d are the rule. Many patients tolerate an alternate-day course of steroids without an increased risk of rejection. A major effect of steroids is on the monocyte–macrophage system, preventing the release of interleukin (IL)-6 and IL-1.

141

CHAPTER 13

Transplantation in the Treatment of Renal Failure

TABLE 13-4

MAINTENANCE IMMUNOSUPPRESSIVE DRUGS

AGENT	PHARMACOLOGY	MECHANISMS	SIDE EFFECTS
Glucocorticoids	Increased bioavailability with hypoalbuminemia and liver disease; prednisone/prednisolone generally used	Binds cytosolic receptors and heat shock proteins. Blocks transcription of IL-1, -2, -3, -6, TNF-α, and IFN-γ	Hypertension, glucose intolerance, dyslipidemia, osteoporosis
Cyclosporine (CsA)	Lipid-soluble polypeptide, variable absorption, microemulsion more predictable	Trimolecular complex with cyclophilin and calcineurin $\rightarrow$ block in cytokine (e.g., IL-2) production; however, stimulates TGF-β production	Nephrotoxicity, hypertension, dyslipidemia, glucose intolerance, hirsutism/hyperplasia of gums
Tacrolimus (FK506)	Macrolide, well absorbed	Trimolecular complex with FKBP-12 and calcineurin $\rightarrow$ block in cytokine (e.g., IL-2) production; may stimulate TGF-β production	Similar to CsA, but hirsutism/hyperplasia of gums unusual, and diabetes more likely
Azathioprine	Mercaptopurine analogue	Hepatic metabolites inhibit purine synthesis	Marrow suppression (WBC > RBC > platelets)
Mycophenolate mofetil (MMF)	Metabolized to mycophenolic acid	Inhibits purine synthesis via inosine monophosphate dehydrogenase	Diarrhea/cramps; dose-related liver and marrow suppression is uncommon
Sirolimus	Macrolide, poor oral bioavailability	Complexes with FKBP-12 and then blocks p70 S6 kinase in the IL-2 receptor pathway for proliferation	Hyperlipidemia, thrombocytopenia

Note: IL, interleukin; TNF, tumor necrosis factor; IFN, interferon; TGF, transforming growth factor; FKBP-12, FK506 binding protein 12; WBC, white blood cells; RBC, red blood cells.

Cyclosporine is a fungal peptide with potent immunosuppressive activity. It acts on the calcineurin pathway to block transcription of mRNA for IL-2 and other proinflammatory cytokines, thereby inhibiting T cell proliferation. Although it works alone, cyclosporine is more effective in conjunction with glucocorticoids and MMF. Clinical results with tens of thousands of renal transplants have been impressive. Of its toxic effects (nephrotoxicity, hepatotoxicity, hirsutism, tremor, gingival hyperplasia, diabetes), only nephrotoxicity presents a serious management problem and is further discussed below.

Tacrolimus (previously called FK506) is a fungal macrolide that has the same mode of action as cyclosporine, as well as a similar side-effect profile; it does not, however, produce hirsutism or gingival hyperplasia. De novo diabetes mellitus is more common with tacrolimus. The drug was first used in liver transplantation and may substitute for cyclosporine entirely or be tried as an alternative in renal patients whose rejections are poorly controlled by cyclosporine.

Sirolimus (previously called rapamycin) is another fungal macrolide but has a different mode of action, i.e., it inhibits T cell growth factor signaling pathways, preventing the response to IL-2 and other cytokines. Sirolimus can be used in conjunction with cyclosporine or tacrolimus, or with MMF, to avoid calcineurin inhibitors. Its use with tacrolimus alone shows promise as a steroid-sparing regimen, especially in patients who would benefit from pancreatic islet cell transplantation, where steroids have an adverse effect on islet survival.

ANTIBODIES TO LYMPHOCYTES

When serum from animals made immune to host lymphocytes is injected into the recipient, a marked suppression of cellular immunity to the tissue graft results. The action on cell-mediated immunity is greater than on humoral immunity. A globulin fraction of serum [antilymphocyte globulin (ALG)] is the agent generally employed. For use in humans, peripheral human lymphocytes, thymocytes, or lymphocytes from spleens or thoracic duct fistulas have been injected into horses, rabbits, or goats to produce antilymphocyte serum, from which the globulin fraction is then separated. A rabbit antithymocyte globulin (Thymoglobulin) is the most common agent currently in use. Monoclonal antibodies against defined lymphocyte subsets offer a more precise and standardized form of therapy. OKT3 is directed to the CD3 molecules that form a portion of the T cell antigen-receptor complex and is thus expressed on all mature T cells.

Another approach to more selective therapy is to target the 55-kDa alpha chain of the IL-2 receptor, expressed only on T cells that have been recently activated. Two such antibodies to the IL-2 receptor, in which either a chimeric protein has been made between mouse Fab with human Fc (basiliximab) or the antibody has been "humanized" by splicing the combining sites of the mouse into a molecule that is 90% human IgG (daclizumab), are in use for prophylaxis of acute rejection in the immediate posttransplant period. They are effective at decreasing the acute rejection rate and have few adverse side effects.

More recently, two new strategies have involved administration of engineered biologic agents: a depleting T cell antibody (alemtuzumab) as induction therapy to minimize maintenance immunosuppression, and a fusion protein (LEA29Y) to block B7 T cell co-stimulatory signals. The latter has shown promise in phase 2 trials and is currently being tested in phase 3 trials in kidney transplantation.

CLINICAL COURSE AND MANAGEMENT OF THE RECIPIENT

Adequate hemodialysis should be performed within 48 h of surgery, and care should be taken that the serum potassium level is not markedly elevated so that intraoperative cardiac arrhythmias can be averted. The diuresis that commonly occurs postoperatively must be carefully monitored; in some instances, it may be massive, reflecting the inability of ischemic tubules to regulate sodium and water excretion; with large diureses, massive potassium losses may occur. Most chronically uremic patients have some excess of extracellular fluid, and it is useful to maintain an expanded fluid volume in the immediate postoperative period. Acute tubular necrosis (ATN) may cause immediate oliguria or may follow an initial short period of graft function. ATN is most likely when cadaveric donors have been underperfused or if the interval between cessation of blood flow and organ harvest (warm ischemic time) is more than a few minutes. Recovery usually occurs within 3 weeks, although periods as long as 6 weeks have been reported. Superimposition of rejection on ATN is common, and the differential diagnosis may be difficult without a graft biopsy. Cyclosporine therapy prolongs ATN, and some patients do not diurese until the dose is drastically reduced. Many centers avoid starting cyclosporine for the first several days, using ALG or a monoclonal antibody along with MMF and prednisone until renal function is established. **Figure 13-2** illustrates an algorithm followed by many transplant centers for early posttransplant management of recipients at high or low risk of early renal dysfunction.

THE REJECTION EPISODE

Early diagnosis of rejection allows prompt institution of therapy to preserve renal function and to prevent irreversible damage. Clinical evidence of rejection is rarely characterized by fever, swelling, and tenderness over the allograft. Rejection may present only with a rise in serum creatinine, with or without a reduction in urine volume. The focus should be on ruling out other causes of functional deterioration.

Doppler ultrasonography or magnetic resonance angiography may be useful in ascertaining changes in the renal vasculature and in renal blood flow, even in the absence of changes in urinary flow. Thrombosis of the renal vein occurs rarely; it may be reversible if caused by technical factors and intervention is prompt. Diagnostic ultrasound is the procedure of choice to rule out urinary obstruction or to confirm the presence of perirenal collections of urine, blood, or lymph. When renal function has been good initially, a rise in the serum creatinine level is the most sensitive and reliable indicator of possible rejection and may be the only sign.

Calcineurin inhibitors (cyclosporine or tacrolimus) may cause deterioration in renal function in a manner similar to a rejection episode. In fact, rejection processes tend to be more indolent with these inhibitors, and the only way to make a diagnosis may be by renal biopsy. Calcineurin inhibitors have an afferent arteriolar constrictor effect on the kidney and may produce permanent vascular and interstitial injury after sustained high-dose therapy. Addition of angiotensin-converting enzyme (ACE) inhibitors or nonsteroidal anti-inflammatory drugs is likely to raise serum creatinine levels. The former are generally safe to use after the early months, while the latter are best avoided in all renal transplant patients. There is no universally accepted lesion that makes a diagnosis of calcineurin inhibitor toxicity, although interstitial fibrosis, isometric tubular vacuolization, and thickening of arteriolar walls have been noted by some. Basically, if the biopsy does not reveal moderate and active cellular rejection activity, the serum creatinine will most likely respond to a reduction in dose. Blood levels of drug can be useful if they are very high or very low but do not correlate precisely with renal function, although serial changes in a patient can be useful. If rejection activity is present in the biopsy, appropriate therapy is indicated. The first rejection episode is usually treated with IV administration of methylprednisolone, 500–1000 mg daily for 3 days. Failure to respond is an indication for antibody therapy, usually with OKT3 or antithymocyte globulin.

Biopsy may be necessary to confirm the presence of rejection; when evidence of antibody-mediated injury is present with endothelial injury and deposition of complement component C4d is detected by fluorescence labeling, one can usually detect the antibody in recipient blood. The prognosis is poor, and aggressive use of plasmapheresis, immunoglobulin infusions, or anti-CD20 monoclonal antibody (rituximab) that targets B lymphocytes is indicated.

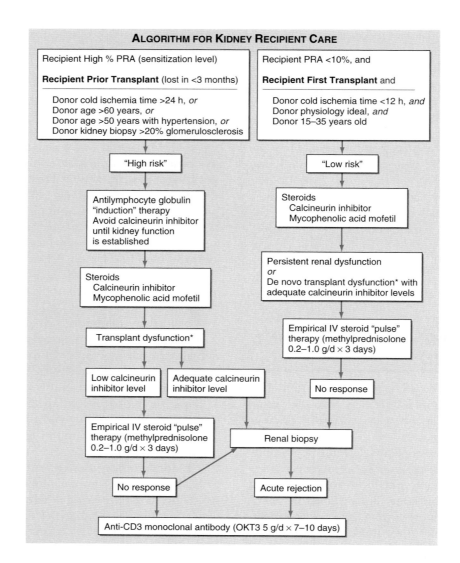

ALGORITHM FOR KIDNEY RECIPIENT CARE

Recipient High % PRA (sensitization level)

Recipient Prior Transplant (lost in <3 months)

Donor cold ischemia time >24 h, *or*
Donor age >60 years, *or*
Donor age >50 years with hypertension, *or*
Donor kidney biopsy >20% glomerulosclerosis

Recipient PRA <10%, and

Recipient First Transplant and

Donor cold ischemia time <12 h, *and*
Donor physiology ideal, *and*
Donor 15–35 years old

"High risk"

"Low risk"

Antilymphocyte globulin "induction" therapy
Avoid calcineurin inhibitor until kidney function is established

Steroids
  Calcineurin inhibitor
  Mycophenolic acid mofetil

Steroids
  Calcineurin inhibitor
  Mycophenolic acid mofetil

Persistent renal dysfunction
or
De novo transplant dysfunction* with adequate calcineurin inhibitor levels

Transplant dysfunction*

Empirical IV steroid "pulse" therapy (methylprednisolone 0.2–1.0 g/d × 3 days)

Low calcineurin inhibitor level

Adequate calcineurin inhibitor level

No response

Empirical IV steroid "pulse" therapy (methylprednisolone 0.2–1.0 g/d × 3 days)

Renal biopsy

No response

Acute rejection

Anti-CD3 monoclonal antibody (OKT3 5 g/d × 7–10 days)

FIGURE 13-2

A typical algorithm for early posttransplant care of the kidney recipient. If any of the recipient or donor "high-risk" factors exist, more aggressive management is called for. Low-risk patients can be treated with a standard immunosuppressive regimen. Patients at higher risk of rejection or early ischemic and nephrotoxic transplant dysfunction are often induced with an antilymphocyte globulin to provide more potent early immunosuppression or to spare calcineurin nephrotoxicity. *When there is early transplant dysfunction, prerenal, obstructive, and vascular causes must be ruled out by ultrasonographic examination. The panel reactive antibody (PRA) is a quantitation of how much antibody is present in a candidate against a panel of cells representing the distribution of antigens in the donor pool.

MANAGEMENT PROBLEMS

The usual clinical manifestations of infection in the posttransplant period are blunted by immunosuppressive therapy. The major toxic effect of azathioprine is bone marrow suppression, which is less likely with MMF, while calcineurin inhibitors have no marrow effects. All drugs predispose to unusual opportunistic infections, however. The typical times after transplantation when the most common opportunistic infections occur are tabulated in Table 13-5. The signs and symptoms of infection may be masked or distorted. Fever without obvious cause is common, and only after days or weeks may it become apparent that it has a viral or fungal origin.

Bacterial infections are most common during the first month after transplantation. The importance of blood cultures in such patients cannot be overemphasized because systemic infection without obvious foci is frequent, although wound infections with or without urinary fistulas are most common. Particularly ominous are rapidly occurring pulmonary lesions, which may result in death within 5 days of onset. When these become apparent, immunosuppressive agents should be discontinued, except for maintenance doses of prednisone.

Aggressive diagnostic procedures, including transbronchial and open lung biopsy, are frequently indicated. In the case of *Pneumocystis carinii* infection, trimethoprim-sulfamethoxazole (TMP-SMX) is the treatment of choice;

TABLE 13-5

THE MOST COMMON OPPORTUNISTIC INFECTIONS IN THE RENAL TRANSPLANT RECIPIENT

Peritransplant (<1 month)	Late (>6 months)
Wound infections	*Aspergillus*
Herpesvirus	*Nocardia*
Oral candidiasis	BK virus (polyoma)
Urinary tract infection	Herpes zoster
Early (1–6 months)	Hepatitis B
Pneumocystis carinii	Hepatitis C
Cytomegalovirus	
Legionella	
Listeria	
Hepatitis B	
Hepatitis C	

amphotericin B has been used effectively in systemic fungal infections. Prophylaxis against *P. carinii* with daily or alternate-day low-dose TMP-SMX is very effective. Involvement of the oropharynx with *Candida* may be treated with local nystatin. Tissue-invasive fungal infections require treatment with systemic agents such as fluconazole. Small doses (a total of 300 mg) of amphotericin given over a period of 2 weeks may be effective in fungal infections refractory to fluconazole. Macrolide antibiotics, especially ketoconazole and erythromycin, and some calcium channel blockers (diltiazem, verapamil) compete with calcineurin inhibitors for P450 catabolism and cause elevated levels of these immunosuppressive drugs. Analeptics, such as phenytoin and carbamazepine, will increase catabolism to result in low levels. *Aspergillus*, *Nocardia*, and especially cytomegalovirus (CMV) infections also occur.

CMV is a common and dangerous DNA virus in transplant recipients. It does not generally appear until the end of the first posttransplant month. Active CMV infection is sometimes associated, or occasionally confused, with rejection episodes. Patients at highest risk for severe CMV disease are those without anti-CMV antibodies who receive a graft from a CMV antibody–positive donor (15% mortality). Valganciclovir is a cost-effective and bioavailable oral form of ganciclovir that has been proven effective in both prophylaxis and treatment of CMV disease. Early diagnosis in a febrile patient with clinical suspicion of CMV disease can be made by determining CMV viral load in the blood. A rise in IgM antibodies to CMV is also diagnostic. Culture of CMV from blood may be less sensitive. Tissue invasion of CMV is common in the gastrointestinal tract and lungs. CMV retinopathy occurs late in the course, if untreated. Treatment of active CMV disease with valganciclovir is always indicated. In many patients immune to CMV, viral activation can occur with major immunosuppressive regimens.

The polyoma group (BK, JC, SV40) is another class of DNA viruses that can become dormant in kidneys and can be activated by immunosuppression. When reactivation occurs with BK there is a 50% chance of progressive fibrosis and loss of the graft within 1 year by the activated virus. The use of tacrolimus has been associated with the highest risk.

Renal biopsy is necessary for the diagnosis. There are promising results with leflunomide and cidofovir, but it is most important to reduce the immunosuppressive load.

The complications of glucocorticoid therapy are well known and include gastrointestinal bleeding, impairment of wound healing, osteoporosis, diabetes mellitus, cataract formation, and hemorrhagic pancreatitis. The treatment of unexplained jaundice in transplant patients should include cessation or reduction of immunosuppressive drugs if hepatitis or drug toxicity is suspected. Therapy in such circumstances often does not result in rejection of a graft, at least for several weeks. Acyclovir is effective in therapy of herpes simplex virus infections.

CHRONIC LESIONS OF THE TRANSPLANTED KIDNEY

While 1-year transplant survival is excellent, most recipients experience progressive decline in kidney function over time thereafter. Chronic renal transplant dysfunction can be caused by recurrent disease, hypertension, cyclosporine or tacrolimus nephrotoxicity, chronic immunologic rejection, secondary focal glomerulosclerosis, or a combination of these pathophysiologies. Chronic vascular changes with intimal proliferation and medial hypertrophy are commonly found. Control of systemic and intrarenal hypertension with ACE inhibitors is thought to have a beneficial influence on the rate of progression of chronic renal transplant dysfunction. Renal biopsy can distinguish subacute cellular rejection from recurrent disease or secondary focal sclerosis.

MALIGNANCY

The incidence of tumors in patients on immunosuppressive therapy is 5–6%, or approximately 100 times greater than that in the general population of the same age range. The most common lesions are cancer of the skin and lips and carcinoma in situ of the cervix, as well as lymphomas such as non-Hodgkin's lymphoma. The risks are increased in proportion to the total immunosuppressive load administered and time elapsed since transplantation. Surveillance for skin and cervical cancers is necessary.

OTHER COMPLICATIONS

Hypercalcemia after transplantation may indicate failure of hyperplastic parathyroid glands to regress. Aseptic necrosis of the head of the femur is probably due to preexisting hyperparathyroidism, with aggravation by glucocorticoid treatment. With improved management of calcium and phosphorus metabolism during chronic dialysis, the incidence of parathyroid-related complications has fallen dramatically. Persistent hyperparathyroid activity may require subtotal parathyroidectomy.

Hypertension may be caused by (1) native kidney disease; (2) rejection activity in the transplant; (3) renal artery stenosis, if an end-to-end anastomosis was constructed with an iliac artery branch; and (4) renal calcineurin inhibitor toxicity. This toxicity may improve with reduction in dose. Whereas ACE inhibitors may be useful, calcium channel blockers are more frequently used initially. Amelioration of hypertension to the range of 120–130/70–80 mmHg should be the goal in all patients.

While most transplant patients have a robust production of erythropoietin and normalization of hemoglobin, *anemia* is commonly seen in the posttransplant period. Often the anemia is attributable to bone marrow–suppressant immunosuppressive medications such as azathioprine, MMF, or sirolimus. Gastrointestinal bleeding is a common side effect of high-dose and long-term steroid administration. Many transplant patients have creatinine clearances of 30–50 mL/min and can be considered in the same way as other patients with chronic renal insufficiency for anemia management, including supplemental erythropoietin.

Chronic hepatitis, particularly when due to hepatitis B virus, can be a progressive, fatal disease over a decade or so. Patients who are persistently hepatitis B surface antigen–positive are at higher risk, according to some studies, but the presence of hepatitis C virus is also a concern when one embarks on a course of immunosuppression in a transplant recipient.

Both chronic dialysis and renal transplant patients have a higher incidence of death from myocardial infarction and stroke than the population at large, and this is particularly true in diabetic patients. Contributing factors are the use of glucocorticoids and sirolimus, as well as hypertension. Recipients of renal transplants have a high prevalence of coronary artery and peripheral vascular diseases. The percentage of deaths from these causes has been slowly rising as the numbers of transplanted diabetic patients and the average age of all recipients increase. More than 50% of renal recipient mortality is attributable to cardiovascular disease. In addition to strict control of blood pressure and blood lipid levels, close monitoring of patients for indications of further medical or surgical intervention is an important part of management.

FURTHER READINGS

CHANDRAKER A et al: Transplantation immunobiology, in *Brenner and Rector's The Kidney*, 7th ed, B Brenner (ed). Philadelphia, Saunders, 2004, pp 2759–2784

DENTON MD et al: Immunosuppressive strategies in renal transplantation. Lancet 353:1083, 1999

HRICIK DE: Comparing early withdrawal or avoidance of steroids with standard steroid therapy in kidney transplant recipients. Nat Clin Pract Nephrol 4:360, 2008

PERCO P et al: Kidney injury molecule-1 as a biomarker of acute kidney injury in renal transplant recipients. Nat Clin Pract Nephrol 4:362, 2008

PESCOVITZ MD, GOVANI M: Sirolimus and mycophenolate mofetil for calcineurin-free immunosuppression in renal transplant recipients. Am J Kidney Dis 38:S16, 2001

RIGOTTI P et al: Outcome of renal transplantation from very old donors. N Engl J Med 360:1464, 2009

SAYEGH MH, CARPENTER CB: Transplantation 50 years later—Progress, challenges and promises. N Engl J Med 351:2761, 2004

VARAGUNAM M et al: C3 polymorphisms and allograft outcome in renal transplantation. N Engl J Med 360:874, 2009

VICENTI F: Immunosuppression minimization: Current and future trends in transplant immunosuppression. J Am Soc Nephrol 14:1940, 2003

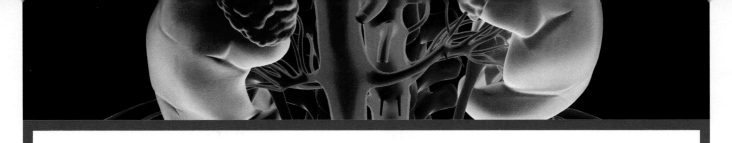

CHAPTER 14

INFECTIONS IN TRANSPLANT RECIPIENTS

Robert Finberg ■ Joyce Fingeroth

The evaluation of infections in transplant recipients involves consideration of both the donor and the recipient of the transplanted organ. Infections following transplantation are complicated by the use of drugs that are necessary to enhance the likelihood of survival of the transplanted organ but that also cause the host to be immunocompromised. Thus, what might have been a latent or asymptomatic infection in an immunocompetent donor or in the recipient prior to therapy can become a life-threatening problem when the recipient becomes immunosuppressed.

PRETRANSPLANTATION EVALUATION

A variety of organisms have been transmitted by organ transplantation (Table 14-1). Careful attention to the sterility of the medium used to process the organ combined with meticulous microbiologic evaluation reduces rates of transmission of bacteria that may be present or grow in the organ culture medium. From 2 to >20% of donor kidneys are estimated to be contaminated with bacteria—in most cases, with the organisms that colonize the skin or grow in the tissue culture medium used to bathe the donor kidney while it awaits implantation. The reported rate of bacterial contamination of transplanted stem cells (bone marrow, peripheral blood, cord blood) is as high as 17%, but is most commonly ~1%. The

use of enrichment columns and monoclonal-antibody depletion procedures results in a higher incidence of contamination. In one series of patients receiving contaminated products, 14% had fever or bacteremia, but none died. Results of cultures performed at the time of cryopreservation and at the time of thawing were helpful in guiding therapy for the recipient.

In many transplantation centers, transmission of infections that may be latent or clinically inapparent in the donor organ has resulted in the development of specific donor-screening protocols. In addition to ordering serologic studies focused on viruses such as herpes-group viruses [herpes simplex virus types 1 and 2 (HSV-1, HSV-2), varicella-zoster virus (VZV), cytomegalovirus (CMV), human herpesvirus (HHV) type 6, Epstein-Barr virus (EBV), and Kaposi's sarcoma–associated herpesvirus (KSHV)] as well as hepatitis B and C viruses, human immunodeficiency virus (HIV), human T cell lymphotropic virus type I, and West Nile virus, donors should be screened for parasites such as *Toxoplasma gondii* and *Trypanosoma cruzi* (the latter particularly in Latin America). Clinicians caring for prospective organ donors should also consider assessing stool for parasites, examine chest radiographs for evidence of granulomatous disease, and perform purified protein derivative (PPD) skin testing or obtain blood for immune cell–based assays that detect active or latent *Mycobacterium tuberculosis* infection. An

ORGANISMS TRANSMITTED BY ORGAN TRANSPLANTATION AND THEIR PRIMARY SITES OF REACTIVATION DISEASE[a]

	BLOOD	LUNGS	HEART	BRAIN	LIVER/SPLEEN	SKIN
Viruses						
Cytomegalovirus[b]	+	+	±	±	+	±
Epstein-Barr virus[c]	+	+	±	±	+	±
Herpes simplex virus		+		±	+	+
Human herpesvirus type 6	+	+		+		+
Kaposi's sarcoma–associated herpesvirus	+	±			±	+
Hepatitis B and C viruses					+	
Rabies virus[d]				+		
West Nile virus	+			+		
Fungi						
Candida albicans	+	+			+	+
Histoplasma capsulatum	+	+			+	+
Cryptococcus neoformans	+	+		+	±	+
Parasites						
Toxoplasma gondii[e]		+	+	+		
Strongyloides stercoralis[f,g]		+				
Trypanosoma cruzi[g]			+			
Plasmodium falciparum[g]	+					
Prion Diseases						
Creutzfeldt-Jakob disease (CJD)[h]				+		
Variant CJD/bovine spongiform encephalopathy[i]				+		

[a]+, well documented; ±, probably occurs.
[b]Cytomegalovirus reactivation is prone to occur in the transplanted organ. The same may be true for Kaposi's sarcoma–associated herpesvirus.
[c]Epstein-Barr virus reactivation usually presents as an extranodal proliferation of transformed B cells and can be present either as a diffuse disease or as a mass lesion in a single organ.
[d]Rabies virus has been transmitted through corneal transplants.
[e]T. gondii usually causes disease in the brain. In hematopoietic stem cell transplant recipients, acute pulmonary disease may also occur. Heart transplant recipients develop disease in the allograft.
[f]Strongyloides "hyperinfection" may present with pulmonary disease—often associated with gram-negative bacterial pneumonia.
[g]While transmission with organs has been described, it is unusual.
[h]CJD (sporadic and familial) has been transmitted with corneal transplants. Whether it can be transmitted with blood is not known.
[i]Variant CJD can be transmitted with transfused non-leukodepleted blood, posing a theoretical risk to transplant recipients.

investigation of the donor's dietary habits (e.g., consumption of raw meat or fish or of unpasteurized dairy products), occupations or avocations (e.g., gardening or spelunking), and travel history (e.g., travel to areas with endemic fungi) is also mandatory. It is expected that the recipient will have been likewise assessed. Because of immune dysfunction resulting from chemotherapy or underlying chronic disease, however, direct testing of the recipient may prove less reliable. This chapter considers aspects of infection unique to various transplantation settings.

INFECTIONS IN SOLID ORGAN TRANSPLANT (SOT) RECIPIENTS

Morbidity and mortality among SOT recipients are reduced by the use of effective antibiotics. The organisms that cause acute infections in recipients of SOT are different from those that infect hematopoietic stem cell transplant (HSCT) recipients because SOT recipients do not go through a period of neutropenia. As the transplantation procedure involves major surgery, however, SOT recipients are subject to infections at anastomotic sites and to wound infections. Compared with HSCT recipients, SOT patients are immunosuppressed for longer periods (often permanently). Thus they are susceptible to many of the same organisms as patients with chronically impaired T cell immunity.

During the early period (<1 month after transplantation), infections are most commonly caused by extracellular bacteria (staphylococci, streptococci, enterococci, *Escherichia coli*, other gram-negative organisms), which often originate in surgical wound or anastomotic sites. The type of transplant largely determines the spectrum of infection.

In subsequent weeks, the consequences of the administration of agents that suppress cell-mediated immunity become apparent, and acquisition or reactivation of viruses and parasites (from the recipient or from the transplanted organ) can occur. CMV infection is often a problem, particularly in the first 6 months after transplantation, and may present as severe systemic disease or as infection of the transplanted organ. HHV-6 reactivation [assessed by plasma polymerase chain reaction (PCR)] occurs within the first 2–4 weeks after transplantation and may be associated with fever, leukopenia, and possibly encephalitis. Data suggest that replication of HHV-6 and HHV-7 may exacerbate CMV-induced disease. CMV is associated not only with generalized immunosuppression but also with organ-specific, rejection-related syndromes: glomerulopathy in kidney transplant recipients, bronchiolitis obliterans in lung transplant recipients, vasculopathy in heart transplant recipients, and the vanishing bile duct syndrome in liver transplant recipients. A complex interplay between increased CMV replication and enhanced graft rejection is well established: increasing immunosuppression leads to increased CMV replication, which is associated with graft rejection. For this reason, considerable attention has been focused on the diagnosis, prophylaxis, and treatment of CMV infection in SOT recipients. Early transmission of West Nile virus to transplant recipients from an organ donor has been reported; however, the risk of West Nile acquisition has been reduced by implementation of screening procedures.

Beyond 6 months after transplantation, infections characteristic of patients with defects in cell-mediated immunity—e.g., infections with *Listeria*, *Nocardia*, *Rhodococcus*, various fungi, and other intracellular pathogens— may be a problem. International patients and global travelers may experience reactivation of dormant infections with trypanosomes, *Leishmania*, *Plasmodium*, *Strongyloides*, and other parasites. Elimination of these late infections will not be possible until the patient develops specific tolerance to the transplanted organ in the absence of drugs that lead to generalized immunosuppression. Meanwhile, vigilance, prophylaxis/preemptive therapy (when indicated), and rapid diagnosis and treatment of infections can be lifesaving in SOT recipients, who, unlike most HSCT recipients, continue to be immunosuppressed.

SOT recipients are susceptible to EBV–B cell lymphoproliferative disease (EBV-LPD) from as early as 2 months to many years after transplantation. The prevalence of this complication is increased by potent and prolonged use of T cell–suppressive drugs. Decreasing the degree of immunosuppression may in some cases reverse the condition. Among SOT patients, those with heart and lung transplants—who receive the most intensive immunosuppressive regimens—are most likely to develop EBV-LPD, particularly in the lungs. Although the disease usually

originates in recipient B cells, several cases of donor origin, particularly in the transplanted organ, have been noted. High organ-specific content of B lymphoid tissues (e.g., bronchial-associated lymphoid tissue in the lung), anatomic factors (e.g., lack of access of host T cells to the transplanted organ because of disturbed lymphatics), and differences in major histocompatibility loci between the host T cells and the organ (e.g., lack of cell migration or lack of effective T cell/macrophage cooperation) may result in defective elimination of EBV-infected B cells. SOT recipients are also highly susceptible to the development of Kaposi's sarcoma and less frequently to the B cell proliferative disorders associated with KSHV, such as primary effusion lymphoma and multicentric Castleman's disease. Kaposi's sarcoma is much more common (in fact, 550–1000 times more common than in the general population), can develop very rapidly after transplantation, and can also occur in the allograft. However, because the seroprevalence of KSHV is very low in Western countries, Kaposi's sarcoma is not often observed.

KIDNEY TRANSPLANTATION

(See Table 14-2.)

Early Infections

Bacteria often cause infections that develop in the period immediately after kidney transplantation. There is a role for perioperative antibiotic prophylaxis, and many centers give cephalosporins to decrease the risk of postoperative complications. Urinary tract infections developing soon after transplantation are usually related to anatomic alterations resulting from surgery. Such early infections may require prolonged treatment (e.g., 6 weeks of antibiotic administration for pyelonephritis). Urinary tract infections that occur >6 months after transplantation may be treated for shorter periods because they do not seem to be associated with the high rate of pyelonephritis or relapse seen with infections that occur in the first 3 months.

Prophylaxis with TMP-SMX [one double-strength tablet (800 mg of sulfamethoxazole, 160 mg of trimethoprim) per day] for the first 4–6 months after transplantation decreases the incidence of early and middle-period infections (Tables 14-2, and 14-3).

Middle-Period Infections

Because of continuing immunosuppression, kidney transplant recipients are predisposed to lung infections characteristic of those in patients with T cell deficiency (i.e., infections with intracellular bacteria, mycobacteria, nocardiae, fungi, viruses, and parasites). The high mortality rates associated with *Legionella pneumophila* infection

TABLE 14-2

COMMON INFECTIONS AFTER KIDNEY TRANSPLANTATION

	PERIOD AFTER TRANSPLANTATION		
INFECTION SITE	**EARLY (<1 MONTH)**	**MIDDLE (1–4 MONTHS)**	**LATE (>6 MONTHS)**
Urinary tract	Bacteria (*Escherichia coli*, *Klebsiella*, Enterobacteriaceae, *Pseudomonas*, *Enterococcus*) associated with bacteremia and pyelonephritis; *Candida*	CMV (fever, bone marrow suppression, hepatitis); BK virus (nephropathy, graft failure, vasculopathy)	Bacteria (late urinary tract infections usually not associated with bacteremia); BK virus (nephropathy, graft failure, generalized vasculopathy)
Lungs	Bacteria (*Legionella* in endemic settings)	CMV disease; *Pneumocystis*; *Legionella*	*Nocardia*; invasive fungi
Central nervous system		*Listeria* (meningitis); *Toxoplasma gondii*	CMV disease; *Listeria* (meningitis); *Cryptococcus* (meningitis); *Nocardia*

Note: CMV, cytomegalovirus.

led to the closing of renal transplant units in hospitals with endemic legionellosis.

About 50% of all renal transplant recipients presenting with fever 1–4 months after transplantation have evidence of CMV disease; CMV itself accounts for the fever in more than two-thirds of cases and thus is the predominant pathogen during this period. CMV infection may also present as arthralgias, myalgias, or organ-specific symptoms. During this period, this infection may represent primary disease (in the case of a seronegative recipient of a kidney from a seropositive donor) or may represent reactivation disease or superinfection. Patients may have atypical lymphocytosis. Unlike immunocompetent patients, however, they often do not have lymphadenopathy or splenomegaly. Therefore, clinical suspicion and laboratory confirmation are necessary for diagnosis. The clinical syndrome may be accompanied by bone marrow suppression (particularly leukopenia). CMV also causes glomerulopathy and is associated with an increased incidence of other opportunistic infections. Because of the frequency and severity of disease, a considerable effort has been made to prevent and treat

TABLE 14-3

PROPHYLAXIS OF INFECTIONS IN TRANSPLANT RECIPIENTS

RISK FACTOR	ORGANISM	PROPHYLACTIC ANTIBIOTICS	EXAMINATION(S)[a]
Travel to or residence in area with known risk of fungal infection	*Coccidioides*, *Histoplasma*, *Blastomyces*	Consider imidazoles	Chest radiography, antigen testing, serology
Latent viruses	HSV, VZV, EBV, CMV	Acyclovir after hematopoietic stem cell transplantation to prevent HSV and VZV; ganciclovir to prevent CMV in some settings	Serologic test for HSV, VZV, CMV, HHV-6, EBV, KSHV
Latent fungi and parasites	*Pneumocystis jiroveci*, *Toxoplasma gondii*	Trimethoprim-sulfamethoxazole (dapsone or atovaquone)	Serology for *Toxoplasma*
History of exposure to tuberculosis or latent tuberculosis	*Mycobacterium tuberculosis*	Isoniazid if recent conversion for positive chest imaging and/or no previous treatment	Chest imaging; PPD and/or cell-based assay

[a]Serologic examination, PPD testing, and interferon assays may be less reliable after transplantation.
Note: CMV, cytomegalovirus; EBV, Epstein-Barr virus; HHV-6, human herpesvirus type 6; HSV, herpes simplex virus; KSHV, Kaposi's sarcoma–associated herpesvirus; PPD, purified protein derivative; VZV, varicella-zoster virus.

CMV infection in renal transplant recipients. An immune globulin preparation enriched with antibodies to CMV was used by many centers in the past in an effort to protect the group at highest risk for severe infection (seronegative recipients of seropositive kidneys). However, with the development of highly effective oral antiviral agents, CMV immune globulin is no longer used. Ganciclovir (valganciclovir) is beneficial when prophylaxis is indicated and for the treatment of serious CMV disease. One study showed a significant (50%) reduction in CMV disease and rejection at 6 months among patients who received prophylactic valacyclovir (an acyclovir congener) for the first 90 days after renal transplantation. Acyclovir (valacyclovir) is less efficacious but also less toxic than ganciclovir (valganciclovir). The availability of valganciclovir and valacyclovir has allowed most centers to move to oral prophylaxis for transplant recipients. Additional oral prophylactic agents, such as maribavir, are in clinical study.

Infection with the other herpes-group viruses may become evident within 6 months after transplantation or later. Early after transplantation, HSV may cause either oral or anogenital lesions that are usually responsive to acyclovir. Large ulcerating lesions in the anogenital area may lead to bladder and rectal dysfunction as well as predisposing to bacterial infection. VZV may cause fatal disseminated infection in nonimmune kidney transplant recipients, but in immune patients reactivation zoster usually does not disseminate outside the dermatome; thus disseminated VZV infection is a less fearsome complication in kidney transplantation than in hematopoietic stem cell transplantation. HHV-6 reactivation may take place and (although usually asymptomatic) may be associated with fever, rash, marrow suppression, or encephalitis.

EBV disease is more serious; it may present as an extranodal proliferation of B cells that invade the central nervous system (CNS), nasopharynx, liver, small bowel, heart, and other organs, including the transplanted kidney. The disease is diagnosed by the finding of a mass of proliferating EBV-positive B cells. The incidence of EBV-LPD is higher among patients who acquire EBV infection from the donor and among patients given high doses of cyclosporine, FK506, glucocorticoids, and anti–T cell antibodies. Disease may regress once immunocompetence is restored. KSHV infection can be transmitted with the donor kidney, although it more often represents latent infection of the recipient. Kaposi's sarcoma often appears within 1 year after transplantation, although the range of onset is wide (1 month to ~20 years). Avoidance of immunosuppressive agents that inhibit calcineurin has been associated with less outgrowth of EBV and less CMV replication. The use of rapamycin (sirolimus) has led to regression of Kaposi's sarcoma.

The papovaviruses BK virus and JC virus (polyomavirus hominis types 1 and 2) have been cultured from the urine of kidney transplant recipients (as they have from that of HSCT recipients) in the setting of profound immunosuppression. High levels of BK virus replication detected by PCR in urine and blood are predictive of pathology, particularly in the setting of renal transplantation. Excretion of BK virus and BK viremia are associated with the development of ureteral strictures, polyomavirus-associated nephropathy (1–10% of renal transplant recipients), and (less commonly) generalized vasculopathy. Timely reduction of immunosuppression is critical and can reduce rates of graft loss related to polyomavirus-associated nephropathy from 90% to 10–30%. A possible role for treatment with cidofovir (given by the IV route and by bladder instillation), leflunomide, quinolones, and (most recently) lactoferrin has been reported, but the efficacy of these agents has not been substantiated through adequate clinical study. JC virus is associated with rare cases of progressive multifocal leukoencephalopathy. Adenoviruses may persist with continued immunosuppression in these patients, but disseminated disease like that which occurs in HSCT recipients is much less common.

Kidney transplant recipients are also subject to infections with other intracellular organisms. These patients may develop pulmonary infections with *Nocardia*, *Aspergillus*, and *Mucor* as well as infections with other pathogens in which the T cell/macrophage axis plays an important role. In patients without IV catheters, *Listeria monocytogenes* is a common cause of bacteremia ≥1 month after renal transplantation and should be seriously considered in renal transplant recipients presenting with fever and headache. Kidney transplant recipients may develop *Salmonella* bacteremia, which can lead to endovascular infections and require prolonged therapy. Pulmonary infections with *Pneumocystis* are common unless the patient is maintained on TMP-SMX prophylaxis. *Nocardia* infection may present in the skin, bones, and lungs or in the CNS, where it usually takes the form of single or multiple brain abscesses. Nocardiosis generally occurs ≥1 month after transplantation and may follow immunosuppressive treatment for an episode of rejection. Pulmonary findings are nonspecific: localized disease with or without cavities is most common, but the disease may disseminate. The diagnosis is made by culture of the organism from sputum or from the involved nodule. As with *Pneumocystis*, prophylaxis with TMP-SMX is often efficacious in the prevention of disease. The occurrence of *Nocardia* infections >2 years after transplantation suggests that a long-term prophylactic regimen may be justified.

Toxoplasmosis can occur in seropositive patients but is less common than in other transplant settings, usually developing in the first few months after kidney transplantation. Again, TMP-SMX is helpful in prevention. In endemic areas, histoplasmosis, coccidioidomycosis, and blastomycosis may cause pulmonary infiltrates or disseminated disease.

Late Infections

Late infections (>6 months after kidney transplantation) may involve the CNS and include CMV retinitis as well as other CNS manifestations of CMV disease. Patients (particularly those whose immunosuppression has been increased) are at risk for subacute meningitis due to *Cryptococcus neoformans*. Cryptococcal disease may present in an insidious manner (sometimes as a skin infection before the development of clear CNS findings). *Listeria* meningitis may have an acute presentation and requires prompt therapy to avoid a fatal outcome.

Patients who continue to take glucocorticoids are predisposed to ongoing infection. "Transplant elbow" is a recurrent bacterial infection in and around the elbow that is thought to result from a combination of poor tensile strength of the skin of steroid-treated patients and steroid-induced proximal myopathy that requires patients to push themselves up with their elbows to get out of chairs. Bouts of cellulitis (usually caused by *Staphylococcus aureus*) recur until patients are provided with elbow protection.

Kidney transplant recipients are susceptible to invasive fungal infections, including those due to *Aspergillus* and *Rhizopus*, which may present as superficial lesions before dissemination. Mycobacterial infection (particularly that with *Mycobacterium marinum*) can be diagnosed by skin examination. Infection with *Prototheca wickerhamii* (an achlorophyllic alga) has been diagnosed by skin biopsy. Warts caused by human papillomaviruses (HPVs) are a late consequence of persistent immunosuppression; imiquimod or other forms of local therapy are usually satisfactory.

Although BK virus replication and virus-associated disease can be detected far earlier, the median time to clinical diagnosis of polyomavirus-associated nephropathy is ~300 days, qualifying it as a late-onset disease. With establishment of better screening procedures (e.g., blood PCR), it is likely that this disease will be detected earlier (see "Middle-Period Infections," earlier in the chapter).

MISCELLANEOUS INFECTIONS IN SOLID ORGAN TRANSPLANTATION

Indwelling IV Catheter Infections

The prolonged use of indwelling IV catheters for administration of medications, blood products, and nutrition is common in diverse transplantation settings and poses a risk of local and bloodstream infections. Significant insertion-site infection is most commonly caused by *S. aureus*. Bloodstream infection most frequently develops within a week of catheter placement or in patients who become neutropenic. Coagulase-negative staphylococci are the most common isolates from the blood.

Tuberculosis

The incidence of tuberculosis occurring within the first 12 months after solid organ transplantation is greater than that observed after hematopoietic stem cell transplantation (0.23–0.79%) and ranges broadly worldwide (1.2–15%), reflecting the prevalences of tuberculosis in local populations. Lesions suggesting prior tuberculosis on chest x-ray, older age, diabetes, chronic liver disease, graft-versus-host disease (GVHD), and intense immunosuppression are predictive of tuberculosis reactivation and development of disseminated disease in a host with latent disease. Tuberculosis has rarely been transmitted from the donor organ. In contrast to the low mortality rate among HSCT recipients, mortality rates among SOT patients are reported to be as high as 30%. Vigilance is indicated, as the presentation of disease is often extrapulmonary (gastrointestinal, genitourinary, central nervous, endocrine, musculoskeletal, laryngeal) and atypical, sometimes manifesting as a fever of unknown origin. A careful history and a direct evaluation of both the recipient and the donor prior to transplantation are optimal. Skin testing of the recipient with PPD may be unreliable because of chronic disease and/or immunosuppression, but newer cell-based assays that measure interferon and/or cytokine production may prove more sensitive in the future. Isoniazid toxicity has not been a significant problem except in the setting of liver transplantation. Therefore, appropriate prophylaxis should proceed. An assessment of the need to treat latent disease should include careful consideration of the possibility of a false-negative test result. Pending final confirmation of suspected tuberculosis, aggressive multidrug treatment in accordance with the guidelines of the Centers for Disease Control and Prevention (CDC), the Infectious Diseases Society of America, and the American Thoracic Society is indicated because of the high mortality rates among these patients. Altered drug metabolism (e.g., upon co-administration of rifampin and certain immunosuppressive agents) can be managed with careful monitoring of drug levels and appropriate dose adjustment. Close follow-up of hepatic enzymes is warranted, particularly during treatment with isoniazid, pyrazinamide, and/or rifampin. Drug-resistant tuberculosis is especially problematic in these individuals.

Virus-Associated Malignancies

In addition to malignancy associated with gammaherpesvirus infection (EBV, KSHV) and simple warts (HPV), other tumors that are virus associated or suspected of being virus associated are more likely to develop in transplant recipients, particularly those who require long-term immunosuppression, than in the general population. The interval to tumor development is usually >1 year. Transplant recipients develop nonmelanoma skin or lip cancers that, in contrast to de novo skin cancers, have a high ratio of squamous cells to basal cells. HPV may play a major role in these lesions. Cervical and vulvar carcinomas, quite clearly associated with HPV, develop with increased frequency in female transplant recipients. Among renal transplant recipients, rates of melanoma are modestly increased and rates of cancers of the kidney and bladder are increased.

VACCINATION OF TRANSPLANT RECIPIENTS

In addition to receiving antibiotic prophylaxis, transplant recipients should be vaccinated against likely pathogens (Table 14-4). In the case of HSCT recipients, optimal responses cannot be achieved until after immune reconstitution, despite previous immunization of both donor and recipient. Recipients of allogeneic HSCTs must be reimmunized if they are to be protected against pathogens. The situation is less clear-cut in the case of autologous transplantation. T and B cells in the peripheral blood may reconstitute the immune response if they are transferred in adequate numbers. However, cancer patients (particularly those with Hodgkin's disease, in whom vaccination has been extensively studied) who are undergoing chemotherapy do not respond normally to immunization, and titers of antibodies to infectious agents fall more rapidly than in healthy individuals. Therefore, even immunosuppressed patients who have not had HSCTs may need booster vaccine injections. If memory cells are specifically eliminated as part of a stem cell "cleanup" procedure, it will be necessary to reimmunize the recipient with a new primary series. Optimal times for immunizations of different transplant

TABLE 14-4

VACCINATION FOR SOLID ORGAN TRANSPLANT (SOT) RECIPIENTS[a]

Streptococcus pneumoniae, Haemophilus influenzae, Neisseria meningitidis	Immunize before transplantation and every 5 years for Pneumovax (others not established) See CDC recommendations
Seasonal influenza	Vaccinate in the fall Vaccinate close contacts
Poliomyelitis	Administer inactivated vaccine
Measles/mumps/rubella	Immunize before transplantation with attenuated vaccine
Tetanus, diphtheria	Immunize before transplantation; give boosters at 10 years or as required; primary series not required
Hepatitis B and A	Immunize before transplantation as appropriate
Human papillomavirus	Recommendations pending

[a]Immunizations should be given before transplantation whenever possible.

populations are being evaluated. Yearly immunization of household and other contacts (including health care personnel) against influenza benefits the patient by preventing local spread.

In the absence of compelling data as to optimal timing, it is reasonable to administer the pneumococcal and *Haemophilus influenzae* type b conjugate vaccines to both autologous and allogeneic HSCT recipients beginning 12 months after transplantation. A series that includes both the 7-valent pneumococcal conjugate vaccine and the 23-valent Pneumovax is now recommended (following CDC guidelines). The pneumococcal and *H. influenzae* type b vaccines are particularly important for patients who have undergone splenectomy. In addition, diphtheria, tetanus, acellular pertussis, and inactivated polio vaccines can all be given at these same intervals (12 months and, as required, 24 months after transplantation). *Neisseria meningitidis* polysaccharide (a new conjugate vaccine) is now available and will probably be recommended in the future. Some authorities recommend a new primary series for tetanus/diphtheria/pertussis and inactivated polio vaccine beginning 12 months after transplantation. Because of the risk of spread, household contacts of HSCT recipients (or of patients immunosuppressed as a result of chemotherapy) should receive only inactivated polio vaccine. Live-virus measles/mumps/rubella (MMR) vaccine can be given to autologous HSCT recipients 24 months after transplantation and to most allogeneic HSCT recipients at the same point if they are not receiving maintenance therapy with immunosuppressive drugs and do not have ongoing GVHD. The risk of spread from a household contact is lower for MMR vaccine than for polio vaccine. Neither patients nor their household contacts should be vaccinated with vaccinia unless they have been exposed to the smallpox virus. Among patients who have active GVHD and/or are taking high maintenance doses of glucocorticoids, it may be prudent to avoid all live-virus vaccines. Vaccination to prevent hepatitis B and hepatitis A also seems advisable.

In the case of SOT recipients, administration of all the usual vaccines and of the indicated booster doses should be completed before immunosuppression, if possible, to maximize responses. For patients taking immunosuppressive agents, the administration of pneumococcal vaccine should be repeated every 5 years. No data are available for the meningococcal vaccine, but it is probably reasonable to administer it along with the pneumococcal vaccine. *H. influenzae* conjugate vaccine is safe and should be efficacious in this population; therefore, its administration before transplantation is recommended. Booster doses of this vaccine are not recommended for adults. SOT recipients who continue to receive immunosuppressive drugs should not receive live-virus vaccines. A person in this group who is exposed to measles should be given immune globulin. Similarly, an immunocompromised patient who is seronegative for varicella and who comes into contact with a person who has chickenpox should be given varicella-zoster immune globulin as soon as possible (and certainly within 96 h) or, if this is not possible, should be started immediately on a 10- to 14-day course of acyclovir therapy. Upon the discontinuation of treatment, clinical disease may still occur in a small number of patients; thus vigilance is indicated. Rapid re-treatment should limit the symptoms of disease. Household contacts of transplant recipients can receive live attenuated VZV vaccine, but vaccinees should avoid direct contact with the patient if a rash develops. Virus-like particle (VLP) vaccines (not live attenuated) have recently been licensed for the prevention of infection with several HPV serotypes most commonly implicated in cervical and anal carcinomas and in anogenital and laryngeal warts. For example, the tetravalent vaccine contains HPV serotypes 6, 11, 16, and 18. At present, no information is available about the safety, immunogenicity, or efficacy of this vaccine in transplant recipients.

Immunocompromised patients who travel may benefit from some but not all vaccines. In general, these patients should receive any killed or inactivated vaccine preparation appropriate to the area they are visiting; this recommendation includes the vaccines for Japanese encephalitis, hepatitis A and B, poliomyelitis, meningococcal infection, and typhoid. The live typhoid vaccines are not recommended for use in most immunocompromised patients, but inactivated or purified polysaccharide typhoid vaccine can be used. Live yellow fever vaccine should not be administered.

On the other hand, primary immunization or boosting with the purified-protein hepatitis B vaccine is indicated if patients are likely to be exposed. Patients who will reside for >6 months in areas where hepatitis B is common (Africa, Southeast Asia, the Middle East, Eastern Europe, parts of South America, and the Caribbean) should receive hepatitis B vaccine. Inactivated hepatitis A vaccine should also be used in the appropriate setting. A combined vaccine is now available that provides dual protection against hepatitis A and hepatitis B. If hepatitis A vaccine is not administered, travelers should consider receiving passive protection with immune globulin (the dose depending on the duration of travel in the high-risk area).

FURTHER READINGS

BIRDWELL KA et al: Decreased antibody response to influenza vaccination in kidney transplant recipients: A prospective cohort study. Am J Kidney Dis 54:112, 2009

HIRSCH HH, SUTHANTHIRAN M: The natural history, risk factors and outcomes of polyomavirus BK–associated nephropathy after renal transplantation. Nat Clin Pract Nephrol 2:240, 2006

HRICIK DE: Comparing early withdrawal or avoidance of steroids with standard steroid therapy in kidney transplant recipients. Nat Clin Pract Nephrol 4:360, 2008

KOTTON CN et al: Prevention of infection in adult travelers after solid organ transplantation. Am J Transplant 5:8, 2004

MUNOZ P et al: *Mycobacterium tuberculosis* infection in recipients of solid organ transplants. Clin Infect Dis 40:581, 2005

SNYDER JJ et al: Rates of first infection following kidney transplant in the United States. Kidney Int 75:317, 2009

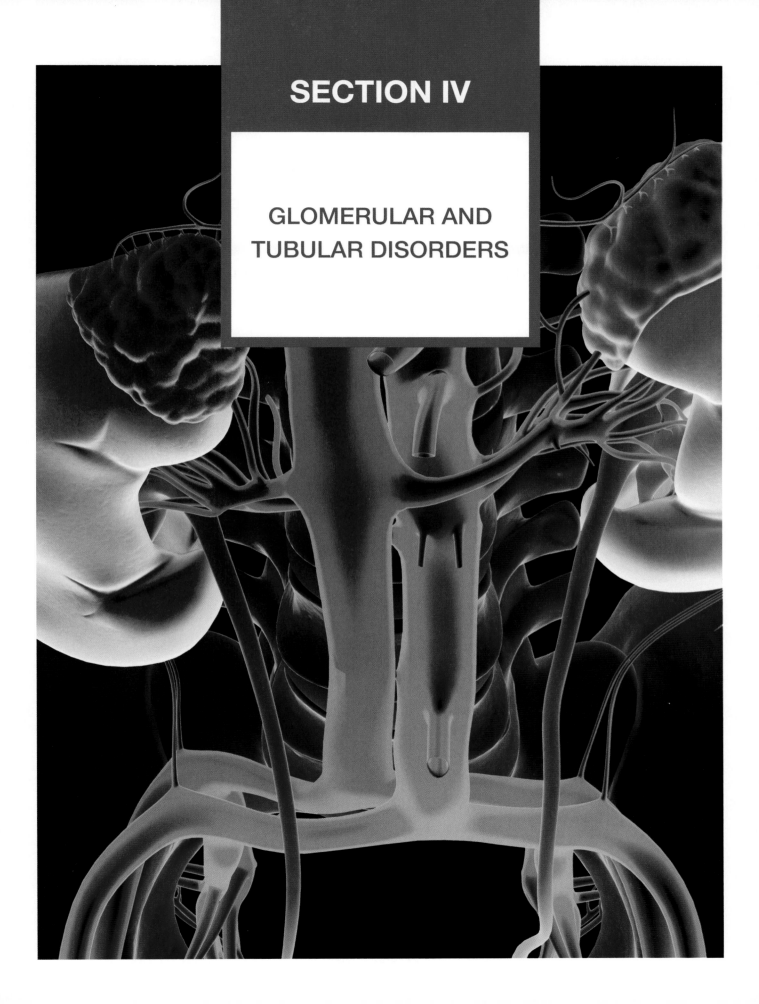

SECTION IV

GLOMERULAR AND TUBULAR DISORDERS

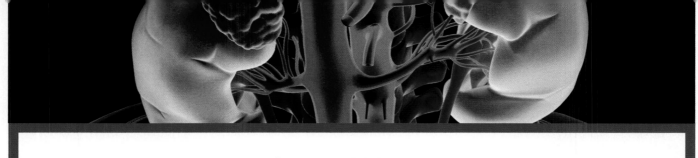

CHAPTER 15

GLOMERULAR DISEASES

Julia B. Lewis ■ Eric G. Neilson

Two human kidneys harbor nearly 1.8 million glomerular capillary tufts. Each glomerular tuft resides within Bowman's space. The capsule circumscribing this space is lined by parietal epithelial cells that transition into tubular epithelia forming the proximal nephron. The glomerular capillary tuft derives from an afferent arteriole that forms a branching capillary bed embedded in mesangial matrix (Fig. 15-1). This capillary network funnels into an efferent arteriole, which passes filtered blood into cortical peritubular capillaries or medullary vasa recta that supply and exchange with a folded tubular architecture. Hence the glomerular capillary tuft, fed and drained by arterioles, represents an arteriolar portal system. Fenestrated endothelial cells resting on a glomerular basement membrane (GBM) line glomerular capillaries. Delicate foot processes extending from epithelial podocytes shroud the outer surface of these capillaries, and

podocytes interconnect to each other by slit-pore membranes forming a selective filtration barrier.

The glomerular capillaries filter 120–180 L/d of plasma water containing various solutes for reclamation or discharge by downstream tubules. Most large proteins and all cells are excluded from filtration by a physicochemical barrier governed by pore size and negative electrostatic charge. The mechanics of filtration and reclamation are quite complicated for many solutes (Chap. 1). For example, in the case of serum albumin, the glomerulus is an imperfect barrier. Although albumin has a negative charge, which would tend to repel the negatively charged GBM, it only has a physical radius of 3.6 nm, while pores in the GBM and slit-pore membranes have a radius of 4 nm. Consequently, considerable amounts of albumin (estimates range from 4000 to 9000 mg/d) inevitably

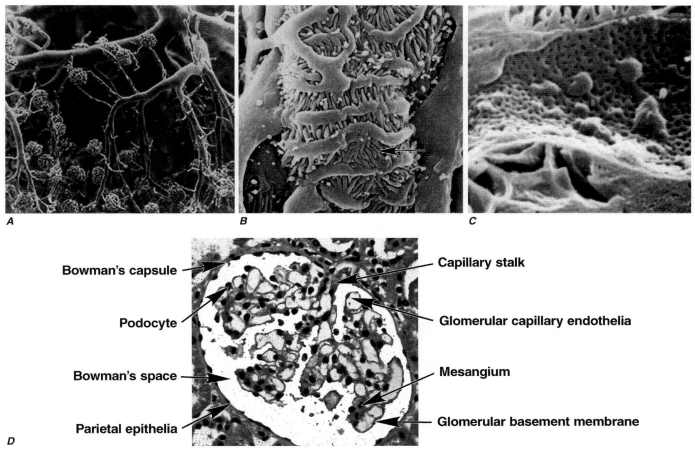

FIGURE 15-1

Glomerular architecture. A. The glomerular capillaries form from a branching network of renal arteries, arterioles, leading to an afferent arteriole, glomerular capillary bed (tuft), and a draining efferent arteriole (modified from Hypertension 5:8–16, 1983). **B.** Scanning electron micrograph of podocytes that line the outer surface of the glomerular capillaries (arrow shows foot process). **C.** Scanning electron micrograph of the fenestrated endothelia lining the glomerular capillary. **D.** The various normal regions of the glomerulus on light microscopy. (A–C, courtesy of Dr. Vincent Gattone, Indiana University; with permission.)

cross the filtration barrier to be reclaimed by megalin and cubilin receptors along the proximal tubule. Remarkably, humans with normal nephrons do not excrete more than 8–10 mg of albumin in daily voided urine. This amount of albumin, and other proteins, can rise to gram quantities following glomerular injury.

The breadth of diseases affecting the glomerulus is expansive because the glomerular capillaries can be injured in a variety of ways, producing many different lesions and several unique changes to the urinalysis. Some order to this vast subject is brought by grouping all of these diseases into a smaller number of clinical syndromes.

PATHOGENESIS OF GLOMERULAR DISEASE

There are many forms of glomerular disease with pathogenesis variably linked to the presence of genetic mutations, infection, toxin exposure, autoimmunity, atherosclerosis,

hypertension, emboli, thrombosis, or diabetes mellitus. Even after careful study, however, the cause often remains unknown, and the lesion is called *idiopathic*. Specific or unique features of pathogenesis are mentioned with the description of each of the glomerular diseases later in this chapter.

Some glomerular diseases result from genetic mutations producing familial disease. (1) Congenital nephrotic syndrome from mutations in *NPHS1* (nephrin) and *NPHS2* (podocin) affect the slit-pore membrane at birth, and *TRPC6* cation channel mutations in adulthood produce *focal segmental glomerulosclerosis* (FSGS). (2) Partial lipodystrophy from mutations in genes encoding lamin A/C or PPARγ cause a metabolic syndrome that can be associated with *membranoproliferative glomerulonephritis* (MPGN), which is sometimes accompanied by dense deposits and C3 nephritic factor. (3) Alport's syndrome, from mutations in the genes encoding for the α3, α4, or α5 chains of type IV collagen, produces *split-basement membranes* with *glomerulosclerosis*. (4) Lysosomal storage diseases, such as

SECTION IV

Glomerular and Tubular Disorders

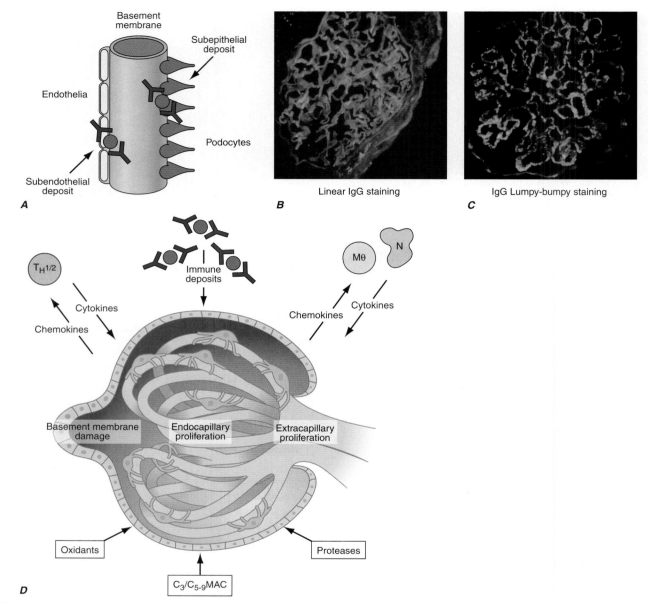

FIGURE 15-2

The glomerulus is injured by a variety of mechanisms. A.
Preformed immune deposits can precipitate from the circulation and collect along the glomerular basement membrane (GBM) in the subendothelial space or can form in situ along the subepithelial space. **B.** Immunofluorescent staining of glomeruli with labeled anti-IgG demonstrating linear staining from a patient with anti-GBM disease or immune deposits from a patient with membranous glomerulonephritis. **C.** The mechanisms of glomerular injury have a complicated pathogenesis.

Immune deposits and complement deposition classically draw macrophages and neutrophils into the glomerulus. T lymphocytes may follow to participate in the injury pattern as well. **D.** Amplification mediators as locally derived oxidants and proteases expand this inflammation, and, depending on the location of the target antigen and the genetic polymorphisms of the host, basement membranes are damaged with either endocapillary or extracapillary proliferation.

α–galactosidase A deficiency causing Fabry's disease and *N*-acetylneuraminic acid hydrolase deficiency causing nephrosialidosis, produce FSGS.

Systemic hypertension and atherosclerosis can produce pressure stress, ischemia, or lipid oxidants that lead to *chronic glomerulosclerosis. Malignant hypertension* can quickly complicate glomerulosclerosis with fibrinoid necrosis of arterioles and glomeruli, thrombotic microangiopathy, and acute

renal failure. *Diabetic nephropathy* is an acquired sclerotic injury associated with thickening of the GBM secondary to the long-standing effects of hyperglycemia, advanced glycosylation end-products, and reactive oxygen species.

Inflammation of the glomerular capillaries is called *glomerulonephritis*. Most glomerular or mesangial antigens involved in *immune-mediated glomerulonephritis* are unknown (**Fig. 15-2**). Glomerular epithelial or mesangial cells may shed them or express epitopes that mimic other immunogenic proteins made elsewhere in the body. Bacteria, fungi, and viruses can directly infect the kidney producing their own antigens. Autoimmune diseases like idiopathic *membranous glomerulonephritis* (MGN) or MPGN are confined to the kidney, while systemic inflammatory diseases like *lupus nephritis* or *Wegener's granulomatosis* spread to the kidney, causing secondary glomerular injury. *Antiglomerular basement membrane disease* producing Goodpasture's syndrome primarily injures both the lung and kidney because of the narrow distribution of the α3 NC1 domain of type IV collagen that is the target antigen.

While the adaptive immune response is similar to that of other tissues, early T cell activation plays an important role in the mechanism of glomerulonephritis. Antigens presented by class II major histocompatibility complex (MHC) molecules on macrophages and dendritic cells in conjunction with associative recognition molecules engage the CD4/8 T cell repertoire. Local activation of Toll-like receptors on glomerular cells, deposition of immune complexes, or complement injury to glomerular structures induces mononuclear cell infiltration, which subsequently leads to an adaptive immune response attracted to the kidney by local release of chemokines. Neutrophils, macrophages, and T cells are drawn by chemokines into the glomerular tuft, where they react with antigens and epitopes on or near somatic cells or their structures, producing more cytokines and proteases that damage the mesangium, capillaries, and/or the GBM.

Mononuclear cells by themselves can injure the kidney, but autoimmune events that damage glomeruli classically produce a humoral immune response. *Poststreptococcal glomerulonephritis*, *lupus nephritis*, and idiopathic *membranous nephritis* typically are associated with immune deposits along the GBM, while anti-GBM antibodies are produced in anti-GBM disease. Preformed circulating immune complexes can precipitate along the subendothelial side of the GBM, while other immune deposits form in situ on the subepithelial side. These latter deposits accumulate when circulating autoantibodies find their antigen trapped along the subepithelial edge of the GBM. Immune deposits in the glomerular mesangium may result from the deposition of preformed circulating complexes or in situ antigen–antibody interactions. Immune deposits can stimulate the release of local proteases and activate the complement cascade, producing C_{5-9} attack complexes. In addition, local oxidants can damage glomerular structures, producing proteinuria and effacement of the podocytes. Overlapping etiologies or pathophysiologic mechanisms can produce similar glomerular lesions, suggesting that downstream molecular and cellular responses often converge towards common patterns of injury.

PROGRESSION OF GLOMERULAR DISEASE

Persistent glomerulonephritis that worsens renal function is always accompanied by interstitial nephritis, renal fibrosis, and tubular atrophy (Fig. 4-25). What is not so obvious, however, is that renal failure in glomerulonephritis best correlates histologically with the appearance of tubulointerstitial nephritis rather than with the type of inciting glomerular injury.

Loss of renal function due to interstitial damage can be explained hypothetically by several mechanisms. The simplest explanation is that urine flow is impeded by tubular obstruction as a result of interstitial inflammation and fibrosis. Thus, obstruction of the tubules with debris or by extrinsic compression results in aglomerular nephrons. A second mechanism suggests that interstitial changes, including interstitial edema or fibrosis, alter tubular and vascular architecture and thereby compromise the normal tubular transport of solutes and water from tubular lumen to vascular space. This failure increases the solute and water content of the tubule fluid, resulting in isosthenuria and polyuria. Adaptive mechanisms related to tubuloglomerular feedback also fail, resulting in a reduction of renin output from the juxtaglomerular apparatus of glomeruli trapped by interstitial inflammation. Consequently, the local vasoconstrictive influence of angiotensin II on the glomerular arterioles decreases, and filtration drops owing to a generalized decrease in arteriolar tone. A third mechanism involves changes in vascular resistance due to damage of peritubular capillaries. The cross-sectional volume of these capillaries is decreased in areas of interstitial inflammation, edema, or fibrosis. These structural alterations in vascular resistance affect renal function through two mechanisms. First, tubular cells are very metabolically active, and, as a result, decreased perfusion could lead to ischemic injury. Second, impairment of glomerular arteriolar outflow leads to increased intraglomerular hypertension in less involved glomeruli; this selective intraglomerular hypertension aggravates and extends *mesangial sclerosis* and *glomerulosclerosis* to less-involved glomeruli. Regardless of the exact mechanism, early *acute tubulointerstitial nephritis* suggests potentially recoverable renal function, while the development of *chronic interstitial fibrosis* prognosticates a permanent loss.

Persistent damage to glomerular capillaries spreads to the tubulointerstitium in association with proteinuria. There is an untested hypothesis that efferent arterioles leading from inflamed glomeruli carry forward inflammatory mediators, which induces downstream interstitial nephritis, resulting in fibrosis. Glomerular filtrate from injured glomerular capillaries adherent to Bowman's capsule may also be misdirected to the periglomerular interstitium. Most nephrologists believe, however, that proteinuric glomerular filtrate forming tubular fluid is the primary route to downstream tubulointerstitial injury, although none of these hypotheses are mutually exclusive.

The simplest explanation for the effect of proteinuria on the development of interstitial nephritis is that increasingly severe proteinuria, carrying activated cytokines and lipoproteins producing reactive oxygen species, triggers a downstream inflammatory cascade in and around epithelial cells lining the tubular nephron. These effects induce T lymphocyte and macrophage infiltrates in the interstitial spaces along with fibrosis and tubular atrophy. The details of this process are described in Chap. 2.

Tubules disappear following direct damage to their basement membranes, leading to decondensation and epithelial–mesenchymal transitions forming more interstitial fibroblasts at the site of injury. Transforming growth factor β (TGF-β), fibroblast growth factor 2, and platelet-derived growth factor (PDGF) are particularly active in this transition. With persistent nephritis, fibroblasts multiply and lay down tenascin and a fibronectin scaffold for the polymerization of new interstitial collagens I/III. These events form scar tissue through a process called fibrogenesis. In experimental studies, bone morphogenetic protein 7 and hematopoietic growth factor can reverse early fibrogenesis and preserve tubular architecture. When fibroblasts outdistance their survival factors, they apoptose, and the permanent renal scar becomes acellular, leading to irreversible renal failure.

Approach to the Patient:
GLOMERULAR DISEASE

Hematuria, Proteinuria, and Pyuria Patients with glomerular disease usually have some hematuria with varying degrees of proteinuria. Hematuria is typically asymptomatic. As little as 3–5 red blood cells in the spun sediment from first voided morning urine is suspicious. The diagnosis of glomerular injury can be delayed because patients will not realize they have *microscopic hematuria*, and only rarely with the exception of IgA nephropathy and sickle cell disease is *gross hematuria* present. When working up microscopic hematuria, perhaps accompanied by minimal proteinuria (<500 mg/24 h), it is important to exclude anatomic lesions, such as malignancy of the urinary tract, particularly in older men. Microscopic hematuria may also appear with the onset of benign prostatic hypertrophy, interstitial nephritis, papillary necrosis, renal stones, cystic kidney diseases, or renal vascular injury. However, when red blood cell casts (Fig. 4-31) or dysmorphic red blood cells are found in the sediment, glomerulonephritis is likely.

Sustained proteinuria >1–2 g/24 h is also commonly associated with glomerular disease. Patients often will not know they have proteinuria unless they become edematous or notice foamy urine on voiding. *Sustained proteinuria* has to be distinguished from lesser amounts of so-called *benign proteinuria* in the normal population (Table 15-1). This latter class of proteinuria is nonsustained, generally <1 g/24 h, and is sometimes called *functional* or *transient proteinuria*. Fever, exercise, obesity, sleep apnea, emotional stress, and congestive heart failure can explain transient proteinuria. Proteinuria only seen with upright posture is called *orthostatic proteinuria*. Occasionally, isolated proteinuria sustained over multiple clinic visits is found in diabetic nephropathy, *nil lesion*, *mesangioproliferative glomerulonephritis*, and FSGS. Proteinuria in most adults with glomerular disease is *nonselective*, containing albumin and a mixture of other serum proteins, while in children with nil lesion from *minimal change disease*, the proteinuria is *selective* and largely composed of albumin.

Some patients with inflammatory glomerular disease, such as acute poststreptococcal glomerulonephritis or MPGN, may have *pyuria* caused by the presence of considerable numbers of leukocytes in the urine. This latter finding has to be distinguished from urine infected with bacteria.

Clinical Syndromes Various forms of glomerular injury can also be parsed into several distinct syndromes on clinical grounds (Table 15-2). These syndromes, however, are not always mutually exclusive. There is an *acute nephritic syndrome* producing 1–2 g/24 h of proteinuria, hematuria with red blood cell casts, pyuria, hypertension, fluid retention, and a rise in serum creatinine associated with a reduction in glomerular filtration. If glomerular inflammation develops slowly, the serum creatinine will rise gradually over many weeks, but if the serum creatinine rises quickly, particularly over a few days, acute nephritis is sometimes called *rapidly progressive glomerulonephritis* (RPGN); the histopathologic term *crescentic glomerulonephritis* refers to the clinical occurrence of RPGN in a patient with this characteristic glomerular lesion. When patients with

TABLE 15-1

URINE ASSAYS FOR ALBUMINURIA/PROTEINURIA

	24-HOUR ALBUMIN[a] (mg/24 h)	ALBUMIN[a]/CREATININE RATIO (mg/g)	DIPSTICK PROTEINURIA	24-HOUR URINE PROTEIN[b] (mg/24 h)
Normal	8–10	<30	–	<150
Microalbuminuria	30–300	30–300	–/Trace/1+	–
Proteinuria	>300	>300	Trace–3+	>150

[a]Albumin detected by radioimmunoassay.
[b]Albumin represents 30–70% of the total protein excreted in the urine.

TABLE 15-2

PATTERNS OF CLINICAL GLOMERULONEPHRITIS

GLOMERULAR SYNDROMES	PROTEINURIA	HEMATURIA	VASCULAR INJURY
Acute Nephritic Syndromes			
Poststreptococcal glomerulonephritis[a]	+/++	++/+++	−
Subacute bacterial endocarditis[a]	+/++	++	−
Lupus nephritis[a]	+/++	++/+++	−
Antiglomerular basement membrane disease[a]	++	++/+++	−
IgA nephropathy[a]	+/++	++/+++[c]	−
ANCA small-vessel vasculitis[a]			
Wegener's granulomatosis	+/++	++/+++	++++
Microscopic polyangiitis	+/++	++/+++	++++
Churg-Strauss syndrome	+/++	++/+++	++++
Henoch-Schönlein purpura[a]	+/++	++/+++	++++
Cryoglobulinemia[a]	+/++	++/+++	++++
Membranoproliferative glomerulonephritis[a]	++	++/+++	−
Mesangioproliferative glomerulonephritis	+	+/++	−
Pulmonary-Renal Syndromes			
Goodpasture's syndrome[a]	++	++/+++	−
ANCA small-vessel vasculitis[a]			
Wegener's granulomatosis	+/++	++/+++	++++
Microscopic polyangiitis	+/++	++/+++	++++
Churg-Strauss syndrome	+/++	++/+++	++++
Henoch-Schönlein purpura[a]	+/++	++/+++	++++
Cryoglobulinemia[a]	+/++	++/+++	++++
Nephrotic Syndromes			
Minimal change disease	++++	−	−
Focal segmental glomerulosclerosis	+++/++++	+	−
Membranous glomerulonephritis	++++	+	−
Diabetic nephropathy	++/++++	−/+	−
AL and AA amyloidosis	+++/++++	+	+/++
Light-chain deposition disease	+++	+	−
Fibrillary-immunotactoid disease	+++/++++	+	+
Fabry's disease	+	+	−
Basement Membrane Syndromes			
Anti-GBM disease[a]	++	++/+++	−
Alport's syndrome	++	++	−
Thin basement membrane disease	+	++	−
Nail-patella syndrome	++/+++	++	−
Glomerular Vascular Syndromes			
Atherosclerotic nephropathy	+	+	+++
Hypertensive nephropathy[b]	+/++	+/++	++
Cholesterol emboli	+/++	++	+++
Sickle cell disease	+/++	++[c]	+++
Thrombotic microangiopathies	++	++	+++
Antiphospholipid syndrome	++	++	+++
ANCA small-vessel vasculitis[a]			
Wegener's granulomatosis	+/++	++/+++	++++
Microscopic polyangiitis	+/++	++/+++	++++
Churg-Strauss syndrome	+++	++/+++	++++
Henoch-Schönlein purpura[a]	+/++	++/+++	++++
Cryoglobulinemia[a]	+/++	++/+++	++++
AL and AA amyloidosis	+++/++++	+	+/++
Infectious Disease–Associated Syndromes			
Poststreptococcal glomerulonephritis[a]	+/++	++/+++	−
Subacute bacterial endocarditis[a]	+/++	++	−

(Continued)

TABLE 15-2 (*CONTINUED*)

PATTERNS OF CLINICAL GLOMERULONEPHRITIS

GLOMERULAR SYNDROMES	PROTEINURIA	HEMATURIA	VASCULAR INJURY
HIV	+++	+/++	–
Hepatitis B and C	+++	+/++	–
Syphilis	+++	+	–
Leprosy	+++	+	–
Malaria	+++	+/++	–
Schistosomiasis	+++	+/++	–

[a]Can present as rapidly progressive glomerulonephritis (RPGN); sometimes called crescentic glomerulonephritis.
[b]Can present as a malignant hypertensive crisis producing an aggressive fibrinoid necrosis in arterioles small arteries with microangiopathic hemolytic anemia.
[c]Can present with gross hematuria.
Note: ANCA, antineutrophil cytoplasmic antibodies; AL, amyloid L; AA, amyloid A; GBM, glomerular basement membrane.

RPGN present with lung hemorrhage from Goodpasture's syndrome, antineutrophil cytoplasmic antibodies (ANCA) small-vessel vasculitis, lupus erythematosus, or cryoglobulinemia, they are often diagnosed as having a *pulmonary-renal syndrome*. *Nephrotic syndrome* describes the onset of heavy proteinuria (>3.0 g/24 h), hypertension, hypercholesterolemia, hypoalbuminemia, edema/anasarca, and microscopic hematuria; if only large amounts of proteinuria are present without clinical manifestations, the condition is sometimes called *nephrotic-range proteinuria*. The glomerular filtration rate (GFR) in these patients may initially be normal or, rarely, higher than normal, but with persistent hyperfiltration and continued nephron loss, it typically declines over months to years. Patients with a *basement membrane syndrome* either have genetically abnormal basement membranes or an autoimmune response to basement membrane collagen IV associated with microscopic hematuria, mild to heavy proteinuria, and hypertension with variable elevations in serum creatinine. *Glomerular-vascular syndrome* describes patients with vascular injury producing hematuria and moderate proteinuria. Affected individuals can have vasculitis, thrombotic microangiopathy, antiphospholipid syndrome, or, more commonly, a systemic disease such as atherosclerosis, cholesterol emboli, hypertension, sickle cell anemia, and autoimmunity. *Infectious diseases-associated syndrome* is most important if one has an international perspective. Save for subacute bacterial endocarditis in the western hemisphere, malaria and schistosomiasis may be the most common causes of glomerulonephritis throughout the world, closely followed by HIV and chronic hepatitis B and C. These infectious diseases produce a variety of inflammatory reactions in glomerular capillaries, ranging from nephrotic syndrome to acute nephritic injury, and yield urinalyses that demonstrate a combination of hematuria and proteinuria.

These six general categories of syndromes are usually determined at the bedside with the help of a history and physical examination, blood chemistries, renal ultrasound, and urinalysis. These initial studies help frame further diagnostic workup that typically involves some testing of the serum for the presence of various proteins (HIV and hepatitis B and C antigens), antibodies (anti-GBM, antiphospholipid, ASO, anti-DNAase, anti-hyaluronidase, ANCA, anti-DNA, cryoglobulins, anti-HIV, and anti–hepatitis B and C antibodies) or depletion of complement components (C_3 and C_4). The bedside history and physical examination can also help determine whether the glomerulonephritis is isolated to the kidney (*primary glomerulonephritis*) or is part of a systemic disease (*secondary glomerulonephritis*). When confronted with an abnormal urinalysis and elevated serum creatinine, with or without edema or congestive heart failure, one must consider whether the glomerulonephritis is *acute* or *chronic*. This assessment is best made by careful history (last known urinalysis or serum creatinine during pregnancy or insurance physical, evidence of infection, or use of medication or recreational drugs); the size of the kidneys on renal ultrasound examination; and how the patient feels at presentation. Chronic glomerular disease often presents with decreased kidney size. Patients who quickly develop renal failure are fatigued and weak; feel miserable; often have uremic symptoms associated with nausea, vomiting, fluid retention, and somnolence. Primary glomerulonephritis presenting with renal failure that has progressed slowly, however, can be remarkably asymptomatic, as are patients with acute glomerulonephritis without much loss in renal function. Once this initial information is collected, selected patients who are clinically stable, have adequate blood clotting parameters, and are willing to receive treatment are encouraged to have a renal biopsy. Biopsies can be done safely with an ultrasound-guided biopsy gun.

RENAL PATHOLOGY

A renal biopsy in the setting of glomerulonephritis can quickly identify the type of glomerular injury and often suggests a course of treatment. The biopsy is processed for light microscopy using stains for *hematoxylin and eosin* (H&E) to assess cellularity and architecture, *periodic acid-Schiff* (PAS) to stain carbohydrate moieties in the membranes of the glomerular tuft and tubules, *Jones-methenamine silver* to enhance basement membrane structure, *Congo red* for amyloid deposits, and *Masson's trichrome* to identify collagen deposition and assess the degree of glomerulosclerosis and interstitial fibrosis. Biopsies are also processed for direct immunofluorescence using conjugated antibodies against IgG, IgM, and IgA to detect the presence of "lumpy-bumpy" immune deposits or "linear" IgG or IgA antibodies bound to GBM, antibodies against trapped complement proteins (C_3 and C_4), or specific antibodies against a relevant antigen. High-resolution electron microscopy can clarify the principal location of immune deposits and the status of the basement membrane.

Each region of a renal biopsy is assessed separately. By light microscopy, glomeruli (at least 10 and ideally 20) are reviewed individually for discrete lesions; <50% involvement is considered *focal*, and >50% is *diffuse*. Injury in each glomerular tuft can be *segmental*, involving a portion of the tuft, or *global*, involving most of the glomerulus. Glomeruli can have *proliferative* characteristics, showing increased cellularity. When cells in the capillary tuft proliferate, it is called *endocapillary*, and when cellular proliferation extends into Bowman's space, it is called *extracapillary*. *Synechiae* are formed when epithelial podocytes attach to Bowman's capsule in the setting of glomerular injury; *crescents*, which in some cases may be the extension of synechiae, develop when fibrocellular/fibrin collections fill all or part of Bowman's space; and *sclerotic* glomeruli show acellular, amorphous accumulations of proteinaceous material throughout the tuft with loss of functional capillaries and normal mesangium. Since *age-related glomerulosclerosis* is common in adults, one can estimate the background percentage of sclerosis by dividing the patient's age in half and subtracting 10. Immunofluorescent and electron microscopy can detect the presence and location of *subepithelial, subendothelial, or mesangial* immune deposits, or *reduplication* or *splitting* of the basement membrane. In the other regions of the biopsy, the vasculature surrounding glomeruli and tubules can show *angiopathy, vasculitis*, the presence of *fibrils*, or *thrombi*. The tubules can be assessed for adjacency to one another; separation can be the result of edema, tubular dropout, or collagen deposition resulting from interstitial fibrosis. Interstitial fibrosis is an ominous sign of irreversibility and progression to renal failure.

ACUTE NEPHRITIC SYNDROMES

Acute nephritic syndromes classically present with hypertension, hematuria, red blood cell casts, pyuria, and mild to moderate proteinuria. Extensive inflammatory damage to glomeruli can cause a fall in GFR and eventually produce uremic symptoms with salt and water retention, leading to edema and hypertension.

POSTSTREPTOCOCCAL GLOMERULONEPHRITIS

Poststreptococcal glomerulonephritis is prototypical for *acute endocapillary proliferative glomerulonephritis*. The incidence of poststreptococcal glomerulonephritis is decreasing in Western countries, and it is typically sporadic. Epidemic cases are still seen, though less commonly. Acute poststreptococcal glomerulonephritis typically affects children between the ages of 2 and 14 years, but 10% of cases are patients older than 40. It is more common in males, and the familial or cohabitant incidence is as high as 40%. Skin and throat infections with particular M types of streptococci (nephritogenic strains) antedate glomerular disease; M types 47, 49, 55, 2, 60, and 57 are seen following impetigo and M types 1, 2, 4, 3, 25, 49, and 12 with pharyngitis. Poststreptococcal glomerulonephritis due to impetigo develops 2–6 weeks after skin infection and 1–3 weeks after streptococcal pharyngitis.

The renal biopsy in poststreptococcal glomerulonephritis demonstrates hypercellularity of mesangial and endothelial cells, glomerular infiltrates of polymorphonuclear leukocytes, granular subendothelial immune deposits of IgG, IgM, C_3, C_4, and C_{5-9}, and subepithelial deposits (which appear as "humps") (Fig. 4-4). Poststreptococcal glomerulonephritis is an immune-mediated disease involving putative streptococcal antigens, circulating immune complexes, and activation of complement in association with cell-mediated injury. Many candidate antigens have been proposed over the years; three such candidates from nephritogenic streptococci are zymogen, a precursor of exotoxin B; glyceraldehyde phosphate dehydrogenase, also known as presorbing antigen (PA-Ag); and streptokinase. All have a biochemical affinity for GBMs, and in this location they may act as a target for antibodies.

The classic presentation is an acute nephritic picture with hematuria, pyuria, red blood cell casts, edema, hypertension, and oliguric renal failure, which may be severe enough to appear as RPGN. Systemic symptoms of headache, malaise, anorexia, and flank pain (due to swelling of the renal capsule) are reported in as many as 50% of cases. Five percent of children and 20% of adults have proteinuria in the nephrotic range. In the first week of symptoms, 90% of patients will have a depressed CH_{50} and decreased levels of C_3 with normal levels of C_4. Positive rheumatoid factor (30–40%), cryoglobulins and circulating immune complexes (60–70%), and ANCA against myeloperoxidase (10%) are also reported. Positive cultures for streptococcal infection are inconsistently present (10–70%), but increased titers of antistreptolysin O (ASO) (30%), anti-DNAase (70%) or antihyaluronidase antibodies (40%) can help confirm the diagnosis. Consequently, the diagnosis of poststreptococcal glomerulonephritis rarely requires a renal biopsy. A subclinical disease is reported in some series to be four to five times as common as clinical nephritis, and these latter cases are characterized by asymptomatic microscopic hematuria with low serum complement levels. Treatment is supportive, with control of hypertension, edema, and dialysis as needed. Antibiotic treatment for streptococcal infection should be given to all patients and their cohabitants. There is no role for immunosuppressive therapy, even in the setting of crescents. Recurrent poststreptococcal glomerulonephritis is rare despite repeated streptococcal infections. Early death is rare in children but does occur in the elderly. Overall, the prognosis is good, with permanent renal failure being very uncommon (1–3%), and even less so in children. Complete resolution of the hematuria and proteinuria in children occurs within 3–6 weeks of the onset of nephritis.

SUBACUTE BACTERIAL ENDOCARDITIS

Endocarditis-associated glomerulonephritis is typically a complication of subacute bacterial endocarditis, particularly in patients who remain untreated for a long time, have negative blood cultures, or have right-sided endocarditis. Glomerulonephritis is unusual in acute bacterial endocarditis because it takes 10–14 days to develop immune complex–mediated injury, by which time the patient has been treated, often with emergent surgery. Grossly, the kidneys in subacute bacterial endocarditis have subcapsular hemorrhages with a "flea-bitten" appearance, and microscopy on renal biopsy reveals a focal proliferation around foci of necrosis associated with abundant mesangial, subendothelial, and subepithelial immune deposits of IgG, IgM, and C_3. Patients who present with a clinical picture of RPGN have crescents. Embolic infarcts or septic abscesses may also be present. The pathogenesis hinges on the renal deposition of circulating immune complexes in the kidney with complement activation. Patients present with gross or microscopic hematuria, pyuria, and mild proteinuria or, less commonly, RPGN with rapid loss of renal function. A normocytic anemia, elevated erythrocyte sedimentation rate, hypocomplementemia, high titers of rheumatoid factor, type III cryoglobulins, and circulating immune complexes are often present. Levels of serum creatinine may be elevated at diagnosis, but with modern therapy there is little progression to chronic renal failure. Primary treatment is eradication of the infection with 4–6 weeks of antibiotics, and if accomplished expeditiously, the prognosis for renal recovery is good.

As variants of persistent bacterial infection in blood, glomerulonephritis can occur in patients with ventriculoatrial and ventriculoperitoneal shunts; pulmonary, intraabdominal, pelvic, or cutaneous infections; and infected vascular prostheses. The clinical presentation of these conditions is variable and includes proteinuria, microscopic hematuria, and acute renal failure. Blood cultures are usually positive and serum complement levels low, and there may be elevated levels of C-reactive proteins, rheumatoid factor, antinuclear antibodies, and cryoglobulins. Renal lesions include membranoproliferative glomerulonephritis (MPGN), diffuse proliferative glomerulonephritis (DPGN), or mesangioproliferative glomerulonephritis, sometimes leading to RPGN. Treatment focuses on eradicating the infection, with most patients treated as if they have endocarditis.

LUPUS NEPHRITIS

Lupus nephritis is a common and serious complication of systemic lupus erythematosus (SLE) and most severe in African-American female adolescents. Thirty to fifty percent of patients will have clinical manifestations of renal disease at the time of diagnosis, and 60% of adults and 80% of children develop renal abnormalities at some point in the course of their disease. Lupus nephritis results from the deposition of circulating immune complexes, which activate the complement cascade leading to complement-mediated damage, leukocyte infiltration, activation of procoagulant factors, and release of various cytokines. In situ immune complex formation following glomerular binding of nuclear antigens may also play a role in renal injury. The presence of antiphospholipid antibodies may trigger a thrombotic microangiopathy in a minority of patients.

The clinical manifestations, course of disease, and treatment of lupus nephritis are closely linked to the renal pathology. The most common clinical sign of renal disease is proteinuria, but hematuria, hypertension, varying degrees of renal failure, and an active urine sediment with red blood cell casts can all be present. Although significant renal pathology can be found on biopsy even in the absence of major abnormalities in the urinalysis, most nephrologists do not biopsy patients until the urinalysis is convincingly abnormal. The extrarenal manifestations of lupus are important in establishing a firm diagnosis of systemic lupus because, while serologic abnormalities are common in lupus nephritis, they are not diagnostic. Anti-dsDNA antibodies that fix complement correlate best with the presence of renal disease. Hypocomplementemia is common in patients with acute lupus nephritis (70–90%) and declining complement levels may herald a flare. Renal biopsy, however, is the only reliable method of identifying the morphologic variants of lupus nephritis.

The World Health Organization (WHO) workshop in 1974 first outlined several distinct patterns of lupus-related glomerular injury; these were modified in 1982. In 2004 the International Society of Nephrology in conjunction with the Renal Pathology Society again updated the classification. This latest version of lesions seen on biopsy (Table 15-3) best defines clinicopathologic correlations, provides valuable prognostic information, and forms the basis for modern treatment recommendations. Class I nephritis describes normal glomerular histology by any

TABLE 15-3

CLASSIFICATION FOR LUPUS NEPHRITIS

Class I	Minimal mesangial	Normal histology with mesangial deposits
Class II	Mesangial proliferation	Mesangial hypercellularity with expansion of the mesangial matrix
Class III	Focal nephritis	Focal endocapillary ± extracapillary proliferation with focal subendothelial immune deposits and mild mesangial expansion
Class IV	Diffuse nephritis	Diffuse endocapillary ± extracapillary proliferation with diffuse subendothelial immune deposits and mesangial alterations
Class V	Membranous nephritis	Thickened basement membranes with diffuse subepithelial immune deposits; may occur with Class III or IV lesions and is sometimes called mixed membranous and proliferative nephritis
Class VI	Sclerotic nephritis	Global sclerosis of nearly all glomerular capillaries

Note: Revised in 2004 by the International Society of Nephrology-Renal Pathology Society Study Group.

technique or normal light microscopy with minimal mesangial deposits on immunofluorescent or electron microscopy. Class II designates mesangial immune complexes with *mesangial proliferation*. Both Class I and II lesions are typically associated with minimal renal manifestation and normal renal function; nephrotic syndrome is rare. Patients with lesions limited to the renal mesangium have an excellent prognosis and generally do not need therapy for their lupus nephritis.

The subject of lupus nephritis is presented under acute nephritic syndromes because of the aggressive and important proliferative lesions seen in Class III–V renal disease. Class III describes *focal lesions with proliferation or scarring*, often involving only a segment of the glomerulus (Fig. 4-10). Class III lesions have the most varied course. Hypertension, an active urinary sediment, and proteinuria are common with nephrotic-range proteinuria in 25–33% of patients. Elevated serum creatinine is present in 25% of patients. Patients with mild proliferation involving a small percentage of glomeruli respond well to therapy with steroids alone, and fewer than 5% progress to renal failure over 5 years. Patients with more severe proliferation involving a greater percentage of glomeruli have a far worse prognosis and may have lower remission rates. Treatment of those patients is the same as that for Class IV lesions, as some nephrologists believe that Class III lesions

are simply an early presentation of Class IV disease. Class IV describes *global, diffuse proliferative lesions* involving the vast majority of glomeruli. Patients with Class IV lesions commonly have high anti-DNA antibody titers, low serum complement, hematuria, red blood cell casts, proteinuria, hypertension, and decreased renal function; 50% of patients have nephrotic-range proteinuria. Patients with crescents on biopsy may have a rapidly progressive decline in renal function. Without treatment, this aggressive lesion has the worst renal prognosis. However, if a remission—defined as a return to near-normal renal function and proteinuria ≤330 mg/dL per day is achieved with treatment, renal outcomes are excellent. Treatment must combine high-dose steroids with either cyclophosphamide or mycophenolate mofetil. Current evidence suggests that inducing a remission with administration of steroids and either cyclophosphamide or mycophenolate mofetil for 2–6 months, followed by maintenance therapy with lower doses of steroids and mycophenolate mofetil, may best balance the likelihood of successful remission with the side effects of therapy. There is no consensus on the use of high-dose intravenous methylprednisolone versus oral prednisone, monthly intravenous cyclophosphamide versus daily oral cyclophosphamide, or other immunosuppressants such as cyclosporine or azathioprine. Nephrologists tend to avoid prolonged use of cyclophosphamide in patients of childbearing age without first banking eggs or sperm.

The Class V lesion describes subepithelial immune deposits producing a *membranous pattern;* a subcategory of Class V lesions is associated with proliferative lesions and is sometimes called *mixed membranous and proliferative disease;* this category of injury is treated like Class IV glomerulonephritis. Sixty percent of patients present with nephrotic syndrome or lesser amounts of proteinuria. Patients with lupus nephritis Class V, like patients with *idiopathic membranous nephropathy*, are predisposed to renal-vein thrombosis and other thrombolic complications. A minority of patients with Class V will present with hypertension and renal dysfunction. There are conflicting data on the clinical course, prognosis, and appropriate therapy for patients with Class V disease, which may reflect the heterogeneity of this group of patients. Patients with severe nephrotic syndrome, elevated serum creatinine, and a progressive course will probably benefit from therapy with steroids in combination with other immunosuppressive agents. Therapy with inhibitors of the renin-angiotensin system also may attenuate the proteinuria.

Patients with any of the above lesions also can transform to another lesion; hence patients often require reevaluation, including repeat renal biopsy. Lupus patients with Class VI lesions have greater than 90% *sclerotic glomeruli* and end-stage renal disease with interstitial fibrosis. As a group, approximately 20% of patients with lupus nephritis will reach end-stage disease, requiring dialysis or transplantation. Systemic lupus tends to become quiescent once there is renal failure, perhaps due to the immunosuppressant effects of uremia. Renal transplantation in renal failure from lupus, usually performed after approximately 6 months of inactive disease, results in allograft survival rates comparable to patients transplanted for other reasons.

ANTIGLOMERULAR BASEMENT MEMBRANE DISEASE

Patients who develop autoantibodies directed against glomerular basement antigens frequently develop a glomerulonephritis termed *antiglomerular basement membrane (anti-GBM) disease*. When they present with lung hemorrhage and glomerulonephritis, they have a pulmonary-renal syndrome called *Goodpasture's syndrome*. The target epitopes for this autoimmune disease lie in the quaternary structure of α3 NC1 domain of collagen IV. MHC-restricted T cells initiate the autoantibody response because humans are not tolerant to the epitopes created by this quaternary structure. The epitopes are normally sequestered in the collagen IV hexamer and can be exposed by infection, smoking, oxidants, or solvents. Goodpasture's syndrome appears in two age groups: in young men in their late 20s and in men and women in their 60–70s. Disease in the younger age group is usually explosive, with hemoptysis, a sudden fall in hemoglobin, fever, dyspnea, and hematuria. Hemoptysis is largely confined to smokers, and those who present with lung hemorrhage as a group do better than older populations who have prolonged, asymptomatic renal injury; presentation with oliguria is often associated with a particularly bad outcome. The performance of an urgent kidney biopsy is important in suspected cases of Goodpasture's syndrome to confirm the diagnosis and assess prognosis. Renal biopsies typically show *focal or segmental necrosis* that later, with aggressive destruction of the capillaries by cellular proliferation, leads to crescent formation in Bowman's space (Fig. 4-12). As these lesions progress, there is concomitant interstitial nephritis with fibrosis and tubular atrophy. The presence of anti-GBM antibodies and complement is recognized on biopsy by linear immunofluorescent staining for IgG (rarely IgA). In testing serum for anti-GBM antibodies, it is particularly important that the α3 NC1 domain of collagen IV alone be used as the target. This is because nonnephritic antibodies against the α1 NC1 domain are seen in paraneoplastic syndromes and cannot be discerned from assays that use whole basement membrane fragments as the binding target. Between 10 and 15% of sera from patients with Goodpasture's syndrome also contain ANCA antibodies against myeloperoxidase. This subset of patients has a vasculitis-associated variant, which has a surprisingly good prognosis with treatment. Prognosis at presentation is worse if there are >50% crescents on renal biopsy with advanced fibrosis, if serum creatinine is >5–6 mg/dL, if oliguria is present, or if there is a need for acute dialysis. Although frequently attempted, most of these latter patients will not respond to plasmapheresis and steroids. Patients with advanced renal failure who present with hemoptysis should still be treated for their lung hemorrhage, as it responds to plasmapheresis and can be lifesaving. Treated patients with less severe disease typically respond to 8–10 treatments of plasmapheresis accompanied by oral prednisone and cyclophosphamide in the first 2 weeks. Kidney transplantation is possible, but because there is risk of recurrence, experience suggests that patients should wait for 6 months and until serum antibodies are undetectable.

IgA NEPHROPATHY

Berger first described the glomerulonephritis termed *IgA nephropathy*. It is classically characterized by episodic hematuria associated with the deposition of IgA in the mesangium. IgA nephropathy is one of the most common forms of glomerulonephritis worldwide. There is a male preponderance, a peak incidence in the second and third decades of life, and rare familial clustering. There are geographic differences in the prevalence of IgA nephropathy, with 30% prevalence along the Asian and Pacific Rim and 20% in southern Europe, compared to lower prevalence in northern Europe and North America. It was initially hypothesized that variation in detection, in part, reflected regional differences in the recognition of asymptomatic microscopic hematuria or the frequency of renal biopsies. With clinical care in nephrology becoming more uniform and regional reports coming largely from larger cities, however, this variation in prevalence more likely reflects true differences among racial and ethnic groups. Clinical and laboratory evidence suggests close similarities between Henoch-Schönlein purpura and IgA nephropathy. Henoch-Schönlein purpura is distinguished clinically from IgA nephropathy by prominent systemic symptoms, a younger age (<20 years old), preceding infection, and abdominal complaints. Deposits of IgA are also found in the glomerular mesangium in a variety of systemic diseases, including chronic liver disease, Crohn's disease, gastrointestinal adenocarcinoma, chronic obstructive bronchiectasis, idiopathic interstitial pneumonia, dermatitis herpetiformis, mycosis fungoides, leprosy, ankylosing spondylitis, relapsing polychondritis, and Sjögren's syndrome. IgA deposition in these entities is not usually associated with clinically significant glomerular inflammation or renal dysfunction and thus is not called IgA nephropathy.

IgA nephropathy is an immune complex-mediated glomerulonephritis defined by the presence of diffuse mesangial IgA deposits often associated with mesangial hypercellularity. IgM, IgG, C_3, or immunoglobulin light chains may be codistributed with IgA. IgA deposited in the mesangium is typically polymeric and of the IgA1 subclass, the pathogenic significance of which is not clear. Abnormalities have been described in IgA production by plasma cells, particularly secretory IgA; in IgA O-glycosylation; in IgA clearance, predominantly by the

SECTION IV

Glomerular and Tubular Disorders

liver; in mesangial IgA clearance and receptors for IgA; and in growth factor and cytokine-mediated events. Despite the presence of elevated serum IgA levels in 20–50% of patients, IgA deposition in skin biopsies in 15–55% of patients, or elevated levels of secretory IgA and IgA-fibronectin complexes, a renal biopsy is necessary to make the diagnosis. Although the immunofluorescent pattern of IgA on renal biopsy defines IgA nephropathy in the proper clinical context, a variety of histologic lesions may be seen on light microscopy (Fig. 4-6), including DPGN; *segmental sclerosis*; and, rarely, *segmental necrosis with cellular crescent formation*, which typically presents as RPGN.

The two most common presentations of IgA nephropathy are recurrent episodes of macroscopic hematuria during or immediately following an upper respiratory infection in children (Henoch-Schönlein purpura) or asymptomatic microscopic hematuria most often seen in adults. Between episodes, the urinalysis is normal. When the hematuria persists, one finds increasing amounts of proteinuria; nephrotic syndrome, however, is uncommon. The presence or absence of proteinuria at the time of diagnosis often determines whether patients with asymptomatic hematuria are biopsied, which reflects the bias in habits of clinical practice. Proteinuria can occur late in the course of the disease. Rarely, patients can present with acute renal failure and a rapidly progressive clinical picture. IgA nephropathy is a benign disease for the majority of patients, with progression to renal failure seen in only 25–30% over 20–25 years; in fact, 5–30% of patients go into complete remission. Risk factors for the loss of renal function include the presence of hypertension or proteinuria, the absence of episodes of macroscopic hematuria, male age, older age of onset, and more severe changes on renal biopsy.

There is no agreement on optimal treatment. Both large studies that include patients with multiple glomerular diseases and small studies of patients with IgA nephropathy support the use of angiotensin-converting enzyme (ACE) inhibitors in patients with proteinuria or declining renal function. Tonsillectomy, steroid therapy, and fish oil have all been suggested in small studies to benefit select patients with IgA nephropathy. When presenting as RPGN, patients typically receive steroids, cytotoxic agents, and plasmapheresis.

ANCA SMALL VESSEL VASCULITIS

A group of patients with small-vessel vasculitis (arterioles, capillaries, and venules; rarely small arteries) and glomerulonephritis have serum ANCA; the antibodies are of two types: anti-proteinase 3 (PR3) or anti-myeloperoxidase (MPO). ANCA are produced with the help of T cells and activate leukocytes and monocytes, which together damage the walls of small vessels. Endothelial injury also attracts more leukocytes and extends the inflammation. Wegener's granulomatosis,

microscopic polyangiitis, and Churg-Strauss syndrome belong to this group because they are ANCA-positive and have a *pauci-immune glomerulonephritis* with few immune complexes in small vessels and glomerular capillaries. Patients with any of these three diseases can have any combination of the above serum antibodies, but anti-PR3 antibodies are more common in Wegener's and anti-MPO antibodies are more common in microscopic polyangiitis or Churg-Strauss. While each of these diseases have some unique clinical features, most features do not predict relapse or progression, and as a group they are generally treated in the same way. Only the presence of upper-airway involvement, persistent pulmonary injury, and anti-PR3 antibodies suggests that the course of disease will be more difficult. Induction therapy usually includes some combination of plasmapheresis, methylprednisolone, and cyclophosphamide. The benefit of plasmapheresis in this setting is uncertain. The steroids are tapered soon after acute inflammation subsides, and patients are maintained on cyclophosphamide or azathioprine for up to a year to minimize the risk of relapse.

Wegener's Granulomatosis

Patients with this disease classically present with fever, purulent rhinorrhea, nasal ulcers, sinus pain, polyarthralgias/arthritis, cough, hemoptysis, shortness of breath, microscopic hematuria, and 0.5–1 g/24 h of proteinuria; occasionally there may be cutaneous purpura and mononeuritis multiplex. Presentation without renal involvement is termed *limited Wegener's granulomatosis*, although some of these patients will show signs of renal injury later. Chest x-ray often reveals nodules and persistent infiltrates, sometimes with cavities. Biopsy of involved tissue will show a small-vessel vasculitis and adjacent noncaseating granulomas. Renal biopsies during active disease demonstrate *segmental necrotizing glomerulonephritis* without immune deposits (Fig. 4-11). The cause of Wegener's granulomatosis is unknown. In case-controlled studies there is greater risk associated with exposure to silica dust. The disease is also more common in patients with α_1 antitrypsin deficiency, which is an inhibitor of PR3.

Microscopic Polyangiitis

Clinically, these patients look somewhat similar to those with Wegener's granulomatosis, except they rarely have significant lung disease or destructive sinusitis. The distinction is made on biopsy where the vasculitis in microscopic polyangiitis is without granulomas. Some patients will also have injury limited to the capillaries and venules.

Churg-Strauss Syndrome

When small-vessel vasculitis is associated with peripheral eosinophilia, cutaneous purpura, mononeuritis, asthma, and allergic rhinitis, a diagnosis of Churg-Strauss syndrome is considered. Hypergammaglobulinemia, elevated levels of serum IgE, or the presence of rheumatoid factor sometimes accompanies the allergic state. Lung inflammation, including fleeting cough and pulmonary infiltrates, often precedes the systemic manifestations of disease by years; lung manifestations are rarely absent. A third of patients may have exudative pleural effusions associated with eosinophils. Small-vessel vasculitis and *focal segmental necrotizing glomerulonephritis* can be seen on renal biopsy, usually absent eosinophils or granulomas. The cause of Churg-Strauss syndrome is autoimmune, but the inciting factors are unknown. Interestingly, some asthma patients treated with leukotriene receptor antagonists will develop this vasculitis.

MEMBRANOPROLIFERATIVE GLOMERULONEPHRITIS

MPGN is sometimes called *mesangiocapillary glomerulonephritis* or *lobar glomerulonephritis*. It is an immune-mediated glomerulonephritis characterized by thickening of the GBM with mesangioproliferative changes; 70% of patients have hypocomplementemia. MPGN is rare in African Americans, and idiopathic disease usually presents in childhood or young adulthood. MPGN is subdivided pathologically into Type I, Type II, and Type III disease. *Type I MPGN* is commonly associated with persistent hepatitis C infections, autoimmune diseases like lupus or cryoglobulinemia, or neoplastic diseases (Table 15–4). *Types II and III MPGN* are usually idiopathic, except in the presence of C_3 nephritic factor and/or in partial lipodystrophy producing Type II disease or complement receptor deficiency in Type III disease.

TABLE 15-4

MEMBRANOPROLIFERATIVE GLOMERULONEPHRITIS
Type I Disease (Most Common)
Idiopathic
Subacute bacterial endocarditis
Systemic lupus erythematosus
Hepatitis C ± cryoglobulinemia
Mixed cryoglobulinemia
Hepatitis B
Cancer: Lung, breast, and ovary (germinal)
Type II Disease (Dense Deposit Disease)
Idiopathic
C_3 nephritic factor-associated
Partial lipodystrophy
Type III Disease
Idiopathic
Complement receptor deficiency

Type I MPGN, the most proliferative of the three types, shows mesangial proliferation with lobular segmentation on renal biopsy and mesangial interposition between the capillary basement membrane and endothelial cells, producing a double contour sometimes called *tram-tracking* (Figs. 4-7 and 4-9). Subendothelial deposits with low serum levels of C_3 are typical, although 50% of patients have normal levels of C_3 and occasional intramesangial deposits. Low serum C_3 and a dense thickening of the GBM containing ribbons of dense deposits and C_3 characterize Type II MPGN, sometimes called *dense deposit disease* (Fig. 4-8). Classically, the glomerular tuft has a lobular appearance; intramesangial deposits are rarely present and subendothelial deposits are generally absent. Proliferation in Type III MPGN is less common than the other two types and is often focal; mesangial interposition is rare, and subepithelial deposits can occur along widened segments of the GBM that appear laminated and disrupted.

Type I MPGN is secondary to glomerular deposition of circulating immune complexes or their in situ formation. Types II and III MPGN may be related to "nephritic factors," which are autoantibodies that stabilize C_3 convertase and allow it to activate serum C_3. Patients with MPGN present with proteinuria, hematuria, and pyuria (30%), systemic symptoms of fatigue and malaise that are most common in children with Type I disease, or an acute nephritic picture with RPGN and a speedy deterioration in renal function in up to 25% of patients. Low serum C_3 levels are common. Fifty percent of patients with MPGN develop end-stage disease 10 years after diagnosis, and 90% have renal insufficiency after 20 years. Nephrotic syndrome, hypertension, and renal insufficiency all predict poor outcome. In the presence of proteinuria, treatment with inhibitors of the renin–angiotensin system is prudent. Evidence for treatment with dipyridamole, coumadin, or cyclophosphamide is not strongly established nor recommended. There is some evidence supporting the efficacy of treatment of *primary MPGN* with steroids, particularly in children. In *secondary MPGN*, treating the associated infection, autoimmune disease, or neoplasms is of demonstrated benefit. Although all primary renal diseases can recur over time in transplanted renal allografts, patients with MPGN are well known to be at risk for this adverse event.

MESANGIOPROLIFERATIVE GLOMERULONEPHRITIS

Mesangioproliferative glomerulonephritis is characterized by expansion of the mesangium, sometimes associated with mesangial hypercellularity; thin, single contoured capillary walls; and mesangial immune deposits. Clinically, it can present with varying degrees of proteinuria and, commonly, hematuria. Mesangioproliferative disease may be seen in IgA nephropathy, malaria, resolving postinfectious glomerulonephritis, and Class II nephritis from lupus, all of which can have a similar histologic appearance. With these secondary entities excluded, the diagnosis of *primary mesangioproliferative glomerulonephritis* is made in less than 15% of renal biopsies. As an immune-mediated renal lesion with deposits of IgM, C1q, and C_3, the clinical course is variable. Patients with isolated hematuria may have a very benign course, and those with heavy proteinuria occasionally progress to renal failure. There is little agreement on treatment, but some clinical reports suggest benefit from use of inhibitors of the renin-angiotensin system, steroid therapy, and even cytotoxic agents.

NEPHROTIC SYNDROME

Nephrotic syndrome classically presents with heavy proteinuria, minimal hematuria, hypoalbuminemia, hypercholesterolemia, edema, and hypertension. If left undiagnosed or untreated, some of these syndromes will progressively damage enough glomeruli to cause a fall in GFR, producing renal failure.

Therapies for various causes of nephrotic syndrome are noted under individual disease headings below. In general, all patients with hypercholesterolemia secondary to nephrotic syndrome should be treated with lipid-lowering agents since they are at increased risk for cardiovascular disease. Edema secondary to salt and water retention can be controlled with the judicious use of diuretics, avoiding intravascular volume depletion. Venous complications secondary to the hypercoagulable state associated with nephrotic syndrome can be treated with anticoagulants. The losses of various serum binding proteins, such as thyroid-binding globulin, lead to alterations in functional tests. Lastly, proteinuria itself is hypothesized to be nephrotoxic, and treatment of proteinuria with inhibitors of the renin-angiotensin system can lower urinary protein excretion.

MINIMAL CHANGE DISEASE

Minimal change disease (MCD), sometimes known as *nil lesion*, causes 70–90% of nephrotic syndrome in childhood but only 10–15% of nephrotic syndrome in adults. MCD usually presents as a primary renal disease but can be associated with several other conditions, including Hodgkin's disease, allergies, or use of nonsteroidal anti-inflammatory agents; significant interstitial nephritis often accompanies cases associated with nonsteroidal use. MCD on renal biopsy shows no obvious glomerular lesion by light microscopy and is negative for deposits by immunofluorescent microscopy, or occasionally shows small amounts of IgM in the mesangium (Fig. 4-1). Electron microscopy, however, consistently demonstrates an effacement of the foot process supporting the epithelial podocytes with weakening of slit-pore membranes. The pathophysiology of this lesion is uncertain. Most agree there is a circulating cytokine, perhaps related to a T cell response that alters capillary charge and podocyte integrity. The evidence for cytokine-related immune injury is circumstantial and is suggested by the presence of preceding allergies, altered cell-mediated immunity during viral infections, and the high frequency of remissions with steroids.

MCD presents clinically with the abrupt onset of edema and nephrotic syndrome accompanied by acellular urinary sediment. Less common clinical features include hypertension (30% in children, 50% in adults), microscopic hematuria (20% in children, 33% in adults), atopy or allergic symptoms (40% in children, 30% in adults), and decreased renal function (<5% in children, 30% in adults). The appearance of acute renal failure in adults is usually caused by intrarenal edema (nephrosarca) that is responsive to intravenous albumin and diuretics. This presentation must be distinguished from acute renal failure secondary to hypovolemia. In children, the abnormal urine principally contains albumin with minimal amounts of higher molecular weight proteins, and is sometimes called *selective proteinuria*. Although up to 30% of children have a spontaneous remission, all children today are treated with steroids; only children who are nonresponders are biopsied in this setting. Primary responders are patients who have a complete remission (<0.2 mg/24 h of proteinuria) after a single course of prednisone; steroid-dependent patients relapse as their steroid dose is tapered. Frequent relapsers have two or more relapses in the 6 months following taper, and steroid-resistant patients fail to respond to steroid therapy. Ninety to 95% of children will develop a complete remission after 8 weeks of steroid therapy, and 80–85% of adults will achieve complete remission, but only after a longer course of 20–24 weeks. Patients with steroid resistance can develop FSGS on repeat biopsy. Some hypothesize that if the first renal biopsy does not have a sample of deeper glomeruli, then the correct early diagnosis of FSGS may be missed.

Relapses occur in 70–75% of children after the first remission, and early relapse predicts multiple subsequent relapses. The frequency of relapses decreases after puberty, although there is an increased risk of relapse following the rapid tapering of steroids in all groups. Relapses are less common in adults but are more resistant to subsequent therapy. Prednisone is first-line therapy, and other immunosuppressive drugs, such as cyclophosphamide, chlorambucil, and mycophenolate mofetil, are saved for frequent relapsers, and steroid-dependent or steroid-resistant patients. Cyclosporine can induce remission, but relapse is also common when cyclosporine is withdrawn. The long-term prognosis in adults is less favorable when acute renal failure or steroid resistance occurs.

FOCAL SEGMENTAL GLOMERULOSCLEROSIS

FSGS refers to a pattern of renal injury characterized by segmental glomerular scars that involve some but not all glomeruli; the clinical findings of FSGS largely manifest as

TABLE 15-5

FOCAL SEGMENTAL GLOMERULOSCLEROSIS

Primary focal segmental glomerulosclerosis
Secondary focal segmental glomerulosclerosis
  Viruses: HIV/Hepatitis B/Parvovirus
  Hypertensive nephropathy
  Reflux nephropathy
  Cholesterol emboli
  Drugs: Heroin/analgesics
  Oligomeganephronia
  Renal dysgenesis
  Alport's syndrome
  Sickle cell disease
  Lymphoma
  Radiation nephritis
  Familial podocytopathies
    NPHS1 mutation/nephrin
    NPHS2 mutation/podocin
    TRPC6 mutation/cation channel
    ACTN4 mutation/Actinin
    α-Galactosidase A deficiency/Fabry's disease
  N-acetylneuraminic acid hydrolase deficiency/
    nephrosialidosis

proteinuria. When the secondary causes of FSGS are eliminated (Table 15-5), the remaining patients are considered to have FSGS. The incidence of this disease is increasing, and it now represents up to one-third of cases of nephrotic syndrome in adults and one-half of cases of nephrotic syndrome in African Americans, in whom it is seen more commonly. The pathogenesis of FSGS is probably multifactorial. Possible mechanisms include a T cell–mediated circulating permeability factor, TGF-β–mediated cellular proliferation and matrix synthesis, and podocyte abnormalities associated with genetic mutations.

The pathologic changes of FSGS are most prominent in glomeruli located at the corticomedullary junction (Fig. 4-2), so if the renal biopsy specimen is from superficial tissue, the lesions can be missed, which sometimes leads to a misdiagnosis of MCD. In addition to focal and segmental scarring, other variants have been described, including cellular lesions with *endocapillary hypercellularity* and heavy proteinuria; *collapsing glomerulopathy* (Fig. 4-3) with segmental or global glomerular collapse and a rapid decline in renal function; or the *glomerular tip lesion*, which seems to have a better prognosis.

FSGS can present with any level of proteinuria, hematuria, hypertension, or renal insufficiency. Nephrotic range proteinuria, African-American race, and renal insufficiency are associated with a poor outcome, with 50% of patients reaching renal failure in 6–8 years. FSGS rarely remits spontaneously, but treatment-induced remission of proteinuria significantly improves prognosis. Treatment of patients with *primary FSGS* should include inhibitors of the renin-angiotensin system. Based on retrospective studies, patients with nephrotic range proteinuria can be

treated with steroids but respond far less often than patients with MCD. Proteinuria remits in only 20–45% of patients receiving a course of steroids over 6–9 months. Limited evidence suggests that the use of cyclosporine in steroid-responsive patients helps ensure remissions, while other cytotoxic agents confer little added benefit over steroid therapy. Primary FSGS recurs in 25–40% of patients given allografts at end-stage disease, leading to graft loss in half of those cases. The treatment of *secondary FSGS* typically involves treating the underlying cause and controlling proteinuria. There is no role for steroids or other immunosuppressive agents in secondary FSGS.

MEMBRANOUS GLOMERULONEPHRITIS

MGN, or *membranous nephropathy* as it is sometimes called, accounts for approximately 30% of cases of nephrotic syndrome in adults, with a peak incidence between the ages of 30 and 50 years and a male-to-female ratio of 2:1. It is rare in childhood and by far the most common cause of nephrotic syndrome in the elderly. In 25–30% of cases, MGN is secondary to malignancy (solid tumors of the breast, lung, colon), infection (hepatitis B, malaria, schistosomiasis), or rheumatologic disorders like lupus or rarely rheumatoid arthritis (Table 15-6).

Uniform thickening of the basement membrane along the peripheral capillary loops is seen by light microscopy on renal biopsy (Fig. 4-5); this thickening needs to be distinguished from that seen in diabetes and amyloidosis. Immunofluorescence demonstrates diffuse granular deposits of IgG and C_3, and electron microscopy typically reveals electron-dense subepithelial deposits. While different stages (I–V) of progressive membranous lesions have been described, some published analyses indicate the degree of tubular atrophy or interstitial fibrosis is more predictive of

TABLE 15-6

MEMBRANOUS GLOMERULONEPHRITIS

Primary/idiopathic membranous glomerulonephritis
Secondary membranous glomerulonephritis
  Infection: Hepatitis B and C, syphilis, malaria,
    schistosomiasis, leprosy, filariasis
  Cancer: Breast, colon, lung, stomach, kidney,
    esophagus, neuroblastoma
  Drugs: gold, mercury, penicillamine, nonsteroidal
    anti-inflammatory agents, probenecid
  Autoimmune diseases: systemic lupus erythematosus,
    rheumatoid arthritis, primary biliary cirrhosis,
    dermatitis herpetiformis, bullous pemphigoid,
    myasthenia gravis, Sjögren's syndrome, Hashimoto's
    thyroiditis
  Other systemic diseases: Fanconi's syndrome, sickle
    cell anemia, diabetes, Crohn's disease, sarcoidosis,
    Guillain-Barré syndrome, Weber-Christian disease,
    angiofollicular lymph node hyperplasia

progression than is the stage of glomerular disease. The presence of subendothelial deposits or the presence of tubuloreticular inclusions strongly points to a diagnosis of membranous lupus nephritis, which may precede the extrarenal manifestations of lupus. Work in Heyman nephritis, an animal model of MGN, suggests that glomerular lesions result from in situ formation of immune complexes with megalin receptor–associated protein as the putative antigen. This antigen is not found in human podocytes, but human antibodies have been described against neutral endopeptidase expressed by podocytes, hepatitis antigens B/C, *Helicobacter pylori* antigens, tumor antigens, and thyroglobulin.

Eighty percent of patients with MGN present with nephrotic syndrome and nonselective proteinuria. Microscopic hematuria is seen in up to 50% of patients. Spontaneous remissions occur in 20–33% of patients and often occur late in the course after years of nephrotic syndrome. One-third of patients continue to have relapsing nephrotic syndrome but maintain normal renal function, and approximately another third of patients develop renal failure or die from the complications of nephrotic syndrome. Male gender, older age, hypertension, and the persistence of proteinuria are associated with worse prognosis. Although thrombotic complications are a feature of all nephrotic syndromes, MGN has the highest reported incidences of renal vein thrombosis, pulmonary embolism, and deep vein thrombosis. Prophylactic anticoagulation is controversial but has been recommended for patients with severe or prolonged proteinuria in the absence of risk factors for bleeding.

In addition to the treatment of edema, dyslipidemia, and hypertension, inhibition of the renin-angiotensin system is recommended. Therapy with immunosuppressive drugs is also recommended for patients with primary MGN and persistent proteinuria (>3.0 g/24 h). The choice of immunosuppressive drugs for therapy is controversial, but current recommendations based on small clinical studies are to treat with steroids and cyclophosphamide, chlorambucil, or cyclosporine. Experience with mycophenolate mofetil or anti-CD20 antibody is even more limited.

DIABETIC NEPHROPATHY

Diabetic nephropathy is the single most common cause of chronic renal failure in the United States, accounting for 45% of patients receiving renal replacement therapy, and is a rapidly growing problem worldwide. The dramatic increase in the number of patients with diabetic nephropathy reflects the epidemic increase in obesity, metabolic syndrome, and Type 2 diabetes mellitus. Approximately 40% of patients with Type 1 or 2 diabetes develop nephropathy, but due to the higher prevalence of Type 2 diabetes (90%) compared to Type 1 (10%), the majority of patients with diabetic nephropathy have Type 2 disease.

Renal lesions are more common in African-American, Native American, Polynesian, and Maori populations. Risk factors for the development of diabetic nephropathy include hyperglycemia, hypertension, dyslipidemia, smoking, a family history of diabetic nephropathy, and gene polymorphisms affecting the activity of the renin-angiotensin–aldosterone axis.

Within 1–2 years after the onset of clinical diabetes, morphologic changes appear in the kidney. Thickening of the GBM is a sensitive indicator for the presence of diabetes but correlates poorly with the presence or absence of clinically significant nephropathy. The composition of the GBM is altered notably with a loss of heparan sulfate moieties that form the negatively charged filtration barrier. This change results in increased filtration of serum proteins into the urine, predominantly negatively charged albumin. The expansion of the mesangium due to the accumulation of extracellular matrix correlates with the clinical manifestations of diabetic nephropathy. This expansion in mesangial matrix can be associated with the development of *mesangial sclerosis*. Some patients also develop eosinophilic, PAS$^+$ nodules called *nodular glomerulosclerosis* or *Kimmelstiel-Wilson nodules*. Immunofluorescence microscopy often reveals the nonspecific deposition of IgG (at times in a linear pattern) or complement staining without immune deposits on electron microscopy. Prominent vascular changes are frequently seen with hyaline and hypertensive arteriosclerosis. This is associated with varying degrees of chronic glomerulosclerosis and tubulointerstitial changes. Renal biopsies from patients with Types 1 and 2 diabetes are largely indistinguishable.

These pathologic changes are the result of a number of postulated factors. Multiple lines of evidence support an important role for increases in glomerular capillary pressure (intraglomerular hypertension) in alterations in renal structure and function. Direct effects of hyperglycemia on the actin cytoskeleton of renal mesangial and vascular smooth-muscle cells as well as diabetes-associated changes in circulating factors such as atrial natriuretic factor, angiotensin II, and insulin-like growth factor (IGF) may account for this. Sustained glomerular hypertension increases matrix production, alterations in the GBM with disruption in the filtration barrier (and hence proteinuria), and glomerulosclerosis. A number of factors have also been identified that alter matrix production, including the accumulation of advanced glycosylation end products, circulating factors including growth hormone, IGF-I, angiotensin II, connective tissues growth factor, TGF-β, and dyslipidemia.

The natural history of diabetic nephropathy in patients with Types 1 and 2 diabetes is similar. However, since the onset of Type 1 diabetes is readily identifiable and the onset of Type 2 diabetes is not, a patient newly diagnosed with Type 2 diabetes may have renal disease for many years before nephropathy is discovered and presents as *advanced diabetic nephropathy*. At the onset of diabetes, renal hypertrophy and glomerular hyperfiltration are present. The degree of glomerular hyperfiltration correlates with the subsequent risk of clinically significant nephropathy. In the approximately 40% of patients with diabetes who develop diabetic nephropathy, the earliest manifestation is an increase in albuminuria detected by sensitive radioimmunoassay (Table 15-1). Albuminuria in the range of 30–300 mg/24 h is called *microalbuminuria*. In patients with Type 1 or 2 diabetes, microalbuminuria appears 5–10 years after the onset of diabetes. It is currently recommended to test patients with Type 1 disease for microalbuminuria 5 years after diagnosis of diabetes and yearly thereafter, and, because the time of onset of Type 2 diabetes is often unknown, to test Type 2 patients at the time of diagnosis of diabetes and yearly thereafter.

Patients with small rises in albuminuria increase their levels of urinary albumin excretion, typically reaching dipstick positive levels of proteinuria (>300 mg albuminuria) 5–10 years after the onset of early albuminuria. Microalbuminuria is a potent risk factor for cardiovascular events and death in patients with Type 2 diabetes. Many patients with Type 2 diabetes and microalbuminuria succumb to cardiovascular events before they progress to proteinuria or renal failure. Proteinuria in frank diabetic nephropathy can be variable, ranging from 500 mg to 25 g/24 h, and is often associated with nephrotic syndrome. More than 90% of patients with Type 1 diabetes and nephropathy have diabetic retinopathy, so the absence of retinopathy in Type 1 patients with proteinuria should prompt consideration of a diagnosis other than diabetic nephropathy; only 60% of patients with Type 2 diabetes with nephropathy have diabetic retinopathy. There is a highly significant correlation between the presence of retinopathy and the presence of Kimmelstiel-Wilson nodules (Fig. 4–18). Also, characteristically, patients with advanced diabetic nephropathy have normal to enlarged kidneys, in contrast to other glomerular diseases where kidney size is usually decreased. Using the above epidemiologic and clinical data, and in the absence of other clinical or serologic data suggesting another disease, diabetic nephropathy is usually diagnosed without a renal biopsy. After the onset of proteinuria >500 mg/24 h, renal function inexorably declines, with 50% of patients reaching renal failure in 5–10 years; thus, from the earliest stages of microalbuminuria, it usually takes 10–20 years to reach end-stage renal disease. Hypertension may predict which patients develop diabetic nephropathy, as the presence of hypertension accelerates the rate of decline in renal function. Once renal failure appears, however, survival on dialysis is far shorter for patients with diabetes compared to other dialysis patients; some diabetics do better clinically if they are started on dialysis before they reach advanced renal failure. Survival is best for patients with Type 1 diabetes who receive a transplant from a living related donor.

Good evidence supports the benefits of blood sugar and blood pressure control as well as inhibition of the renin-angiotensin system in retarding the progression of diabetic nephropathy. In patients with Type 1 diabetes, intensive control of blood sugar clearly prevents the development or progression of diabetic nephropathy. The evidence in patients with Type 2 disease, although less compelling, also supports intensive control of blood sugar. Controlling systemic blood pressure to levels of 130/80 mmHg or less decreases renal and cardiovascular adverse events in this high-risk population. The vast majority of patients with diabetic nephropathy require three or more antihypertensive drugs to achieve this goal. Drugs that inhibit the renin-angiotensin system, independent of their effects on systemic blood pressure, have been repeatedly shown to slow the progression of diabetic nephropathy at early (microalbuminuria) and late (proteinuria with reduced glomerular filtration) stages, independent of any effect they may have on systemic blood pressure.

Since angiotensin II increases efferent arteriolar resistance and, hence, glomerular capillary pressure, one key mechanism for the efficacy of ACE inhibitors or angiotensin receptor blockers (ARBs) is reducing glomerular hypertension. Patients with Type 1 diabetes for 5 years who develop albuminuria or declining renal function should be treated with ACE inhibitors. Patients with Type 2 diabetes and microalbuminuria or proteinuria may be treated with ACE inhibitors or ARBs.

GLOMERULAR DEPOSITION DISEASES

Plasma cell dyscrasias producing excess light chain immunoglobulin sometimes lead to the formation of glomerular and tubular deposits that cause heavy proteinuria and renal failure; the same is true for the accumulation of serum amyloid A protein fragments seen in several inflammatory diseases. This broad group of proteinuric patients has *glomerular deposition disease.*

Light-Chain Deposition Disease

The biochemical characteristics of nephrotoxic light chains produced in light-chain malignancies typically confers a specific pattern of renal injury in each individual patient; that of either cast nephropathy (Fig. 4-15), which causes renal failure but not heavy proteinuria, amyloidosis, or *light-chain deposition disease* (Fig. 4-14), which produce nephrotic syndrome with renal failure. These latter patients produce kappa light chains that do not have the biochemical features necessary to form amyloid fibrils. Instead, they self-aggregate and form granular deposits along the glomerular capillary and mesangium, tubular basement membrane, and Bowman's capsule. When predominant in glomeruli, nephrotic syndrome develops, and about 70% of patients progress to dialysis. Light-chain deposits are not fibrillar and do not stain with Congo red, but they are easily detected with anti–light-chain antibody using immunofluorescence, or as granular deposits on electron microscopy. A combination of the light-chain rearrangement, self-aggregating properties at neutral pH, and abnormal metabolism probably contribute to the deposition. Treatment for light-chain deposition disease is treatment of the primary disease. As so many patients with light-chain deposition disease progress to renal failure, the overall prognosis is grim.

Renal Amyloidosis

Most *renal amyloidosis* is either the result of primary fibrillar deposits of immunoglobulin light chains [amyloid L (AL)], or secondary to fibrillar deposits of serum amyloid A (AA) protein fragments. Even though both occur for different reasons, their clinicopathophysiology is quite similar and will be discussed together. Amyloid infiltrates the liver, heart, peripheral nerves, carpal tunnel, upper pharynx, and kidney, producing restrictive cardiomyopathy, hepatomegaly, macroglossia, and heavy proteinuria sometimes associated with renal vein thrombosis. In systemic AL amyloidosis, also called *primary amyloidosis*, light chains produced in excess by clonal plasma cell dyscrasias are made into fragments by macrophages so they can self-aggregate at acid pH. A disproportionate number of these light chains (75%) are of the *lambda* class. About 10% of these patients have overt myeloma with lytic bone lesions and infiltration of the bone marrow with >30% plasma cells; nephrotic syndrome is common, and about 20% of patients progress to dialysis. AA amyloidosis is sometimes called *secondary amyloidosis* and also affects the kidney with nephrotic syndrome. It is due to deposition of β-pleated sheets of serum amyloid A protein, an acute phase reactant whose physiologic function is unknown. Forty percent of patients with AA amyloid have rheumatoid arthritis, and another 10% have ankylosing spondylitis or psoriatic arthritis; the rest derive from other lesser causes. Less common in Western countries but more common in Mediterranean regions, particularly in Sephardic and Iraqi Jews, is familial Mediterranean fever (FMF). FMF is caused by a mutation in the gene encoding pyrin, while Muckle-Wells syndrome, a related disorder, results from a mutation in cryropyrin; both proteins are important in the apoptosis of leukocytes early in inflammation. Receptor mutations in tumor necrosis factor receptor (TNFR)-1–associated periodic syndrome also produce chronic inflammation and secondary amyloidosis. Fragments of serum amyloid A protein increase and self-aggregate by attaching to receptors for advanced glycation end products in the extracellular environment; nephrotic syndrome is common, and about 40–60% of patients progress to dialysis. AA and AL amyloid fibrils are detectable with Congo red or in more detail with electron microscopy (Fig. 4-13). Biopsy of involved liver or kidney is diagnostic 90% of the time when the pretest probability is high; abdominal fat pad aspirates are positive about 70% of the time, but apparently less so when looking for AA amyloid. Amyloid deposits are distributed along blood vessels and in the mesangial regions of the kidney. The treatment for primary amyloidosis is not particularly effective; melphalan and autologous hematopoietic stem cell transplantation can delay the course of disease in about 30% of patients. Secondary amyloidosis is also relentless unless the primary disease can be controlled. Some new drugs in development that disrupt the formation of fibrils may be available in the future.

Fibrillary-Immunotactoid Glomerulopathy

There is no agreement on whether *fibrillary glomerulonephritis* and *immunotactoid glomerulonephritis* are different or one and the same. Both are hard to distinguish by clinical presentation but have some apparent differences with electron microscopy. Fibrillar/microtubular deposits of oligoclonal or oligotypic immunoglobulins and complement appear in the mesangium and along the glomerular capillary wall. In fibrillary glomerulonephritis the fibrils are smaller and more randomly distributed than in immunotactoid glomerulonephritis. Congo red stains are negative in both disorders. The cause of this "nonamyloid" glomerulopathy is mostly idiopathic; reports of immunotactoid glomerulonephritis describe an occasional association with chronic lymphocytic leukemia or B cell lymphoma. Both disorders appear in adults in the fourth decade with moderate to heavy proteinuria, hematuria, and a wide variety of histologic lesions, including DPGN, MPGN, MGN, or mesangioproliferative glomerulonephritis. Nearly half of patients will develop renal failure over a few years. There is no consensus on treatment of this uncommon disorder.

FABRY'S DISEASE

Fabry's disease is an X-linked inborn error of globotriaosylceramide metabolism secondary to deficient lysosomal α-galactosidase A activity, resulting in excessive intracellular storage of globotriaosylceramide. Affected organs include the vascular endothelium, heart, brain, and kidneys. Classically, Fabry's disease presents in childhood in males with multi-organ involvement. Hemizygotes with hypomorphic mutations sometimes present in the fourth to sixth decade with single organ involvement. Rarely, dominant-negative α-galactosidase A mutations or female heterozygotes with unfavorable X inactivation present with mild single-organ involvement. Renal biopsy reveals enlarged glomerular visceral epithelial cells packed with small clear vacuoles containing globotriaosylceramide; vacuoles may also be found in parietal and tubular epithelia (Fig. 4-16). These vacuoles of electron-dense materials in parallel arrays (zebra bodies) are easily seen on electron microscopy. Ultimately, glomeruli develop FSGS. The nephropathy of Fabry's disease typically presents in the third decade as mild to moderate proteinuria, sometimes with microscopic hematuria or nephrotic syndrome. Urinalysis may reveal oval fat bodies and birefringent glycolipid globules under polarized light (Maltese cross). Renal biopsy is necessary for definitive diagnosis. Progression to renal failure occurs by the fourth or fifth decade. Treatment with recombinant α-galactosidase A has been demonstrated to clear microvascular endothelial deposits of globotriaosylceramide from the kidneys, heart, and skin.

PULMONARY-RENAL SYNDROMES

Several diseases can present with catastrophic hemoptysis and glomerulonephritis associated with varying degrees of renal failure. The usual causes include Goodpasture's syndrome, Wegener's granulomatosis, microscopic polyangiitis, Churg-Strauss vasculitis, and, rarely, Henoch-Schönlein purpura or cryoglobulinemia. Each of these diseases can also present without hemoptysis and are discussed in detail in "Acute Nephritic Syndromes" earlier in the chapter. Pulmonary bleeding in this setting is life-threatening and often results in airway intubation, and acute renal failure requires dialysis in the intensive care unit. Diagnosis is difficult initially because biopsies and serologic testing take time. Treatment with plasmapheresis and methylprednisolone is often empiric and temporizing until results of testing are available.

BASEMENT MEMBRANE SYNDROMES

All kidney epithelia, including podocytes, rest on basement membranes assembled into a planar surface through the interweaving of collagen IV with laminins, nidogen, and sulfated proteoglycans. Structural abnormalities in GBMs associated with hematuria are characteristic of several familial disorders related to the expression of collagen IV genes. The extended family of collagen IV contains six chains, which are expressed in different tissues at different stages of embryonic development. All epithelial basement membranes early in human development are composed of interconnected triple-helical protomers rich in $\alpha1.\alpha1.\alpha2(IV)$ collagen. Some specialized tissues undergo a developmental switch replacing $\alpha1.\alpha1.\alpha2(IV)$ protomers with an $\alpha3.\alpha4.\alpha5(IV)$ collagen network; this switch occurs in the kidney (glomerular and tubular basement membrane), lung, testis, cochlea, and eye, while an $\alpha5.\alpha5.\alpha6(IV)$ network appears in skin, smooth muscle, and esophagus and along Bowman's capsule in the kidney. This switch probably occurs because the $\alpha3.\alpha4.\alpha5(IV)$ network is more resistant to proteases and ensures the structural longevity of critical tissues. When basement membranes are the target of glomerular disease, they produce moderate proteinuria, some hematuria, and progressive renal failure.

ANTI-GBM DISEASE

Autoimmune disease where antibodies are directed against the α3 NC1 domain of collagen IV produces an anti-GBM disease often associated with RPGN and/or a pulmonary-renal syndrome called Goodpasture's syndrome. Discussion of this disease is covered in "Acute Nephritic Syndromes" earlier in the chapter.

ALPORT'S SYNDROME

Classically, patients with Alport's syndrome develop hematuria, thinning and splitting of the GBMs, mild proteinuria (<1–2 g/24 h), and chronic glomerulosclerosis, leading to renal failure in association with sensorineural deafness. Some patients develop lenticonus of the anterior lens capsule and, rarely, mental retardation or leiomyomatosis. Approximately 85% of patients with Alport's syndrome have an X-linked inheritance of mutations in the α5(IV) collagen chain on chromosome Xq22–24. Female carriers have variable penetrance depending on the type of mutation or the degree of mosaicism created by X inactivation. Fifteen percent of patients have autosomal recessive disease of the α3(IV) or α4(IV) chains on chromosome 2q35–37. Rarely, some kindred have an autosomal dominant inheritance of dominant-negative mutations in α3(IV) or α4(IV) chains.

Pedigrees with this syndrome are quite variable in their rate and frequency of tissue damage leading to organ failure. Patients with nonsense or missense mutations, reading frame shifts, or large deletions generally develop renal failure and sensorineural deafness by age 30 (juvenile form), while patients with splice variants, exon skipping, or missense mutations of α-helical glycines generally deteriorate after the age of 30 (adult form) with mild or late deafness. Early, severe deafness or lenticonus suggest a poorer prognosis.

Alport's patients early in their disease typically have thin basement membranes on renal biopsy (Fig. 4-17), which thicken over time into multilamellations surrounding lucent areas that often contain granules of varying density—the so-called split basement membrane. In any Alport kidney there are areas of thinning mixed with splitting of the GBM. Tubules drop out, glomeruli scar, and the kidney eventually succumbs to interstitial fibrosis. Primary treatment is control of systemic hypertension and use of ACE inhibitors to slow renal progression. Although patients who receive renal allografts usually develop anti-GBM antibodies directed toward the collagen epitopes absent in their native kidney, overt Goodpasture's syndrome is uncommon and graft survival is good.

THIN BASEMENT MEMBRANE DISEASE

Some variants of Alport's syndrome are now recognized as a subpopulation of patients with *thin basement membrane disease*. Thin basement membranes are found in 5–10% of the so-called normal population. These subclinical patients have normal blood pressure and little proteinuria, and they rarely progress to renal failure. If

SECTION IV

Glomerular and Tubular Disorders

they present with hematuria, they are often given the diagnosis of *benign familial hematuria*. Many of these patients have mutations in the same α3(IV) or α4(IV) collagen genes associated with autosomal recessive or dominant Alport's syndrome. Clearly, the boundary between nonprogressive Alport's syndrome and benign familial hematuria is quite variable, as there is a spectrum of clinical penetrance.

NAIL-PATELLA SYNDROME

Patients with nail-patella syndrome develop iliac horns on the pelvis and dysplasia of the dorsal limbs involving the patella, elbows, and nails, variably associated with neural-sensory hearing impairment, glaucoma, and abnormalities of the GBM and podocytes, leading to hematuria, proteinuria, and FSGS. The syndrome is autosomal-dominant, with haploinsufficiency for the LIM homeodomain transcription factor LMX1B; pedigrees are extremely variable in the penetrance for all features of the disease. LMX1B regulates the expression of genes encoding α3 and α4 chains of collagen IV, interstitial type III collagen, podocin, and CD2AP that help form the slit-pore membranes connecting podocytes. Mutations in the LIM domain region of LMX1B are associated with glomerulopathy, and renal failure appears in as many as 30% of patients. Proteinuria or isolated hematuria is discovered throughout life, but usually by the third decade, and is inexplicably more common in females. On renal biopsy there is lucent damage to the lamina densa of the GBM, an increase in collagen III fibrils along glomerular capillaries and in the mesangium, and damage to the slit-pore membrane, producing heavy proteinuria not unlike that seen in congenital nephrotic syndrome. Patients with renal failure do well with transplantation.

GLOMERULAR-VASCULAR SYNDROMES

A variety of diseases result in classic vascular injury to the glomerular capillaries. Most of these processes also damage blood vessels elsewhere in the body. The group of diseases discussed here lead to vasculitis, renal endothelial injury, thrombosis, ischemia, and/or lipid-based occlusions.

ATHEROSCLEROTIC NEPHROPATHY

Aging in the developed world is commonly associated with the occlusion of coronary and systemic blood vessels. The reasons for this include obesity, insulin resistance, smoking, hypertension, and diets rich in lipids that deposit in the arterial and arteriolar circulation, producing local inflammation and fibrosis of small blood vessels. When the renal arterial circulation is involved, the glomerular microcirculation is damaged, leading to chronic nephrosclerosis. Patients with GFRs <60 mL/min have more cardiovascular events and hospitalizations than those with higher filtration rates. Several aggressive

lipid disorders can accelerate this process, but most of the time atherosclerotic progression to chronic nephrosclerosis is associated with poorly controlled hypertension. Approximately 10% of glomeruli are normally sclerotic by age 40, rising to 20% by age 60 and 30% by age 80. Serum lipid profiles in humans are greatly affected by *apolipoprotein E* polymorphisms; the E4 allele is accompanied by increases in serum cholesterol and is more closely associated with atherogenic profiles in patients with renal failure. Mutations in E2 alleles, particularly in Japanese patients, produce a specific renal abnormality called *lipoprotein glomerulopathy* associated with glomerular lipoprotein thrombi and capillary dilation.

HYPERTENSIVE NEPHROSCLEROSIS

Uncontrolled systemic hypertension causes permanent damage to the kidneys in about 6% of patients with elevated blood pressure. As many as 27% of patients with end-stage kidney disease have hypertension as a primary cause. Although there is not a clear correlation between the extent or duration of hypertension and the risk of end-organ damage, *hypertensive nephrosclerosis* is fivefold more frequent in African Americans than Caucasians. Associated risk factors for progression to end-stage kidney disease include age, sex, race, smoking, hypercholesterolemia, duration of hypertension, low birth weight, and preexisting renal injury. Kidney biopsies in patients with hypertension, microhematuria, and moderate proteinuria demonstrate arteriolosclerosis, chronic nephrosclerosis, and interstitial fibrosis in the absence of immune deposits (Fig. 4-19). Today, based on a careful history, physical examination, urinalysis, and some serologic testing, the diagnosis of chronic nephrosclerosis is usually inferred without a biopsy. Treating hypertension is the best way to avoid progressive renal failure; most guidelines recommend lowering blood pressure to <130/80 mmHg if there is preexisting diabetes or kidney disease. In the presence of kidney disease, most patients begin therapy with two drugs, classically a thiazide diuretic and an ACE inhibitor; many will require three drugs. There is strong evidence in African Americans with hypertensive nephrosclerosis that therapy initiated with an ACE inhibitor can slow the rate of decline in renal function independent of systemic blood pressure. Patients with lower levels of hypertension are usually started on a thiazide diuretic or an ACE inhibitor alone. Malignant acceleration of hypertension can complicate the course of chronic nephrosclerosis, particularly in the setting of scleroderma (Fig. 4-22) or cocaine use. The hemodynamic stress of malignant hypertension causes fibrinoid necrosis of small blood vessels, thrombotic microangiography, a nephritic urinalysis, and acute renal failure. In the setting of renal failure, chest pain, or papilledema, the condition is treated as a hypertensive emergency. Slightly lowering the blood pressure often produces an immediate reduction in GFR that improves as the vascular injury attenuates and autoregulation of blood vessel tone is restored.

CHOLESTEROL EMBOLI

Aging patients with clinical complications from atherosclerosis sometimes shower cholesterol crystals into the circulation—either spontaneously or, more commonly, following an endovascular procedure with manipulation of the aorta—or with use of systemic anticoagulation. Spontaneous emboli may shower acutely or shower subacutely and somewhat more silently. Irregular emboli trapped in the microcirculation produce ischemic damage that induces an inflammatory reaction. Depending on the location of the atherosclerotic plaques releasing these cholesterol fragments, one may see cerebral transient ischemic attacks; livedo reticularis in the lower extremities; Hollenhorst plaques in the retina with visual field cuts; necrosis of the toes; and acute glomerular capillary injury leading to *focal glomerulosclerosis* sometimes associated with hematuria, mild proteinuria, and loss of renal function, which typically progresses over a few years. Occasional patients have fever, eosinophilia, or eosinophiluria. A skin biopsy of an involved area may be diagnostic. Since tissue fixation dissolves the cholesterol, one typically sees only residual, biconvex clefts in the vessel (Fig. 4-20). There is no therapy to reverse embolic occlusions, and steroids do not help. Controlling blood pressure and lipids and cessation of smoking are usually recommended for prevention.

SICKLE CELL DISEASE

Although individuals with SA-hemoglobin are usually asymptomatic, most will gradually develop hyposthenuria due to subclinical infarction of the renal medulla, thus predisposing them to volume depletion. Patients with homozygous SS-sickle cell disease develop chronic vasoocclusive disease in many organs. Polymers of deoxygenated SS-hemoglobin distort the shape of red blood cells. These cells attach to endothelia and obstruct small blood vessels, producing frequent, random, and painful sickle cell crises over time. Vessel occlusions in the kidney produce glomerular hypertension, FSGS, interstitial nephritis, and renal infarction associated with hyposthenuria, microscopic hematuria, and even gross hematuria; some patients also present with MPGN. By the second or third decade of life, persistent vasoocclusive disease in the kidney leads to varying degrees of renal failure, and some patients end up on dialysis. Treatment is directed toward reducing the frequency of painful crises and administering ACE inhibitors in the hope of delaying a progressive decline in renal function. Sickle cell patients can have transplantations, and renal graft survival is comparable to African Americans given transplantations for other reasons.

THROMBOTIC MICROANGIOPATHIES

Thrombotic thrombocytopenic purpura (TTP) and *hemolytic-uremic syndrome* (HUS) represent a spectrum of thrombotic microangiopathies. TTP and HUS share the general features of idiopathic thrombocytopenic purpura, hemolytic anemia, fever, renal failure, and neurologic disturbances. When patients have more evidence of renal injury, their condition tends to be called HUS, and when there is more neurologic disease, it is considered to be TTP. In adults there is often a mixture of both, which is why they are often called TTP/HUS. On examination of kidney tissue there is evidence of *glomerular capillary endotheliosis* associated with platelet thrombi, damage to the capillary wall, and formation of fibrin material in and around glomeruli (Fig. 4-21). These tissue findings are similar to what is seen in preeclampsia/HELLP (hemolysis, elevated liver enzymes, and low platelet count syndrome), malignant hypertension, and the antiphospholipid syndrome. TTP/HUS is also seen in pregnancy; with the use of oral contraceptives or quinine; in renal transplant patients given OKT3 for rejection; in patients taking the calcineurin inhibitors cyclosporine and tacrolimus or in patients taking the antiplatelet agents ticlopidine and clopidogrel; or following HIV infection.

Although there is no agreement on how much they share a final common pathophysiology, two general groups of patients are recognized: childhood HUS associated with enterohemorrhagic diarrhea and TTP/HUS in adults. Childhood HUS is caused by a toxin released by *Escherichia coli* O157:H7 and occasionally by *Shigella dysenteriae*. This shiga toxin (veratoxin) directly injures endothelia, enterocytes, and renal cells, causing apoptosis, platelet clumping, and intravascular hemolysis by binding to the glycolipid receptors (Gb3). These receptors are more abundant along endothelia in children compared to adults. In familial cases of adult TTP/HUS, there is a genetic deficiency of the ADAMTS13 metalloprotease that cleaves large multimers of von Willebrand's factor. Absent ADAMTS13, these large multimers cause platelet clumping and intravascular hemolysis. An antibody to ADAMTS13 is found in many sporadic cases of adult TTP/HUS, but not all; many patients also have antibodies to the thrombospondin receptor on selected endothelial cells in small vessels or increased levels of plasminogen-activator inhibitor 1 (PAI-1). The treatment of childhood HUS or adult TTP/HUS is daily plasmapheresis, which can be lifesaving. Plasmapheresis is given until the platelet count rises, but in relapsing patients it may need to be continued well after the platelet count improves, and in resistant patients twice-daily exchange may be helpful. Most patients respond within 2 weeks of daily plasmapheresis. Since TTP/HUS often has an autoimmune basis, there is an anecdotal role in relapsing patients for using splenectomy, steroids, immunosuppressive drugs, or anti-CD20 antibody. Patients with childhood HUS from infectious diarrhea are not given antibiotics, as antibiotics are thought to accelerate the release of the toxin and the diarrhea is usually self-limited.

ANTIPHOSPHOLIPID SYNDROME

Antiphospholipid syndrome develops in patients expressing antibodies to anionic phospholipids, particularly β_2 glycoprotein 1. Half of the patients have no obvious cause, a few are pregnant, some are already receiving hemodialysis or have a renal allograft, and the rest have a primary glomerulonephritis (nil lesion or membranous nephropathy) or a rheumatologic disease such as SLE. Lupus patients often also coexpress a lupus anticoagulant, with elevation in the activated partial tissue thromboplastin time. Clinical presentation of the catastrophic form of antiphospholipid syndrome appears as mixed thrombosis of the arterial and venous circulation with varying degrees of thrombocytopenia, hemolytic anemia, deep vein thrombosis, transient ischemic attacks, pulmonary embolism, and spontaneous abortions; lesser degrees of disease are more common. The kidneys are injured in this syndrome in approximately 25% of patients, particularly those with IgG antibodies. Some patients develop acute renal failure, while others suffer subclinical damage over time. Patients who present with acute flank pain and renal vein thrombosis in the setting of proteinuria should always be checked for antiphospholipid antibodies. Clinically, the antiphospholipid syndrome can wax and wane, and many patients have recurrences; <10% present with catastrophic multi-organ involvement and acute renal failure. Dialysis patients with antiphospholipid syndrome experience frequent occlusion of their arteriovenous graft. The urinalysis in most patients typically shows a mixed picture of moderate proteinuria (1–2 g/24 h) and hematuria. Glomerular capillaries and large and small renal arteries and veins occlude, accompanied by ischemic mesangiolysis and vessel hyperplasia, leading eventually to chronic glomerulosclerosis and interstitial fibrosis. Evidence of antiphospholipid syndrome on biopsy can usually be distinguished as an added complication of an underlying renal disease, particularly lupus nephritis. The mainstay of treatment for antiphospholipid syndrome is warfarin. There is also evidence of vasculitis in many patients due to complement-fixing antiphospholipid antibodies, which responds to the addition of steroids. Acute renal failure sometimes responds to removal of antiphospholipid antibodies with plasmapheresis and adjustment of immunosuppression where clinically indicated.

INFECTIOUS DISEASE–ASSOCIATED SYNDROMES

A number of infectious diseases will injure the glomerular capillaries as part of a systemic reaction producing an immune response or from direct infection of renal tissue. Evidence of this immune response is collected by glomeruli in the form of immune deposits that damage the kidney, producing moderate proteinuria and hematuria. Some of these infectious diseases represent the most common causes of glomerulonephritis worldwide.

POSTSTREPTOCOCCAL GLOMERULONEPHRITIS

This form of glomerulonephritis is one of the classic complications of streptococcal infection. The discussion of this disease can be found in the section "Acute Nephritic Syndromes."

SUBACUTE BACTERIAL ENDOCARDITIS

Renal injury from persistent bacteremia absent the continued presence of a foreign body, regardless of cause, is treated presumptively as if the patient has endocarditis. The discussion of this disease can be found in "Acute Nephritic Syndromes" earlier in the chapter.

HUMAN IMMUNODEFICIENCY VIRUS

HIV-associated nephropathy is seen after an interval of approximately 2.5 years from discovery of HIV, and many patients have low CD4 counts. Most lesions on renal biopsy show FSGS followed by MPGN. Other less common renal lesions include DPGN, IgA nephropathy, MCD, and membranous or mesangioproliferative glomerulonephritis. The disease affects up to 10% of HIV-infected patients and is more commonly seen in African-American men than in Caucasians, and in intravenous drug users or homosexuals. The FSGS characteristically reveals collapse of the glomerular capillary tuft called *collapsing glomerulopathy*, visceral epithelial cell swelling, microcystic dilatation of renal tubules, and tubuloreticular inclusions. Renal epithelial cells express replicating HIV virus, but host immune responses also play a role in the pathogenesis. MPGN and DPGN have been reported more commonly in HIV-infected Caucasians and in patients co-infected with hepatitis B or C. HIV-associated TTP has also been reported.

HIV patients with FSGS typically present with nephrotic-range proteinuria and hypoalbuminemia, but unlike patients with other etiologies for nephrotic syndrome, they do not commonly have hypertension, edema, or hyperlipidemia. Renal ultrasound also reveals large, echogenic kidneys, and renal function in some patients declines rapidly. Treatment with inhibitors of the renin-angiotensin system decreases the proteinuria. Although evidence from large, well-designed clinical trials is lacking, many feel that effective antiretroviral therapy benefits both the patient and the kidney. Dismal survival once renal failure is reached has improved, and many centers now offer renal allografts to select HIV patients.

HEPATITIS B AND C

Chronic hepatitis B infection can be associated with polyarteritis nodosa, more commonly in adults than children. Typically, however, infected patients only present with microscopic hematuria, nonnephrotic or nephrotic-range proteinuria, and hypertension. Alternatively, the hepatitis B carrier state can produce an MGN that is more common in children than adults or MPGN that is more common in adults than in children. Renal histology is indistinguishable from idiopathic MGN or Type I MPGN. There are no good treatment guidelines, but interferon α and lamivudine have been used to some effect in small studies. Children have a good prognosis, with 66% achieving spontaneous remission within 3 years. In contrast, 30% of adults have renal insufficiency and 10% have renal failure 5 years after diagnosis.

Up to 30% of patients with chronic hepatitis C infection have some renal manifestations. Patients often present with cryoglobulinemia and nephrotic syndrome, microscopic hematuria, abnormal liver function tests, depressed C_3 levels, anti-hepatitis C virus antibodies, and viral RNA in the blood. The renal lesions most commonly seen, in order of decreasing frequency, are *cryoglobulinemic glomerulonephritis, MGN,* and *Type I MPGN.* Treatment aims at reducing the level of the infection.

OTHER VIRUSES

Other viral infections are occasionally associated with glomerular lesions, but cause and effect are not well established. These viral infections and their respective glomerular lesions include cytomegalovirus producing MPGN; influenza and anti-GBM disease; measles-associated endocapillary proliferative glomerulonephritis, with measles antigen in the capillary loops and mesangium; parvovirus causing mild proliferative or mesangioproliferative glomerulonephritis; mumps and mesangioproliferative glomerulonephritis; Epstein-Barr virus producing MPGN, diffuse proliferative nephritis, or IgA nephropathy; dengue hemorrhagic fever causing endocapillary proliferative glomerulonephritis; and coxsackie virus producing *focal glomerulonephritis* or DPGN.

SYPHILIS

Secondary syphilis, with rash and constitutional symptoms, develops weeks to months after the chancre first appears and occasionally presents with the nephrotic syndrome from MGN caused by subepithelial immune deposits containing treponemal antigens. The diagnosis is confirmed with non-treponemal and treponemal tests for *Treponema pallidum.* The renal lesion responds to treatment with penicillin or an alternative drug, if allergic. Additional testing for other sexually transmitted diseases is an important part of disease management.

LEPROSY

Despite aggressive eradication programs, approximately 400,000 new cases of leprosy appear annually worldwide. The diagnosis is best made in patients with multiple skin lesions accompanied by sensory loss in affected areas, using skin smears showing paucibacillary or multibacillary infection (WHO criteria). Leprosy is caused by infection with *Mycobacterium leprae* and can be classified by Ridley-Jopling criteria into various types: tuberculoid, borderline tuberculoid, mid-borderline and borderline lepromatous, and lepromatous. In some series, all cases with borderline lepromatous and lepromatous types of leprosy have various forms of glomerulonephritis. Most common is focal glomerulonephritis followed by mesangioproliferative glomerulonephritis or renal amyloidosis; much less common are the renal lesions of DPGN and MPGN. Treatment with dapsone, rifampicin, and clofazimine can irradiate the infection in nearly all patients.

MALARIA

There are 300–500 million incident cases of malaria each year worldwide, and the kidney is commonly involved. Glomerulonephritis is due to immune complexes containing malarial antigens that are implanted in the glomerulus. In malaria from *P. falciparum,* mild proteinuria is associated with subendothelial deposits, mesangial deposits, and mesangioproliferative glomerulonephritis that usually resolve with treatment. In quartan malaria from infection with *Plasmodium malariae,* children are more commonly affected and renal involvement is more severe. Transient proteinuria and microscopic hematuria can resolve with treatment of the infection. However, resistant nephrotic syndrome with progression to renal failure over 3–5 years does happen, as <50% of patients respond to steroid therapy. Affected patients with nephrotic syndrome have thickening of the glomerular capillary walls, with subendothelial deposits of IgG, IgM, and C_3 associated with a sparse membranoproliferative lesion. The rare mesangioproliferative glomerulonephritis reported with *Plasmodium vivax* or *Plasmodium ovale* typically has a benign course.

SCHISTOSOMIASIS

Schistosomiasis affects more than 300 million people worldwide and primarily involves the urinary and gastrointestinal tracts. Glomerular involvement varies with the specific strain of schistosomiasis; *Schistosoma mansoni* is most commonly associated with clinical renal disease, and the glomerular lesions can be classified: Class I is a *mesangioproliferative glomerulonephritis*; Class II is an *extracapillary proliferative glomerulonephritis*; Class III is a *membranoproliferative glomerulonephritis*; Class IV is a *focal segmental glomerulonephritis*; and Class V lesions have *amyloidosis*. Classes I–II often remit with treatment of the infection, but Classes III and IV lesions are associated with IgA immune deposits and progress despite antiparasitic and/or immunosuppressive therapy.

OTHER PARASITES

Renal involvement with toxoplasmosis infections is rare. When it occurs, patients present with nephrotic syndrome and have a histologic picture of MPGN. Fifty percent of patients with leishmaniasis will have mild to moderate proteinuria and microscopic hematuria, but renal insufficiency is rare. Acute DPGN, MGN, and mesangioproliferative glomerulonephritis have all been observed on biopsy. The nematodes, filariasis and trichinosis, can be associated with glomerular injury presenting with proteinuria, hematuria, and a variety of histologic lesions that typically resolve with eradication of the infection.

FURTHER READINGS

APPEL AS et al: An update on the use of mycophenolate mofetil in lupus nephritis and other primary glomerular diseases. Nat Clin Pract Nephrol 5:132, 2009

CHADBAN SJ, ATKINS RC: Glomerulonephritis. Lancet 365:1797, 2005

CUNARD R, KELLY CJ: Immune-mediated renal disease. J Allergy Clin Immunol 111:S637, 2003

GUBLER MC: Inherited diseases of the glomerular basement membrane. Nat Clin Pract Nephrol 4:24, 2008

HEYMANN F et al: Kidney dendritic cell activation is required for progression of renal disease in a mouse model of glomerular injury. J Clin Invest 119:1286, 2009

HUDSON BG et al: Alport and Goodpasture syndromes and the type IV collagen family. N Engl J Med 348:2543, 2003

HURTADO A, JOHNSON RJ: Hygiene hypothesis and the prevalence of glomerulonephritis. Kidney Int 68:S62, 2005

LEBLEU VS et al: Stem cell-based therapy for glomerular diseases: An evolving concept. J Am Soc Nephrol 19:1621, 2008

STOKES MB et al: Glomerular disease related to anti-VEGF therapy. Kidney Int 74:1487, 2008

TRYGGVASON K et al: Hereditary proteinuria syndromes and mechanisms of proteinuria. N Engl J Med 354:1387, 2006

CHAPTER 15

Glomerular Diseases

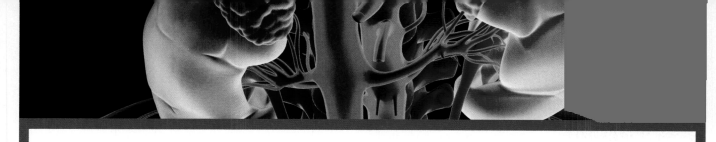

CHAPTER 16

POLYCYSTIC KIDNEY DISEASE AND OTHER INHERITED TUBULAR DISORDERS

David J. Salant ■ Parul S. Patel

INTRODUCTION

The polycystic kidney diseases are among the most common life–threatening inherited diseases worldwide. They are equally prevalent in all ethnic and racial groups. Progressive expansion of numerous fluid-filled cysts results in massive enlargement of the kidneys (Fig. 16-1) and frequently causes kidney failure. Autosomal dominant polycystic kidney disease (ADPKD) is seen predominantly in adults, whereas autosomal recessive polycystic kidney disease (ARPKD) is mainly a disease of childhood. As shown in Table 16-1, renal cysts are also seen in several other hereditary kidney diseases, some of which may have defects in a common signaling pathway with ADPKD and ARPKD. Table 16-2 summarizes the gene defects and functional abnormalities in inherited tubular diseases that manifest primarily with alterations in fluid, electrolyte, acid–base, and mineral balance.

AUTOSOMAL DOMINANT POLYCYSTIC KIDNEY DISEASE

Etiology and Pathogenesis

ADPKD is a systemic disorder resulting from mutations in either the *PKD-1* or *PKD-2* gene. The *PKD-1* encoded protein, polycystin-1, is a large receptor-like molecule, whereas the *PKD-2* gene product, polycystin-2, has features of an ion-channel protein. Both are transmembrane proteins present throughout all segments of the nephron and are localized to the luminal surface of tubular cells in primary cilia, on the basal surface in focal adhesion complexes, and on the lateral surface in adherens junctions. The proteins are thought to function independently, or as a complex, to regulate fetal and adult epithelial cell gene transcription, apoptosis, differentiation, and cell-matrix interactions. Disruption of these processes leads to epithelial dedifferentiation, unregulated proliferation and apoptosis,

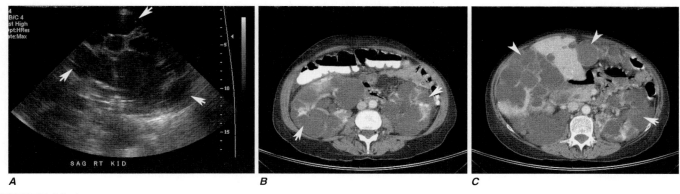

FIGURE 16-1

Renal ultrasonogram and contrast-enhanced abdominal CT scan in a 56-year-old woman with autosomal dominant polycystic kidney disease. **A.** Sonogram of the right kidney showing numerous cysts of varying sizes (arrows). **B.** Abdominal CT scan demonstrating bilaterally enlarged kidneys with large cysts (arrows). **C.** Multiple liver cysts (arrowheads) and renal cysts (arrow) are seen in an upper abdominal image.

altered cell polarity, disorganization of surrounding extracellular matrix, excessive fluid secretion, and abnormal expression of several genes, including some that encode growth factors. Vasopressin-mediated elevation of cyclic AMP (cAMP) levels in cyst epithelia plays a major role in cystogenesis by stimulating cell proliferation and fluid secretion into the cyst lumen through apical chloride and aquaporin channels. Cyst formation begins in utero from any point along the nephron, although <5% of total nephrons are thought to be involved. As the cysts accumulate fluid, they enlarge, separate entirely from the nephron, compress the neighboring renal parenchyma, and progressively compromise renal function.

GENETIC CONSIDERATIONS

ADPKD occurs in 1:400–1:1000 individuals worldwide and accounts for ~4% of end-stage renal disease (ESRD) in the United States. Over 90% of cases are inherited as an autosomal dominant trait, with the remainder likely representing spontaneous mutations. Mutations in the *PKD-1* gene on chromosome 16 (ADPKD-1) account for 85% of cases, whereas mutations in the *PKD-2* gene on chromosome 4 (ADPKD-2) represent the remainder. A few families appear to have a defect at a site that is different from either of these loci. Direct mutation analysis of isolated cysts suggests there is loss of heterozygosity, whereby a somatic mutation in the normal "wild-type" allele of a small number of tubular epithelial cells leads to unregulated clonal proliferation of the cells that ultimately form the cyst lining.

Clinical Features

Phenotypic heterogeneity is a hallmark of ADPKD, as evidenced by family members who share the same mutation but have a different clinical course. Affected individuals are often asymptomatic into the fourth or fifth decade. Presenting symptoms and signs include abdominal discomfort, hematuria, urinary tract infection, incidental discovery of hypertension, abdominal mass, elevated serum creatinine, or cystic kidneys on imaging studies (Fig. 16-1*A* and *B*). Frequently the diagnosis is made prior to the onset of symptoms, when asymptomatic members in affected families request screening. In most patients, renal function declines progressively over the course of 10–20 years from the time of diagnosis, but not everyone with ADPKD develops ESRD; it occurs in about 60% of patients by age 70. Those with ADPKD-2 tend to have later onset and slower progression. Hypertension is common and often precedes renal dysfunction, perhaps mediated by increased activity of the renin-angiotensin system. There is only mild proteinuria, and impaired urinary concentrating ability manifests early as polyuria and nocturia. Risk factors for progressive kidney disease include younger age at diagnosis, black race, male gender, presence of polycystin-1 mutation, and hypertension. There is a close correlation between the rate of kidney expansion and the rate of decline in kidney function. Dull, persistent flank and abdominal pain and early satiety and gastroesophageal reflux symptoms are common due to the mass effect of the enlarged kidneys. Cyst rupture or hemorrhage into a cyst may produce acute flank pain or symptoms and signs of localized peritonitis. Hematuria may result from cyst rupture into the collecting system or from uric acid or calcium oxalate kidney stones. Nephrolithiasis occurs in about 20% of patients. Urinary tract infection, including acute pyelonephritis, occurs with increased frequency in ADPKD. Infection in a kidney or liver cyst is a particularly serious complication. It is most often due to gram-negative bacteria and presents with pain, fever, and chills. Blood cultures are frequently positive, but urine culture may be negative because infected kidney cysts do not communicate directly with the collecting system. Distinguishing between infection and cyst hemorrhage is often a challenge, and the diagnosis relies mainly on clinical and

TABLE 16-1

INHERITED CYSTIC KIDNEY DISEASES

DISEASE (OMIM)	MODE OF INHERITANCE	LOCUS	GENE	PROTEIN	RENAL ABNORMALITIES	EXTRA-RENAL ABNORMALITIES
Autosomal dominant polycystic kidney disease (601313, 173910)	AD	16p13	*PKD1*	polycystin-1	Cortical and medullary cysts	Cerebral aneurysms; liver cysts, other[a]
	AD	4q21	*PKD2*	polycystin-2	Cortical and medullary cysts	Cerebral aneurysms; liver cysts, other[a]
Autosomal recessive polycystic kidney disease (263200)	AR	6p21	*PKDH1*	fibrocystin	Distal tubule and collecting duct cysts	Hepatic fibrosis; Caroli syndrome
Nephronophthisis I (Juvenile/ Adolescent, 256100)	AR	2q13	*NPHP1*	nephrocystin	Small fibrotic kidneys; medullary cysts	Retinitis pigmentosa
Nephronophthisis II (Infantile, 602088)	AR	9q31	*INVS*	inversin	Large kidneys; widespread cysts	Situs inversus
Nephronophthisis III (Juvenile/ Adolescent, 604387)	AR	3q22	*NPHP3*	nephrocystin-3	Small fibrotic kidneys; medullary cysts	Retinitis pigmentosa; hepatic fibrosis
Nephronophthisis IV (Juvenile/ Adolescent, 606966)	AR	1p36	*NPHP4*	nephrocystin-4	Small fibrotic kidneys; medullary cysts	Retinitis pigmentosa
Nephronophthisis V (Juvenile/ Adolescent)	AR	3q13	*NPHP5*	nephrocystin-5	Small fibrotic kidneys; medullary cysts	Amaurosis
Medullary cystic kidney disease (174000, 603860)	AD	1q21	*MCKD1*	unknown	Small fibrotic kidneys; medullary cysts	None
	AD	16p12	*UMOD*	uromodulin (Tamm-Horsfall protein)	Small fibrotic kidneys; medullary cysts	Hyperuricemia and gout
Tuberous sclerosis (191100)	AD	9q34	*TSC1*	tuberin	Renal cysts; angiomyo-lipomas; renal cell carcinoma	Adenoma sebaceum; CNS hamartomas
	AD	16p13	*TSC1*	hamartin	Renal cysts; angiomyo-lipomas; renal cell carcinoma	Adenoma sebaceum; CNS hamartomas
Von Hippel-Lindau disease (608537)	AD	3p26-p25	*VHL*	pVHL	Renal cysts; renal cell carcinoma	Retinal angiomas; CNS hemangioblastomas; pheochromocytomas

Note: AD, autosomal dominant; AR, autosomal recessive; OMIM, online Mendelian inheritance in man.
[a]See text for details.

TABLE 16-2

INHERITED TABULAR DISORDERS

DISEASE (OMIM)	MODE OF INHERITANCE	LOCUS	GENE	PROTEIN	RENAL ABNORMALITIES	EXTRA-RENAL ABNORMALITIES
Bartter's syndrome						
Type 1 (601678)	AR	15q15	SLC12A1	NKCC2	Salt wasting; hypokalemia	
Type 2 (41200)	AR	11q24	KCNJ1	ROMK	Salt wasting; hypokalemia	
Type 3 (607364)	AR	1p36	ClCNKb	CLCNKb	Salt wasting; hypokalemia	
Type 4 (602023)	AR	1p31	BSND	Barttin	Salt wasting; hypokalemia	Sensorineural deafness
Type 5 (601199)	AD	3q13	CaSR	CaSR	Salt wasting; hypokalemia	
Gitelman's syndrome (263800)	AR	16q13	SLC12A3	NCCT	Salt wasting; hypokalemia hypomagnesemia	
Pseudohypoaldosteronism Type 1 (264350, 177735)	AR	16p13 16p13 12p13	SCNN1B SCNN1G SCNN1A	α, β, or γ subunits of ENaC	Hyperkalemia; salt wasting	Increased lung secretions and lung infections
	AD	4q31	NR3C2	Mineralocorticoid receptor (type I)	Hyperkalemia; salt wasting	
Primary hypomagnesemia (FHHNC, 248250)	AR	3q27	CLDN16	Claudin 16 (Paracellin - 1)	Hypomagnesemia; nephrocalcinosis	
Hypomagnesemia with secondary hypocalcemia (602014)	AR	9q22	TRPM6	TRPM6	Hypomagnesemia; hypocalcemia	
Renal magnesium wasting (154020)	AD	11q23	FXYD2	FXYD2	Hypomagnesemia; hypocalciuria	
Autosomal dominant hypoparathyroidism (601199)	AD	3q13	CaSR	CaSR	Hypocalcemia; hypercalciuria; hypomagnesemia	
Liddle's syndrome (177200)	AD	16p13	SCNN1B	β and γ subunits of ENaC	Hypertension; hypokalemia; alkalosis	
Pseudohypoaldosteronism Type II (Gordon syndrome, 145260)	AD	12p13 17q21	WNK1 Wnk4	WNK 1 WNK 4	Hypertension; hyperkalemia	
Nephrogenic DI Type 1 (304800)	XL	Xq28	AVPR2	AVPR2	Renal concentrating defect	
Nephrogenic DI Type 2 (125800)	AR, AD	12q13	AQP2	AQP2	Renal concentrating defect	
Nephrogenic syndrome of inappropriate antidiuresis (300539)	XL	Xq28	AVPR2	AVPR2	Hyponatremia	
Distal renal tubular acidosis (267300, 602722, 259730, 179800)	AR	2cenq13 7q33	ATP6B1 ATP6A4	H⁺-ATPase (B1) H⁺-ATPase (α4)	Hyperchloremic metabolic acidosis; nephrocalcinosis	Sensorineural deafness (B1 defect only); grwoth retardation
	AR AD	8q22 17q21	CA2 SLC4A1	CA2 AE1	Proximal and distal RTA Distal RTA	

(Continued)

TABLE 16-2 (CONTINUED)

INHERITED TABULAR DISORDERS

DISEASE (OMIM)	MODE OF INHERITANCE	LOCUS	GENE	PROTEIN	RENAL ABNORMALITIES	EXTRA-RENAL ABNORMALITIES
Proximal renal tubular acidosis (604278)	AR	4q21	SLC4A4	NBC-1	Moderate hyperchloremic metabolic acidosis	Glaucoma; band keratopathy
Cystinuria (220100)	AR	2p16 19q13	SLC3A1 SLC7A9	rBAT b⁰+AT	Cystine stones; dibasic aminoaciduria	
Hartnup disease (234500)	AR	5p15	SLC6A19	B⁰AT1	Neutral aminoaciduria	Rash, dermatitis, ataxia; dementia
Dent's disease (300009)	XL	Xp11	CLCN5	CLC5	Proximal tubular dysfunction; nephrocalcinosis	Osteomalacia; rickets
Renal glucosuria (233100)	AR	16p11	SLC5A2	SGLT2	Glucosuria	
Hereditary hypophos-phatemic rickets with hypercalciuria (HHRH, 241530)	AR	9q34	SLC34A3	Sodium-phosphate co-transporter	Hypophosphatemia; hypercalciuria	Rickets
Vitamin D-dependent rickets type I (VDDR I, 264700)	AR	12q14	CYP27B1	25-vitamin D3-1-α-hydroxylase	Hypocalcemia	Rickets

Note: OMIM, online Mendelian inheritance in man; AD, autosomal dominant; AR, autosomal recessive; XL, X-linked; DI, diabetes insipidus; NKCC2, Na-K-2Cl co-transporter; ROMK, renal outer medullary potassium channel; CLCNKb, chloride channel Kb; CaSR, calcium-sensing receptor; NCCT, thiazide-sensitive Na-Cl co-transporter; ENaC, amiloride-sensitive epithelial sodium channel; FHHNC, familial hypomagnesemia with hypercalciuria and nephrocalcinosis; TRPM6, transient receptor potential cation channel, subfamily M, member 6; WNK, with no lysine (K); AVPR2, arginine vasopressin receptor 2; CA2, carbonic anhydrase II; AE1, anion exchanger 1; NBC, sodium–bicarbonate co-transporter; rBAT, renal basic amino acid transport glycoprotein; AT1, amino acid transporter; CLC5, chloride channel 5; SGLT2, sodium/glucose co-transporter.

bacteriological findings. Radiological and nuclear imaging studies are generally not helpful.

Numerous extrarenal manifestations of ADPKD highlight the systemic nature of the disease and likely reflect a generalized abnormality in collagen and extracellular matrix. Patients with ADPKD have a fourfold increased risk of subarachnoid or cerebral hemorrhage from a ruptured intracranial aneurysm as compared to the general population. Saccular aneurysms of the anterior cerebral circulation may be detected in up to 10% of asymptomatic patients on magnetic resonance angiogram (MRA) screening, but most are small, have a low risk of spontaneous rupture, and do not merit the risk of intervention. In general, hemorrhage tends to occur before the age of 50 years in patients with a family history of intracranial hemorrhage, and those who have survived a previous bleed, have aneurysms larger than 10 mm, and have uncontrolled hypertension. Other vascular abnormalities include aortic root and annulus dilatation. Cardiac valvular abnormalities occur in 25% of patients, most commonly mitral valve prolapse and aortic regurgitation. Although most valvular lesions are asymptomatic, some may progress over time and warrant valve replacement. The incidence of hepatic cysts rises progressively up to 40% in patients over the age of 60 years. Most patients are asymptomatic with normal liver function tests, but hepatic cysts may bleed, become infected, rupture, and cause pain. Although the frequency of liver cysts is equal between genders, women are more likely to have massive cysts (Fig. 16–1C). Colonic diverticulae are common, with a higher incidence of perforation in patients with ADPKD. Abdominal wall and inguinal hernias also occur with a higher frequency than in the general population.

Diagnosis and Screening

The sensitivity of renal ultrasonography for the detection of ADPKD is 100% for subjects 30 years or older with a positive family history. Diagnostic criteria require two or more cysts in one kidney and at least one cyst in the contralateral kidney in young subjects, but four or more in subjects older than 60 years because of the increased frequency of benign simple cysts. Most often, the diagnosis is made from a positive family history and imaging studies showing large kidneys with multiple bilateral cysts and possibly liver cysts (Fig. 16–1). Before the age of 30 years, CT scan or T2–weighted MRI is more sensitive for detecting presymptomatic disease because the sensitivity of ultrasound falls to 95% for ADPKD type 1 and <70% for ADPKD type 2. Genetic linkage analysis and mutational screening for *ADPKD-1* and *ADPKD-2* is available for equivocal cases, especially when a young adult from an affected family is being considered as a potential kidney donor. Genetic counseling is essential for those being screened. It is recommended that screening for asymptomatic intracranial

aneurysms should be restricted to patients with a personal or family history of intracranial hemorrhage and those in high-risk occupations. Intervention should be limited to aneurysms larger than 10 mm.

Treatment:
℞ AUTOSOMAL DOMINANT POLYCYSTIC KIDNEY DISEASE

At present, treatment is largely supportive, as there is no single therapy that has been shown to prevent the decline in kidney function. Hypertension control with a target blood pressure of 130/85 mmHg or less is recommended according to Joint National Committee (JNC) VII guidelines; however, lower levels have been reported to slow the rate of loss of kidney function. A multidrug approach that includes agents to inhibit the renin-angiotensin system is frequently required. There is no compelling evidence to recommend a low-protein diet, especially in patients with advanced kidney dysfunction where optimizing nutritional status is important. Lipid-soluble antimicrobials, such as trimethoprim-sulfamethoxazole and quinolone antibiotics that have good tissue permeation, are the preferred therapy for infected kidney and liver cysts. Pain management occasionally requires cyst drainage by percutaneous aspiration, sclerotherapy with alcohol or, rarely, surgical drainage. Patients with ADPKD appear to have a survival advantage on either peritoneal dialysis or hemodialysis compared to patients with other causes of ESRD. Those undergoing kidney transplantation may require bilateral nephrectomy if the kidneys are massively enlarged or have been the site of infected cysts. Posttransplantation survival rates are similar to those of patients with other causes of kidney failure, but patients remain at risk for the extrarenal complications of ADPKD. Studies in animal models of inherited cystic diseases have identified promising therapeutic strategies, including vasopressin V_2 receptor antagonists that suppress cyst growth by lowering intracellular cAMP and inhibitors of cell signaling that target the epidermal growth factor receptor tyrosine kinase to control cell proliferation.

AUTOSOMAL RECESSIVE POLYCYSTIC KIDNEY DISEASE

GENETIC CONSIDERATIONS

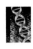 ARPKD is primarily a disease of infants and children. The incidence is 1:20,000 births. The kidneys are enlarged, with small cysts, <5 mm, limited to the collecting tubules.

The ARPKD gene on chromosome 6p21, *PKHD1* (polycystic kidney and hepatic disease 1), encodes several alternatively spliced transcripts (Table 16–1). The largest transcript produces a multidomain transmembrane protein termed *fibrocystin (polyductin)* that is found in the cortical and medullary collecting ducts and thick ascending limb of Henle's loop in the kidney as well as in biliary and pancreatic duct epithelia. Like the polycystins, fibrocystin has receptor-like features and may be involved in cell-cell and cell-matrix interactions. Fibrocystin, the polycystins, and several proteins involved in animal models of PKD are located in association with primary cilia on the tubular epithelial cell apical surface, which suggests that they may cooperate in a mechanosensory pathway. A large number of different mutations have been identified throughout *PKHD1* and are unique to individual families. Most patients are compound heterozygotes. Those with two truncating mutations frequently die shortly after birth, whereas those that survive beyond the neonatal period generally have at least one missense mutation. Mutations in *PKHD1* have also been identified in about 30% of children with congenital hepatic fibrosis (Caroli syndrome) without evident kidney involvement.

Clinical Features

The clinical presentation of ARPKD is highly variable. Up to 50% of affected neonates die of pulmonary hypoplasia, the result of oligohydramnios from severe intrauterine kidney disease. About 80% of those who survive the neonatal period are still alive after 10 years; however, one-third of them will have developed ESRD. Enlarged kidneys may be detected soon after birth as bilateral abdominal masses. Impaired urinary concentrating ability and metabolic acidosis ensue as tubular function deteriorates. Hypertension often occurs in the first few years of life. Kidney function deteriorates progressively from childhood into early adult life. Longer-term survivors frequently develop portal hypertension, esophageal varices, and hypersplenism from periportal fibrosis.

Diagnosis

Ultrasonography reveals large, echogenic kidneys. The diagnosis can be made in utero after 24 weeks of gestation in severe cases, but cysts generally become visible only after birth. The absence of renal cysts in either parent on ultrasonography helps to distinguish ARPKD from ADPKD in older patients. The wide range of different mutations and the large size of the gene complicate molecular diagnosis, although prenatal diagnosis is possible by gene linkage to the *PKHD1* locus in families with a previous confirmed ARPKD birth.

Treatment:
℞ AUTOSOMAL RECESSIVE POLYCYSTIC KIDNEY DISEASE

No specific therapy exists for ARPKD. Improvements in mechanical ventilation, neonatal support, blood pressure management, dialysis, and kidney transplantation have led to survival well into adulthood. Complications of hepatic fibrosis may necessitate liver transplantation. Future therapies may target aberrant cell signaling mechanisms, as in ADPKD.

NEPHRONOPHTHISIS

Genetics and Pathogenesis

Nephronophthisis (NPHP) is the most common genetic cause of ESRD in childhood and adolescence. Five distinct genetic mutations with autosomal recessive inheritance have been identified (Table 16-1). Although their precise functions are unclear, the defective protein products, named nephrocystins and inversin, localize to the primary cilium and associated basal body of renal epithelial cells, similar to the polycystins and fibrocystin. NPHP is classified into infantile, juvenile, and adolescent forms based on the age of ESRD onset. In juvenile NPHP, the most common form, the kidneys are shrunken and histology shows tubular atrophy, thickening of tubular basement membranes, diffuse interstitial fibrosis, and microscopic medullary cysts. In the infantile form, the kidneys are large and histology is similar to the juvenile form, except that medullary cysts are more prominent and develop earlier.

Clinical Features

In juvenile NPHP, symptoms typically appear after one year of age. Impaired tubular function causes salt wasting and defective urinary concentration and acidification. Patients may present with polyuria, polydipsia, volume depletion, or systemic acidosis. Progressive kidney failure leads to growth retardation, anemia, and symptoms of uremia. On average, ESRD occurs by age 5 in the infantile form, age 13 in the juvenile form, and age 19 in the adolescent form. Up to 15% of patients with juvenile NPHP have extrarenal manifestations (Table 16-1), most commonly retinitis pigmentosa (Senior-Loken syndrome). Other abnormalities include blindness from amaurosis, oculomotor apraxia, cerebellar ataxia, mental retardation, hepatic fibrosis, and ventricular septal defect. Situs inversus is seen in some cases of infantile NPHP, consistent with mutation in *INVS*, a gene that is critical for left-right patterning in the embryo.

Diagnosis

The diagnosis of NPHP should be considered in patients with a family history of kidney disease, early-onset progressive renal failure, and a bland urine sediment with minimal proteinuria. Ultrasonography reveals small hyperechoic kidneys in juvenile NPHP and large kidneys with cysts in the infantile form.

R_x Treatment: NEPHRONOPHTHISIS

No specific therapy exists to prevent loss of kidney function in NPHP. Salt and water replacement are required for patients with salt wasting and polyuria. Therapy should include sodium bicarbonate or citrate for acidosis, control of secondary hyperparathyroidism, erythropoietin for anemia, and timely institution of dialysis and transplantation.

MEDULLARY CYSTIC KIDNEY DISEASE

GENETIC CONSIDERATIONS

The medullary cystic kidney diseases (MCKD) generally present in young adults. Two genetic loci have been defined, both with autosomal dominant transmission (Table 16-1). The locus for MCKD1 has been mapped to chromosome 1q21. Mutations in the uromodulin gene (UMOD) that encodes the Tamm-Horsfall mucoprotein on chromosome 16p12 have been identified in MCKD2.

Clinical Features

Like NPHP, patients with MCKD have atrophic kidneys with diffuse interstitial fibrosis, cysts restricted to the renal medulla, salt wasting, and polyuria. Disease onset is later than NPHP. Consequently, there is no growth retardation, salt wasting is milder, and ESRD occurs later, usually between the ages of 20 and 60. There are no extrarenal manifestations in MCKD1. Most patients with MCKD2 and the genetically related familial juvenile hyperuricemic nephropathy also have severe hyperuricemia and precocious onset of gout.

Diagnosis

The diagnosis of MCKD should be considered in young adults presenting with a family history suggesting dominant inheritance of kidney disease, progressive renal failure, bland urinalysis with little or no proteinuria, and small, dense kidneys with medullary cysts on ultrasonography or CT. The presence of hyperuricemia and gout are further clues to the diagnosis of MCKD2. MCKD2 can be confirmed by mutation analysis of UMOD.

R_x Treatment: MEDULLARY CYSTIC KIDNEY DISEASE

There is no specific therapy for MCKD. Allopurinol is indicated for patients with gout and makes sense for those with presymptomatic hyperuricemia, although there is no evidence that it prevents progressive renal failure in MCKD2. Dialysis and transplantation outcomes appear to be favorable.

TUBEROUS SCLEROSIS

Tuberous sclerosis (TS) is an autosomal dominant disorder affecting 1 out of 6000 people. It results from inactivating mutations in either the TSC1 gene encoding tuberin or the TSC2 gene encoding hamartin (Table 16-1). Hamartin and tubulin form a complex that is thought to negatively regulate the cell cycle. The presence of either mutation produces uncontrolled proliferation in numerous tissues, including the skin, central nervous system (CNS), heart, skeleton, and kidneys. CNS hamartomas can cause seizures, mental retardation, and autism. Expressivity is highly variable, but the kidneys are affected in 80% of patients. Renal TS occurs in three forms: renal cysts, renal angiomyolipomas, and renal cell carcinoma. Cysts are usually asymptomatic and are not evident on imaging studies until adulthood. Cysts may be large and numerous, sometimes leading to ESRD and producing a clinical scenario that can be confused with ADPKD, especially if there are few other systemic manifestations of TS. Angiomyolipomas are the most common renal abnormality, occur bilaterally, are often multiple, and are usually asymptomatic. Spontaneous bleeding can produce flank pain, nausea and vomiting, hematuria, and even life-threatening retroperitoneal hemorrhage. Large lesions, >4 cm, are most likely to cause pain and bleeding, and may require surgical excision. Multicentric renal cell carcinomas have been reported to occur with increased frequency in TS. Patients with TS should be screened for renal involvement at initial diagnosis with ultrasound or CT. Those with cysts or angiomyolipomas require regular imaging to monitor for the development of renal cell carcinoma.

VON HIPPEL-LINDAU DISEASE

Von Hippel-Lindau disease (VHL) is a rare autosomal dominant disease characterized by abnormal angiogenesis with benign and malignant tumors affecting multiple tissues. The disease is inherited as a mutation in one allele of the VHL tumor suppressor gene. Somatic mutation of the normal allele leads to retinal angiomas, CNS hemangioblastomas, pheochromocytomas and multicentric clear cell cysts, hemangiomas, and adenomas of the kidney. The kidneys are affected in three-quarters of patients, and half develop clear cell carcinomas in the renal cysts. Ten percent of patients present with symptoms of clear cell carcinoma. It is noteworthy that VHL mutations also account for 60% of spontaneous clear cell carcinomas of the kidney. The diagnosis of renal cell carcinoma in VHL disease is made at a mean age of 44 years, while 70% of patients who survive to age 60 develop renal carcinoma. The high risk of renal cell carcinoma mandates periodic surveillance (usually yearly in adults) by either CT or MRI. Routine screening and awareness of the natural history of lesions has enabled renal-sparing approaches to disease management. Tumors <3 cm in size require careful monitoring for growth, while partial nephrectomy is indicated in those >3 cm in the absence of metastasis. Nonsurgical renal-sparing strategies, including percutaneous radiofrequency ablation and selective arterial embolization, have shown promise in short-term trials.

MEDULLARY SPONGE KIDNEY

Pathology and Clinical Features

Medullary sponge kidney (MSK) is a common, benign condition of unknown cause characterized by ectasia of the papillary collecting ducts of one or both kidneys. Urinary stasis in the dilated ducts, hypocitraturia, and, occasionally, incomplete distal renal tubular acidosis (dRTA) contribute to the formation of small calcium-containing calculi. Most cases are asymptomatic or are discovered during investigation of asymptomatic hematuria. Symptomatic patients typically present as young adults with renal colic and the passage of stones or recurrent urinary tract infections; however, MSK may cause hematuria and nephrolithiasis in children. Most cases are sporadic, although MSK has been found rarely in association with other congenital anomalies of the urinary tract and with congenital hepatic ductal ectasia and fibrosis (Caroli disease).

■ Diagnosis

In patients with nephrolithiasis, MSK is characteristically seen as hyperdense papillae with clusters of small stones on renal ultrasonography or abdominal x-ray (**Fig. 16-2**). The classical "paintbrush-like" features of MSK, representing the ectatic collecting ducts, are best seen on intravenous urography. However, this procedure has been supplanted in many radiology departments by contrast-enhanced, high-resolution helical CT with digital reconstruction (Fig. 16-2).

℞ **Treatment:**
MEDULLARY SPONGE KIDNEY

No treatment is necessary in asymptomatic individuals aside from maintaining high fluid intake to reduce the risk of nephrolithiasis. Recurrent stone formation should prompt a metabolic evaluation and treatment as in any stone former (Chap. 9). In those patients with hypocitraturia and incomplete distal renal tubular acidosis, treatment with potassium citrate helps prevent new stone formation. Urinary tract infections should be treated promptly.

SECTION IV

Glomerular and Tubular Disorders

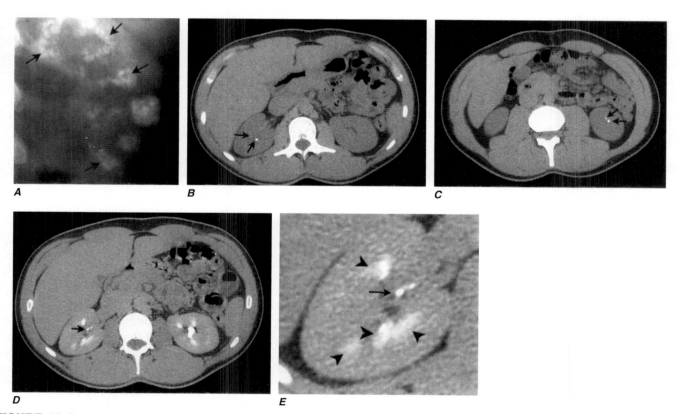

FIGURE 16-2

Radiographs of medullary sponge kidney disease. A. Plain x-ray film of a patient with a history of recurrent nephrolithiasis showing clusters of stones in the papillae (arrows). **B–E.** CT scan of an 18-year-old male patient investigated for persistent microscopic hematuria. **B** and **C.** CT without contrast showing a few small stones in the papillae (arrows). **D** and **E.** Contrast-enhanced CT of the same region shown in B. In addition to the stone (arrow), a blush of contrast is seen filling the ectatic collecting ducts (arrowheads).

HEREDITARY DISORDERS OF SODIUM, POTASSIUM, AND MAGNESIUM HANDLING WITHOUT HYPERTENSION

Inherited forms of hypochloremic metabolic alkalosis and hypokalemia without hypertension are due to genetic mutations of various ion transporters and channels of the thick ascending limb (TAL) of Henle's loop and distal convoluted tubule (DCT) (Table 16-2 and Fig. 16-3). In 1962 Bartter and colleagues described two African–American patients with a syndrome of metabolic alkalosis, hypovolemia, hyposthenuria, and failure to thrive associated with juxtaglomerular apparatus hyperplasia, hyperaldosteronism, and normal blood pressure. Subsequently, Gitelman and colleagues identified a similar but milder syndrome accompanied by severe hypomagnesemia from urinary magnesium wasting and presenting in later childhood and adolescence. These disorders are now known to occur sporadically or from genetically heterogenous loss-of-function autosomal recessive mutations that cause salt-losing tubulopathy.

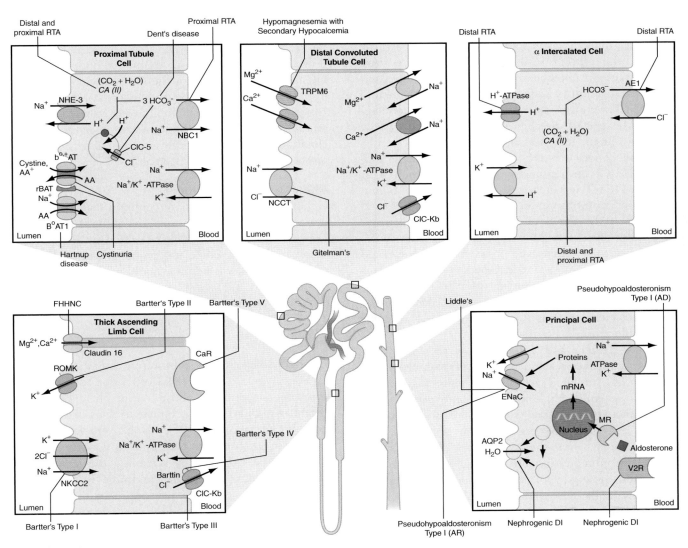

FIGURE 16-3

Schematic representation of channels, transporters, and enzymes associated with hereditary renal tubular disorders. AD, autosomal dominant; AR, autosomal recessive; DI, diabetes insipidus; NKCC2, Na-K-2Cl co-transporter; ROMK, renal outer medullary potassium channel; ClC-Kb, chloride channel Kb; CaR, calcium-sensing receptor 1; FHHNC, familial hypomagnesemia with hypercalciuria and nephrocalcinosis; NCCT, thiazide-sensitive Na-Cl co-transporter; ENaC, amiloride-sensitive epithelial sodium channel; TRPM6, transient receptor potential cation channel, subfamily M, member 6; WNK, with no lysine (K); V2R, arginine vasopressin receptor 2; MR, mineralocorticoid receptor; RTA, renal tubular acidosis; CA2, carbonic anhydrase II; AE1, anion exchanger 1; NBC1, sodium-bicarbonate co-transporter 1; rBAT, renal basic amino acid transport glycoprotein; AT1, amino acid transporter 1; CLC5, chloride channel 5; AA, amino acids; AA+, basic AA.

BARTTER'S SYNDROME AND GITELMAN'S SYNDROME

Genetics and Pathogenesis

Bartter's syndrome may result from mutations affecting any of four ion transport proteins in the TAL. The proteins affected include the apical loop-diuretic sensitive sodium-potassium–chloride co-transporter NKCC2 (type 1), the apical potassium channel ROMK (type 2), and the baso-lateral chloride channel ClC-Kb (type 3). Bartter type 4 results from mutations in barttin, an essential subunit of ClC-Ka and ClC-Kb that enables transport of the chlo-ride channels to the cell surface. Barttin is also expressed in the inner ear, which accounts for the deafness invariably associated with Bartter type 4. The TAL transporters func-tion in an integrated manner to maintain both the electri-cal potential difference and sodium gradient between the lumen and the cell (Fig. 16-3). Loss of the lumen-positive electrical transport potential that normally drives the para-cellular reabsorption of sodium, calcium, and magnesium causes NaCl wasting, hypercalciuria, and mild hypomag-nesemia. As expected, the clinical syndrome mimics a state induced by chronic ingestion of a loop diuretic.

Gitelman's syndrome is due to mutations in the thiazide-sensitive Na-Cl co-transporter (NCCT) in the DCT. Defects in NCCT in Gitelman's syndrome impair sodium and chloride reabsorption in the DCT (Fig. 16-3) and, thus, resemble the effects of thiazide diuretics. It remains unclear how this defect leads to severe magnesium wast-ing. A Bartter-like phenotype (type 5) with associated hypocalcemia has also been described in a few patients with autosomal dominant gain-of-function mutations in the extracellular calcium-sensing receptor (CaSR). Unreg-ulated activation of this G-protein–coupled receptor inhibits sodium reabsorption in the TAL.

In both Bartter's and Gitelman's syndromes, hypov-olemia from impaired sodium and chloride reabsorption in either the TAL or DCT activates the renin-angiotensin-aldosterone system (RAS). The consequent hyperaldostero-nism, together with increased distal flow and sodium deliv-ery, stimulates increased sodium reabsorption in the collecting tubules via the epithelial sodium channel (ENaC). This promotes increased potassium and hydrogen ion secretion, causing hypokalemia and metabolic alkalosis. Additionally, in Bartter's syndrome, RAS activation causes increased levels of cyclooxygenase 2 (COX-2) and marked overproduction of renal prostaglandins (PGE$_2$), which exacerbates the polyuria and electrolyte abnormalities.

Clinical Features

Bartter's Syndrome

Bartter's syndrome is a rare disease that most often presents in the neonatal period or early childhood with polyuria, polydipsia, salt craving, and growth retardation. Blood pressure is normal or low. Metabolic abnormalities include hypokalemia, hypochloremic metabolic alkalosis, decreased urinary concentrating and diluting ability, hypercalciuria with nephrocalcinosis, mild hypomagnesemia, and increased urinary prostaglandin excretion. Hyperprostaglandin E syndrome is a particularly severe form of Bartter's syndrome in which neonates present with pronounced volume depletion and failure to thrive, as well as fever, vomiting, and diarrhea from PGE$_2$ overproduction. In the antenatal period, fetal polyuria may cause maternal poly-hydramnios and premature labor. Sensorineural deafness occurs in those cases with barttin gene mutations. Patients with severe Bartter's syndrome that survive early child-hood may develop chronic renal failure from nephrocalci-nosis or from tubular atrophy and interstitial fibrosis from severe persistent hypokalemia. Patients with Bartter's syn-drome type 3 have a phenotype intermediate between Bartter's and Gitelman's syndromes, consistent with muta-tion of the ClC-Kb chloride channel in both the TAL and DCT with preservation of the ClC-Ka chloride channel in the TAL. This disease occurs predominantly in African-American patients and resembles most closely the classical syndrome described by Bartter. Onset is generally later in childhood, patients have mild or no nephrocalcinosis, and prostaglandin excretion is normal.

Gitelman's Syndrome

Gitelman's syndrome is more common than Bartter's syn-drome and has a generally milder clinical course with later age of presentation. It is characterized by hypocalciuria, severe hypomagnesemia, and prominent muscular symp-toms and signs, including fatigue, weakness, carpopedal spasm, cramps, and tetany. Excess prostaglandin production does not typically occur in Gitelman's syndrome.

Diagnosis

Hypokalemia and hypochloremic metabolic alkalosis without hypertension is more often due to surreptitious vomiting or diuretic abuse rather than Bartter's or Gitelman's syndromes. In contrast to the salt-losing tubu-lopathies, urinary chloride levels are very low or unde-tectable in patients with surreptitious vomiting. Diuretic abuse can be excluded by screening the urine for the offending drugs. Gitelman's syndrome is distinguished from most forms of Bartter's syndrome by the presence of severe hypomagnesemia and hypocalciuria.

Treatment:
R$_X$ BARTTER'S SYNDROME AND GITELMAN'S SYNDROME

Both conditions require lifelong therapy with potassium and magnesium supplements and liberal salt intake. High doses of spironolactone or amiloride are necessary to treat the hypokalemia, alkalosis, and magnesium wasting. Nonsteroidal anti-inflammatory drugs (NSAIDs) reduce the polyuria and salt wasting in Bartter's syndrome but are ineffective in Gitelman's syndrome. They may be lifesaving in hyperprostaglandin E syndrome. COX-2 inhibitors are effective and justified because of the gastrointestinal complications that may arise from the long-term use of high doses of NSAIDs. In Gitelman's syndrome, magnesium repletion is essential to correct the hypokalemia and control muscle weakness, tetany, and metabolic alkalosis; however, it may prove difficult in patients wasting large amounts of magnesium.

PSEUDOHYPOALDOSTERONISM TYPE I

Patients with type I pseudohypoaldosteronism present with severe renal salt wasting and hyperkalemia. Although these findings resemble mineralocorticoid deficiency, plasma renin activity and aldosterone levels are elevated. Defective salt handling is the result of autosomal recessive loss-of-function mutations of the α, β, or γ subunits of the ENaC or autosomal dominant mutations of one allele of the mineralocorticoid receptor (Table 16-2 and Fig. 16-3). The autosomal recessive form is a multisystem disorder with a severe phenotype, often manifesting in the neonatal period with renal salt wasting, vomiting, hyponatremia, hyperkalemia, acidosis, and failure to thrive. Impaired channel activity in the skin and lungs can produce excess sodium and chloride loss in sweat, excess fluid in the airways, and a propensity for lower respiratory tract infections mimicking cystic fibrosis. In contrast, the autosomal dominant form of type I pseudohypoaldosteronism has a more benign course that is limited mainly to renal salt wasting and hyperkalemia. Aggressive salt replacement and management of hyperkalemia can lead to survival into adulthood, and symptoms may become less severe with time, especially in the dominant form. In the latter, high-dose fludrocortisone or carbenoxolone provides additional benefit by raising intracellular mineralocorticoid activity and partly restoring the functional defect in the mutant receptor.

MAGNESIUM WASTING DISORDERS

In addition to Gitelman's syndrome, there are several hereditary disorders that cause urinary magnesium wasting (Table 16-2 and Fig. 16-3). These include autosomal recessive familial hypomagnesemia with hypercalciuria and nephrocalcinosis (FHHNC), autosomal recessive hypomagnesemia with secondary hypocalcemia (HSH), autosomal dominant hypomagnesemia, and autosomal dominant hypoparathyroidism. Common clinical features are the early onset of spasms, tetany, and seizures, as well as associated or secondary disturbances in calcium homeostasis.

Familial Hypomagnesemia with Hypercalciuria and Nephrocalcinosis

FHHNC (also known as primary hypomagnesemia) is the first example of a disorder attributable to a defective protein involved in paracellular ion transport. *CLDCN16* encodes claudin 16 (previously known as paracellin-1), a member of the claudin family of proteins that are involved in tight junction formation. Claudin 16 is expressed in the TAL of Henle's loop and the DCT. Claudin 16 is thought to be an essential component of the paracellular pathway for Mg, and Ca to a lesser extent, reabsorption in the TAL. Clinical manifestations begin in infancy and include hypomagnesemia that is refractory to oral supplementation, hypercalciuria, and nephrocalcinosis. Recurrent urinary tract infections and nephrolithiasis have also been observed, and some patients manifest ocular defects, including corneal calcifications and chorioretinitis.

Hypomagnesemia with Secondary Hypocalcemia

Hypomagnesemia in HSH results from a defect in the TRPM6 channel, a member of the transient receptor potential (TRP) family of proteins that are involved in cation transport. TRPM6 is expressed in intestinal epithelia and renal tubules and is thought to mediate transepithelial magnesium transport. Affected individuals have presented with symptoms attributable to hypomagnesemia with secondary impairment of parathyroid function and hypocalcemia. Seizures and muscle spasms occur in infancy, and restoration of magnesium and calcium levels requires high doses of oral magnesium supplementation.

Other Hereditary Hypomagnesemic Disorders

Mutations of the sodium-potassium-ATPase γ-subunit can cause an autosomal dominant form of hypomagnesemia. Activating mutations of the CaSR in autosomal dominant hypoparathyroidism primarily manifests as hypocalcemia, but hypomagnesemia has been reported in 50% of patients.

HEREDITARY TUBULAR DISORDERS CAUSING HYPERTENSION DUE TO SALT RETENTION

LIDDLE'S SYNDROME

Liddle's syndrome mimics a state of aldosterone excess by the presence of early and severe hypertension, often accompanied by hypokalemia and metabolic alkalosis, but plasma aldosterone and renin levels are low. This disorder is due to unregulated sodium reabsorption by an overactive ENaC in the cortical collecting duct (Fig. 16-3). Deletional mutations of the intracellular domain of the β or γ subunit of ENaC (Table 16-2) prevent recycling from the apical membrane and an inability to downregulate the number of channels despite a high intracellular sodium concentration. Increased potassium and hydrogen ion secretion follow the lumen-negative electrical potential that results from chloride-independent sodium reabsorption. Amiloride or triamterene block ENaC and, combined with salt restriction, provide effective therapy for hypertension and hypokalemia.

FAMILIAL HYPERKALEMIC HYPERTENSION (PSEUDOHYPOALDOSTERONISM TYPE II; GORDON SYNDROME)

Familial hyperkalemic hypertension (FHHt) is a rare autosomal dominant disease that manifests in adolescence or early adulthood with thiazide-responsive low-renin hypertension, hyperkalemia, and metabolic acidosis with normal renal function. In some families, mutations have been identified in the WNK kinases 1 and 4 that lead to increased activity of the thiazide-sensitive sodium chloride co-transporter, NCCT. This causes hypertension from enhanced salt reabsorption in the DCT and impaired distal secretion of potassium and hydrogen ion, all of which can be corrected with thiazide diuretics.

INHERITED DISORDERS OF WATER HANDLING

HEREDITARY NEPHROGENIC DIABETES INSIPIDUS

Hereditary nephrogenic diabetes insipidus (NDI) is a rare monogenic disease that usually presents in infancy with severe vasopressin-resistant polyuria, dehydration, failure to thrive, and dilute urine despite the presence of hypernatremia.

Genetics and Pathogenesis

Vasopressin [antidiuretic hormone (ADH)]-stimulated water reabsorption in the collecting duct is mediated by the type 2 vasopressin receptor (V2R) on the basal surface of principal cells. Activation of the adenylyl cyclase-cAMP pathway phosphorylates vesicle-associated aquaporin-2 (AQP2) water channels and stimulates their insertion into the apical plasma membrane. Water enters the cells from the tubular lumen through AQP2 and exits along an osmotic gradient into the hypertonic medulla and vasa rectae via basal AQP3/4 channels (Fig. 16-3). X-linked mutations of V2R account for about 90% of cases of NDI, such that the expression of the receptor on the cell surface is impaired. The remaining cases are due to various autosomal recessive or dominant mutations of AQP2 that cause the water channels to be retained within the cytosol (Table 16-2). The effect of these mutations is an inability to concentrate the urine and conserve water despite high plasma levels of vasopressin. Penetrance is variable in heterozygous female carriers of X-linked NDI, and some have a moderate concentrating defect.

Clinical Features

Whereas NDI in adults is most often acquired from conditions such as hypercalcemia, lithium therapy, and partial chronic urinary obstruction, hereditary NDI typically presents in infancy. Unlike other polyuric syndromes such as Bartter's and Gitelman's syndromes, conservation of electrolytes is normal, and hypernatremia is entirely from the loss of water. Recurrent episodes of dehydration and hypernatremia can lead to seizures and mental retardation. Although renal function is otherwise normal, chronically high urine flow causes dilatation of the ureters and bladder and may cause bladder dysfunction and obstructive uropathy.

Diagnosis

The diagnosis in infants and children with hereditary NDI is usually apparent from the family history and clinical presentation. The diagnosis can be confirmed by the presence of high plasma levels of vasopressin in the face of polyuria and hypotonic urine. This may be especially useful in adults with partial NDI to distinguish the polyuric state from central diabetes insipidus or psychogenic polydipsia. Genetic screening for mutations in *AVPR2* and *AQP2* is available in research centers and should be performed to identify affected infants from families at risk of NDI in order to begin treatment and avoid dehydration and its consequences.

Treatment:
℞ HEREDITARY NEPHROGENIC DIABETES INSIPIDUS

In families with high awareness of the condition, early diagnosis and treatment with abundant water intake has enabled many patients to live to adulthood with normal mental and physical development. Exogenous vasopressin is ineffective, and because these patients can excrete up to 20 L of urine per day, maintaining adequate water intake is challenging. Thiazide diuretics and salt restriction can reduce urine output by inducing a state of mild volume contraction, thereby promoting increased proximal reabsorption of isotonic fluid and inhibiting the generation of free water. A combination thiazide-amiloride formulation will avoid thiazide-induced hypokalemia and alkalosis, and indomethacin may further reduce urine output by inhibiting prostaglandin synthesis.

NEPHROGENIC SYNDROME OF INAPPROPRIATE ANTIDIURESIS

Activating mutations of the V2R were recently described in two boys who presented with irritability and seizures within the first three months of life. Laboratory evaluation was significant for hyponatremia with inappropriately elevated urinary osmolality and undetectable vasopressin levels. Genomic analysis revealed missense mutations of *AVPR2* causing constitutive activation of V2R and inappropriate water reabsorption.

INHERITED RENAL TUBULAR ACIDOSIS

Nonanion gap (hyperchloremic) metabolic acidosis from proximal tubular bicarbonate wasting or impaired distal net acid excretion may be a primary (sporadic or inherited) tubular disorder or acquired secondary to a variety of conditions (Chap. 5). There are three forms of renal tubular acidosis (RTA). Types 1 and 2 may be acquired or primary, whereas the most common form, type 4 RTA, is usually acquired in association with moderate renal dysfunction and is characterized by hyperkalemia.

TYPE 1 (DISTAL) RTA

Clinical Features and Diagnosis

In primary distal RTA (dRTA), the kidneys are unable to acidify the urine to pH <5.5 in the presence of systemic metabolic acidosis or after acid loading as a result of impaired hydrogen ion secretion or bicarbonate reabsorption in the distal nephron. Other features are hypokalemia, hypocitraturia, hypercalciuria, nephrocalcinosis, and/or nephrolithiasis. Chronic untreated acidosis may cause rickets or osteomalacia. Inheritance of primary dRTA includes autosomal dominant and autosomal recessive forms with a broad spectrum of clinical expression. Autosomal recessive dRTA most often presents in infancy with severe acidosis, failure to thrive, impaired growth, and impaired kidney function from nephrocalcinosis. Many patients with autosomal dominant dRTA, and some with recessive disease, are asymptomatic, and RTA is discovered incidentally in adolescence or adulthood during evaluation for kidney stones. In the absence of systemic acidosis, the diagnosis of incomplete dRTA is suggested by hypocitraturia and hypercalciuria and can be confirmed by failure of the urine to acidify to pH <5.5 after acid loading with oral ammonium chloride or calcium chloride.

Genetics and Pathophysiology

Primary dRTA may be hereditary or sporadic. Several kindreds with hereditary dRTA have been identified in Southeast Asia and in areas of the world where parental consanguinity is high. The cellular basis for dRTA lies in dysfunction at the level of the α type intercalated cell of

the cortical collecting duct (Fig. 16-3). Mutations affecting subunits of the H^+-ATPase proton pump on the luminal surface impair hydrogen ion secretion, account for most forms of autosomal recessive dRTA, and are often associated with early-onset sensorineural hearing loss (Table 16-2). Autosomal dominant dRTA results from mutations involving the chloride-bicarbonate exchanger AE1, the gateway for bicarbonate exit into the blood. Anion exchange by the mutant AE1 is normal, but aberrant targeting of AE1 from the basal to apical plasma membrane is believed to cause bicarbonate loss into the urine instead of recovery. Bi-allelic mutations of AE1 may impair transport activity and account for some cases of recessive disease, sometimes associated with late-onset hearing loss (Table 16-2). A syndrome of osteopetrosis, short stature, and mental retardation, so-called "marble-brain disease" with dRTA, is due to mutations in carbonic anhydrase II. Urinary potassium wasting and defective urinary concentration are characteristic of dRTA, but the precise mechanisms are unclear. Calcium is released from bone in the process of buffering of acid and results in hypercalciuria. Enhanced proximal citrate absorption accounts for hypocitraturia and, together with hypercalciuria, predisposes to nephrocalcinosis and calcium phosphate stone formation.

℞ **Treatment:**
TYPE 1 (DISTAL) RTA

Early initiation of alkali replacement at doses equivalent to 1–3 mmol/kg per day of bicarbonate in divided doses will usually correct the acidosis, hypokalemia, and hypocitraturia, maintaining growth and preventing bone disease in early-onset dRTA. Citrate is generally tolerated better than sodium bicarbonate and can be given as potassium or sodium salt, depending on the severity of hypokalemia. In patients who present later with kidney stones, large fluid intake and sufficient alkali to restore normal acid-base balance corrects the hypocitraturia and reduces hypercalciuria, thereby inhibiting the formation of new stones.

TYPE 2 (PROXIMAL) RTA

Proximal RTA (pRTA) is the result of impaired bicarbonate reabsorption in the proximal tubule where the bulk of filtered bicarbonate is recovered (Fig. 16-3). It is most often secondary to various autoimmune, drug-induced, infiltrative, or other tubulopathies (Chap. 5) or a result of tubular injury from inherited diseases in which endogenous metabolites accumulate and produce tubular injury. Such inherited disorders include Wilson's disease, cystinosis, tyrosinemia, galactosemia, hereditary fructose intolerance, glycogen storage disease type I, and Lowe's syndrome. In this situation pRTA is but one of several abnormalities that constitute Fanconi syndrome. Other features are hyperphosphaturia, hyperuricosuria, hypercalciuria, nonselective aminoaciduria, and glycosuria. In addition to hyperchloremic acidosis, rickets or osteomalacia are the predominant effects of Fanconi syndrome.

A rare infantile form of primary pRTA with isolated proximal tubular bicarbonate wasting is due to homozygous mutations of the proximal tubule basolateral sodium-bicarbonate exchanger NBC1 (Table 16-2). This exchanger is the main mechanism by which bicarbonate moves from the proximal tubule cell back into the blood. Other manifestations include short stature and mental retardation. An ocular phenotype that includes bilateral glaucoma, cataracts, and band keratopathy reflects a role of NBC1 in maintaining normal fluid balance in the eye and clarity of the lens.

Patients with pRTA have severe metabolic acidosis, and it is difficult to restore normal acid-base balance despite large amounts of alkali. This is a consequence of their continuing to waste bicarbonate (fractional excretion >15%) until the serum level falls below a threshold level, usually about 15–17 mmol/L, at which time bicarbonate is completely reabsorbed and the urine is maximally acidified with pH <5.5. When the serum bicarbonate is raised above the threshold with alkali therapy, bicarbonate wasting recurs and causes hypokalemia by flooding the distal nephron with a nonreabsorbable anion.

℞ **Treatment:**
TYPE 2 (PROXIMAL) RTA

Treatment of pRTA requires 5–15 mmol/kg per day of bicarbonate together with supplemental potassium and vitamin D.

OTHER MONOGENIC DISORDERS OF PROXIMAL TUBULAR FUNCTION

(See Fig. 16-3)

CYSTINURIA

Cystinuria is an autosomal recessive disorder of cystine and dibasic amino acid (ornithine, arginine, and lysine) transport in the proximal tubule and intestinal epithelial cells. With a prevalence of about 1 in 7000, it represents one of the more common heritable diseases. Impaired tubular absorption leads to high concentrations of cystine, which is insoluble in the acid environment of the renal tubules. Clinical severity varies from asymptomatic cystine crystalluria in heterozygous carriers to the frequent passage of gravel and cystine stones, ureteral obstruction, recurrent urinary infections, and progressive

kidney failure in homozygotes. The disease is due to mutations in one of two genes, *SLC3A1* and *SLC7A9* (Table 16-2). *SLC3A1* encodes rBAT, a high-affinity, sodium-independent transporter for dibasic amino acids. The protein product of *SLC7A9*, $b^{0,+}AT$, is a catalytic subunit that associates with rBAT to form the active transporter. Diagnosis of cystinuria is established by a positive family history, the finding of hexagonal cystine crystals on urinalysis, and 24-hour urinary cystine excretion that exceeds 400 mg (normal less than 30 mg/d). Genetic analysis will probably become commonly available.

℞ **Treatment:**
CYSTINURIA

The mainstay of treatment is hydration to achieve a urine output of 2.5 L/d or more to reduce urine cystine concentration to <300 mg/L, together with urine alkalinization to pH 7.0–7.5 with potassium citrate, and sodium restriction. Cystine is an oxidized dimer formed by linking two cysteine residues via a disulfide bond between the -SH groups. Thus, in intractable cases, thiol derivatives like penicillamine, captopril, and tiopronin may be added as second-line chelation therapy to dissociate the cystine molecule into more soluble disulfide compounds. Various stone removal and urinary drainage procedures are often required.

HARTNUP DISEASE

Hartnup disease is an autosomal recessive condition caused by a defect in intestinal and renal transport of neutral amino acids. The major clinical manifestations are cerebellar ataxia and pellagra-like skin lesions. Other than aminoaciduria, the kidneys are unaffected. The defective gene *SLC6A19* encodes a sodium-dependent and chloride-independent neutral amino acid transporter, which is expressed predominately in the intestine and renal tubules (Table 16-2). Amino acids such as tryptophan that are retained in the intestinal lumen are converted to indole compounds that are toxic to the CNS. Abnormal tryptophan metabolism also leads to niacin deficiency that accounts for the skin manifestations. Symptoms are aggravated by a protein-deficient diet and alleviated with a high-protein diet and nicotinamide supplements.

DENT'S DISEASE

Dent's disease and X-linked recessive nephrolithiasis are unusual forms of Fanconi syndrome due to X-linked recessive mutations of the gene encoding CLCN5, a channel belonging to a family of voltage-gated chloride channels (Table 16-2). The disorders are characterized by childhood onset of low-molecular-weight proteinuria, hypercalciuria, nephrocalcinosis and nephrolithiasis. Rickets or osteomalacia occurs in 30% of patients, and progressive renal failure from interstitial fibrosis, tubular atrophy, and glomerulosclerosis commonly develops in adulthood. CLCN5 serves to maintain the electrical gradient and acid environment established in proximal tubular cell endosomes by proton-ATPase, which is necessary for the degradation of low-molecular-weight proteins normally filtered by the glomerulus. Defects in CLCN5 appear to disrupt this process and lead to tubular cell dysfunction.

℞ **Treatment:**
DENT'S DISEASE

Treatment is directed at controlling hypercalciuria by dietary salt restriction and thiazide diuretics, which favor calcium reabsorption. Restriction of dietary calcium is not recommended.

RENAL GLUCOSURIA

Isolated glucosuria in the presence of a normal blood glucose concentration is due to mutations in *SLC5A2*, the gene encoding the high-capacity sodium-glucose co-transporter SGLT2 in the proximal renal tubule (Table 16-2). Subjects with this disorder are usually asymptomatic and do not have other features of proximal tubular dysfunction. Depending on the severity of the defect, the tubular maximum for glucose reabsorption may fall well within normal blood glucose levels and lead to >50 g/d of glucosuria. Such patients may have polyuria from osmotic diuresis.

RENAL PHOSPHATE WASTING

Renal phosphate wasting resulting in hypophosphatemia and rickets or osteomalacia may be part of a generalized disorder of proximal tubular function, as in Fanconi syndrome, or an isolated phenomenon. Isolated phosphaturia is most often due to the inhibition of renal tubular phosphate reabsorption by one or other phosphaturic hormone. An exception is hereditary hypophosphatemic rickets with hypercalciuria (HHRH). HHRH is an autosomal recessive disorder due to mutations in *SLC34A3*, the gene encoding the proximal tubule sodium-phosphate co-transporter (Table 16-2). Defective phosphate reabsorption causes renal phosphate wasting and leads to stunted growth from rickets. The low serum phosphorus levels appropriately stimulate 1-hydroxylation of vitamin D,

which increases intestinal calcium absorption, suppresses parathyroid hormone (PTH) secretion, and results in hypercalciuria. High levels of 1,25-dihydroxyvitamin D help distinguish HHRH from hormonal causes of hyperphosphaturia. Treatment is directed at phosphate repletion.

VITAMIN D–DEPENDENT RICKETS

Vitamin D–dependent rickets exists in two forms that manifest with hypocalcemia, hypophosphatemia, elevated PTH levels, and the skeletal abnormalities of rickets and osteomalacia. Tetany may be present in severe cases. Vitamin D–dependent rickets type I is an autosomal recessive disease resulting from mutations in *CYP27B1*, the gene that encodes $25(OH)D_3$-1α-hydroxylase, an enzyme in the proximal tubule that catalyzes the hydroxylation and activation of $25(OH)D_3$ into $1,25(OH)_2D_3$ (Table 16-2). It can be treated with physiologic replacement doses of $1,25(OH)_2D_3$. In contrast, vitamin D–dependent rickets type II is due to end-organ resistance to $1,25(OH)_2D_3$ as a result of mutations in the vitamin D receptor.

FURTHER READINGS

GOFFIN E et al: Is peritoneal dialysis a suitable renal replacement therapy in autosomal dominant polycystic kidney disease? Nat Clin Pract Nephrol 5:122, 2009

GRANTHAM JJ: Clinical practice. Autosomal dominant polycystic kidney disease. N Engl J Med 359:1477, 2008

GUAY-WOODFORD L: Other cystic kidney diseases, in *Comprehensive Clinical Nephrology*, 2d ed, RJ Johnson and J Feehally (eds). New York, Saunders, 2003

HART TC et al: Mutations of the UMOD gene are responsible for medullary cystic kidney disease 2 and familial juvenile hyperuricaemic nephropathy. J Med Genet 39:882, 2002

JECK N et al: Salt handling in the distal nephron: Lessons learned from inherited human disorders. Am J Physiol Regul Integr Comp Physiol 288:R782, 2005

KISTLER AD et al: Identification of a unique urinary biomarker profile in patients with autosomal dominant polycystic kidney disease. Kidney Int 76:89, 2009

KUMAR S et al: Long term outcome of patients with autosomal dominant polycystic kidney diseases receiving peritoneal dialysis. Kidney Int 74:946, 2008

LAING CM et al: Renal tubular acidosis: Developments in our understanding of the molecular basis. Int J Biochem Cell Biol 37:1151, 2005

SANDS JM, BICHET DG: Nephrogenic diabetes insipidus. Ann Intern Med 144:186, 2006

SAUNIER S et al: Nephronophthisis. Curr Opin Genet Dev 15:324, 2005

TORRES VE et al: Autosomal dominant polycystic kidney disease: The last 3 years. Kidney Int 76:149, 2009

———, HARRIS PC: Mechanisms of disease: Autosomal dominant and recessive polycystic kidney diseases. Nat Clin Pract Nephrol 2:40, 2006

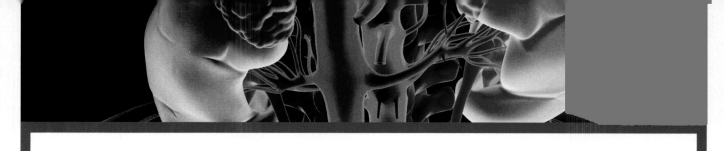

CHAPTER 17

TUBULOINTERSTITIAL DISEASES OF THE KIDNEY

Alan S. L. Yu ■ Barry M. Brenner

Primary tubulointerstitial diseases of the kidney are characterized by histologic and functional abnormalities that involve the tubules and interstitium to a greater degree than the glomeruli and renal vasculature (Table 17-1). Secondary tubulointerstitial disease occurs as a consequence of progressive glomerular or vascular injury. Morphologically, acute forms of these disorders are characterized by interstitial edema, often associated with cortical and medullary infiltration by both mononuclear cells and polymorphonuclear leukocytes, and patchy areas of tubule cell necrosis. In more chronic forms, interstitial fibrosis predominates, inflammatory cells are typically mononuclear, and abnormalities of the tubules tend to be more widespread, as evidenced by atrophy, luminal dilatation, and thickening of tubule basement membranes. Because of the nonspecific nature of the histology, particularly in chronic tubulointerstitial diseases, biopsy specimens rarely provide a specific diagnosis. The urine sediment is also unlikely to be diagnostic, except in allergic forms of acute tubulointerstitial disease in which eosinophils may predominate in the urinary sediment.

Defects in renal function often accompany these alterations of tubule and interstitial structure (Table 17-2). Proximal tubule dysfunction may be manifested as selective reabsorptive defects leading to hypokalemia, aminoaciduria, glycosuria, phosphaturia, uricosuria, or bicarbonaturia [proximal or type II renal tubular acidosis (RTA); Chap. 16]. In combination, these defects constitute the *Fanconi syndrome*. Proteinuria, predominantly of low-molecular-weight proteins, is usually modest, rarely >2 g/d.

Defects in urinary acidification and concentrating ability often represent the most troublesome of the tubule dysfunctions encountered in patients with tubulointerstitial disease. Hyperchloremic metabolic acidosis often develops at a relatively early stage in the course. Patients with this finding generally elaborate urine of maximal acidity (pH ≤ 5.3). In such patients the defect in acid excretion is usually caused by a reduced capacity to generate and excrete ammonia due to the reduction in renal mass. Preferential damage to the collecting ducts, as in amyloidosis or chronic obstructive uropathy, may also predispose to distal or type I RTA, characterized by high urine pH (≥ 5.5) during spontaneous or NH_4Cl-induced metabolic acidosis. Patients with tubulointerstitial diseases affecting predominantly medullary and papillary structures (such as analgesic nephropathy and sickle cell disease) may also exhibit concentrating defects, with resultant nocturia and polyuria.

TABLE 17-1

PRINCIPAL CAUSES OF TUBULOINTERSTITIAL DISEASE OF THE KIDNEY

Acute Interstitial Nephritis

Drugs[a]
  Antibiotics (β-lactams, sulfonamides, quinolones, vancomycin, erythromycin, minocycline, rifampin, ethambutol, acyclovir)
  Nonsteroidal anti-inflammatory drugs, cyclooxygenase 2 inhibitors
  Diuretics (thiazides, furosemide, triamterene)
  Anticonvulsants (phenytoin, phenobarbital, carbamazepine, valproic acid)
  Miscellaneous (captopril, H_2 receptor blockers, proton pump inhibitors, mesalazine, indinavir, allopurinol)
Infection
  Bacteria (*Streptococcus*, *Staphylococcus*, *Legionella*, *Salmonella*, *Brucella*, *Yersinia*, *Corynebacterium diphtheriae*)
  Viruses (Epstein-Barr virus, cytomegalovirus, hantavirus, polyomavirus, HIV)
  Miscellaneous (*Leptospira*, *Rickettsia*, *Mycoplasma*)
Idiopathic
  Tubulointerstitial nephritis–uveitis syndrome
  Anti-tubule basement membrane disease
  Sarcoidosis

Chronic Tubulointerstitial Diseases

Hereditary renal diseases
  Polycystic kidney disease[a] (Chap. 16)
  Medullary cystic disease (Chap. 16)
  Medullary sponge kidney (Chap. 16)
Exogenous toxins
  Analgesic nephropathy[a]
  Lead nephropathy
  Miscellaneous nephrotoxins (e.g., lithium,[a] cyclosporine,[a] heavy metals, slimming regimens with Chinese herbs)
Metabolic toxins
  Hyperuricemia[a]
  Hypercalcemia
  Miscellaneous metabolic toxins (e.g., hypokalemia, hyperoxaluria, cystinosis, Fabry's disease)
Autoimmune disorders
  Sjögren's syndrome
Neoplastic disorders
  Leukemia
  Lymphoma
  Multiple myeloma[a]
Miscellaneous disorders
  Sickle cell nephropathy
  Chronic pyelonephritis
  Chronic urinary tract obstruction
  Vesicoureteral reflux[a]
  Radiation nephritis
  Balkan nephropathy
  Tubulointerstitial disease secondary to glomerular and vascular disease

[a]Common.

TOXINS

Although the kidney is vulnerable to toxic injury, renal damage by a variety of nephrotoxins often goes unrecognized because the manifestations of such injury are usually nonspecific in nature and insidious in onset. Diagnosis largely depends on a history of exposure to a certain toxin. Particular attention should be paid to the occupational history, as well as to an assessment of exposure—current and remote—to drugs, especially antibiotics and analgesics, and to dietary supplements or herbal remedies. The recognition of a potential association between a patient's renal disease and exposure to a nephrotoxin is crucial because, unlike many other forms of renal disease, progression of the functional and morphologic abnormalities associated with toxin-induced nephropathies may be prevented, and even reversed, by eliminating additional exposure.

EXOGENOUS TOXINS

Analgesic Nephropathy

A distinct syndrome has been described in heavy users of analgesic mixtures containing phenacetin (banned in the United States since 1983) in combination with aspirin,

TABLE 17-2

FUNCTIONAL CONSEQUENCES OF TUBULOINTERSTITIAL DISEASE

DEFECT	CAUSE(S)
Reduced glomerular filtration rate[a]	Obliteration of microvasculature and obstruction of tubules
Fanconi syndrome	Damage to proximal tubular reabsorption of glucose, amino acids, phosphate, and bicarbonate
Hyperchloremic acidosis[a]	1. Reduced ammonia production
	2. Inability to acidify the collecting duct fluid (distal renal tubular acidosis)
	3. Proximal bicarbonate wasting
Tubular or small-molecular-weight proteinuria[a]	Failure of proximal tubule protein reabsorption
Polyuria, isosthenuria[a]	Damage to medullary tubules and vasculature
Hyperkalemia[a]	Potassium secretory defects including aldosterone resistance
Salt wasting	Distal tubular damage with impaired sodium reabsorption

[a]Common.

SECTION IV

Glomerular and Tubular Disorders

acetaminophen, or caffeine. Morphologically, analgesic nephropathy is characterized by papillary necrosis and tubulointerstitial inflammation. At an early stage, damage to the vascular supply of the inner medulla (vasa recta) leads to a local interstitial inflammatory reaction and, eventually, to papillary ischemia, necrosis, fibrosis, and calcification. The susceptibility of the renal papillae to damage by phenacetin is believed to be related to the establishment of a renal gradient for its acetaminophen metabolite, resulting in papillary tip concentrations tenfold higher than those in renal cortex.

In analgesic nephropathy, renal function usually declines gradually. Occasionally, papillary necrosis may be associated with hematuria and even renal colic owing to obstruction of a ureter by necrotic tissue. More than half of patients have sterile pyuria. Patients with analgesic nephropathy are usually unable to generate maximally concentrated urine, reflecting the underlying medullary and papillary damage. An acquired form of distal RTA (Chap. 16) may contribute to the development of *nephrocalcinosis*. The occurrence of anemia out of proportion to the degree of renal failure may also provide a clue to the diagnosis. When analgesic nephropathy has progressed to renal insufficiency, the kidneys usually appear bilaterally shrunken on intravenous pyelography, and the calyces are deformed. A "ring sign" on the pyelogram is pathognomonic of papillary necrosis and represents the radiolucent sloughed papilla surrounded by the radiodense contrast material in the calyx. CT may reveal papillary calcifications surrounding the central sinus complex in a "garland" pattern (**Fig. 17-1**). Transitional cell carcinoma may develop in the urinary pelvis or ureters as a late complication of analgesic abuse.

Whether non-phenacetin analgesics, alone or in combination, cause renal disease is controversial. Recent cohort studies in individuals with normal baseline renal function suggest that the risk of moderate analgesic use, if any, is low. Until conclusive evidence is available, however, physicians should consider screening heavy users of acetaminophen and nonsteroidal anti-inflammatory drugs

(NSAIDs) for evidence of renal disease and discouraging their use of these drugs.

Lead Nephropathy

Lead intoxication may produce a chronic tubulointerstitial renal disease. Children who repeatedly ingest lead-based paints (pica) may develop kidney disease as adults. Significant occupational exposure may occur in workplaces where lead-containing metals or paints are heated to high temperatures, such as battery factories, smelters, salvage yards, and weapon firing ranges.

Tubule transport processes enhance the accumulation of lead within renal cells, particularly in the proximal convoluted tubule, leading to cell degeneration, mitochondrial swelling, and eosinophilic intranuclear inclusion bodies rich in lead. In addition, lead nephropathy is associated with ischemic changes in the glomeruli, fibrosis of the adventitia of small renal arterioles, and focal areas of cortical scarring. Eventually, the kidneys become atrophic.

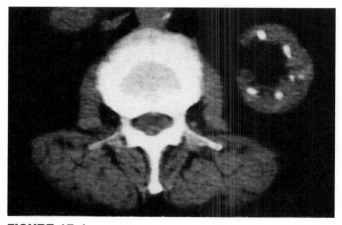

FIGURE 17-1

Radiologic appearance of analgesic nephropathy. A non-contrast CT scan shows an atrophic left kidney with papillary calcifications in a garland pattern. *(Reprinted by permission from Macmillan Publishers Ltd, MM Elseviers et al, Kidney International 48:1316, 1995.)*

Urinary excretion of lead, porphyrin precursors such as δ-aminolevulinic acid and coproporphyrin, and urobilinogen may be increased. Patients with chronic lead nephropathy are characteristically *hyperuricemic*, a consequence of enhanced reabsorption of filtered urate. Acute gouty arthritis (so-called saturnine gout) develops in about 50% of patients with lead nephropathy, in striking contrast to other forms of chronic renal failure in which de novo gout is rare (Chap. 8). Hypertension is also a complication. Therefore, in any patient with slowly progressive renal failure, atrophic kidneys, gout, and hypertension, the diagnosis of lead intoxication should be considered. Features of acute lead intoxication (abdominal colic, anemia, peripheral neuropathy, and encephalopathy) are usually absent.

The diagnosis may be suspected by finding elevated serum levels of lead. However, because blood levels may not be elevated even in the presence of a toxic total-body burden of lead, the quantitation of lead excretion following infusion of the chelating agent calcium disodium edetate is a more reliable indicator of serious lead exposure. Urinary excretion of >0.6 mg/d of lead is indicative of overt toxicity, but even lead burdens of 0.08–0.6 mg/d may cause progressive loss of renal function.

Rx **Treatment:**
LEAD NEPHROPATHY

Treatment includes removing the patient from the source of exposure and augmenting lead excretion with a chelating agent such as calcium disodium edetate.

Lithium

Use of lithium salts for bipolar disorder is associated with chronic tubulointerstitial nephropathy, generally manifest as the insidious development of chronic renal insufficiency. Nephrogenic diabetes insipidus, which may occur alone or in association with the renal insufficiency, is common. It manifests as polyuria and polydipsia and is due to lithium-induced downregulation of the vasopressin-regulated water channels in the collecting duct. Mild proteinuria and hypercalcemia due to lithium-induced hyperparathyroidism are common. The predominant finding on renal biopsy is tubular atrophy and interstitial fibrosis out of proportion to the extent of glomerular or vascular disease. Tubular cysts are common, and concomitant focal segmental glomerulosclerosis can be observed.

Renal function should be followed in patients taking this drug, and caution should be exercised if lithium is employed in patients with underlying renal disease. Once renal impairment occurs, lithium therapy should be stopped and an alternative agent substituted. Despite discontinuation of lithium, chronic renal disease in such patients is often irreversible and can progress to end-stage renal failure.

Miscellaneous Nephrotoxins

The immunosuppressant *cyclosporine* causes both acute and chronic renal injury. The acute injury and the use of cyclosporine in transplantation are discussed in Chap. 13. The chronic injury results in an irreversible reduction in glomerular filtration rate (GFR), with mild proteinuria and arterial hypertension. Hyperkalemia is a relatively common complication and results, in part, from tubule resistance to aldosterone. The histologic changes in renal tissue include patchy interstitial fibrosis and tubular atrophy. In addition, the intrarenal vasculature often demonstrates hyalinosis, and focal segmental glomerular sclerosis can be present as well. In patients receiving this drug for renal transplantation (Chap. 13), chronic graft dysfunction and recurrence of the primary disease may coincide with chronic cyclosporine injury, and, on clinical grounds, distinction among these may be difficult. Dose reduction appears to mitigate cyclosporine-associated renal fibrosis but may increase the risk of rejection and graft loss. Treatment of any associated arterial hypertension may lessen renal injury.

Chinese herbs nephropathy is characterized by rapidly progressive interstitial renal fibrosis in young women due to ingestion of weight-reduction pills containing Chinese herbs; at least one of the culprit ingredients is aristolochic acid. Clinically, patients present with progressive chronic renal insufficiency with sterile pyuria and anemia that is disproportionately severe relative to the level of renal function. The pathologic findings are interstitial fibrosis and tubular atrophy that affects the cortex in preference to the medulla, fibrous intimal thickening of the interlobular arteries, and a relative paucity of cellular infiltrates.

Metabolic Toxins

Acute Uric Acid Nephropathy

(See also Chap. 8.) Acute overproduction of uric acid and extreme hyperuricemia often lead to a rapidly progressive renal insufficiency, so-called acute uric acid nephropathy. This tubulointerstitial disease is usually seen as part of the tumor lysis syndrome in patients given cytotoxic drugs for the treatment of lymphoproliferative or myeloproliferative disorders, but may also occur in these patients before such treatment is begun. The pathologic changes are largely the result of deposition of uric acid crystals in the kidneys and their collecting systems, leading to partial or complete obstruction of collecting ducts, renal pelvis, or ureter. Since obstruction is often bilateral, patients typically follow the clinical course of acute renal failure, characterized by oliguria and rapidly rising serum creatinine concentration. In the early phase, uric acid crystals can be found in urine, usually in association with microscopic or gross hematuria. Hyperuricemia can also be a consequence of renal failure of any etiology. The finding of a urine uric acid/creatinine ratio >1 mg/mg (0.7 mol/mol) distinguishes acute uric acid nephropathy from other causes of renal failure.

Prevention of hyperuricemia in patients at risk by treatment with allopurinol in doses of 200–800 mg/d prior to cytotoxic therapy reduces the danger of acute uric acid nephropathy. Once hyperuricemia develops, however, efforts should be directed to preventing deposition of uric acid within the urinary tract. Increasing urine volume with potent diuretics (furosemide or mannitol) effectively lowers intratubular uric acid concentrations, and alkalinization of the urine to pH ≥7 with sodium bicarbonate and/or a carbonic anhydrase inhibitor (acetazolamide) enhances uric acid solubility. If these efforts, together with allopurinol therapy, are ineffective in preventing acute renal failure, dialysis should be instituted to lower the serum uric acid concentration as well as to treat the acute manifestations of uremia.

Gouty Nephropathy

(See also Chap. 8.) Patients with less severe but prolonged forms of hyperuricemia are predisposed to a more chronic tubulointerstitial disorder, often referred to as *gouty nephropathy*. The severity of renal involvement correlates with the duration and magnitude of the elevation of the serum uric acid concentration. Histologically, the distinctive feature of gouty nephropathy is the presence of crystalline deposits of uric acid and monosodium urate salts in kidney parenchyma. These deposits not only cause intrarenal obstruction but also incite an inflammatory response, leading to lymphocytic infiltration, foreign-body giant cell reaction, and eventual fibrosis, especially of medullary and papillary regions of the kidney. Since patients with gout frequently suffer from hypertension and hyperlipidemia, degenerative changes of the renal arterioles may constitute a striking feature of the histologic abnormality, often out of proportion to other morphologic defects. Clinically, gouty nephropathy is an insidious cause of renal insufficiency. Early in its course, GFR may be near normal, often despite focal morphologic changes in medullary and cortical interstitium, proteinuria, and diminished urinary concentrating ability. Whether reducing serum uric acid levels with allopurinol exerts a beneficial effect on the kidney remains to be demonstrated. Although such undesirable consequences of hyperuricemia as gout and uric acid stones respond well to allopurinol, use of this drug in asymptomatic hyperuricemia has not been shown to improve renal function consistently. Uricosuric agents such as probenecid, which may increase uric acid stone production, are clearly contraindicated.

Hypercalcemic Nephropathy

Chronic hypercalcemia, as occurs in primary hyperparathyroidism, sarcoidosis, multiple myeloma, vitamin D intoxication, or metastatic bone disease, can cause tubulointerstitial damage and progressive renal insufficiency. The earliest lesion is a focal degenerative change in renal epithelia, primarily in collecting ducts, distal convoluted tubules, and loops of Henle. Tubule cell necrosis leads to nephron obstruction and stasis of intrarenal urine, favoring local precipitation of calcium salts and infection. Dilatation and atrophy of tubules eventually occur, as do interstitial fibrosis, mononuclear leukocyte infiltration, and interstitial calcium deposition (nephrocalcinosis). Calcium deposition may also occur in glomeruli and the walls of renal arterioles.

Clinically, the most striking defect is an inability to concentrate the urine maximally, resulting in polyuria and nocturia. Reduced collecting duct responsiveness to vasopressin and defective transport of NaCl in the ascending limb of Henle's loop are responsible for this. Reductions in GFR and renal blood flow also occur, both in acute severe hypercalcemia and with prolonged hypercalcemia of lesser severity. Eventually, uncontrolled hypercalcemia leads to severe tubulointerstitial damage and overt renal failure. Abdominal x-rays may demonstrate nephrocalcinosis as well as nephrolithiasis, the latter due to the hypercalciuria that often accompanies hypercalcemia.

℞ **Treatment:**
HYPERCALCEMIC NEPHROPATHY

Treatment consists of reducing the serum calcium concentration toward normal and correcting the primary abnormality of calcium metabolism. Renal dysfunction of acute hypercalcemia may be completely reversible. Gradual, progressive renal insufficiency related to chronic hypercalcemia, however, may not improve even with correction of the calcium disorder.

RENAL PARENCHYMAL DISEASE ASSOCIATED WITH EXTRARENAL NEOPLASM

Except for the glomerulopathies associated with lymphomas and several solid tumors (Chap. 15), the renal manifestations of primary extrarenal neoplastic processes are confined mainly to the interstitium and tubules. Although metastatic renal involvement by solid tumors is unusual, the kidneys are often invaded by neoplastic cells in hematologic malignancies. In postmortem studies of patients with *lymphoma* and *leukemia*, renal involvement is found in approximately half. Diffuse infiltration of the renal parenchyma with malignant cells is seen most commonly. There may be flank pain, and x-rays may show enlargement of one or both kidneys. Renal insufficiency occurs in a minority, and treatment of the primary disease may improve renal function in these cases.

Plasma Cell Dyscrasias

Several glomerular and tubulointerstitial disorders may occur in association with plasma cell dyscrasias. Infiltration of the kidneys with myeloma cells is infrequent. When it occurs, the process is usually focal, so renal insufficiency from this cause is also uncommon. The more usual lesion is *myeloma kidney*, characterized histologically by atrophic tubules, many with eosinophilic intraluminal casts, and numerous multinucleated giant cells within tubule walls and in the interstitium (Fig. 17-2). Bence-Jones proteins are thought to cause myeloma kidney through direct toxicity to renal tubule cells. In addition, Bence-Jones proteins may precipitate within the distal nephron where the high concentrations of these proteins and the acid composition of the tubule fluid favor intraluminal cast formation and intrarenal obstruction. Further precipitation of Bence-Jones proteins can be induced by dehydration, which should, therefore, be avoided. Multiple myeloma may also affect the kidneys indirectly. Hypercalcemia or hyperuricemia may lead to the nephropathies described above. Proximal tubule disorders are also seen occasionally, including type II proximal RTA and the Fanconi syndrome.

Amyloidosis

(See also Chap. 15.) Glomerular pathology usually predominates and leads to heavy proteinuria and azotemia. However, tubule function may also be deranged, giving rise to a nephrogenic diabetes insipidus and to distal (type I) RTA. In several cases these functional abnormalities correlated with peritubular deposition of amyloid, particularly in areas surrounding vasa rectae, loops of Henle, and collecting ducts. Bilateral enlargement of the kidneys, especially in a patient with massive proteinuria and tubule dysfunction, should raise the possibility of amyloid renal disease.

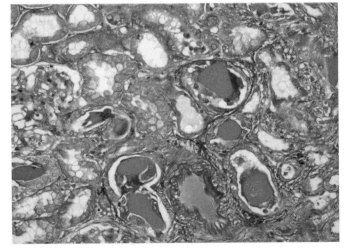

FIGURE 17-2

Histologic appearance of myeloma cast nephropathy. A hematoxylin-eosin–stained kidney biopsy shows many atrophic tubules filled with eosinophilic casts (consisting of Bence-Jones protein), which are surrounded by giant cell reactions. *(Courtesy of Dr. Michael N. Koss, University of Southern California Keck School of Medicine; with permission.)*

Allergic Interstitial Nephritis

An acute diffuse tubulointerstitial reaction may result from hypersensitivity to a number of drugs, including β-lactams, sulfonamides, fluoroquinolone antibiotics, and the antituberculous drugs isoniazid and rifampin. Acute tubulointerstitial damage has also occurred after use of thiazide and loop diuretics, allopurinol, NSAIDs, and cyclooxygenase 2 (COX-2) inhibitors. Of note, the tubulointerstitial nephropathy that develops in some patients taking NSAIDs and COX-2 inhibitors may be associated with nephrotic-range proteinuria and histologic evidence of either minimal change or membranous glomerulopathy. Proton-pump inhibitors are an increasingly recognized culprit and have recently been implicated in up to half of cases of biopsy-proven acute tubulointerstitial nephritis. The use of mesalazine for the treatment of inflammatory bowel disease is associated with a more subacute disorder in which a severe indolent interstitial nephritis occurs several months after the initiation of the drug. Grossly, the kidneys are usually enlarged. Histologically, the interstitium of the kidney reveals pronounced edema and infiltration with polymorphonuclear leukocytes, lymphocytes, plasma cells, and, in some cases, large numbers of eosinophils. If the process is severe, tubule cell necrosis and regeneration may also be apparent. Immunofluorescence studies have either been unrevealing or demonstrated a linear pattern of immunoglobulin and complement deposition along tubule basement membranes.

Most patients require several weeks of drug exposure before developing evidence of renal injury. Rare cases have occurred after only a few doses or after a year or more of use. Renal failure is usually present; a triad of fever, skin rash, and peripheral blood eosinophilia is highly suggestive of acute tubulointerstitial nephritis but is present in only 10% of patients. Examination of the urine sediment reveals hematuria and often pyuria; occasionally, eosinophils may be present. Proteinuria is usually mild to moderate, except in cases of NSAID- or COX-2 inhibitor–associated glomerulopathy. The clinical picture may be confused with acute glomerulonephritis, but when acute renal failure and hematuria are accompanied by eosinophilia, skin rash, and a history of drug exposure, acute tubulointerstitial nephritis should be regarded as the leading diagnostic possibility. Discontinuation of the drug usually results in complete reversal of the renal injury; rarely, renal damage may be irreversible. Glucocorticoids may accelerate renal recovery, but their value has not been definitively established.

Sjögren's Syndrome

When the kidneys are involved in this disorder, the predominant histologic findings are those of chronic tubulointerstitial disease. Interstitial infiltrates are composed primarily of lymphocytes, causing the histology of the renal parenchyma in these patients to resemble that of the salivary and lacrimal glands. Renal functional defects include diminished urinary concentrating ability and distal (type I) RTA. Urinalysis may show pyuria (predominantly lymphocyturia) and mild proteinuria.

Tubulointerstitial Abnormalities Associated with Glomerulonephritis

Primary glomerulopathies are often associated with damage to tubules and the interstitium. Occasionally, the primary disorder may affect glomeruli and tubules directly. For example, in more than half of patients with the nephropathy of systemic lupus erythematosus, deposits of immune complexes can be identified in tubule basement membranes, usually accompanied by an interstitial mononuclear inflammatory reaction. Similarly, in many patients with glomerulonephritis associated with anti-glomerular basement membrane antibody, the same antibody is reactive against tubule basement membranes as well. More frequently, tubulointerstitial damage is a secondary consequence of glomerular dysfunction. The extent of tubulointerstitial fibrosis correlates closely with the degree of renal impairment. Potential mechanisms by which glomerular disease might cause tubulointerstitial injury include glomerular leak of plasma proteins toxic to epithelial cells, activation of tubule epithelial cells by glomerulus-derived cytokines, reduced peritubular blood flow leading to downstream tubulointerstitial ischemia, and hyperfunction of remnant tubules.

MISCELLANEOUS DISORDERS

Vesicoureteral Reflux

(See also Chap. 21.) When the function of the ureterovesical junction is impaired, urine may reflux into the ureters due to the high intravesical pressure that develops during voiding. Clinically, reflux is often detected on the voiding and postvoiding films obtained during intravenous pyelography, although voiding cystourethrography may be required for definitive diagnosis. Bladder infection may ascend the urinary tract to the kidneys through incompetent ureterovesical sphincters. Not surprisingly, therefore, reflux is often discovered in patients with acute and/or chronic urinary tract infections. With more severe degrees of reflux, characterized by dilatation of ureters and renal pelves, progressive renal damage often appears. Uncertainty exists as to the necessity of infection in producing the scarred kidney of reflux nephropathy. Substantial proteinuria is often present, and glomerular lesions similar to those of idiopathic focal glomerulosclerosis (Chap. 15) are often found in addition to the changes of chronic tubulointerstitial disease. Surgical correction of reflux is usually

necessary only with the more severe degrees of reflux since renal damage correlates with the extent of reflux. Obviously, if extensive glomerulosclerosis already exists, urologic repair may no longer be warranted.

Radiation Nephritis

Renal dysfunction can be expected to occur if ≥ 23 Gy (2300 rad) of x-ray irradiation is administered to both kidneys. Histologic examination of the kidneys reveals hyalinized glomeruli and arterioles, atrophic tubules, and extensive interstitial fibrosis. Radiation nephritis can present acutely or chronically with renal failure, moderate to malignant hypertension, anemia, and proteinuria that may reach the nephrotic range. Malignant hypertension without renal failure may follow unilateral renal irradiation and resolve with ipsilateral nephrectomy. Radiation nephritis has all but vanished because of heightened awareness of its pathogenesis by radiotherapists.

GLOBAL CONSIDERATIONS

The spectrum of causes of chronic tubulointerstitial nephritis shows marked geographical variation. Chinese herb nephropathy has mostly been reported in Belgium and in parts of Asia. Analgesic nephropathy has been found worldwide but is a particularly frequent cause of chronic renal failure in Scotland, Belgium, and Australia. Balkan endemic nephropathy is a chronic, slowly progressive tubulointerstitial disease of unknown etiology that is exclusively confined to Bulgaria, Serbia, Croatia, Bosnia, and Romania. These differences in incidence probably reflect geographical variation in exposure to particular nephrotoxins, but could also be explained by genetic factors or differing diagnostic criteria.

FURTHER READINGS

Baker RJ, Pusey CD: The changing profile of acute tubulointerstitial nephritis. Nephrol Dial Transplant 19:8, 2004

Bateman V: Proximal tubular injury in myeloma. Contrib Nephrol 153:87, 2007

Curhan GC et al: Lifetime non-narcotic analgesic abuse and decline in renal function in women. Arch Intern Med 164:1519, 2004

Gonzalez E et al: Early steroid treatment improves the recovery of renal function in patients with drug-induced acute interstitial nephritis. Kidney Int 73:940, 2008

Kelly CJ, Neilson EG: Tubulointerstitial diseases, in *Brenner and Rector's The Kidney*, 7th ed, BM Brenner (ed). Philadelphia, Saunders, 2004, pp 1483–1512

Lin JL et al: Environmental lead exposure and progression of chronic renal diseases in patients without diabetes. N Engl J Med 348:277, 2003

Presne C et al: Lithium-induced nephropathy: Rate of progression and prognostic factors. Kidney Int 64:585, 2003

Roser M et al: Gitelman syndrome. Hypertension 53:893, 2009

Waters AM et al: Tubulointerstitial nephritis as an extraintestinal manifestation of Crohn's disease. Nat Clin Pract Nephrol 4:693, 2008

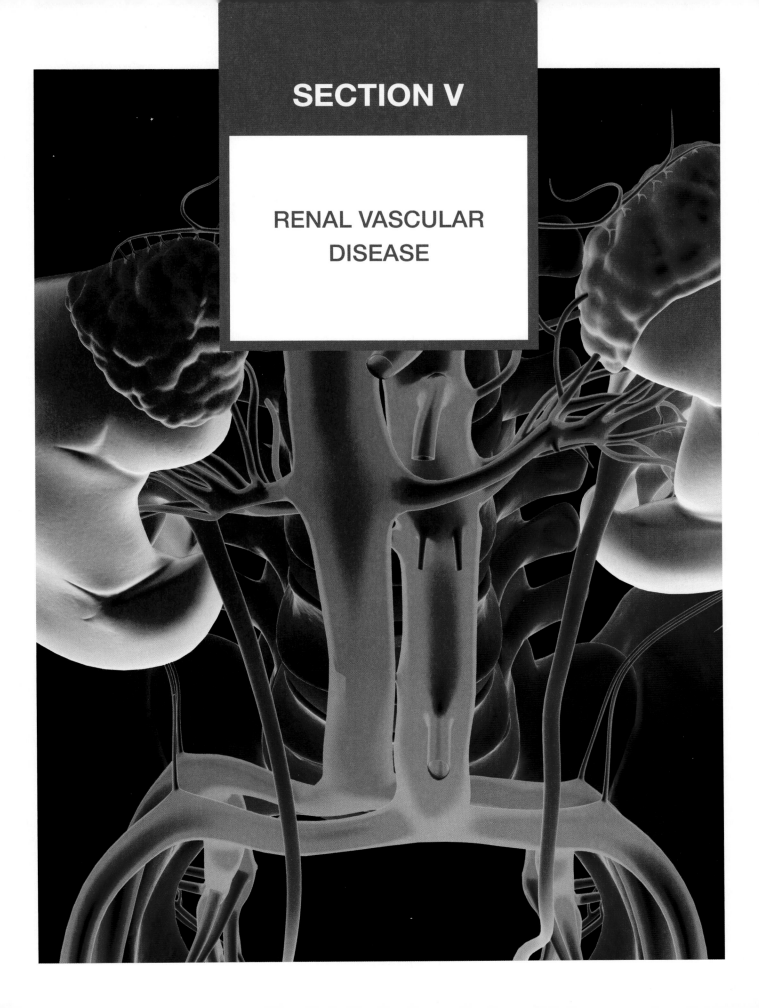

SECTION V

RENAL VASCULAR DISEASE

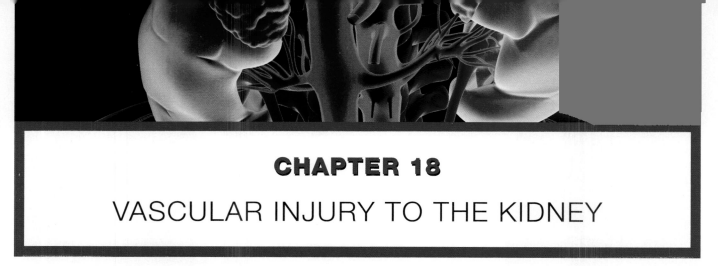

CHAPTER 18

VASCULAR INJURY TO THE KIDNEY

Kamal F. Badr ■ Barry M. Brenner

Renal vasculature is commonly involved in atherosclerotic, hypertensive, embolic, inflammatory, and hematologic vascular disorders. Adequate delivery of blood to the glomerular capillary network is crucial for glomerular filtration and overall salt and water balance. Thus, in addition to threatening the viability of renal tissue, vascular injury to the kidney may compromise the maintenance of body fluid volume and composition. It is important to keep in mind the unique nature of the renal microvasculature, in particular the presence of a large network of (glomerular) capillaries that subserves the process of glomerular filtration.

ATHEROSCLEROSIS

Renal Vascular Injury in Systemic Atherosclerotic Vascular Disease (AVD)

■ Macrovascular Atherosclerotic Disease

As is the case in other vascular beds, the renal artery and its branches are potential sites for plaque formation, which may lead to ischemic renal disease and hypertension.

■ Microvascular Atherosclerotic Disease

Numerous trials in cardiovascular medicine have focused attention on the clinical significance of the rate of urinary albumin excretion (UAE) as an early and powerful predictor of systemic AVD. As illustrated in **Fig. 18-1**, while both systemic and renal endothelial beds are subject to oxidant stress, inflammation, and hemodynamic injury, a measurable response (elevated UAE) is detectable in the renal microcirculation years before the emergence of systemic disease and/or adverse events in other vascular beds. The strong correlation between UAE and cardiovascular risk, and the parallel improvements noted in both with pharmacologic therapy, support the emerging concept of the renal circulation as an early detection site for atherosclerotic endothelial injury and an integrated marker of cardiovascular risk.

Atherosclerotic Renovascular Disease (ARVD) (Renal Artery Stenosis and Ischemic Nephropathy)

It is estimated that ~5% of cases of hypertension are caused by renal artery stenosis (RAS). In population-based studies, significant (>60%) stenosis is found in 9.1% of men and 5.5% of women over 65. The incidence, however, is considerably higher in those being studied for coronary (19%) or peripheral (35–50%) vascular disease. Autopsy studies in patients dying of stroke revealed that at least 1 renal artery is >75% stenosed in 10% of the patients studied. The common cause in the middle-aged and elderly is an atheromatous plaque at the origin of the renal artery. Bilateral involvement is

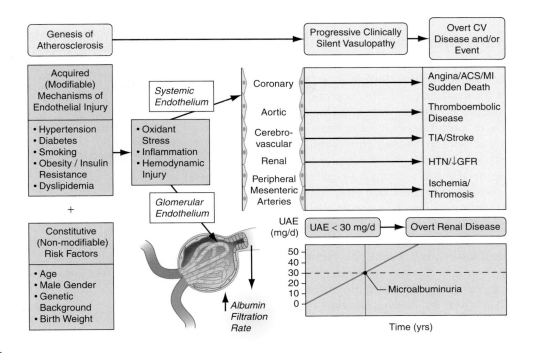

FIGURE 18-1

Comparative pathophysiology and clinical consequences of atherosclerosis-associated endothelial cell injury in systemic versus renal circulations. In contrast to the systemic endothelial bed in which early atherosclerotic injury is undetectable, the high volume of fluid filtered across the glomerular endothelium (140–180 L/d) markedly amplifies the functional consequence (increased albumin filtration) of early endothelial (and podocyte) injury in the glomerulus. The emergence of microalbuminuria thus unmasks systemic endothelial injury likely occurring simultaneously in other vascular beds, progressing silently to overt disease years later. CV, cardiovascular; ACS, acute coronary syndrome; MI, myocardial infarction; TIA, transient ischemic attack; HTN, hypertension; GFR, glomerular filtration rate; UAE, urinary albumin excretion.

present in half of the affected cases. Established plaques progress in >50% of cases over 5 years (15% to total occlusion). Renal hypotrophy is detectable in 20% of affected kidneys. In younger women (15–50 years), stenosis is due to intrinsic structural abnormalities of the arterial wall caused by *fibromuscular dysplasia.*

In addition to stimulation of renin release, renovascular disease is associated with increased sympathetic neural activity, resulting in frequently described flushing, loss of nocturnal blood pressure (BP) decrease, autonomic instability, and rapid BP swings. In most patients being evaluated for RAS, glomerular filtration rate (GFR) is <60 mL/min, with 85% having stage 3–5 chronic kidney disease. GFR in these ranges is a strong independent predictor of cardiovascular risk. Thus, patients with ARVD are more likely to suffer from stroke, heart failure, or myocardial infarction than to progress to end-stage renal disease.

Diagnosis

Diagnostic evaluation for significant RAS should begin with noninvasive approaches. An initial screening test is Doppler ultrasonography, which provides information on blood-flow velocity and pressure waveforms in the renal arteries and, when positive, is helpful (sensitivity is 70% at best). Its limitations, however, include significant operator dependence, technical difficulty in obese patients, and poor sensitivity in the presence of multiple renal arteries, distal stenoses, and total occlusion. Measurement of the intrarenal resistance index (RI) provides valuable information on the extent of parenchymal disease and, hence, on the prognosis for functional recovery following revascularization procedures. Absence of compensatory hypertrophy in the contralateral kidney should raise the suspicion of bilateral stenosis or superimposed parenchymal renal disease, most commonly hypertensive or diabetic nephropathy. Because angiotensin-converting enzyme (ACE) inhibitors magnify the impairment in renal blood flow and GFR caused by functionally significant renal artery stenosis, use of these drugs in association with ^{99m}Tc-labeled pentetic acid (DTPA) or ^{99m}Tc-labeled mertiatide (MAG$_3$) renography enhances diagnostic precision and is of additional predictive value. Gadolinium-enhanced three-dimensional magnetic resonance angiography (MRA) has replaced previous modalities as the most sensitive (>90%) and specific (95%) test for the diagnosis of RAS. The most definitive diagnostic procedure is contrast-enhanced arteriography. Intraarterial digital subtraction techniques minimize the requirements for contrast, reducing the risk of renal toxicity.

℞ **Treatment:**
RENAL ARTERY STENOSIS

When blood pressure is controlled and renal function is preserved, expectant therapy and careful follow-up form the best approach for managing RAS. This approach is justified by the devastating consequences of atheroembolic complications of percutaneous revascularization, including loss of renal function. Despite enthusiasm for revascularization procedures for tight RAS in the early to mid-1990s, the past decade has witnessed a significant change in management strategies, stressing more conservative approaches. Medical therapy is aimed at controlling BP and preserving GFR, and includes typically at least three drugs. Angiotensin antagonists (ACE inhibitors or angiotensin receptor blockers) and diuretics are required in most patients. When goal BPs are achieved, clinical outcomes and survival are comparable for medical and revascularization therapies. Revascularization therapy (angioplasty with stent placement) may improve the chances of attaining goal BP, but should be considered only after optimal medical therapy has failed to achieve goal BP, or resulted in a >30% increase in serum creatinine. BP control and preservation of renal function following revascularization should not be expected when the RI of the targeted kidney is >80%. In experienced hands, the complications of angioplasty or stenting are acceptably low. Clinical studies suggest that percutaneous revascularization prevents additional deterioration or even improves renal function in selected patients. Despite technical advances in percutaneous renal revascularization, optimal technique is still evolving. Embolic protection devices may prove useful. Table 18-1 lists current indications for revascularization in patients with RAS. Because of safety, cost, and long-term efficacy, surgical repair is now rarely indicated.

Success rates with conventional percutaneous transluminal angioplasty in young patients with fibromuscular dysplasia are 50% cure and improvement in BP control in another 30%.

Atheroembolic Renovascular Disease

Atheroembolic renal disease is part of a systemic syndrome characterized by cholesterol crystal embolization. Renal damage results from embolization of cholesterol crystals from atherosclerotic plaques present in large arteries, such as the aorta, to small arteries in the renal vasculature. Atheroembolic renal disease is an increasingly common and often underdiagnosed cause of renal insufficiency in the elderly. Autopsy studies identify cholesterol emboli in 2.4–4% of renal tissue samples, but the incidence increases significantly in elderly individuals, especially in those who had undergone abdominal arteriography or surgery. Male gender, older age, hypertension,

TABLE 18-1

INDICATIONS AND PREREQUISITES FOR REVASCULARIZATION IN RENAL ARTERY STENOSIS
Indications
Uncontrolled BP despite maximal therapy
Progressive rise in creatinine (other causes excluded)
Intolerance to ACE-Is, ARBs (>30% increase in creatinine or severe hyperkalemia)
Recurrent pulmonary edema, CHF, or volume overload
Prerequisites
Experienced operator
Presence of two kidneys
RI <0.80 in target kidney(s)

Note: BP, blood pressure; ACE-Is, angiotensin-converting enzyme inhibitors; ARBs, angiotensin receptor blockers; CHF, congestive heart failure; RI, renal index.

and diabetes mellitus are important predisposing factors, present in 85% of cases. Patients with cholesterol embolization syndrome also often have a history of ischemic cardiovascular disease, aortic aneurysm, cerebrovascular disease, congestive heart failure, or renal insufficiency. A significant association is present between RAS and atheroembolic renal disease. Inciting events, which include vascular surgery, arteriography, angioplasty, anticoagulation with heparin, and thrombolytic therapy, can be identified in ~50% of cases. Arteriographic procedures constitute the most common cause of cholesterol embolization.

Clinical manifestations usually appear 1–14 days after an inciting event, but their onset can be more insidious. Systemic manifestations occur in fewer than half of patients and include fever, myalgias, headache, and weight loss. Cutaneous manifestations, such as livedo reticularis, "purple" toes, and toe gangrene, occur in 50–90% of patients and constitute the most common extrarenal findings. Other targets of cholesterol embolization include the retina, musculoskeletal system, nervous system, and gut. Accelerated or labile hypertension is present in one-half of patients; malignant hypertension has been described. Renal insufficiency is usually subacute and advances in a stepwise fashion over a period of several weeks. Renal failure, however, can be acute and oliguric. Uremic signs and symptoms requiring dialytic therapy develop in 40% of patients, only half of whom recover sufficient renal function to discontinue dialysis after 1 year. Renal infarction secondary to cholesterol embolization is rare. Cholesterol embolic disease in renal allografts has been reported and can be of donor or of recipient origin.

Laboratory Findings

In addition to rising blood urea nitrogen (BUN) and creatinine, laboratory findings may include eosinophilia (60–80%), eosinophiluria, leukocytosis, elevated sedimentation rate, anemia, and hypocomplementemia.

Antemortem diagnosis of atherosclerotic renal emboli is difficult. The demonstration of cholesterol emboli in the retina is helpful, but a firm diagnosis is established only by renal biopsy. Histologic examination of the occluded vessels reveals biconvex needle-shaped clefts representing the sites of cholesterol crystal deposition. The cholesterol crystals themselves are removed by the usual solvents of tissue fixation but can be visualized in frozen sections of fresh tissue as birefringent crystals under polarized light. They may also be seen in asymptomatic skeletal muscle or skin. Atheroembolic renal disease is associated with a 64–81% mortality rate.

Rx **Treatment:**
ATHEROEMBOLIC RENAL DISEASE

No effective therapy for atheroembolic renal disease is available. Withdrawal of anticoagulation may be beneficial. In some patients, kidney function improved even after a prolonged period of renal insufficiency. Cholesterol-lowering agents may also improve outcome. An aggressive therapeutic approach with patient-tailored supportive measures may be associated with more favorable clinical outcome. Numerous reports suggest a beneficial effect for steroid therapy, but controlled studies are lacking.

Thromboembolic Renovascular Disease

Thrombosis of the major renal arteries or their branches is an important cause of deterioration of renal function, especially in the elderly. It is often difficult to diagnose, and therefore requires a high index of suspicion. Thrombosis may occur as a result of intrinsic pathology in the renal vessels (posttraumatic, atherosclerotic, or inflammatory) or as a result of emboli originating in distant vessels, most commonly fat emboli, emboli originating in the left heart (mural thrombi following myocardial infarction, bacterial endocarditis, or aseptic vegetations), or "paradoxical" emboli passing from the right side of the circulation via a patent foramen ovale or atrial septal defect. Renal emboli are bilateral in 15–30% of cases.

The clinical presentation is variable, depending on the time course and the extent of the occlusive event. Acute thrombosis and infarction, such as follows embolization, may result in sudden onset of flank pain and tenderness, fever, hematuria, leukocytosis, nausea, and vomiting. If infarction occurs, liver enzymes may be elevated, namely aspartate aminotransferase (AST), lactate dehydrogenase (LDH), and alkaline phosphatase, which rise and fall in the order listed. Urinary LDH and alkaline phosphatase may also increase after infarction. Renal function deteriorates acutely, leading in bilateral

thrombosis to acute oliguric renal failure. More gradual (i.e., atherosclerotic) occlusion of a single renal artery may go undetected. A spectrum of clinical presentations lies between these two extremes. Hypertension usually follows renal infarction and results from renin release in the peri-infarction zone. Hypertension is usually transient but may be persistent. Diagnosis is established by renal arteriography.

Rx **Treatment:**
ACUTE RENAL ARTERIAL THROMBOSIS

Management options for *acute* renal arterial thrombosis include surgical intervention, anticoagulant therapy, intrarenal tissue plasminogen activator, percutaneous rheolytic thrombectomy, conservative and supportive therapy, and control of hypertension. The choice of treatment depends mainly on (1) the condition of the patient, in particular the patient's ability to withstand major surgery; and (2) the extent of renovascular occlusion and amount of renal mass at risk of infarction. In general, supportive care and anticoagulant therapy are indicated in unilateral disease. In *acute* bilateral thrombosis, medical and surgical therapies yield comparable results. About 25% of patients die during the acute episode, usually from extrarenal complications.

RENAL VASCULAR INJURY IN HYPERTENSION

Whether it is "essential" or of known etiology, hypertension results in development of intrinsic lesions of the renal arterioles (hyaline arteriolosclerosis) that eventually lead to loss of function (nephrosclerosis).

"Essential" Hypertension (Arteriolar Nephrosclerosis)

Arteriolar nephrosclerosis is seen in patients who are hypertensive (BP >150/90 mmHg) for an extended period of time but whose hypertension has not progressed to a malignant form. Such patients, usually in the older age group, are often discovered to be hypertensive on routine physical examination or as a result of nonspecific symptomatology (e.g., headaches, weakness, palpitations).

The characteristic pathology is in the afferent arterioles, which have thickened walls due to deposition of homogeneous eosinophilic material (hyaline arteriolosclerosis). Narrowing of vascular lumina results, with consequent ischemic injury to glomeruli and tubules.

Physical examination may reveal changes in retinal vessels (arteriolar narrowing and/or flame-shaped hemorrhages), cardiac hypertrophy, and possibly signs of congestive heart failure. Renal disease may manifest as a mild to moderate elevation of serum creatinine concentration, microalbuminuria, or proteinuria.

"Malignant" Hypertension

Patients with long-standing hypertension or patients not previously known to be hypertensive may develop malignant hypertension characterized by a sudden (accelerated) elevation of BP (diastolic BP often >130 mmHg) accompanied by papilledema, central nervous system manifestations, cardiac decompensation, and acute progressive deterioration of renal function. The absence of papilledema does not rule out the diagnosis in a patient with markedly elevated BP and rapidly declining renal function. The kidneys are characterized by a flea-bitten appearance resulting from hemorrhages in surface capillaries. Histologically, two distinct vascular lesions can be seen. The first, affecting arterioles, is fibrinoid necrosis, i.e., infiltration of arteriolar walls with eosinophilic material including fibrin, thickening of vessel walls, and, occasionally, an inflammatory infiltrate (necrotizing arteriolitis). The second lesion, involving the interlobular arteries, is a concentric hyperplastic proliferation of the cellular elements of the vascular wall with deposition of collagen to form a hyperplastic arteriolitis (onion-skin lesion). Fibrinoid necrosis occasionally extends into the glomeruli, which may also undergo proliferative changes or total necrosis. Most glomerular and tubular changes are secondary to ischemia and infarction. The sequence of events leading to the development of malignant hypertension is poorly defined. Two pathophysiologic alterations appear central in its initiation and/or perpetuation: (1) increased permeability of vessel walls to invasion by plasma components, particularly fibrin, which activates clotting mechanisms leading to a microangiopathic hemolytic anemia, thus perpetuating the vascular pathology; and (2) activation of the renin-angiotensin-aldosterone system at some point in the disease process, which contributes to the acceleration and maintenance of BP elevation and, in turn, to vascular injury.

Malignant hypertension is most likely to develop in a previously hypertensive individual, usually in the third or fourth decade of life. There is a higher incidence among black men. Presenting symptoms are usually neurologic (dizziness, headache, blurring of vision, altered states of consciousness, and focal or generalized seizures). Cardiac decompensation and renal failure appear thereafter. Renal abnormalities include a rapid rise in serum creatinine, hematuria (at times macroscopic), proteinuria, and red and white blood cell casts in the sediment. Nephrotic syndrome may be present. Elevated plasma aldosterone levels cause hypokalemic metabolic alkalosis in the early phase. Uremic acidosis

and hyperkalemia eventually obscure these early findings. Hematologic indices of microangiopathic hemolytic anemia (i.e., schistocytes) are often seen.

℞ **Treatment:**
HYPERTENSION

Control of hypertension is the principal goal of therapy. The time of initiation of therapy, its effectiveness, and patient compliance are crucial factors in arresting the progression of benign nephrosclerosis. Untreated, most of these patients succumb to the extrarenal complications of hypertension. In contrast, malignant hypertension is a medical emergency; its natural course includes a death rate of 80–90% within 1 year of onset, almost always due to uremia. Supportive measures should be instituted to control the neurologic, cardiac, and other complications of acute renal failure, but the mainstay of therapy is prompt and aggressive reduction of BP, which, if successful, can reverse all complications in the majority of patients. Presently, 5-year survival is 50%, and some patients have evidence of partial reversal of the vascular lesions and a return of renal function to near-normal levels.

RENAL VASCULAR INJURY IN SYSTEMIC DISEASES

Hemolytic Uremic Syndrome (HUS) and Thrombotic Thrombocytopenic Purpura (TTP)

HUS and TTP, consumptive coagulopathies characterized by microangiopathic hemolytic anemia and thrombocytopenia, have a particular predilection for the kidney and the central nervous system. Previously, the overlap in clinical manifestations had prompted investigators to regard the two syndromes as a continuum of a single disease entity. Recent evidence, however, points to a clearly distinct molecular basis for their pathophysiology.

Renal Involvement

Evidence of renal involvement is present in the majority of patients with HUS/TTP. Microscopic hematuria (78%) and subnephrotic proteinuria (75%) are the most consistent findings. Male sex, hypertension, prolonged anuria, and hemoglobin levels <10 g/L at onset are associated with a higher risk of renal sequelae in children. Gross hematuria is rare. More than 90% of patients with HUS have significant renal failure, one-third of whom are anuric. The mean duration of renal failure is 2 weeks. Severe acute renal failure or anuria occurs in <10% of cases of classic TTP. The degree of elevation of

BUN on presentation may be a prognostic indicator in patients with HUS/TTP.

Pathology

The characteristic lesion in HUS/TTP is thrombotic microangiopathy. Microthrombi are demonstrated in renal arterioles and capillaries. In TTP, microthrombi are composed predominantly of platelet aggregates and a thin layer of fibrin, and stain strongly for von Willebrand factor (vWF), which has been implicated in its pathogenesis. In contrast, microthrombi in HUS contain predominantly fibrin. Subendothelial hyaline deposits and endothelial cell swelling also contribute to vascular occlusion. Glomerular lesions are ischemic. The glomerular capillary walls are wrinkled, the glomerular tuft may be atrophied, and the Bowman capsule is thickened. Acute cortical or tubular necrosis may occur. Immunofluorescence studies invariably demonstrate fibrinogen along the glomerular capillary walls and in arterial thrombi. Granular deposits of C3 and IgM may be observed in vessel walls and glomeruli. Electron-microscopic studies demonstrate swelling of the glomerular endothelial cells and detachment from the glomerular basement membrane.

Etiology HUS

Two forms of HUS have been described: (1) Diarrhea-associated HUS (D + HUS), the most common form in children, is associated with infection by Shiga toxin–producing *Escherichia coli* (most commonly O157:H7). This form has an excellent prognosis. Most cases occur in summer and autumn. (2) In contrast, non-Shiga toxin–associated HUS (D − HUS) typically affects adults but can occur at any age. It occurs in sporadic or familial forms, is noninfective, and is usually precipitated by drugs and pregnancy. Several studies have demonstrated genetic predisposition in atypical HUS, involving two regulatory proteins of the complement alternative pathway: factor H (FH) and membrane cofactor protein (MCP, or CD46).

TTP

ADAMTS 13 is a member of the recently recognized ADAMTS (a disintegrin with thrombospondin type 1 motifs) zinc metalloproteinase family that cleaves vWF complexes and prevents vWF-platelet interaction. A *severe deficiency of ADAMTS 13* has been described in patients with TTP. Two forms have been identified: (1) In sporadic TTP, the deficiency appears to be *autoimmune suppression* of ADAMTS 13 by circulating IgG antibodies to the protein. (2) Schulman-Upshaw syndrome (a hereditary deficiency) is characterized by thrombocytopenia and microangiopathic hemolysis soon after birth, responding to plasma infusion. Most patients require plasma infusions every 2–4 weeks. Relapses are often triggered by fever, infection, pregnancy, or surgery.

Drug-induced HUS/TTP is well recognized in patients receiving chemotherapeutic agents, most commonly mitomycin C (cumulative dose of ≥20–30 mg/m^2). The onset of hemolytic anemia and renal failure is usually sudden, and mortality rate is high despite supportive therapy. Treatment with plasma exchange, glucocorticoids, immunosuppressive agents, and staphylococcal protein A immunoadsorption, however, are successful in some cases. Ticlopidine and clopidogrel use has also been associated with the disease. Cyclosporine-induced TTP was first reported following bone marrow transplantation but is more common in patients receiving renal transplants and other solid organs. In renal allograft recipients, cyclosporine-induced HUS occurs during the first week after transplantation as drug toxicity is dose related. Renal failure reverses with the cessation of cyclosporine or reduction in its dose.

HUS/TTP may occur after bone marrow transplantation independent of prior radiation or cyclosporine therapy. TTP is commonly associated with pregnancy. Approximately 10–25% of patients with TTP are women who are either near-term pregnant or in the postpartum period; this is also the time for thrombotic events and the occurrence of preeclampsia, eclampsia, and HELLP syndrome (*h*emolysis, *e*levated *l*iver enzymes, and *l*ow *p*latelet count). These syndromes are difficult to distinguish from TTP-HUS. Decreased activity of ADAMTS 13 in late pregnancy may be an additional risk. Finally, thrombotic microangiopathy has been described in conjunction with vascular tumors, acute promyelocytic leukemia, and prostatic, gastric, and pancreatic carcinomas.

℞ Treatment:
HEMOLYTIC UREMIC SYNDROME

Supportive measures—including dialysis, antihypertensive medications, blood transfusions, and management of neurologic complications—have improved survival in patients with HUS/TTP. Adequate fluid balance and bowel rest are important in treating typical HUS associated with diarrhea. Antibiotics to treat infection caused by Shiga toxin–producing *E. coli* O157:H7 have been found to increase the risk of overt HUS by 17-fold, likely by favoring the acute release of large amounts of preformed toxin or by providing selective advantage to *E. coli* O157. Among the therapeutic modalities used to treat patients with HUS/TTP, plasma exchange (plasmapheresis combined with fresh-frozen plasma replacement) is currently the treatment of choice and is superior to plasma infusion alone. Plasmapheresis may remove the recently identified inhibitory autoantibodies against vWF protease from the circulation and supply larger amounts of the protease enzyme. Plasma exchange should be performed daily until remission is achieved, remission being normalization of platelet count, or resolution of neurologic symptoms, or both. Hemoglobin level, percent schistocytosis, reticulocyte count, and renal indices do not appear to be determinants of initial response to therapy, as they may be abnormal for an undefined period after remission. Continuation of plasma exchange for several sessions after remission has been advocated to prevent relapses. Severe renal insufficiency resulting from HUS/TTP often requires dialysis. Renal transplantation has also been performed. HUS/TTP may recur in up to 17% of transplanted patients, independent of cyclosporine use. Higher recurrence rates have been reported for familial HUS.

SCLERODERMA (PROGRESSIVE SYSTEMIC SCLEROSIS)

Renal involvement in scleroderma can present in one of two ways, depending on whether malignant hypertension is superimposed on the renal pathology: (1) *Persistent urinary abnormalities* and an indolent clinical course characterized by proteinuria (15–36%), hypertension (24%), and mild azotemia (15%). Anti-RNA POL3 antibodies are strongly associated with scleroderma renal disease. (2) *Scleroderma renal crisis* (SRC) is a rapid deterioration in renal function, usually accompanied by malignant hypertension, oliguria, proteinuria, fluid retention, microangiopathic hemolytic anemia, and central nervous system involvement. It occurs in 10% of patients, most commonly in the first 4 years following diagnosis, particularly in patients with diffuse cutaneous involvement, 25% of whom develop SRC. SRC may occur in patients with previously indemonstrable or slowly progressive renal disease. Untreated, it leads to chronic renal failure within days to months. A significant association exists between antecedent glucocorticoid therapy and the development of SRC.

℞ **Treatment:**
SCLERODERMA

In SRC, ACE inhibitors have improved 5-year survival from 10 to 65%. Some 60% of SRC patients who receive ACE inhibitors require no dialysis (or temporary dialysis) with a survival rate at 8 years of 80–85%, similar to scleroderma patients who do not develop renal crisis. More than half of patients with SRC who require dialysis and are treated aggressively with ACE inhibitors are able to discontinue dialysis 3–18 months later, suggesting that patients should continue ACE inhibitor therapy even after beginning dialysis. Angiotensin receptor antagonists have not proven to be a satisfactory substitute for ACE inhibitors in patients with SRC. SRC patients who

progress to end-stage renal disease can undergo hemodialysis or peritoneal dialysis, the latter being occasionally limited by compromised peritoneal clearance. A decrease in graft and overall survival has been noted in scleroderma patients following renal transplantation, as well as recurrence of progressive sclerosis in the transplanted kidney, particularly in patients with aggressive disease.

SICKLE CELL NEPHROPATHY

Sickle cell disease causes renal complications as a result of sickling of red blood cells in the microvasculature. The hypertonic and relatively hypoxic environment of the renal medulla, coupled with the slow blood flow in the vasa recta, favors sickling of red blood cells, with resultant local infarction (papillary necrosis). Functional tubule defects in patients with sickle cell disease are likely the result of partial ischemic injury to the renal tubules.

In addition to the intrarenal microvascular pathology described above, the sickle cell disease in young patients is characterized by renal hyperperfusion, glomerular hypertrophy, and hyperfiltration. Many of these individuals eventually develop a glomerulopathy leading to glomerular proteinuria (present in as many as 30%) and, in some, the nephrotic syndrome. Co-inheritance of microdeletions in the α-globin gene (α thalassemia) appears to protect against the development of nephropathy and is associated with lower mean arterial pressure and less proteinuria.

Mild azotemia and hyperuricemia can also develop. Advanced renal failure and uremia occur in 10% of cases. Pathologic examination reveals the typical lesion of "hyperfiltration nephropathy," namely, focal segmental glomerular sclerosis. This finding has led to the suggestion that anemia-induced hyperfiltration in childhood is the principal cause of the adult glomerulopathy. Nephron loss secondary to ischemic injury also contributes to the development of azotemia in these patients.

In addition to the glomerulopathy described above, renal complications of sickle cell disease include *cortical infarcts* leading to loss of function, persistent hematuria, and perinephric hematomas. *Papillary infarcts*, demonstrable radiographically in 50% of patients with sickle trait, lead to an increased risk of bacterial infection in the scarred renal tissues and functional tubule abnormalities. Painless gross hematuria occurs with a higher frequency in sickle trait than in sickle cell disease and likely results from infarctive episodes in the renal medulla. *Functional tubule abnormalities* such as nephrogenic diabetes insipidus result from marked reduction in vasa recta blood flow, combined with ischemic tubule injury. This concentrating defect places these patients at increased risk of dehydration and, hence, sickling crises. The concentrating defect also occurs in individuals with sickle trait. Other tubule defects involve potassium and hydrogen ion excretion, occasionally leading to hyperkalemic metabolic acidosis and a defect in uric acid excretion which, combined with increased purine synthesis in the bone marrow, results in hyperuricemia.

Management of sickle nephropathy is not separate from that of overall patient management. In addition, however, the use of ACE inhibitors has been associated with improvement of the hyperfiltration glomerulopathy. Three-year graft and patient survival in renal transplant recipients with sickle nephropathy is diminished as compared to those with other causes of end-stage renal disease.

RENAL VEIN THROMBOSIS (RVT)

Thrombosis of one or both main renal veins occurs in a variety of settings (Table 18-2). Nephrotic syndrome accompanying membranous glomerulopathy and certain carcinomas seems to predispose to the development of RVT, which occurs in 10–50% of patients with these disorders. RVT may exacerbate preexisting proteinuria but is infrequently the cause of the nephrotic syndrome.

The clinical manifestations depend on the severity and abruptness of its occurrence. Acute cases occur typically in children and are characterized by sudden loss of renal function, often accompanied by fever, chills, lumbar tenderness (with kidney enlargement), leukocytosis, and hematuria. Hemorrhagic infarction and renal rupture may lead to hypovolemic shock. In young adults RVT is usually suspected from an unexpected and relatively acute or subacute deterioration of renal function and/or exacerbation of proteinuria and hematuria in the appropriate clinical setting. In cases of gradual thrombosis, usually occurring in the elderly, the only manifestation may be recurrent pulmonary emboli or development of hypertension. A Fanconi-like syndrome and proximal renal tubular acidosis have been described. RVT is a potential cause of early graft dysfunction following renal transplantation, and its incidence may be decreased with prophylactic low-dose aspirin. The definitive diagnosis can only be established through selective renal venography with visualization of the occluding thrombus. Short of angiography, Doppler ultrasound, contrast-enhanced CT, and MRI often provide evidence of thrombus.

Rx Treatment:
RENAL VEIN THROMBOSIS

Treatment consists of anticoagulation, the main purpose of which is prevention of pulmonary embolization, although some authors have also claimed improvement in renal function and proteinuria. Encouraging reports have appeared concerning the use of streptokinase. Spontaneous recanalization with clinical improvement has also been observed. Anticoagulant therapy is more rewarding in the acute thrombosis seen in younger individuals. Nephrectomy is advocated in infants with life-threatening renal infarction. Percutaneous mechanical thrombectomy is effective in some cases.

BILATERAL CORTICAL NECROSIS

Acute bilateral cortical necrosis is associated with septic abortions, abruptio placentae, and preeclampsia. Coagulation in cortical vessels and arterioles leads to renal tissue necrosis. Anuria and renal failure ensue and may be irreversible. In other cases, renal function returns partially, but on long-term follow-up most patients slowly progress to uremia.

FURTHER READINGS

Bax L et al: Stent placement in patients with atherosclerotic renal artery stenosis and impaired renal function: A randomized trial. Ann Intern Med 150:840, 2009

Chonchol M, Linas S: Diagnosis and management of ischemic nephropathy. Clin J Am Soc Nephrol 1:172, 2006

Garovic VD, Textor SC: Renovascular hypertension and ischemic nephropathy. Circulation 112:1362, 2005

Krumme B: Comparing the cost-effectiveness of various approaches to the management of suspected renal artery stenosis. Nat Clin Pract Nephrol 4:70, 2008

Lammle B et al: Thrombotic thrombocytopenic purpura. J Thromb Haemost 3:1663, 2005

Michael M et al: Interventions for hemolytic uremic syndrome and thrombotic thrombocytopenic purpura: A systematic review of randomized controlled trials. Am J Kidney Dis 53:259, 2009

Steen VD: Scleroderma renal crisis. Rheum Dis Clin North Am 29:315, 2003

Textor SC: Renovascular hypertension update. Curr Hypertens Rep 8:521, 2006

Wysokinski WE et al: Clinical characteristics and long-term follow-up of patients with renal vein thrombosis. Am J Kidney Dis 51:224, 2008

TABLE 18-2

CONDITIONS ASSOCIATED WITH RENAL VEIN THROMBOSIS
Trauma
Extrinsic compression (lymph nodes, aortic aneurysm, tumor)
Invasion by renal cell carcinoma
Dehydration (infants)
Nephrotic syndrome
Pregnancy or oral contraceptives

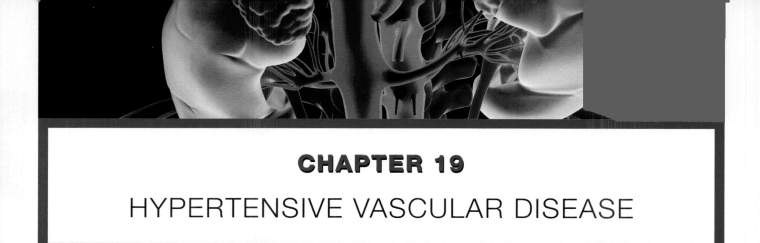

CHAPTER 19

HYPERTENSIVE VASCULAR DISEASE

Theodore A. Kotchen

Hypertension doubles the risk of cardiovascular diseases, including coronary heart disease (CHD), congestive heart failure (CHF), ischemic and hemorrhagic stroke, renal failure, and peripheral arterial disease. Hypertension is often associated with additional cardiovascular disease risk factors, and the risk of cardiovascular disease increases with the total burden of risk factors. Although antihypertensive therapy clearly reduces the risks of cardiovascular and renal disease, large segments of the hypertensive population are either untreated or inadequately treated.

EPIDEMIOLOGY

Blood pressure levels, the rate of age-related blood pressure increase, and the prevalence of hypertension vary among countries and among subpopulations within a country. Hypertension is present in all populations except for a small number of individuals living in primitive, culturally isolated societies. It has been estimated that hypertension accounts for 6% of deaths worldwide. In industrialized societies, blood pressure increases steadily during the first two decades. In children and adolescents, blood pressure is associated with growth and maturation. Blood pressure "tracks" over time in children and between adolescence and young adulthood. In the United States, average systolic blood pressure is higher for men than for women during early adulthood, although among older individuals the age-related rate of rise is steeper for women. Consequently, among individuals age 60 and older, systolic blood pressures of women are higher than those of men. Among adults, diastolic blood pressure also increases progressively with age until ~55 years, after which it tends to decrease. The consequence is a widening of pulse pressure (the difference between systolic and diastolic blood pressure) beyond age 60.

In the United States, based on results of the National Health and Nutrition Examination Survey (NHANES), 28.7% (age-adjusted prevalence) of U.S. adults, or ~58.4 million individuals, have hypertension (defined as any one of the following: systolic blood pressure ≥140 mmHg; diastolic blood pressure ≥90 mmHg; taking antihypertensive medications). Hypertension prevalence is 33.5% in non-Hispanic blacks, 28.9% in non-Hispanic whites, and 20.7% in Mexican Americans. The burden of hypertension increases with age, and among individuals aged ≥60, hypertension prevalence is 65.4%. Recent evidence suggests that the prevalence of hypertension in the United States may be increasing, possibly as a consequence of increasing obesity. The prevalence of hypertension and stroke mortality rates is higher in the southeastern United States than in other regions. In African Americans, hypertension appears earlier, is generally more severe, and results in higher rates of morbidity and mortality from stroke, left ventricular hypertrophy, CHF, and end-stage renal disease (ESRD) than in Caucasian Americans.

Both environmental and genetic factors may contribute to regional and racial variations of blood pressure and hypertension prevalence. Studies of societies undergoing "acculturation" and studies of migrants from a less to a more urbanized setting indicate a profound environmental contribution to blood pressure. Obesity and weight gain are strong, independent risk factors for hypertension. It has been estimated that 60% of hypertensives are >20% overweight. Among populations, hypertension prevalence is related to dietary NaCl intake, and the age-related increase of blood pressure may be augmented by a high NaCl intake. Low dietary intakes of calcium and potassium may also contribute to the risk of hypertension. Additional environmental factors that may contribute to hypertension include alcohol consumption, psychosocial stress, and low levels of physical activity.

Adoption, twin, and family studies document a significant heritable component to blood pressure levels and hypertension. Family studies controlling for a common environment indicate that blood pressure heritabilities are in the range of 15–35%. In twin studies, heritability estimates of blood pressure are ~60% for males and 30–40% for females. High blood pressure before age 55 occurs 3.8 times more frequently among persons with a positive family history of hypertension. Although specific genetic etiologies have been identified for relatively rare causes of hypertension, this has not been the case for the large majority of hypertensive patients. For most individuals, it is likely that hypertension represents a polygenic disorder in which a single gene or combination of genes act in concert with environmental exposures to contribute only a modest effect on blood pressure.

GENETIC CONSIDERATIONS

Although specific genetic variants have been identified in rare Mendelian forms of hypertension (Table 19-5), these variants are not applicable to the vast majority (>98%) of patients with essential hypertension. Blood pressure levels reflect the contributions of many susceptibility genes interacting with each other and with the environment. Essential hypertension is a polygenic disorder, and different patients may carry different subsets of genes that lead to elevated blood pressure and to different phenotypes associated with hypertension, e.g., obesity, dyslipidemia, insulin resistance.

Several strategies are being utilized in the search for specific hypertension-related genes. Animal models (including selectively bred rats and congenic rat strains) provide a powerful approach for evaluating genetic loci and genes associated with hypertension. Comparative mapping strategies allow for the identification of syntenic genomic regions between the rat and human genome that may be involved in blood pressure regulation. In linkage studies, polymorphic genetic markers are examined at regular distances along each chromosome. Linkage information is gathered family by family, and the minimum family unit comprises at least two relatives, often a pair of siblings. To date, genome scans for hypertension have yielded inconsistent results. In complementary association studies, different alleles (or combinations of alleles at different loci) of specific genes or chromosomal regions are compared in hypertensive patients and normotensive control subjects. Current evidence suggests that genes encoding components of the renin-angiotensin-aldosterone system, and angiotensinogen and angiotensin-converting enzyme (ACE) polymorphisms, may be related to hypertension and to blood pressure sensitivity to dietary NaCl. The (α-adducin gene is also thought to be associated with increased renal tubular absorption of sodium, and variants of this gene may also be associated with hypertension and salt sensitivity of blood pressure. Other genes possibly related to hypertension include genes encoding the angiotensin II type 1 (AT_1) receptor, aldosterone synthase, and the β_2-adrenoreceptor.

Preliminary evidence suggests that there may also be genetic determinants of target organ damage attributed to hypertension. Family studies indicate significant heritability of left ventricular mass, and there is considerable individual variation in the responses of the heart to hypertension. Family studies and variations in candidate genes associated with renal damage suggest that genetic factors may also contribute to hypertensive nephropathy. Specific genetic variants have been linked to CHD and stroke.

In the future, it is possible that DNA analysis will predict individual risk for hypertension and target organ damage and will identify responders to specific classes of antihypertensive agents. However, with the exception of the rare, monogenic hypertensive diseases, the genetic variants associated with hypertension remain to be confirmed, and the intermediate steps by which these variants affect blood pressure remain to be determined.

MECHANISMS OF HYPERTENSION

To provide a framework for understanding the pathogenesis and treatment options of hypertensive disorders, it is useful to understand factors involved in the regulation

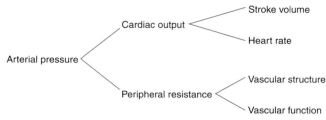

FIGURE 19-1
Determinants of arterial pressure.

of both normal and elevated arterial pressure. Cardiac output and peripheral resistance are the two determinants of arterial pressure (**Fig. 19-1**). Cardiac output is determined by stroke volume and heart rate; stroke volume is related to myocardial contractility and to the size of the vascular compartment. Peripheral resistance is determined by functional and anatomic changes in small arteries (lumen diameter 100–400 μm) and arterioles.

INTRAVASCULAR VOLUME

Vascular volume is a primary determinant of arterial pressure over the long term. Although the extracellular fluid space is composed of vascular and interstitial spaces, in general, alterations in total extracellular fluid volume are associated with proportional changes of blood volume. Sodium is predominantly an extracellular ion and is a primary determinant of the extracellular fluid volume. When NaCl intake exceeds the capacity of the kidney to excrete sodium, vascular volume initially expands and cardiac output increases. However, many vascular beds (including kidney and brain) have the capacity to autoregulate blood flow, and if constant blood flow is to be maintained in the face of increased arterial pressure, resistance within that bed must increase, since:

$$\text{Blood flow} = \frac{\text{pressure across the vascular bed}}{\text{vascular resistance}}$$

The initial elevation of blood pressure in response to vascular volume expansion is related to an increase of cardiac output; however, over time, peripheral resistance increases and cardiac output reverts toward normal. The effect of sodium on blood pressure is related to the provision of sodium with chloride; non-chloride salts of sodium have little or no effect on blood pressure. As arterial pressure increases in response to a high NaCl intake, urinary sodium excretion increases and sodium balance is maintained at the expense of an increase in arterial pressure. The mechanism for this "pressure-natriuresis" phenomenon may involve a subtle increase of glomerular filtration rate, decreased absorbing capacity of the renal tubules, and possibly hormonal factors such as atrial natriuretic factor. In individuals with an impaired capacity to excrete sodium, greater increases of arterial pressure are required to achieve natriuresis and sodium balance.

NaCl-dependent hypertension may be a consequence of a decreased capacity of the kidney to excrete sodium, due to either intrinsic renal disease or to increased production of a salt-retaining hormone (mineralocorticoid) resulting in increased renal tubular reabsorption of sodium. Renal tubular sodium reabsorption may also be augmented by increased neural activity to the kidney. In each of these situations, a higher arterial pressure may be required to achieve sodium balance, i.e., the pressure-natriuresis phenomenon. Conversely, salt-wasting disorders are associated with low blood pressure levels. ESRD is an extreme example of volume-dependent hypertension. In ~80% of these patients, vascular volume and hypertension can be controlled with adequate dialysis; in the other 20%, the mechanism of hypertension is related to increased activity of the renin-angiotensin system and is likely to be responsive to pharmacologic blockade of renin-angiotensin.

AUTONOMIC NERVOUS SYSTEM

The autonomic nervous system maintains cardiovascular homeostasis via pressure, volume, and chemoreceptor signals. Adrenergic reflexes modulate blood pressure over the short term, and adrenergic function, in concert with hormonal and volume-related factors, contributes to the long-term regulation of arterial pressure. The three endogenous catecholamines are norepinephrine, epinephrine, and dopamine. All three play important roles in tonic and phasic cardiovascular regulation. Adrenergic neurons synthesize norepinephrine and dopamine (a precursor of norepinephrine), which are stored in vesicles within the neuron. When the neuron is stimulated, these neurotransmitters are released into the synaptic cleft and to receptor sites on target tissues. Subsequently, the transmitter is either metabolized or taken up into the neuron by an active reuptake process. Epinephrine is synthesized in the adrenal medulla and released into the circulation upon adrenal stimulation.

The activities of the adrenergic receptors are mediated by guanosine nucleotide-binding regulatory proteins (G proteins) and by intracellular concentrations of downstream second messengers. In addition to receptor affinity and density, physiologic responsiveness to catecholamines may also be altered by the efficiency of receptor-effector coupling at a site "distal" to receptor binding. The receptor sites are relatively specific both for the transmitter substance and for the response that occupancy of the receptor site elicits. Norepinephrine and epinephrine are agonists for all adrenergic receptor subtypes, although with varying affinities. Based on their physiology and pharmacology, adrenergic receptors have been divided into two principal types: α and β. These types have been further differentiated into α_1, α_2, β_1, and β_2 receptors. Recent molecular cloning studies have identified several additional subtypes. α Receptors are more avidly occupied and activated by norepinephrine than by epinephrine, and the reverse is true for β receptors. α_1 Receptors are located on postsynaptic cells in smooth muscle and elicit vasoconstriction. α_2 Receptors are localized on presynaptic membranes of postganglionic nerve terminals that synthesize norepinephrine. When activated by catecholamines, α_2 receptors act as negative feedback controllers, inhibiting further norepinephrine release. Different classes of antihypertensive agents either inhibit α_1 receptors or act as agonists of α_2 receptors and reduce systemic sympathetic outflow. Activation of myocardial β_1 receptors stimulates the rate and strength of cardiac contraction, and consequently increases cardiac output. β_1 Receptor activation also stimulates renin release from the kidney. Another class of antihypertensive agents acts by inhibiting β_1 receptors. Activation of β_2 receptors by epinephrine relaxes vascular smooth muscle and results in vasodilation.

Circulating catecholamine concentrations may affect the number of adrenoreceptors in various tissues. Downregulation of receptors may be a consequence of sustained high levels of catecholamines and provides an explanation for decreasing responsiveness, or tachyphylaxis, to catecholamines. For example, orthostatic hypotension is frequently observed in patients with pheochromocytoma, possibly due to the lack of norepinephrine-induced vasoconstriction with assumption of the upright posture. Conversely, with chronic reduction of neurotransmitter substances, adrenoreceptors may increase in number, or be upregulated, resulting in increased responsiveness to the neurotransmitter. Chronic administration of agents that block adrenergic receptors may result in upregulation, and withdrawal of these agents may produce a condition of temporary hypersensitivity to sympathetic stimuli. For example, clonidine is an antihypertensive agent that is a centrally acting α_2 agonist that inhibits sympathetic outflow. Rebound hypertension may occur with the abrupt cessation of clonidine therapy, probably as a consequence of upregulation of α_1 receptors.

Several reflexes modulate blood pressure on a minute-to-minute basis. One arterial baroreflex is mediated by stretch-sensitive sensory nerve endings located in the carotid sinuses and the aortic arch. The rate of firing of these baroreceptors increases with arterial pressure, and the net effect is a decrease of sympathetic outflow, resulting in decreases of arterial pressure and heart rate. This is a primary mechanism for rapid buffering of acute fluctuations of arterial pressure that may occur during postural changes, behavioral or physiologic stress, and changes in blood volume. However, the activity of the baroreflex declines or adapts to sustained increases of arterial pressure such that the baroreceptors are reset to higher pressures. Patients with autonomic neuropathy and impaired baroreflex function may have extremely labile blood pressures with difficult-to-control episodic blood pressure spikes.

Pheochromocytoma is the most obvious example of hypertension related to increased catecholamine production, in this instance by a tumor. Blood pressure can be reduced by surgical excision of the tumor or by pharmacologic treatment with an α_1 receptor antagonist or with an inhibitor of tyrosine hydroxylase, the rate-limiting step in catecholamine biosynthesis. Increased sympathetic activity may contribute to other forms of hypertension. Drugs that block the sympathetic nervous system are potent antihypertensive agents, indicating that the sympathetic nervous system plays a permissive, although perhaps not a causative, role in the maintenance of increased arterial pressure.

RENIN-ANGIOTENSIN-ALDOSTERONE

The renin-angiotensin-aldosterone system contributes to the regulation of arterial pressure primarily via the vasoconstrictor properties of angiotensin II and the sodium-retaining properties of aldosterone. Renin is an aspartyl protease that is synthesized as an enzymatically inactive precursor, prorenin. Most renin in the circulation is synthesized in the segment of the renal afferent renal arteriole (juxtaglomerular cells) that abuts the glomerulus and a group of sensory cells located at the distal end of the loop of Henle, the macula densa. Prorenin may be secreted directly into the circulation or may be activated within secretory cells and released as active renin. Although human plasma contains two- to fivefold times more prorenin than renin, there is no evidence that prorenin contributes to the physiologic activity of this system. There are three primary stimuli for renin secretion: (1) decreased NaCl transport in the thick ascending limb of the loop of Henle (macula densa mechanism), (2) decreased pressure or stretch within the renal afferent arteriole (baroreceptor mechanism), and (3) sympathetic nervous system stimulation of renin-secreting cells via β_1 adrenoreceptors. Conversely, renin secretion is inhibited by increased NaCl transport in the thick ascending limb of the loop of Henle, by increased stretch within the renal afferent arteriole, and by β_1 receptor blockade. In addition, renin secretion may be modulated by a number of humoral factors, including angiotensin II. Angiotensin II directly inhibits renin secretion due to angiotensin II type 1 receptors on juxtaglomerular cells, and renin secretion increases in response to pharmacologic blockade of either ACE or angiotensin II receptors.

Once released into the circulation, active renin cleaves a substrate, angiotensinogen, to form an inactive decapeptide, angiotensin I (**Fig. 19-2**). A converting

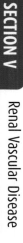

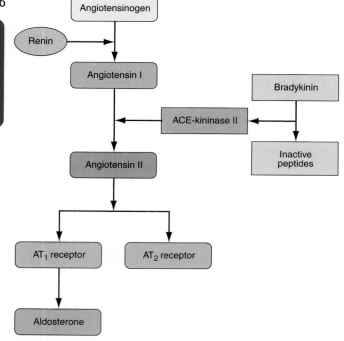

FIGURE 19-2
Renin-angiotensin-aldosterone axis.

enzyme, located primarily but not exclusively in the pulmonary circulation, converts angiotensin I to the active octapeptide, angiotensin II, by releasing the C-terminal histidyl-leucine dipeptide. The same converting enzyme cleaves a number of other peptides, including and thereby inactivating the vasodilator bradykinin. Acting primarily through angiotensin II type 1 (AT_1) receptors located on cell membranes, angiotensin II is a potent pressor substance, the primary trophic factor for the secretion of aldosterone by the adrenal zona glomerulosa, and a potent mitogen stimulating vascular smooth-muscle cell and myocyte growth. Independent of its hemodynamic effects, angiotensin II may play a role in the pathogenesis of atherosclerosis through a direct cellular action on the vessel wall. An angiotensin II type 2 (AT_2) receptor has been characterized. It is widely distributed in the kidney and has the opposite functional effects of the AT_1 receptor. The AT_2 receptor induces vasodilation, sodium excretion, and inhibition of cell growth and matrix formation. Experimental evidence suggests that the AT_2 receptor improves vascular remodeling by stimulating smooth-muscle cell apoptosis and contributes to the regulation of glomerular filtration rate. AT_1 receptor blockade induces an increase in AT_2 receptor activity. Currently, the AT_2 receptor has a less well defined functional role than the AT_1 receptor.

Renin-secreting tumors are clear examples of renin-dependent hypertension. In the kidney, these include benign hemangiopericytomas of the juxtaglomerular

apparatus, and infrequently renal carcinomas, including Wilms' tumors. Renin-producing carcinomas have also been described in lung, liver, pancreas, colon, and adrenals. In these instances, in addition to excision and/or ablation of the tumor, treatment of hypertension includes pharmacologic therapies targeted to inhibit angiotensin II production or action. Renovascular hypertension is another renin-mediated form of hypertension. Obstruction of the renal artery leads to decreased renal perfusion pressure, thereby stimulating renin secretion. Over time, as a consequence of secondary renal damage, this form of hypertension may become less renin dependent.

Angiotensinogen, renin, and angiotensin II are also synthesized locally in many tissues, including the brain, pituitary, aorta, arteries, heart, adrenal glands, kidneys, adipocytes, leukocytes, ovaries, testes, uterus, spleen, and skin. Angiotensin II in tissues may be formed by the enzymatic activity of renin or by other proteases, e.g., tonin, chymase, and cathepsins. In addition to regulating local blood flow, tissue angiotensin II is a mitogen that stimulates growth and contributes to modeling and repair. Excess tissue angiotensin II may contribute to atherosclerosis, cardiac hypertrophy, and renal failure and consequently may be a target for pharmacologic therapy to prevent target organ damage.

Angiotensin II is the primary trophic factor regulating the synthesis and secretion of aldosterone by the zona glomerulosa of the adrenal cortex. Aldosterone synthesis is also dependent on potassium, and aldosterone secretion may be decreased in potassium-depleted individuals. Although acute elevations of adrenocorticotropic hormone (ACTH) levels also increase aldosterone secretion, ACTH is not an important trophic factor for the chronic regulation of aldosterone.

Aldosterone is a potent mineralocorticoid that increases sodium reabsorption by amiloride-sensitive epithelial sodium channels (ENaC) on the apical surface of the principal cells of the renal cortical collecting duct (Chap. 1). Electric neutrality is maintained by exchanging sodium for potassium and hydrogen ions. Consequently, increased aldosterone secretion may result in hypokalemia and alkalosis. Because potassium depletion may inhibit aldosterone synthesis, clinically, hypokalemia should be corrected before evaluating a patient for hyperaldosteronism.

Mineralocorticoid receptors are also expressed in the colon, salivary glands, and sweat glands. Cortisol also binds to these receptors but normally functions as a less potent mineralocorticoid than aldosterone because cortisol is converted to cortisone by the enzyme 11 β-hydroxysteroid dehydrogenase type 2. Cortisone has no affinity for the mineralocorticoid receptor. Primary aldosteronism is a compelling example of mineralocorticoid-mediated hypertension. In this disorder, adrenal aldosterone synthesis and release are independent of renin-angiotensin, and renin release is suppressed by the resulting volume expansion.

Aldosterone also has effects on nonepithelial targets. Independent of a potential effect on blood pressure, aldosterone may also play a role in cardiac hypertrophy and CHF. Aldosterone acts via mineralocorticoid receptors within the myocardium to enhance extracellular matrix and collagen deposition. In animal models, high circulating aldosterone levels stimulate cardiac fibrosis and left ventricular hypertrophy, and spironolactone (an aldosterone antagonist) prevents aldosterone-induced myocardial fibrosis. Pathologic patterns of left ventricular geometry have also been associated with elevations of plasma aldosterone concentration in patients with essential hypertension, as well as in patients with primary aldosteronism. In patients with CHF, low-dose spironolactone reduces the risk of progressive heart failure and sudden death from cardiac causes by 30%. Owing to a renal hemodynamic effect, in patients with primary aldosteronism, high circulating levels of aldosterone may also cause glomerular hyperfiltration and albuminuria. These renal effects are reversible after removal of the effects of excess aldosterone by adrenalectomy or spironolactone.

Increased activity of the renin-angiotensin-aldosterone axis is not invariably associated with hypertension. In response to a low-NaCl diet or to volume contraction, arterial pressure and volume homeostasis may be maintained by increased activity of the renin-angiotensin-aldosterone axis. Secondary aldosteronism (i.e., increased aldosterone secondary to increased renin-angiotensin), but not hypertension, is also observed in edematous states such as CHF and liver disease.

VASCULAR MECHANISMS

Vascular radius and compliance of resistance arteries are also important determinants of arterial pressure. Resistance to flow varies inversely with the fourth power of the radius, and consequently small decreases in lumen size significantly increase resistance. In hypertensive patients, structural, mechanical, or functional changes may reduce lumen diameter of small arteries and arterioles. Remodeling refers to geometric alterations in the vessel wall without changing vessel volume. Hypertrophic (increased cell number, increased cell size, and increased deposition of intercellular matrix) or eutrophic (no change in the amount of material in the vessel wall) vascular remodeling results in decreased lumen size and hence contributes to increased peripheral resistance. Apoptosis, low-grade inflammation, and vascular fibrosis also contribute to remodeling. Lumen diameter is also related to elasticity of the vessel. Vessels with a high degree of elasticity can accommodate an increase of volume with relatively little change of pressure, whereas in a semi-rigid vascular system, a small increment in volume induces a relatively large increment of pressure.

Hypertensive patients have stiffer arteries, and arteriosclerotic patients may have particularly high systolic blood pressures and wide pulse pressures as a consequence of decreased vascular compliance due to structural changes in the vascular wall. Recent evidence suggests that arterial stiffness has independent predictive value for cardiovascular events. Clinically, a number of devices are available to evaluate arterial stiffness or compliance, including ultrasound and MRI.

Ion transport by vascular smooth-muscle cells may contribute to hypertension-associated abnormalities of vascular tone and vascular growth, both of which are modulated by intracellular pH (pH_i). Three ion transport mechanisms participate in the regulation of pH_i: (1) Na^+-H^+ exchange, (2) Na^+-dependent HCO_3^--Cl^- exchange, and (3) cation-independent HCO_3^--Cl^- exchange. Based on measurements in cell types that are more accessible than vascular smooth muscle (e.g., leukocytes, erythrocytes, platelets, skeletal muscle), activity of the Na^+-H^+ exchanger is increased in hypertension, and this may result in increased vascular tone by two mechanisms. First, increased sodium entry may lead to increased vascular tone by activating Na^+-Ca^{2+} exchange and thereby increasing intracellular calcium. Second, increased pH_i enhances calcium sensitivity of the contractile apparatus, leading to an increase in contractility for a given intracellular calcium concentration. Additionally, increased Na^+-H^+ exchange might stimulate vascular smooth-muscle cell growth by enhancing sensitivity to mitogens.

Vascular endothelial function also modulates vascular tone. The vascular endothelium synthesizes and releases a spectrum of vasoactive substances, including nitric oxide, a potent vasodilator. Endothelium-dependent vasodilation is impaired in hypertensive patients. This impairment is often assessed with high-resolution ultrasonography as flow-mediated vasodilation of the brachial artery. Alternatively, endothelium-dependent vasodilation may be assessed with venous occlusion plethysmography in response to an intraarterially infused endothelium-dependent vasodilator, e.g., acetylcholine.

Presently, it is not known if these hypertension-related vascular abnormalities of ion transport and endothelial function are primary alterations or secondary consequences of elevated arterial pressure. Limited evidence suggests that vascular compliance and endothelium-dependent vasodilation may be improved by aerobic exercise, weight loss, and antihypertensive agents. It remains to be determined whether these interventions affect arterial structure and stiffness via a blood pressure–independent mechanism and whether different classes of antihypertensive agents preferentially affect vascular structure and function.

PATHOLOGIC CONSEQUENCES OF HYPERTENSION

Hypertension is a risk factor for all clinical manifestations of atherosclerosis. It is an independent predisposing factor for heart failure, coronary artery disease, stroke, renal disease, and peripheral arterial disease (PAD).

HEART

Heart disease is the most common cause of death in hypertensive patients. Hypertensive heart disease is the result of structural and functional adaptations leading to left ventricular hypertrophy, diastolic dysfunction, CHF, abnormalities of blood flow due to atherosclerotic coronary artery disease and microvascular disease, and cardiac arrhythmias.

Both genetic and hemodynamic factors contribute to left ventricular hypertrophy. Clinically, left ventricular hypertrophy can be diagnosed by electrocardiogram, although echocardiography provides a more sensitive measure of left ventricular wall thickness. Individuals with left ventricular hypertrophy are at increased risk for CHD, stroke, CHF, and sudden death. Aggressive control of hypertension can regress or reverse left ventricular hypertrophy and reduce the risk of cardiovascular disease. It is not clear if different classes of antihypertensive agents have an added impact on reducing left ventricular mass, independent of their blood pressure–lowering effect.

Abnormalities of diastolic function, ranging from asymptomatic heart disease to overt heart failure, are common in hypertensive patients. Patients with diastolic heart failure have a preserved ejection fraction, which is a measure of systolic function. Approximately one-third of patients with CHF have normal systolic function but abnormal diastolic function. Diastolic dysfunction is an early consequence of hypertension-related heart disease and is exacerbated by left ventricular hypertrophy and ischemia. Clinically, cardiac catheterization provides the most accurate assessment of diastolic function; however, this is an invasive procedure and generally not indicated for the assessment of diastolic function. Alternatively, diastolic function can be evaluated by several noninvasive methods, including echocardiography and radionuclide angiography.

BRAIN

Hypertension is an important risk factor for brain infarction and hemorrhage. Approximately 85% of strokes are due to infarction and the remainder are due to hemorrhage, either intracerebral hemorrhage or subarachnoid hemorrhage. The incidence of stroke rises progressively with increasing blood pressure levels, particularly systolic blood pressure in individuals >65 years. Treatment of hypertension convincingly decreases the incidence of both ischemic and hemorrhagic strokes.

Hypertension is also associated with impaired cognition in an aging population, and longitudinal studies support an association between mid-life hypertension and late-life cognitive decline. Hypertension-related cognitive impairment and dementia may be a consequence of a single infarct due to occlusion of a "strategic" larger vessel or multiple lacunar infarcts due to occlusive small vessel disease resulting in subcortical white matter ischemia. Several clinical trials suggest that antihypertensive therapy has a beneficial effect on cognitive function, although this remains an active area of investigation.

Cerebral blood flow remains unchanged over a wide range of arterial pressures (mean arterial pressure of 50–150 mmHg) through a process termed *autoregulation* of blood flow. In patients with the clinical syndrome of malignant hypertension, encephalopathy is related to failure of autoregulation of cerebral blood flow at the upper pressure limit, resulting in vasodilation and hyperperfusion. Signs and symptoms of hypertensive encephalopathy may include severe headache, nausea and vomiting (often of a projectile nature), focal neurologic signs, and alterations in mental status. Untreated, hypertensive encephalopathy may progress to stupor, coma, seizures, and death within hours. It is important to distinguish hypertensive encephalopathy from other neurologic syndromes that may be associated with hypertension, e.g., cerebral ischemia, hemorrhagic or thrombotic stroke, seizure disorder, mass lesions, pseudotumor cerebri, delirium tremens, meningitis, acute intermittent porphyria, traumatic or chemical injury to the brain, and uremic encephalopathy.

KIDNEY

Primary renal disease is the most common etiology of secondary hypertension. Conversely, hypertension is a risk factor for renal injury and ESRD. The increased risk associated with high blood pressure is graded, continuous, and present throughout the entire distribution of blood pressure above optimal. Renal risk appears to be more closely related to systolic than to diastolic blood pressure, and black men are at greater risk than white men for developing ESRD at every level of blood pressure.

The atherosclerotic, hypertension-related vascular lesions in the kidney primarily affect the preglomerular arterioles, resulting in ischemic changes in the glomeruli and postglomerular structures. Glomerular injury may also be a consequence of direct damage to the glomerular capillaries due to glomerular hyperperfusion. Glomerular pathology progresses to glomerulosclerosis, and eventually the renal tubules may also become ischemic and gradually atrophic. The renal lesion associated with malignant hypertension consists of fibrinoid necrosis of the afferent arterioles, sometimes extending into the glomerulus, and may result in focal necrosis of the glomerular tuft.

Clinically, macroalbuminuria (a random urine albumin/creatinine ratio >300 mg/g) or microalbuminuria (a random urine albumin/creatinine ratio 30–300 mg/g) are early markers of renal injury. These are also risk factors for renal disease progression and for cardiovascular disease.

PERIPHERAL ARTERIES

In addition to contributing to the pathogenesis of hypertension, blood vessels may be a target organ for atherosclerotic disease secondary to long-standing elevated blood pressure. Hypertensive patients with arterial disease of the lower extremities are at increased risk for future cardiovascular disease. Although patients with stenotic lesions of the lower extremities may be asymptomatic, intermittent claudication is the classic symptom of PAD. This is characterized by aching pain in the calves or buttocks while walking that is relieved by rest. The ankle-brachial index is a useful approach for evaluating PAD and is defined as the ratio of noninvasively assessed ankle to brachial (arm) systolic blood pressure. An ankle-brachial index <0.90 is considered diagnostic of PAD and is associated with >50% stenosis in at least one major lower limb vessel. Several studies suggest that an ankle-brachial index <0.80 is associated with elevated blood pressure, particularly systolic blood pressure.

DEFINING HYPERTENSION

From an epidemiologic perspective, there is no obvious level of blood pressure that defines hypertension. In adults, there is a continuous, incremental risk of cardiovascular disease, stroke, and renal disease across levels of both systolic and diastolic blood pressure. The Multiple Risk Factor Intervention Trial (MRFIT), which included >350,000 male participants, demonstrated a continuous and graded influence of both systolic and diastolic blood pressure on CHD mortality, extending down to systolic blood pressures of 120 mmHg. Similarly, results of a meta-analysis involving almost 1 million participants indicate that ischemic heart disease mortality, stroke mortality, and mortality from other vascular causes are directly related to the height of the blood pressure, beginning at 115/75 mmHg, without evidence of a threshold. Cardiovascular disease risk doubles for every 20-mmHg increase in systolic and 10-mmHg increase in diastolic pressure. Among older individuals, systolic blood pressure and pulse pressure are more powerful predictors of cardiovascular disease than diastolic blood pressure.

Clinically, hypertension might be defined as that level of blood pressure at which the institution of therapy reduces blood pressure–related morbidity and mortality. Current clinical criteria for defining hypertension are

TABLE 19-1

BLOOD PRESSURE CLASSIFICATION

BLOOD PRESSURE CLASSIFICATION	SYSTOLIC, mmHg	DIASTOLIC, mmHg
Normal	<120	and <80
Prehypertension	120–139	or 80–89
Stage 1 hypertension	140–159	or 90–99
Stage 2 hypertension	≥160	or ≥100
Isolated systolic hypertension	≥140	and <90

Source: Adapted from Chobanian et al.

generally based on the average of two or more seated blood pressure readings during each of two or more outpatient visits. A recent classification recommends blood pressure criteria for defining normal blood pressure, prehypertension, hypertension (stages I and II), and isolated systolic hypertension, which is a common occurrence among the elderly (Table 19-1). In children and adolescents, hypertension is generally defined as systolic and/or diastolic blood pressure consistently >95th percentile for age, gender, and height. Blood pressures between the 90th and 95th percentiles are considered prehypertensive and are an indication for lifestyle interventions.

Home blood pressure and average 24-h ambulatory blood pressure measurements are generally lower than clinic blood pressures. Because ambulatory blood pressure recordings yield multiple readings throughout the day and night, they provide a more comprehensive assessment of the vascular burden of hypertension than a limited number of office readings. Increasing evidence suggests that home blood pressures, including 24-h blood pressure recordings, more reliably predict target organ damage than office blood pressures. Blood pressure tends to be higher in the early morning hours, soon after waking, than at other times of day. Myocardial infarction and stroke are more frequent in the early morning hours. Nighttime blood pressures are generally 10–20% lower than daytime blood pressures, and an attenuated nighttime blood pressure "dip" is associated with increased cardiovascular disease risk. Blunting of the day-night blood pressure pattern occurs in several clinical conditions, including sleep apnea and autonomic neuropathy, and in certain populations, including African Americans. Recommended criteria for a diagnosis of hypertension are average awake blood pressure ≥135/85 mmHg and asleep blood pressure ≥120/75 mmHg. These levels approximate a clinic blood pressure of 140/90 mmHg.

Approximately 15–20% of patients with stage 1 hypertension (as defined in Table 19-1) based on office blood pressures have average ambulatory readings <135/85 mmHg. This phenomenon, so-called white coat hypertension, may also be associated with an increased risk of target organ damage (e.g., left ventricular hypertrophy, carotid atherosclerosis, overall cardiovascular morbidity), although to a lesser extent than individuals with elevated office and ambulatory readings. Individuals with white coat hypertension are also at increased risk for developing sustained hypertension.

CLINICAL DISORDERS OF HYPERTENSION

Depending on methods of patient ascertainment, ~80–95% of hypertensive patients are diagnosed as having "essential" hypertension (also referred to as primary or idiopathic hypertension). In the remaining 5–20% of hypertensive patients, a specific underlying disorder causing the elevation of blood pressure can be identified (Tables 19-2 and 19-3). In individuals with "secondary" hypertension, a specific mechanism for the blood pressure elevation is often more apparent.

ESSENTIAL HYPERTENSION

Essential hypertension tends to be familial and is likely to be the consequence of an interaction between environmental and genetic factors. The prevalence of essential hypertension increases with age, and individuals with relatively high blood pressures at younger ages are at increased risk for the subsequent development of hypertension. It is likely that essential hypertension represents a spectrum of disorders with different underlying pathophysiologies. In the majority of patients with established hypertension, peripheral resistance is increased and cardiac output is normal or decreased; however, in younger patients with mild or labile hypertension, cardiac output may be increased and peripheral resistance may be normal.

When plasma renin activity (PRA) is plotted against 24-h sodium excretion, ~10–15% of hypertensive patients have high PRA and 25% have low PRA. High-renin patients may have a vasoconstrictor form of hypertension, whereas low-renin patients may have a volume-dependent hypertension. Inconsistent associations between

TABLE 19-2

SYSTOLIC HYPERTENSION WITH WIDE PULSE PRESSURE
1. Decreased vascular compliance (arteriosclerosis)
2. Increased cardiac output
a. Aortic regurgitation
b. Thyrotoxicosis
c. Hyperkinetic heart syndrome
d. Fever
e. Arteriovenous fistula
f. Patent ductus arteriosus

TABLE 19-3

SECONDARY CAUSES OF SYSTOLIC AND DIASTOLIC HYPERTENSION	
Renal	Parenchymal diseases, renal cysts (including polycystic kidney disease), renal tumors (including renin-secreting tumors), obstructive uropathy
Renovascular	Arteriosclerotic, fibromuscular dysplasia
Adrenal	Primary aldosteronism, Cushing's syndrome, 17α- hydroxylase deficiency, 11β- hydroxylase deficiency, 11- hydroxysteroid dehydrogenase deficiency (licorice), pheochromocytoma
Aortic coarctation	
Obstructive sleep apnea	
Preeclampsia/ eclampsia	
Neurogenic	Psychogenic, diencephalic syndrome, familial dysautonomia, polyneuritis (acute porphyria, lead poisoning), acute increased intracranial pressure, acute spinal cord section
Miscellaneous endocrine	Hypothyroidism, hyperthyroidism, hypercalcemia, acromegaly
Medications	High-dose estrogens, adrenal steroids, decongestants, appetite suppressants, cyclosporine, tricyclic antidepressants, monamine oxidase inhibitors, erythropoietin, nonsteroidal anti-inflammatory agents, cocaine
Mendelian forms of hypertension	See Table 19-4

plasma aldosterone and blood pressure have been described in patients with essential hypertension. The association between aldosterone and blood pressure is more striking in African Americans, and PRA tends to be low in hypertensive African Americans. This raises the possibility that subtle increases of aldosterone may contribute to hypertension in at least some groups of patients who do not have overt primary aldosteronism. Furthermore, spironolactone, an aldosterone antagonist, may be a particularly effective antihypertensive agent for some patients with essential hypertension, including some patients with "drug-resistant" hypertension.

METABOLIC SYNDROME

Hypertension and dyslipidemia frequently occur together and in association with resistance to insulin-stimulated glucose uptake. This clustering of risk factors is often, but not invariably, associated with obesity, particularly abdominal obesity. Insulin resistance is also associated with an unfavorable imbalance in the endothelial production of mediators that regulate platelet aggregation, coagulation, fibrinolysis, and vessel tone. When these risk factors cluster, the risks for CHD, stroke, diabetes, and cardiovascular disease mortality are further increased.

Depending on the populations studied and the methodologies for defining insulin resistance, ~25–50% of non-obese, non-diabetic hypertensive persons are insulin resistant. The constellation of insulin resistance, hypertension, and dyslipidemia has been designated as the *metabolic syndrome*. As a group, first-degree relatives of patients with essential hypertension are also insulin resistant, and hyperinsulinemia (a surrogate marker of insulin resistance) may predict the eventual development of hypertension and cardiovascular disease. Although the metabolic syndrome may in part be heritable as a polygenic condition, the expression of the syndrome is modified by environmental factors, such as degree of physical activity and diet. Insulin sensitivity increases and blood pressure decreases in response to weight loss. The recognition that cardiovascular disease risk factors tend to cluster within individuals has important implications for the evaluation and treatment of hypertension. Evaluation of both hypertensive patients and individuals at risk for developing hypertension should include assessment of overall cardiovascular disease risk. Similarly, introduction of lifestyle modification strategies and drug therapies should address overall risk, and not simply focus on hypertension.

RENAL PARENCHYMAL DISEASES

Virtually all disorders of the kidney may cause hypertension (Table 19-3), and renal disease is the most common cause of secondary hypertension. Hypertension is present in >80% of patients with chronic renal failure. In general, hypertension is more severe in glomerular diseases than in interstitial diseases, such as chronic pyelonephritis. Conversely, hypertension may cause nephrosclerosis, and in some instances it may be difficult to determine whether hypertension or renal disease was the initial disorder. Proteinuria >1000 mg/d and an active urine sediment are indicative of primary renal disease. In either instance, the goals are to control blood pressure and retard the rate of progression of renal dysfunction.

Renovascular Hypertension

Hypertension due to obstruction of a renal artery, renovascular hypertension, is a potentially curable form of hypertension. The mechanism of hypertension is generally related to activation of the renin-angiotensin system. Two groups of patients are at risk for this disorder: older arteriosclerotic patients who have a plaque obstructing

the renal artery, frequently at its origin, and patients with fibromuscular dysplasia. Although fibromuscular dysplasia may occur at any age, it has a strong predilection for young Caucasian women. The prevalence in females is eightfold that in males. There are several histologic variants of fibromuscular dysplasia, including medial fibroplasia, perimedial fibroplasia, medial hyperplasia, and intimal fibroplasia. Medial fibroplasia is the most common variant and accounts for approximately two-thirds of patients. The lesions of fibromuscular dysplasia are frequently bilateral, and in contrast to atherosclerotic renovascular disease, tend to affect more distal portions of the renal artery.

In addition to the age and gender of the patient, several clues from the history and physical examination suggest a diagnosis of renovascular hypertension. Patients should first be evaluated for evidence of atherosclerotic vascular disease. Although response to antihypertensive therapy does not exclude the diagnosis, severe or refractory hypertension, recent loss of hypertension control or recent onset of moderately severe hypertension, and unexplained deterioration of renal function or deterioration of renal function associated with an ACE inhibitor should raise the possibility of renovascular hypertension. Approximately 50% of patients with renovascular hypertension have an abdominal or flank bruit, and the bruit is more likely to be hemodynamically significant if it lateralizes or extends throughout systole into diastole.

If blood pressure is adequately controlled with a simple antihypertensive regimen and renal function remains stable, there may be little impetus to pursue an evaluation for renal artery stenosis, particularly in an older patient with atherosclerotic disease and comorbid conditions. Patients with long-standing hypertension, advanced renal insufficiency, or diabetes mellitus are less likely to benefit from renal vascular repair. The most effective medical therapies include an ACE inhibitor or an angiotensin II receptor blocker; however, these agents decrease glomerular filtration rate in the stenotic kidney owing to efferent renal arteriolar dilation. In the presence of bilateral renal artery stenosis or renal artery stenosis to a solitary kidney, progressive renal insufficiency may result from the use of these agents. Importantly, the renal insufficiency is generally reversible following discontinuation of the offending drug.

If renal artery stenosis is suspected, and if the clinical condition warrants an intervention such as percutaneous transluminal renal angioplasty (PTRA), placement of a vascular endoprosthesis (stent), or surgical renal revascularization, imaging studies should be the next step in the evaluation. As a screening test, renal blood flow may be evaluated with a radionuclide [^{131}I]-orthoiodohippurate (OIH) scan or glomerular filtration rate may be evaluated with [^{99m}Tc]-diethylenetriamine pentaacetic acid (DTPA) scan, before and after a single dose of captopril (or other ACE inhibitor). The following are consistent with a positive study: (1) decreased relative uptake by the involved kidney, which contributes <40% of total renal function; (2) delayed uptake on the affected side; or (3) delayed washout on the affected side. In patients with normal, or near-normal, renal function, a normal captopril renogram essentially excludes functionally significant renal artery stenosis; however, its usefulness is limited in patients with renal insufficiency (creatinine clearance <20 mL/min) or bilateral renal artery stenosis. Additional imaging studies are indicated if the scan is positive. Doppler ultrasound of the renal arteries produces reliable estimates of renal blood flow velocity and offers the opportunity to track a lesion over time. Positive studies are usually confirmed at angiography, whereas false-negative results occur frequently, particularly in obese patients. Gadolinium-contrast magnetic resonance angiography offers clear images of the proximal renal artery but may miss distal lesions. An advantage is the opportunity to image the renal arteries with an agent that is not nephrotoxic. Contrast arteriography remains the "gold standard" for evaluation and identification of renal artery lesions. Potential risks include nephrotoxicity, particularly in patients with diabetes mellitus or preexisting renal insufficiency.

Some degree of renal artery obstruction may be observed in almost 50% of patients with atherosclerotic disease, and there are several approaches for evaluating the functional significance of such a lesion to predict the effect of vascular repair on blood pressure control and renal function. Each approach has varying degrees of sensitivity and specificity, and no single test is sufficiently reliable to determine a causal relationship between a renal artery lesion and hypertension. On angiography, the presence of collateral vessels to the ischemic kidney suggests a functionally significant lesion. A lateralizing renal vein renin ratio (ratio >1.5 of affected side/contralateral side) has a 90% predictive value for a lesion that would respond to vascular repair; however, the false-negative rate for blood pressure control is 50–60%. Measurement of the pressure gradient across a renal artery lesion does not reliably predict the response to vascular repair.

In the final analysis, a decision concerning vascular repair vs. medical therapy and the type of repair procedure should be individualized for each patient. Patients with fibromuscular disease have more favorable outcomes than patients with atherosclerotic lesions, presumably owing to their younger age, shorter duration of hypertension, and less systemic disease. Because of its low risk-versus-benefit ratio and high success rate (improvement or cure of hypertension in 90% of patients and restenosis rate of 10%), PTRA is the initial treatment of choice for these patients. Surgical revascularization may be undertaken if PTRA is unsuccessful or if a branch lesion is present. In atherosclerotic patients, vascular repair should be considered if blood pressure cannot be adequately controlled with medical therapy or if renal function deteriorates. Surgery may be the preferred initial approach for younger atherosclerotic patients without comorbid conditions; however, for most atherosclerotic patients, depending on the location of the lesion, the initial approach may be PTRA and/or stenting. Surgical revascularization may be indicated if these approaches are unsuccessful, if the vascular lesion is not amenable to PTRA or stenting, or if concomitant aortic surgery is required, e.g., to repair an aneurysm.

PRIMARY ALDOSTERONISM

Excess aldosterone production due to primary aldosteronism is a potentially curable form of hypertension. In patients with primary aldosteronism, increased aldosterone production is independent of the renin-angiotensin system, and the consequences are sodium retention, hypertension, hypokalemia, and low PRA. The reported prevalence of this disorder varies from <2% to ~15% of hypertensive individuals. In part, this variation is related to the intensity of screening and to the criteria for establishing the diagnosis.

History and physical examination provide little information about the diagnosis. The age at the time of diagnosis is generally in the third through fifth decades. Hypertension is usually mild to moderate but occasionally may be severe; primary aldosteronism should be considered in all patients with refractory hypertension. Hypertension in these patients may be associated with glucose intolerance. Most patients are asymptomatic, although, infrequently, polyuria, polydipsia, paresthesias, or muscle weakness may be present as a consequence of hypokalemic alkalosis. The simplest screening test is measurement of serum potassium concentration. In a hypertensive patient with unprovoked hypokalemia (i.e., unrelated to diuretics, vomiting, or diarrhea), the prevalence of primary aldosteronism approaches 40–50%. In patients on diuretics, serum potassium <3.1 mmol/L (<3.1 meq/L) also raises the possibility of primary aldosteronism; however, serum potassium is an insensitive and nonspecific screening test. On initial presentation, serum potassium is normal in ~25% of patients subsequently found to have an aldosterone-producing adenoma, and higher percentages of patients with other etiologies of primary aldosteronism are not hypokalemic. Additionally, hypokalemic hypertension may be a consequence of secondary aldosteronism, other mineralocorticoid- and glucocorticoid-induced hypertensive disorders, and pheochromocytoma.

The ratio of plasma aldosterone to plasma renin activity (PA/PRA) is a useful screening test. These measurements are preferably obtained in ambulatory patients in the morning. A ratio >30:1 in conjunction with a plasma aldosterone concentration >555 pmol/L (>20 ng/dL) reportedly has a sensitivity of 90% and a specificity of 91% for an aldosterone-producing adenoma. In a Mayo Clinic series, an aldosterone-producing adenoma was subsequently surgically confirmed in >90% of hypertensive patients with a PA/PRA ratio ≥20 and a plasma aldosterone concentration ≥415 pmol/L (≥15 ng/dL). There are, however, several caveats to interpreting the ratio. The cutoff for a "high" ratio is laboratory and assay dependent. Although some antihypertensive agents may affect the ratio (e.g., aldosterone antagonists, angiotensin receptor antagonists, and ACE inhibitors may increase renin; aldosterone antagonists may increase aldosterone), the ratio has been reported to be useful as a screening test in measurements obtained with patients taking their usual antihypertensive medications. A high ratio in the absence of an elevated plasma aldosterone level is considerably less specific for primary aldosteronism since many patients with essential hypertension have low renin levels in this setting, particularly African Americans and elderly patients. In patients with renal insufficiency, the ratio may also be elevated because of decreased aldosterone clearance. In patients with an elevated PA/PRA ratio, the diagnosis of primary aldosteronism can be confirmed by demonstrating failure to suppress plasma aldosterone to <277 pmol/L (<10 ng/dL) after IV infusion of 2 L of isotonic saline over 4 h.

Several adrenal abnormalities may culminate in the syndrome of primary aldosteronism, and appropriate therapy depends on the specific etiology. Some 60–70% of patients have an aldosterone-producing adrenal adenoma. The tumor is almost always unilateral, and most measure <3 cm in diameter. Most of the remainder have bilateral adrenocortical hyperplasia (idiopathic hyperaldosteronism). Rarely, primary aldosteronism may be caused by an adrenal carcinoma or an ectopic malignancy, e.g., ovarian arrhenoblastoma. Most aldosterone-producing carcinomas, in contrast to adrenal adenomas and hyperplasia, produce excessive amounts of other adrenal steroids in addition to aldosterone. Functional differences in hormone secretion may assist in the differential diagnosis. Aldosterone biosynthesis is more responsive to ACTH in patients with adenoma and more responsive to angiotensin in patients with hyperplasia. Consequently, patients with adenoma tend to have higher plasma aldosterone in the early morning that decreases during the day, reflecting the diurnal rhythm of ACTH, whereas plasma aldosterone tends to increase with upright posture in patients with hyperplasia, reflecting the normal postural response of the renin-angiotensin-aldosterone axis.

Adrenal CT or MRI should be carried out in all patients diagnosed with primary aldosteronism. High-resolution CT may identify tumors as small as 0.3 cm and is positive for an adrenal tumor 90% of the time. If the CT or MRI is not diagnostic, an adenoma may be detected by adrenal scintigraphy with 6 β-[I[131]] iodomethyl-19-norcholesterol after dexamethasone suppression (0.5 mg every 6 h for 7 days); however, this technique has decreased sensitivity for adenomas <1 cm. When results of functional and anatomic studies are inconclusive, bilateral adrenal venous sampling for aldosterone and cortisol levels in response to ACTH stimulation should be carried out. An ipsilateral/contralateral aldosterone ratio >10, with symmetric ACTH-stimulated cortisol levels, is diagnostic of an aldosterone-producing adenoma.

Hypertension is generally responsive to surgery in patients with adenoma but not in patients with bilateral adrenal hyperplasia. Unilateral adrenalectomy, often done via a laparoscopic approach, is curative in 40–70% of patients with an adenoma. Surgery should be undertaken after blood pressure has been controlled and hypokalemia corrected. Transient hypoaldosteronism may occur for up to 3 months postoperatively, resulting in hyperkalemia. Potassium should be monitored during this time, and hyperkalemia should be treated with potassium-wasting diuretics and with fludrocortisone, if needed. Patients with bilateral hyperplasia should be treated medically. The drug regimen for these patients, as well as for patients with an adenoma who are poor surgical candidates, should include an aldosterone antagonist and, if necessary, other potassium-sparing diuretics.

Glucocorticoid-remediable hyperaldosteronism is a rare, monogenic autosomal dominant disorder characterized by moderate to severe hypertension, often at an early age. Hypokalemia is usually mild or absent. Normally, angiotensin II stimulates aldosterone production by the adrenal zona glomerulosa, whereas ACTH stimulates cortisol production in the zona fasciculata. Owing to a chimeric gene on chromosome 8, ACTH also regulates aldosterone secretion by the zona fasciculata in patients with glucocorticoid-remediable hyperaldosteronism. The consequence is overproduction in the zona fasciculata of both aldosterone and hybrid steroids (18-hydroxycortisol and 18-oxocortisol) due to oxidation of cortisol. The diagnosis may be established by urine excretion rates of these hybrid steroids that are twenty to thirty times normal or by direct genetic testing. Therapeutically, suppression of ACTH with low-dose glucocorticoids corrects the hyperaldosteronism, hypertension, and hypokalemia. Spironolactone is also a therapeutic option.

CUSHING'S SYNDROME

Hypertension occurs in 75–80% of patients with Cushing's syndrome. The mechanism of hypertension may be related to stimulation of mineralocorticoid receptors by cortisol and increased secretion of other adrenal steroids. If clinically suspected, in patients not taking exogenous glucocorticoids, laboratory screening may be carried out with measurement of 24-h excretion rates of urine free cortisol or an overnight dexamethasone-suppression test. Recent evidence suggests that late night salivary cortisol is a sensitive and convenient screening test. Further evaluation is required to confirm the diagnosis and to identify the specific etiology of Cushing's syndrome. Appropriate therapy depends on the etiology.

PHEOCHROMOCYTOMA

Catecholamine-secreting tumors are located in the adrenal medulla (pheochromocytoma) or in extra-adrenal paraganglion tissue (paraganglioma) and account for hypertension in ~0.05% of patients. Approximately 20%

of pheochromocytomas are familial with an autosomal dominant inheritance. Inherited pheochromocytomas may be associated with multiple endocrine neoplasia (MEN) type 2A and type 2B (Table 19-4). If unrecognized, pheochromocytoma may result in lethal cardiovascular consequences. Clinical manifestations, including hypertension, are primarily related to increased circulating catecholamines, although some of these tumors may secrete a number of other vasoactive substances. In a small percent of patients, epinephrine is the predominant catecholamine secreted by the tumor, and these patients may present with hypotension rather than hypertension. The initial suspicion of the diagnosis is based on symptoms and/or the association of pheochromocytoma with other

TABLE 19-4

RARE MENDELIAN FORMS OF HYPERTENSION

DISEASE	PHENOTYPE	GENETIC CAUSE
Glucocorticoid-remediable hyperaldosteronism	Autosomal dominant Absent or mild hypokalemia	Chimeric 11β-hydroxylase/aldoterone gene on chromosome 8
17α-hydroxylase deficiency	Autosomal recessive Males: pseudohermaphroditism Females: primary amenorrhea, absent secondary sexual characteristics	Random mutations of the CYP17 gene on chromosome 10
11β-hydroxylase deficiency	Autosomal recessive Masculinization	Mutations of the CYP11B1 gene on chromosome 8q21-q22
11β-hydroxysteroid dehydrogenase deficiency (apparent mineralo-corticoid excess syndrome)	Autosomal recessive Hypokalemia, low renin, low aldosterone	Mutations in the 11β-hydroxysteroid dehydrogenase gene
Liddle's syndrome	Autosomal dominant Hypokalemia, low renin, low aldosterone	Mutation subunits of the epithelial sodium channel SCNN1B and SCNN1C genes
Pseudohypoaldosteronism type II (Gordon's syndrome)	Autosomal dominant Hyperkalemia, normal glomerular filtration rate	Linkage to chromosomes 1q31-q42 and 17p11-q21
Hypertension exacerbated in pregnancy	Autosomal dominant Severe hypertension in early pregnancy	Missense mutation with substitution of leucine for serine at codon 810 (MR$_{L810}$)
Polycystic kidney disease	Autosomal dominant Large cystic kidneys, renal failure, liver cysts, cerebral aneurysms, valvular heart disease	Mutations in the PKD1 gene on chromosome 16 and PKD2 gene on chromosome 4
Pheochromocytoma	Autosomal dominant	
	(a) Multiple endocrine neoplasia, type 2A Medullary thyroid carcinoma, hyperparathyroidism	(a) Mutations in the RET protooncogene
	(b) Multiple endocrine neoplasia, type 2B Medullary thyroid carcinoma, mucosal neuromas, thickened corneal nerves, alimentary ganglioneuromatoses, marfanoid habitus	(b) Mutations in the RET protooncogene
	(c) von Hippel–Lindau disease Retinal angiomas, hemangioblastomas of the cerebellum and spinal cord, renal cell carcinoma	(c) Mutations in the VHL tumor-suppressor gene
	(d) Neurofibromatosis type 1 Multiple neurofibromas, café au lait spots	(d) Mutations in the NF1 tumor-suppressor gene

disorders (Table 19-4). Laboratory testing consists of measuring catecholamines in either urine or plasma. Genetic screening is also available for evaluating patients and relatives suspected of harboring a pheochromocytoma associated with a familial syndrome. Surgical excision is the definitive treatment of pheochromocytoma and results in cure in ~90% of patients.

MISCELLANEOUS CAUSES OF HYPERTENSION

Hypertension due to *obstructive sleep apnea* is being recognized with increasing frequency. Independent of obesity, hypertension occurs in >50% of individuals with obstructive sleep apnea, the severe end of the sleep-disordered breathing syndrome. The severity of hypertension correlates with the severity of sleep apnea. Approximately 70% of patients with obstructive sleep apnea are obese. Hypertension related to obstructive sleep apnea should also be considered in patients with drug-resistant hypertension and in patients with a history of snoring. The diagnosis can be confirmed by polysomnography. In obese patients, weight loss may alleviate or cure sleep apnea and related hypertension. Continuous positive airway pressure (CPAP) administered during sleep is an effective therapy for obstructive sleep apnea. With CPAP, patients with apparently drug-resistant hypertension may be more responsive to antihypertensive agents.

Coarctation of the aorta is the most common congenital cardiovascular cause of hypertension. The incidence is 1–8 per 1000 live births. It is usually sporadic but occurs in 35% of children with Turner's syndrome. Even when the anatomic lesion is surgically corrected in infancy, up to 30% of patients develop subsequent hypertension and are at risk of accelerated coronary artery disease and cerebrovascular events. Patients with less severe lesions may not be diagnosed until young adulthood. The physical findings are diagnostic, and include diminished and delayed femoral pulses and a systolic pressure gradient between the right arm and the legs, and, depending on the location of the coarctation, between the right and left arms. A blowing systolic murmur may be heard in the posterior left interscapular areas. The diagnosis may be confirmed by chest x-ray and transesophageal echocardiogram. Therapeutic options include surgical repair or balloon angioplasty, with or without placement of an intravascular stent. Subsequently, many patients do not have a normal life expectancy but may have persistent hypertension with death due to ischemic heart disease, cerebral hemorrhage, or aortic aneurysm.

Several additional endocrine disorders, including *thyroid diseases* and *acromegaly*, cause hypertension. Mild diastolic hypertension may be a consequence of hypothyroidism, whereas hyperthyroidism may result in systolic hypertension. *Hypercalcemia* of any etiology, the most common being primary hyperparathyroidism, may result in

hypertension. Hypertension may also be related to a number of prescribed or over-the-counter *medications*.

MONOGENIC HYPERTENSION

A number of rare forms of monogenic hypertension have been identified (Table 19-4). These disorders may be recognized by their characteristic phenotypes, and in many instances the diagnosis may be confirmed by genetic analysis. Several inherited defects in adrenal steroid biosynthesis and metabolism result in mineralocorticoid-induced hypertension and hypokalemia. In patients with a 17α-hydroxylase deficiency, synthesis of sex hormones and cortisol is decreased (Fig. 19-3). Consequently, these individuals do not mature sexually; males may present with pseudohermaphroditism and females with primary amenorrhea and absent secondary sexual characteristics. Because cortisol-induced negative feedback on pituitary ACTH production is diminished, ACTH-stimulated adrenal steroid synthesis proximal to the enzymatic block is increased. Hypertension and hypokalemia are consequences of increased synthesis of mineralocorticoids proximal to the enzymatic block, particularly desoxycorticosterone. Increased steroid production and, hence, hypertension may be treated with low-dose glucocorticoids. An 11β-hydroxylase deficiency results in a salt-retaining adrenogenital syndrome, occurring in 1 in 100,000 live births. This enzymatic defect results in decreased cortisol synthesis, increased synthesis of mineralocorticoids (e.g., desoxycorticosterone), and shunting of steroid biosynthesis into the androgen pathway. In the severe form, the syndrome may present early in life, including the newborn period, with virilization and ambiguous genitalia in females and penile enlargement in males, or in older children as precocious puberty and short stature. Acne, hirsutism, and menstrual irregularities may be the presenting features when the disorder is first recognized in adolescence or early adulthood. Hypertension is less common in the late-onset forms. Patients with an 11β-hydroxysteroid dehydrogenase deficiency have an impaired capacity to metabolize cortisol to its inactive metabolite, cortisone, and hypertension is related to activation of mineralocorticoid receptors by cortisol. This defect may be inherited or acquired, due to licorice-containing glycyrrhizic acid. This same substance is present in the paste of several brands of chewing tobacco. The defect in Liddle's syndrome (Chap. 6) results from constitutive activation of amiloride-sensitive epithelial sodium channels (ENaC) on the distal renal tubule, resulting in excess sodium reabsorption; the syndrome is ameliorated by amiloride. Hypertension exacerbated in pregnancy is due to activation of the mineralocorticoid receptor by progesterone. Approximately 20% of pheochromocytomas are familial and may be associated with distinctive phenotypes.

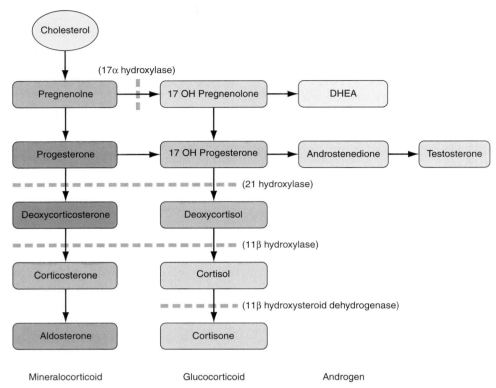

FIGURE 19-3
Adrenal enzymatic defects.

Approach to the Patient:
HYPERTENSION

HISTORY The initial assessment of the hypertensive patient should include a complete history and physical examination to confirm a diagnosis of hypertension, screen for other cardiovascular disease risk factors, screen for secondary causes of hypertension, identify cardiovascular consequences of hypertension and other comorbidities, assess blood pressure–related lifestyles, and determine the potential for intervention.

Most patients with hypertension have no specific symptoms referable to their blood pressure elevation. Although popularly considered a symptom of elevated arterial pressure, headache generally occurs only in patients with severe hypertension. Characteristically, a "hypertensive headache" occurs in the morning and is localized to the occipital region. Other nonspecific symptoms that may be related to elevated blood pressure include dizziness, palpitations, easy fatigability, and impotence. When symptoms are present, they are generally related to hypertensive cardiovascular disease or to manifestations of secondary hypertension. Table 19–5 lists salient features that should be addressed in obtaining a history from a hypertensive patient.

TABLE 19-5

PATIENT'S RELEVANT HISTORY
Duration of hypertension
Previous therapies: responses and side effects
Family history of hypertension and cardiovascular disease
Dietary and psychosocial history
Other risk factors: weight change, dyslipidemia, smoking, diabetes, physical inactivity
Evidence of secondary hypertension: history of renal disease; change in appearance; muscle weakness; spells of sweating, palpitations, tremor; erratic sleep, snoring, daytime somnolence; symptoms of hypo- or hyperthyroidism; use of agents that may increase blood pressure
Evidence of target organ damage: history of TIA, stroke, transient blindness; angina, myocardial infarction, congestive heart failure; sexual function
Other comorbidities

Note: TIA, transient ischemic attack.

MEASUREMENT OF BLOOD PRESSURE Reliable measurements of blood pressure depend on attention to the details of the technique and conditions of the measurement. Owing to recent regulations preventing the use of mercury because of concerns about its potential toxicity, most office measurements are made with aneroid instruments. The accuracy of automated blood pressure instruments should be confirmed. Before taking the blood pressure measurement, the individual should be seated quietly for 5 min in a private, quiet setting with a comfortable room temperature. The center of the cuff should be at heart level, and the width of the bladder cuff should equal at least 40% of the arm circumference; the length of the cuff bladder should encircle at least 80% of the arm circumference. It is important to pay attention to cuff placement, stethoscope placement, and the rate of deflation of the cuff (2 mmHg/s). Systolic blood pressure is the first of at least two regular "tapping" Korotkoff sounds, and diastolic blood pressure is the point at which the last regular Korotkoff sound is heard. In current practice, a diagnosis of hypertension is generally based on seated, office measurements.

Currently available ambulatory monitors are fully automated, use the oscillometric technique, and typically are programmed to take readings every 15–30 min. Ambulatory blood pressure monitoring is not, however, routinely used in clinical practice and is generally reserved for patients in whom white coat hypertension is suspected. The Seventh Report of the Joint National Committee on Prevention, Detection, Evaluation, and Treatment of High Blood Pressure (JNC 7) has also recommended ambulatory monitoring for treatment resistance, symptomatic hypotension, autonomic failure, and episodic hypertension.

PHYSICAL EXAMINATION Body habitus, including weight and height, should be noted. At the initial examination, blood pressure should be measured in both arms, and preferably in the supine, sitting, and standing positions to evaluate for postural hypotension. Even if the femoral pulse is normal to palpation, arterial pressure should be measured at least once in the lower extremity in patients in whom hypertension is discovered before age 30. Heart rate should also be recorded. Hypertensive individuals have an increased prevalence of atrial fibrillation. The neck should be palpated for an enlarged thyroid gland, and patients should be assessed for signs of hypo- and hyperthyroidism. Examination of blood vessels may provide clues about underlying vascular disease and should include funduscopic examination, auscultation for bruits over the carotid and femoral arteries, and palpation of femoral and pedal pulses. The retina is the only tissue in which arteries and arterioles can be examined directly. With increasing severity of hypertension and atherosclerotic disease, progressive funduscopic changes include increased arteriolar light reflex, arteriovenous crossing defects, hemorrhages and exudates and, in patients with malignant hypertension, papilledema. Examination

of the heart may reveal a loud second heart sound due to closure of the aortic valve and an S_4 gallop, attributed to atrial contraction against a noncompliant left ventricle. Left ventricular hypertrophy may be detected by an enlarged, sustained, and laterally displaced apical impulse. An abdominal bruit, particularly a bruit that lateralizes and extends throughout systole into diastole, raises the possibility of renovascular hypertension. Kidneys of patients with polycystic kidney disease may be palpable in the abdomen. The physical examination should also include evaluation for signs of CHF and a neurologic examination.

LABORATORY TESTING Table 19-6 lists recommended laboratory tests in the initial evaluation of hypertensive patients. Repeat measurements of renal function, serum electrolytes, fasting glucose, and lipids may be obtained after introducing a new antihypertensive agent and then annually, or more frequently if clinically indicated. More extensive laboratory testing is appropriate for patients with apparent drug-resistant hypertension or when the clinical evaluation suggests a secondary form of hypertension.

℞ Treatment:
HYPERTENSION

LIFESTYLE INTERVENTIONS Implementation of lifestyles that favorably affect blood pressure has implications for both the prevention and treatment of hypertension. Health-promoting lifestyle modifications are recommended for individuals with pre-hypertension and as an adjunct to drug therapy in hypertensive individuals. These interventions should address overall cardiovascular disease risk. Although the impact of lifestyle interventions on blood pressure is more pronounced in persons with hypertension, in short-term trials, weight loss and

TABLE 19-6

BASIC LABORATORY TESTS FOR INITIAL EVALUATION	
SYSTEM	**TEST**
Renal	Microscopic urinalysis, albumin excretion, serum BUN and/or creatinine
Endocrine	Serum sodium, potassium, calcium, ?TSH
Metabolic	Fasting blood glucose, total cholesterol, HDL and LDL (often computed) cholesterol, triglycerides
Other	Hematocrit, electrocardiogram

Note: BUN, blood urea nitrogen; TSH, thyroid-stimulating hormone; HDL/LDL, high-/low-density lipoprotein.

reduction of dietary NaCl have also been shown to prevent the development of hypertension. In hypertensive individuals, even if these interventions do not produce a sufficient reduction of blood pressure to avoid drug therapy, the number of medications or dosages required for blood pressure control may be reduced. Dietary modifications that effectively lower blood pressure are weight loss, reduced NaCl intake, increased potassium intake, moderation of alcohol consumption, and an overall healthy dietary pattern (Table 19-7).

Prevention and treatment of obesity are important for reducing blood pressure and cardiovascular disease risk. In short-term trials, even modest weight loss can lead to a reduction of blood pressure and an increase of insulin sensitivity. Average blood pressure reductions of 6.3/3.1 mmHg have been observed with a reduction in mean body weight of 9.2 kg. Regular physical activity facilitates weight loss, decreases blood pressure, and reduces the overall risk of cardiovascular disease. Blood pressure may be lowered by 30 min of moderately intense physical activity, such as brisk walking, 6–7 days a week, or by more intense, less frequent workouts.

There is individual variability in the sensitivity of blood pressure to NaCl, and this variability may have a genetic basis. Based on results of meta-analyses, lowering of blood pressure by limiting daily NaCl intake to 4.4–7.4 g (75–125 meq) results in blood pressure reductions of 3.7–4.9/0.9–2.9 mmHg in hypertensive and lesser reductions in normotensive individuals. Diets deficient in potassium, calcium, and magnesium are associated with higher blood pressures and a higher prevalence of hypertension. The urine sodium-to-potassium ratio is a stronger correlate of blood pressure than either sodium or potassium alone. Potassium and calcium supplementation have inconsistent, modest antihypertensive effects, and, independent of blood pressure, potassium supplementation may be associated with reduced stroke

mortality. Alcohol use in persons consuming three or more drinks per day (a standard drink contains ~14 g ethanol) is associated with higher blood pressures, and a reduction of alcohol consumption is associated with a reduction of blood pressure. Mechanisms by which dietary potassium, calcium, or alcohol may affect blood pressure have not been established.

The DASH (Dietary Approaches to Stop Hypertension) trial convincingly demonstrated that over an 8-week period a diet high in fruits, vegetables, and low-fat dairy products lowers blood pressure in individuals with high-normal blood pressures or mild hypertension. Reduction of daily NaCl intake to <6 g (100 meq) augmented the effect of this diet on blood pressure. Fruits and vegetables are enriched sources of potassium, magnesium, and fiber, and dairy products are an important source of calcium.

PHARMACOLOGIC THERAPY Drug therapy is recommended for individuals with blood pressures ≥140/90 mmHg. The degree of benefit derived from antihypertensive agents is related to the magnitude of the blood pressure reduction. Lowering systolic blood pressure by 10–12 mmHg and diastolic blood pressure by 5–6 mmHg confers relative risk reductions of 35–40% for stroke and 12–16% for CHD within 5 years of initiating treatment. Risk of heart failure is reduced by >50%. There is considerable variation in individual responses to different classes of antihypertensive agents, and the magnitude of response to any single agent may be limited by activation of counterregulatory mechanisms that oppose the hypotensive effect of the agent. Selection of antihypertensive agents, and combinations of agents, should be individualized, taking into account age, severity of hypertension, other cardiovascular disease risk factors, comorbid conditions, and practical considerations related to cost, side effects, and frequency of dosing (Table 19-8).

Diuretics Low-dose thiazide diuretics are often used as first-line agents, alone or in combination with other antihypertensive drugs. Thiazides inhibit the Na^+/Cl^- pump in the distal convoluted tubule and, hence, increase sodium excretion. Long term, they may also act as vasodilators. Thiazides are safe, efficacious, and inexpensive, and reduce clinical events. They provide additive blood pressure–lowering effects when combined with beta blockers, ACE inhibitors, or angiotensin receptor blockers. In contrast, addition of a diuretic to a calcium channel blocker is less effective. Usual doses of hydrochlorothiazide range from 6.25–50 mg/d. Owing to an increased incidence of metabolic side effects (hypokalemia, insulin resistance, increased cholesterol), higher doses are generally not recommended. Two potassium-sparing diuretics, amiloride and triamterene, act by inhibiting epithelial sodium channels in the distal

TABLE 19-7

LIFESTYLE MODIFICATIONS TO MANAGE HYPERTENSION	
Weight reduction	Attain and maintain BMI <25 kg/m²
Dietary salt reduction	<6 g NaCl/d
Adapt DASH-type dietary plan	Diet rich in fruits, vegetables, and low-fat dairy products with reduced content of saturated and total fat
Moderation of alcohol consumption	For those who drink alcohol, consume ≤2 drinks/day in men and ≤1 drink/day in women
Physical activity	Regular aerobic activity, e.g., brisk walking for 30 min/d

Note: BMI, body mass index; DASH, Dietary Approaches to Stop Hypertension (trial).

TABLE 19-8

EXAMPLES OF ORAL DRUGS USED IN TREATMENT OF HYPERTENSION

DRUG CLASS	EXAMPLES	USUAL TOTAL DAILY DOSE[a] (DOSING FREQUENCY/DAY)	OTHER INDICATIONS	CONTRAINDICATIONS/ CAUTIONS
Diuretics				
Thiazides	Hydrochlorothiazide	6.25–50 mg (1–2)		Diabetes, dyslipidemia, hyperuricemia, gout, hypokalemia
	Chlorthalidone	25–50 mg (1)		
Loop diuretics	Furosemide	40–80 mg (2–3)	CHF, renal failure	Diabetes, dyslipidemia, hyperuricemia, gout, hypokalemia
	Ethacrynic acid	50–100 mg (2–3)		
Aldosterone antagonists	Spironolactone	25–100 mg (1–2)	CHF, primary aldosteronism	Renal failure, hyperkalemia
	Eplerenone	50–100 mg (1–2)		
K+ retaining	Amiloride	5–10 mg (1–2)		Renal failure, hyperkalemia
	Triamterene	50–100 mg (1–2)		
Beta blockers				Asthma, COPD, 2nd or 3rd degree heart block, sick-sinus syndrome
Cardioselective	Atenolol	25–100 mg (1)	Angina, CHF, post-MI, sinus tachycardia, ventricular tachyarrhythmias	
	Metoprolol	25–100 mg (1–2)		
Nonselective	Propranolol	40–160 mg (2)		
	Propranolol LA	60–180 (1)		
Combined alpha/beta	Labetalol	200–800 mg (2)	? Post-MI, CHF	
	Carvedilol	12.5–50 mg (2)		
Alpha antagonists				
Selective	Prazosin	2–20 mg (2–3)	Prostatism	
	Doxazosin	1–16 mg (1)		
	Terazosin	1–10 mg (1–2)		
Nonselective	Phenoxybenzamine	20–120 mg (2–3)	Pheochromocytoma	
Sympatholytics				
Central	Clonidine	0.1–0.6 mg (2)		
	Clonidine patch	0.1–0.3 mg (1/week)		
	Methyldopa	250–1000 mg (2)		
	Reserpine	0.05–0.25 mg (1)		
	Guanfacine	0.5–2 mg (1)		
ACE inhibitors	Captopril	25–200 mg (2)	Post-MI, CHF, nephropathy	Renal failure, bilateral renal artery stenosis, pregnancy, hyperkalemia
	Lisinopril	10–40 mg (1)		
	Ramipril	2.5–20 mg (1–2)		
Angiotensin II antagonists	Losartan	25–100 mg (1–2)	CHF, diabetic nephropathy, ACE inhibitor cough	Renal failure, bilateral renal artery stenosis, pregnancy, hyperkalemia
	Valsartan	80–320 mg (1)		
	Candesartan	2–32 mg (1–2)		
Calcium antagonists				Heart failure, 2d or 3d degree heart block
Dihydropyridines	Nifedipine (long acting)	30–60 mg (1)	Angina	
Nondihydropyridines	Verapamil (long acting)	120–360 mg (1–2)	Post-MI, supraventricular tachycardias, angina	
	Diltiazem (long-acting)	180-420 mg (1)		
Direct vasodilators	Hydralazine	25–100 mg (2)		Severe coronary artery disease
	Minoxidil	2.5–80 mg (1–2)		

[a]At the initiation of therapy, lower doses may be preferable for elderly patients and for select combinations of antihypertensive agents.
Note: CHF, congestive heart failure; COPD, chronic obstructive pulmonary disease; MI, myocardial infarction; ACE, angiotensin-converting enzyme.

nephron. These agents are weak antihypertensive agents but may be used in combination with a thiazide to protect against hypokalemia. The main pharmacologic target for loop diuretics is the Na^+-K^+-$2Cl^-$ cotransporter in the thick ascending limb of the loop of Henle. Loop diuretics are generally reserved for hypertensive patients with reduced glomerular filtration rates [reflected in serum creatinine >220 µmol/L (>2.5 mg/dL)], CHF, or sodium retention and edema for some other reason such as treatment with a potent vasodilator, e.g., minoxidil.

Blockers of the Renin-Angiotensin System

ACE inhibitors decrease the production of angiotensin II, increase bradykinin levels, and reduce sympathetic nervous system activity. Angiotensin II receptor blockers provide selective blockade of AT_1 receptors, and the effect of angiotensin II on unblocked AT_2 receptors may augment the hypotensive effect. Both classes of agents are effective antihypertensive agents that may be used as monotherapy or in combination with diuretics, calcium antagonists, and alpha-blocking agents. Side effects of ACE inhibitors and angiotensin receptor blockers include functional renal insufficiency due to efferent renal arteriolar dilatation in a kidney with a stenotic lesion of the renal artery. Additional predisposing conditions to renal insufficiency induced by these agents include dehydration, CHF, and use of nonsteroidal anti-inflammatory drugs. Dry cough occurs in ~15% of patients, and angioedema occurs in <1% of patients taking ACE inhibitors. Angioedema occurs most commonly in individuals of Asian origin and more commonly in African Americans than in Caucasians. Hyperkalemia due to hypoaldosteronism is an occasional side effect of both ACE inhibitors and angiotensin receptor blockers.

Aldosterone Antagonists Spironolactone is a nonselective aldosterone antagonist that may be used alone or in combination with a thiazide diuretic. It may be a particularly effective agent in patients with low-renin essential hypertension, resistant hypertension, and primary aldosteronism. In patients with CHF, low-dose spironolactone reduces mortality and hospitalizations for heart failure when given in addition to conventional therapy with ACE inhibitors, digoxin, and loop diuretics. Because spironolactone binds to progesterone and androgen receptors, side effects may include gynecomastia, impotence, and menstrual abnormalities. These side effects are circumvented by a newer agent, eplerenone, which is a selective aldosterone antagonist. Eplerenone has recently been approved in the United States for the treatment of hypertension.

Beta Blockers β-Adrenergic receptor blockers lower blood pressure by decreasing cardiac output, due to a reduction of heart rate and contractility. Other proposed mechanisms by which beta blockers lower blood pressure include a central nervous system effect, and inhibition of renin release. Beta blockers are particularly effective in hypertensive patients with tachycardia, and their hypotensive potency is enhanced by coadministration with a diuretic. In lower doses, some beta blockers selectively inhibit cardiac $β_1$ receptors and have less influence on $β_2$ receptors on bronchial and vascular smooth muscle cells; however, there seems to be no difference in the antihypertensive potencies of cardio-selective and non-selective beta blockers. Certain beta blockers have intrinsic sympathomimetic activity, and it is uncertain whether this constitutes an overall advantage or disadvantage in cardiac therapy. Beta blockers without intrinsic sympathomimetic activity decrease the rate of sudden death, overall mortality, and recurrent myocardial infarction. In patients with CHF, beta blockers have been shown to reduce the risks of hospitalization and mortality. Carvedilol and labetalol block both β receptors and peripheral α-adrenergic receptors. The potential advantages of combined β- and α-adrenergic blockade in treating hypertension remain to be determined.

α-Adrenergic Blockers Postsynaptic, selective α-adrenoreceptor antagonists lower blood pressure by decreasing peripheral vascular resistance. They are effective antihypertensive agents, used either as monotherapy or in combination with other agents. However, in clinical trials of hypertensive patients, alpha blockade has not been shown to reduce cardiovascular morbidity and mortality or to provide as much protection against CHF as other classes of antihypertensive agents. These agents are also effective in treating lower urinary tract symptoms in men with prostatic hypertrophy. Nonselective α-adrenoreceptor antagonists bind to postsynaptic and presynaptic receptors and are primarily used for the management of patients with pheochromocytoma.

Sympatholytic Agents Centrally acting $α_2$ sympathetic agonists decrease peripheral resistance by inhibiting sympathetic outflow. They may be particularly useful in patients with autonomic neuropathy who have wide variations in blood pressure due to baroreceptor denervation. Drawbacks include somnolence, dry mouth, and rebound hypertension on withdrawal. Peripheral sympatholytics decrease peripheral resistance and venous constriction by depleting nerve terminal norepinephrine. Although they are potentially effective antihypertensive agents, their usefulness is limited by orthostatic hypotension, sexual dysfunction, and numerous drug-drug interactions.

Calcium Channel Blockers Calcium antagonists reduce vascular resistance through L-channel blockade, which reduces intracellular calcium and blunts vasoconstriction. This is a heterogeneous group of agents that includes drugs in the following three classes: phenylalkylamines (verapamil), benzothiazepines (diltiazem), and 1,4-dihydropyridines (nifedipine-like). Used alone and in combination with other agents (ACE inhibitors, beta blockers, α_1-adrenergic blockers), calcium antagonists effectively lower blood pressure; however, it is unclear if adding a diuretic to a calcium blocker results in a further lowering of blood pressure. Side effects of flushing, headache, and edema with dihydropyridine use are related to their potencies as arteriolar dilators; edema is due to an increase in transcapillary pressure gradients, not to net salt and water retention.

Direct Vasodilators These agents decrease peripheral resistance and concomitantly activate mechanisms that defend arterial pressure, notably the sympathetic nervous system, the renin-angiotensin-aldosterone system, and sodium retention. Usually, they are not considered first-line agents but are most effective when added to a combination that includes a diuretic and a beta blocker. Hydralazine is a potent direct vasodilator that has antioxidant and nitric-oxide enhancing actions, and minoxidil is a particularly potent agent and is most frequently used in patients with renal insufficiency who are refractory to all other drugs. Hydralazine may induce a lupus-like syndrome, and side effects of minoxidil include hypertrichosis and pericardial effusion.

COMPARISONS OF ANTIHYPERTENSIVES

Based on pooling results from clinical trials, meta-analyses of the efficacy of different classes of antihypertensive agents suggest essentially equivalent blood pressure–lowering effects of the following six major classes of antihypertensive agents when used as monotherapy: thiazide diuretics, beta blockers, ACE inhibitors, angiotensin II receptor blockers, calcium antagonists, and α_2 blockers. On average, standard doses of most antihypertensive agents reduce blood pressure by 8–10/4–7 mmHg; however, there may be subgroup differences in responsiveness. Younger patients may be more responsive to beta blockers and ACE inhibitors, whereas patients over age 50 may be more responsive to diuretics and calcium antagonists. There is a limited relationship between plasma renin and blood pressure response. Patients with high-renin hypertension may be more responsive to ACE inhibitors and angiotensin II receptor blockers than to other classes of agents, whereas patients with low-renin hypertension are more responsive to diuretics and calcium antagonists. Hypertensive African Americans tend to have low renin and may require higher doses of ACE inhibitors and angiotensin II receptor blockers than whites for optimal blood pressure control, although this difference is abolished when these agents are combined with a diuretic. Beta blockers also appear to be less effective than thiazide diuretics in African Americans than in non-African Americans.

A number of clinical trials have evaluated the possibility that different classes of antihypertensive agents have cardiovascular and renal protective effects not totally accounted for by their capacity to lower blood pressure. ACE inhibitors may have particular advantages, beyond that of blood pressure control, in reducing cardiovascular and renal outcomes. ACE inhibitors and angiotensin II receptor blockers decrease proteinuria and retard the rate of progression of renal insufficiency in both diabetic and nondiabetic renal diseases. The renoprotective effect of these agents, compared with other antihypertensive drugs, is less obvious at lower blood pressures. In both hypertensive and normotensive individuals, ACE inhibitors improve symptomatology and risk of death from CHF and reduce morbidity and mortality in the post-myocardial infarction patient. Similar benefits in cardiovascular morbidity and mortality in patients with CHF have also been observed with the use of angiotensin II receptor blockers. ACE inhibitors provide better coronary protection than calcium channel blockers, whereas calcium channel blockers provide more stroke protection than either ACE inhibitors or beta blockers.

In most patients with hypertension and heart failure due to systolic and/or diastolic dysfunction, the use of diuretics, ACE inhibitors or angiotensin II receptor antagonists, and beta blockers is recommended to improve survival. Although the optimal target blood pressure in patients with heart failure has not been established, a reasonable goal is the lowest blood pressure that is not associated with evidence of hypoperfusion.

A recent summary compared the results of 15 large clinical trials on the effects of antihypertensive treatment with different classes of agents on cardiovascular morbidity and mortality. In 13 of these trials, the incidence of cardiovascular events was similar between treatment groups, and in the remaining two trials, the difference was only marginally significant. It is possible that drug-related differences in cardiovascular outcomes are minimized in these large trials because of patient dropout, unplanned crossover of patients between groups, and insufficient statistical power to detect subgroup differences. Nevertheless, it is clear that the greatest cardiovascular and renal protective effects of antihypertensive therapy are related to adequate control of hypertension.

BLOOD PRESSURE GOALS OF ANTIHYPERTENSIVE THERAPY Based on clinical trial data, the maximum protection against combined cardiovascular endpoints is achieved with pressures <135–140 mmHg for systolic blood pressure and <80–85 mmHg for diastolic blood pressure; however, treatment has not reduced cardiovascular disease risk to the level in nonhypertensive individuals. More aggressive blood pressure targets for blood pressure control (e.g., office or clinic blood pressure <130/80 mmHg) may be appropriate for patients with diabetes, CHD, chronic kidney disease, or with additional cardiovascular disease risk factors. In diabetic patients, effective blood pressure control reduces the risk of cardiovascular events and death as well as the risk for microvascular disease (nephropathy, retinopathy). Risk reduction is greater in diabetic than in nondiabetic individuals.

To achieve recommended blood pressure goals, the majority of individuals with hypertension will require treatment with more than one drug. Three or more drugs are frequently needed in patients with diabetes and renal insufficiency. For most agents, reduction of blood pressure at half-standard doses is only ~20% less than at standard doses. Appropriate combinations of agents at these lower doses may have additive or almost additive effects on blood pressure with a lower incidence of side effects.

Despite theoretical concerns about decreasing cerebral, coronary, and renal blood flow by overly aggressive antihypertensive therapy, clinical trials have found no evidence for a "J-curve" phenomenon, i.e., at blood pressure reductions achieved in clinical practice, there does *not* appear to be a lower threshold for increasing cardiovascular risk. Even among patients with isolated systolic hypertension, further lowering of the diastolic blood pressure does not result in harm. However, relatively little information is available concerning the risk/benefit ratio of antihypertensive therapy in individuals >80 years, and, in this population, gradual blood pressure reduction to less aggressive target levels of control may be appropriate.

The term *resistant hypertension* refers to patients with blood pressures persistently >140/90 mmHg despite taking three or more antihypertensive agents, including a diuretic, in reasonable combination and at full doses. Resistant or difficult-to-control hypertension is more common in patients >60 years than in younger patients. Resistant hypertension may be related to "pseudoresistance" (high office blood pressures and lower home blood pressures), nonadherence to therapy, identifiable causes of hypertension (including obesity and excessive alcohol intake), and use of any of a number of nonprescription and prescription drugs (Table 19-3). Rarely, in older patients, pseudohypertension may be related to the inability to measure blood pressure accurately in severely sclerotic arteries. This condition is suggested if the radial pulse remains palpable despite occlusion of the brachial artery by the cuff (Osler maneuver). The actual blood pressure can be determined by direct intraarterial measurement. Evaluation of patients with resistant hypertension might include home blood pressure monitoring to determine if office blood pressures are representative of the usual blood pressure. A more extensive evaluation for a secondary form of hypertension should be undertaken if no other explanation for hypertension resistance becomes apparent.

HYPERTENSIVE EMERGENCIES   Probably due to the widespread availability of antihypertensive therapy, in the United States there has been a decline in the numbers of patients presenting with "crisis levels" of blood pressure. Most patients who present with severe hypertension are chronically hypertensive, and in the absence of acute, end-organ damage, precipitous lowering of blood pressure may be associated with significant morbidity and should be avoided. The key to successful management of severe hypertension is to differentiate hypertensive crises from hypertensive urgencies. The degree of target organ damage, rather than the level of blood pressure alone, determines the rapidity with which blood pressure should be lowered. Tables 19-9 and 19-10 list a number of hypertension-related emergencies and recommended therapies.

Malignant hypertension is a syndrome associated with an abrupt increase of blood pressure in a patient with underlying hypertension or related to the sudden onset of hypertension in a previously normotensive individual. The absolute level of blood pressure is not as important as its rate of rise. Pathologically, the syndrome is associated with diffuse necrotizing vasculitis, arteriolar thrombi, and fibrin deposition in arteriolar walls. Fibrinoid necrosis has been observed in arterioles of kidney, brain, retina, and other organs. Clinically, the syndrome is recognized by progressive retinopathy (arteriolar spasm, hemorrhages, exudates, and papilledema), deteriorating renal function with proteinuria, microangiopathic hemolytic anemia, and encephalopathy. In

TABLE 19-9

PREFERRED PARENTERAL DRUGS FOR SELECTED HYPERTENSIVE EMERGENCIES	
Hypertensive encephalopathy	Nitroprusside, nicardipine, labetalol
Malignant hypertension (when IV therapy is indicated)	Labetalol, nicardipine, nitroprusside, enalaprilat
Stroke	Nicardipine, labetalol, nitroprusside
Myocardial infarction/ unstable angina	Nitroglycerin, nicardipine, labetalol, esmolol
Acute left ventricular failure	Nitroglycerin, enalaprilat, loop diuretics
Aortic dissection	Nitroprusside, esmolol, labetalol
Adrenergic crisis	Phentolamine, nitroprusside
Postoperative hypertension	Nitroglycerin, nitroprusside, labetalol, nicardipine
Preeclampsia/eclampsia of pregnancy	Hydralazine, labetalol, nicardipine

Source: Adapted from DG Vidt, in S Oparil, MA Weber (eds): Hypertension, 2d ed. Philadelphia, Elsevier Saunders, 2005.

TABLE 19-10

USUAL INTRAVENOUS DOSES OF ANTIHYPERTENSIVE AGENTS USED IN HYPERTENSIVE EMERGENCIES[a]

ANTIHYPERTENSIVE AGENT	INTRAVENOUS DOSE
Nitroprusside	Initial 0.3 $(\mu g/kg)/min$; usual 2–4 $(\mu g/kg)/min$; maximum 10 $(\mu g/kg)/min$ for 10 min
Nicardipine	Initial 5 mg/h; titrate by 2.5 mg/h at 5–15 min intervals; max 15 mg/h
Labetalol	2 mg/min up to 300 mg or 20 mg over 2 min, then 40–80 mg at 10-min intervals up to 300 mg total
Enalaprilat	Usual 0.625–1.25 mg over 5 min every 6–8 h; maximum 5 mg/dose
Esmolol	Initial 80–500 $\mu g/kg$ over 1 min, then 50–300 $(\mu g/kg)/min$
Phentolamine	5–15 mg bolus
Nitroglycerin	Initial 5 $\mu g/min$, then titrate by 5 $\mu g/min$ at 3–5 min intervals; if no response is seen at 20 $\mu g/min$, incremental increases of 10–20 $\mu g/min$ may be used
Hydralazine	10–50 mg at 30-min intervals

[a]Constant blood pressure monitoring is required. Start with the lowest dose. Subsequent doses and intervals of administration should be adjusted according to the blood pressure response and duration of action of the specific agent.

these patients, historic inquiry should include questions about the use of monamine oxidase inhibitors and recreational drugs (e.g., cocaine, amphetamines).

Although blood pressure should be lowered rapidly in patients with hypertensive encephalopathy, there are inherent risks of overly aggressive therapy. In hypertensive individuals, the upper and lower limits of autoregulation of cerebral blood flow are shifted to higher levels of arterial pressure, and rapid lowering of blood pressure to below the lower limit of autoregulation may precipitate cerebral ischemia or infarction as a consequence of decreased cerebral blood flow. Renal and coronary blood flows may also decrease with overly aggressive acute therapy. The initial goal of therapy is to reduce mean arterial blood pressure by no more than 25% within minutes to 2 h or to a blood pressure in the range of 160/100–110 mmHg. This may be accomplished with IV nitroprusside, a short-acting vasodilator with a rapid onset of action that allows for minute-to-minute control of blood pressure. Parenteral labetalol and nicardipine are also effective agents for the treatment of hypertensive encephalopathy.

In patients with malignant hypertension without encephalopathy or some other catastrophic event,

it is preferable to reduce blood pressure over hours or longer rather than minutes. This goal may effectively be achieved initially with frequent dosing of short-acting oral agents, such as captopril, clonidine, or labetalol.

Acute, transient blood pressure elevations, lasting days to weeks, frequently occur following thrombotic and hemorrhagic strokes. Autoregulation of cerebral blood flow is impaired in ischemic cerebral tissue, and higher arterial pressures may be required to maintain cerebral blood flow. Although specific blood pressure targets have not been defined for patients with acute cerebrovascular events, aggressive reductions of blood pressure are to be avoided. With the increasing availability of improved methods for measuring cerebral blood flow (using CT technology), studies are in progress to evaluate the effects of different classes of antihypertensive agents on both blood pressure and cerebral blood flow following an acute stroke. Currently, in the absence of other indications for acute therapy, for patients with cerebral infarction who are not candidates for thrombolytic therapy, one recommended guideline is to institute antihypertensive therapy only for those patients with a systolic blood pressure >220 mmHg or a diastolic blood pressure >130 mmHg. If thrombolytic therapy is to be used, the recommended goal blood pressure is <185 mmHg systolic pressure and <110 mmHg diastolic pressure. In patients with hemorrhagic stroke, suggested guidelines for initiating antihypertensive therapy are systolic >180 mmHg or diastolic pressure >130 mmHg. The management of hypertension after subarachnoid hemorrhage is controversial. Cautious reduction of blood pressure is indicated if mean arterial pressure is >130 mmHg.

In addition to pheochromocytoma, an adrenergic crisis due to catecholamine excess may be related to cocaine or amphetamine overdose, clonidine withdrawal, acute spinal cord injuries, and an interaction of tyramine-containing compounds with monamine oxidase inhibitors. These patients may be treated with phentolamine or nitroprusside.

FURTHER READINGS

ADROGUE JH, MADIAS NE: Sodium and potassium in the pathogenesis of hypertension. N Engl J Med 356:1966, 2007

ALLHAT COLLABORATIVE RESEARCH GROUP: Major outcomes in high-risk hypertensive patients randomized to angiotensin converting enzyme inhibitor or calcium channel blocker vs. diuretic: The Antihypertensive and Lipid-Lowering Treatment to Prevent Heart Attack Trial (ALLHAT). JAMA 288:2981, 2002

APPEL LJ et al: Dietary approaches to prevent and treat hypertension: A scientific statement from the American Heart Association. Hypertension 47:296, 2006

Blood Pressure Lowering Treatment Trialists' Collaboration: Effects of ACE inhibitors, calcium antagonists, and other blood pressure-lowering drugs: Results of prospectively designed overviews of randomised trials. Lancet 355:1955, 2000

Casas JP et al: Effect of inhibitors of the renin-angiotensin system and other antihypertensive drugs on renal outcomes: Systematic review and meta-analysis. Lancet 366:2026, 2005

Chobanian AV et al: The Seventh Report of the Joint National Committee on Prevention, Detection, Evaluation, and Treatment of High Blood Pressure: The JNC 7 Report. JAMA 289:2560, 2003

Mancia G: Role of outcome trials in providing information on antihypertensive treatment: Importance and limitations. Am J Hypertens 19:1, 2006

Moser M, Setano JF: Resistant or difficult-to-control hypertension. N Engl J Med 355:385, 2006

Pickering TG et al: Ambulatory blood-pressure monitoring. N Engl J Med 3554:2368, 2006

Wu J et al: A summary of the effects of antihypertensive medications on measured blood pressure. Am J Hypertens 18:935, 2005

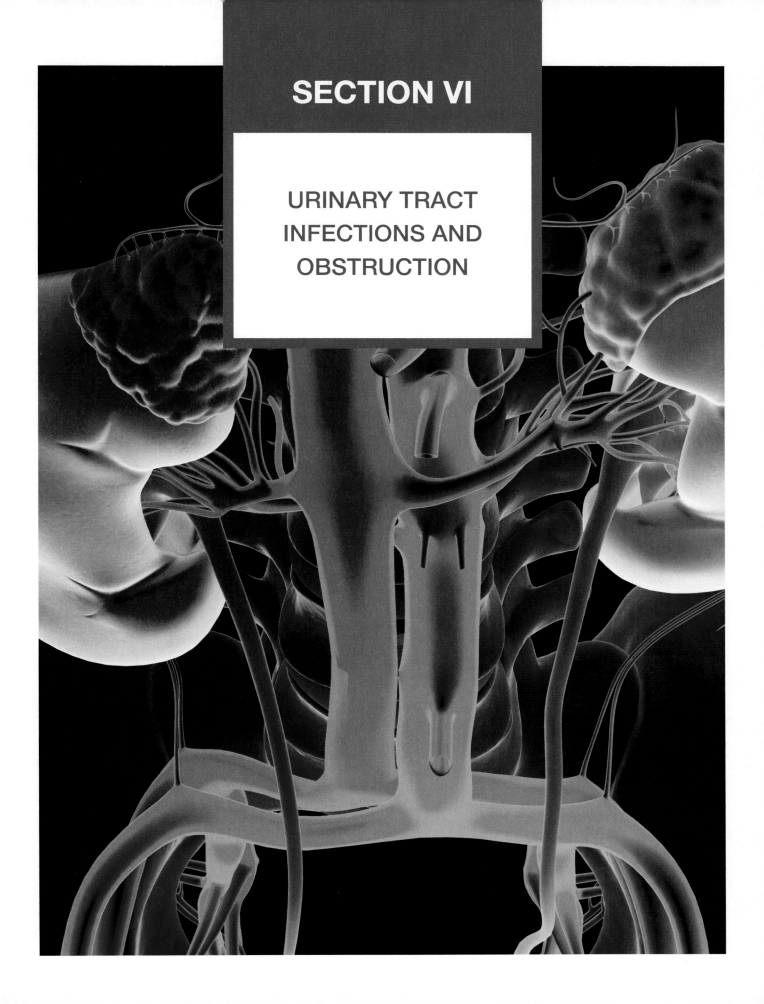

SECTION VI

URINARY TRACT INFECTIONS AND OBSTRUCTION

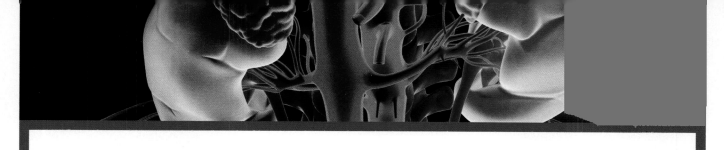

CHAPTER 20

URINARY TRACT INFECTIONS, PYELONEPHRITIS, AND PROSTATITIS

Walter E. Stamm

DEFINITIONS

Acute infections of the urinary tract fall into two general anatomic categories: lower tract infection (urethritis and cystitis) and upper tract infection (acute pyelonephritis, prostatitis, and intrarenal and perinephric abscesses). Infections at various sites may occur together or independently and may either be asymptomatic or present as one of the clinical syndromes described in this chapter. Infections of the urethra and bladder are often considered superficial (or mucosal) infections, while prostatitis, pyelonephritis, and renal suppuration signify tissue invasion.

From a microbiologic perspective, urinary tract infection (UTI) exists when pathogenic microorganisms are detected in the urine, urethra, bladder, kidney, or prostate. In most instances, growth of $\geq 10^5$ organisms per milliliter from a properly collected midstream "clean-catch" urine sample indicates infection. However, significant bacteriuria is lacking in some cases of true UTI. Especially in symptomatic patients, fewer bacteria (10^2–10^4/mL) may signify infection. In urine specimens obtained by suprapubic aspiration or "in-and-out" catheterization, and in samples from a patient with an indwelling catheter, colony counts of 10^2–10^4/mL generally indicate infection. Conversely, colony counts of $>10^5$/mL in midstream urine are occasionally due to specimen contamination, which is especially likely when multiple bacterial species are found.

Infections that recur after antibiotic therapy can be due to the persistence of the originally infecting strain (as judged by species, antibiogram, serotype, and molecular type) or to reinfection with a new strain. "Same-strain" recurrent infections that become evident within 2 weeks of cessation of therapy can be the result of unresolved renal or prostatic infection (termed *relapse*) or of persistent vaginal or intestinal colonization leading to rapid reinfection of the bladder.

Symptoms of dysuria, urgency, and frequency that are unaccompanied by significant bacteriuria have been termed the *acute urethral syndrome*. Although widely used, this term lacks anatomic precision because many cases so designated are actually bladder infections. Moreover, since the pathogen can usually be identified, the term *syndrome*—implying unknown causation—is inappropriate.

Chronic pyelonephritis refers to chronic interstitial nephritis believed to result from bacterial infection of the kidney (Chap. 17). Many noninfectious diseases also cause an interstitial nephritis that is indistinguishable pathologically from chronic pyelonephritis.

ACUTE UTIs: URETHRITIS, CYSTITIS, AND PYELONEPHRITIS

EPIDEMIOLOGY

Epidemiologically, UTIs are subdivided into catheter-associated (or nosocomial) infections and non–catheter-associated (or community-acquired) infections. Infections in either category may be symptomatic or asymptomatic. Acute community-acquired UTIs are very common and account for more than 7 million office visits annually in the United States. In the female population, these infections occur in 1–3% of schoolgirls and then increase markedly in incidence with the onset of sexual activity in adolescence. The vast majority of acute symptomatic infections involve young women; a prospective study demonstrated an annual incidence of 0.5–0.7 infections per patient-year in this group. In the male population, acute symptomatic UTIs occur in the first year of life (often in association with urologic abnormalities); thereafter, UTIs are unusual in male patients under the age of 50. The development of asymptomatic bacteriuria parallels that of symptomatic infection, and is rare among men under 50 but common among women between 20 and 50. Asymptomatic bacteriuria is more common among elderly men and women, with rates as high as 40–50% in some studies. The incidence of acute uncomplicated pyelonephritis among community-dwelling women 18–49 years of age is 28 cases per 10,000 women.

ETIOLOGY

Many microorganisms can infect the urinary tract, but by far the most common agents are the gram-negative bacilli. *Escherichia coli* causes ~80% of acute infections (both cystitis and pyelonephritis) in patients without catheters, urologic abnormalities, or calculi. Other gram-negative rods, especially *Proteus* and *Klebsiella* spp. and occasionally *Enterobacter* spp., account for a smaller proportion of uncomplicated infections. These organisms, along with *Serratia* spp. and *Pseudomonas* spp., assume increasing importance in recurrent infections and in infections associated with urologic manipulation, calculi, or obstruction. They play a major role in nosocomial, catheter-associated infections. *Proteus* spp. (through the production of urease) and *Klebsiella* spp. (through the production of extracellular slime and polysaccharides) predispose to stone formation and are isolated more frequently from patients with calculi.

Gram-positive cocci play a lesser role in UTIs. However, *Staphylococcus saprophyticus*—a novobiocin-resistant, coagulase-negative species—accounts for 10–15% of acute symptomatic UTIs in young female patients. Enterococci occasionally cause acute uncomplicated cystitis in women. More commonly, enterococci and *Staphylococcus aureus* cause infections in patients with renal stones or with previous instrumentation or surgery. Isolation of *S. aureus* from the urine should arouse suspicion of bacteremic infection of the kidney. *Staphylococcus epidermidis* is a common cause of catheter-associated UTI.

About one-third of women with dysuria and frequency have either an insignificant number of bacteria in midstream urine cultures or completely sterile cultures, and have been previously defined as having the urethral syndrome. About three-quarters of these women have pyuria, while one-quarter have no pyuria and little objective evidence of infection. In the women with pyuria, two groups of pathogens account for most infections. Low counts (10^2–10^4/mL) of typical bacterial uropathogens such as *E. coli*, *S. saprophyticus*, *Klebsiella*, or *Proteus* are found in midstream urine specimens from most of these women. These bacteria are probably the causative agents in these infections because they can usually be isolated from a suprapubic aspirate, are associated with pyuria, and respond to appropriate antimicrobial therapy. In other women with acute urinary symptoms, pyuria, and urine that is sterile (even when obtained by suprapubic aspiration), sexually transmitted urethritis-producing agents such as *Chlamydia trachomatis*, *Neisseria gonorrhoeae*, and herpes simplex virus (HSV) are etiologically important. These agents are found most frequently in young, sexually active women with new sexual partners.

The causative role of several more unusual bacterial and nonbacterial pathogens in UTIs remains poorly defined. *Ureaplasma urealyticum* has frequently been isolated from the urethra and urine of patients with acute dysuria and frequency, but is also found in specimens from many patients without urinary symptoms. Ureaplasmas and *Mycoplasma genitalium* probably account for some cases of urethritis and cystitis. *U. urealyticum* and *Mycoplasma hominis* have been isolated from prostatic and renal tissues of patients with acute prostatitis and pyelonephritis, respectively, and are probably responsible for some of these infections as well. Adenoviruses cause acute hemorrhagic cystitis in children and in some young adults, often in epidemics. Although other viruses can be isolated from urine (e.g., cytomegalovirus), they are thought not to cause acute UTI. Colonization of the urine of catheterized or diabetic patients by *Candida* and other fungal species is common and sometimes progresses to symptomatic invasive infection.

PATHOGENESIS AND SOURCES OF INFECTION

The urinary tract should be viewed as a single anatomic unit that is united by a continuous column of urine extending from the urethra to the kidney. In the vast majority of UTIs, bacteria gain access to the bladder via the urethra. Ascent of bacteria from the bladder may follow and is probably the pathway for most renal parenchymal infections.

The vaginal introitus and distal urethra are normally colonized by diphtheroids, streptococcal species, lactobacilli, and staphylococcal species, but not by the enteric gram-negative bacilli that commonly cause UTIs. In females prone to the development of cystitis, however, enteric gram-negative organisms residing in the bowel colonize the introitus, the periurethral skin, and the distal urethra before and during episodes of bacteriuria. The factors that predispose to periurethral colonization with gram-negative bacilli remain poorly understood, but alteration of the normal vaginal flora by antibiotics, other genital infections, or contraceptives (especially spermicide) appears to play an important role. Loss of the normally dominant H_2O_2-producing lactobacilli from the vaginal flora appears to facilitate colonization by E. coli. Small numbers of periurethral bacteria probably gain entry to the bladder frequently, and this process is facilitated in some cases by urethral massage during intercourse. Whether bladder infection ensues depends on interacting effects of strain pathogenicity, inoculum size, and local and systemic host defense mechanisms. Recent data from both animal models and human studies indicate that E. coli sometimes invades the bladder epithelium, forming intracellular colonies (biofilms) that may persist and become a source of recurrent infection.

Under normal circumstances, bacteria placed in the bladder are rapidly cleared, partly through the flushing and dilutional effects of voiding, but also as a result of the antibacterial properties of urine and the bladder mucosa. Owing mostly to a high urea concentration and high osmolarity, the bladder urine of many healthy persons inhibits or kills bacteria. Prostatic secretions possess antibacterial properties as well. Bladder epithelial cells secrete cytokines and chemokines—primarily interleukin (IL) 6 and IL-8—upon interaction with bacteria, causing polymorphonuclear leukocytes to enter the bladder epithelium and the urine soon after infection arises and play a role in clearing bacteriuria. The role of locally produced antibody remains unclear.

Hematogenous pyelonephritis occurs most often in debilitated patients who are either chronically ill or receiving immunosuppressive therapy. Metastatic staphylococcal or candidal infections of the kidney may follow bacteremia or fungemia, spreading from distant foci of infection in the bone, skin, or vasculature, or elsewhere.

CONDITIONS AFFECTING PATHOGENESIS
Gender and Sexual Activity

The female urethra appears to be particularly prone to colonization with colonic gram-negative bacilli because of its proximity to the anus, its short length (~4 cm), and its termination beneath the labia. Sexual intercourse causes the introduction of bacteria into the bladder and is temporally associated with the onset of cystitis; it thus appears to be important in the pathogenesis of UTIs in both pre- and postmenopausal women. Voiding after intercourse reduces the risk of cystitis, probably because it promotes the clearance of bacteria introduced during intercourse. Use of spermicidal compounds with a diaphragm or cervical cap or use of spermicide-coated condoms dramatically alters the normal introital bacterial flora and has been associated with marked increases in vaginal colonization with E. coli and in the risk of both cystitis and acute pyelonephritis. In healthy, community-dwelling postmenopausal women, the risk of UTI (both cystitis and pyelonephritis) is increased by a history of recent sexual activity, recent UTI, diabetes mellitus, and incontinence.

In male patients who are <50 years old and who have no history of heterosexual or homosexual insertive rectal intercourse, UTI is exceedingly uncommon, and this diagnosis should be questioned in the absence of clear documentation. An important factor predisposing to bacteriuria in men is urethral obstruction due to prostatic hypertrophy. Insertive rectal intercourse is also associated with an increased risk of cystitis in men. Men (and women) who are infected with HIV and who have CD4+ T cell counts of <200/μL are at increased risk of both bacteriuria and symptomatic UTI. Finally, lack of circumcision has been identified as a risk factor for UTI in both male neonates and young men.

Pregnancy

UTIs are detected in 2–8% of pregnant women. Symptomatic upper tract infections, in particular, are unusually common during pregnancy; fully 20–30% of pregnant women with asymptomatic bacteriuria subsequently develop pyelonephritis. This predisposition to upper tract infection during pregnancy results from decreased ureteral tone, decreased ureteral peristalsis, and temporary incompetence of the vesicoureteral valves. Bladder catheterization during or after delivery causes additional infections. Increased incidences of low birth weight, premature delivery, and neonatal death result from UTIs (particularly upper tract infections) during pregnancy.

Obstruction

Any impediment to the free flow of urine—tumor, stricture, stone, or prostatic hypertrophy—results in hydronephrosis and a greatly increased frequency of UTI. Infection superimposed on urinary tract obstruction may lead to rapid destruction of renal tissue. It is of utmost importance, therefore, when infection is present, to identify and repair obstructive lesions. On the other hand, when an obstruction is minor and is not progressive or associated with infection, great caution should be exercised in attempting surgical correction. The introduction of infection in such cases may be more damaging than an uncorrected minor obstruction that does not significantly impair renal function.

Neurogenic Bladder Dysfunction

Interference with bladder enervation, as in spinal cord injury, tabes dorsalis, multiple sclerosis, diabetes, and other diseases, may be associated with UTI. The infection may be initiated by the use of catheters for bladder drainage and is favored by the prolonged stasis of urine in the bladder. An additional factor often operative in these cases is bone demineralization due to immobilization, which causes hypercalciuria, calculus formation, and obstructive uropathy.

Vesicoureteral Reflux

Defined as reflux of urine from the bladder cavity up into the ureters and sometimes into the renal pelvis, vesicoureteral reflux occurs during voiding or with elevation of pressure in the bladder. In practice, this condition is detected as retrograde movement of radiopaque or radioactive material during a voiding cystourethrogram. An anatomically impaired vesicoureteral junction facilitates reflux of bacteria and thus upper tract infection. However, since—even in the healthy urinary system—a fluid connection between the bladder and the kidneys always exists, some retrograde movement of bacteria probably takes place during infection but is not detected by radiologic techniques.

Vesicoureteral reflux is common among children with anatomic abnormalities of the urinary tract or with anatomically normal but infected urinary tracts. In the latter group, reflux disappears with advancing age and is probably attributable to factors other than UTI. Longterm follow-up of children with UTI who have reflux has established that renal damage correlates with marked reflux, not with infection. Thus, it appears reasonable to search for reflux in children with unexplained failure of renal growth or with renal scarring, because UTI per se is an insufficient explanation for these abnormalities. On the other hand, it is doubtful that all children who have recurrent UTIs but whose urinary tract appears normal on pyelography should be subjected to voiding cystoureterography merely for the detection of the rare patient with marked reflux not revealed by intravenous pyelography.

Bacterial Virulence Factors

Not all strains of E. coli are equally capable of infecting the intact urinary tract. Bacterial virulence factors markedly influence the likelihood that a given strain, once introduced into the bladder, will cause UTI. Most E. coli strains that cause symptomatic UTIs in noncatheterized patients belong to a small number of specific O, K, and H serogroups. These uropathogenic clones have accumulated a number of virulence genes that are often closely linked on the bacterial chromosome in "pathogenicity islands." Bacterial adherence to uroepithelial cells is a critical first step in the initiation of infection (**Fig. 20-1**). For both E. coli and Proteus spp., fimbriae (hairlike proteinaceous surface appendages) mediate bacterial attachment to specific receptors on epithelial cells, which in turn initiates important events in the mucosal epithelial cell, including secretion of IL-6 and IL-8 (with subsequent chemotaxis of leukocytes to the bladder mucosa) and induction of apoptosis and epithelial cell desquamation. Besides fimbriae, uropathogenic E. coli strains usually produce cytotoxins, hemolysin, and aerobactin (a siderophore for scavenging iron) and are resistant to the bactericidal action of human serum. Nearly all E. coli strains causing acute pyelonephritis and most of those causing acute cystitis are uropathogenic strains possessing pathogenicity islands. In contrast, infections in patients with structural or functional abnormalities of the urinary tract are generally caused by bacterial strains that lack these uropathogenic properties; the implication is that these properties are not needed for infection of the compromised urinary tract.

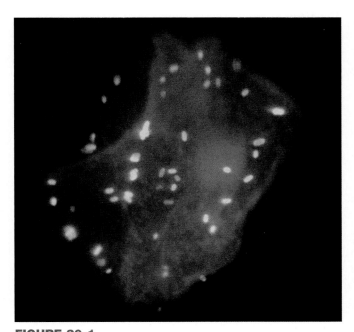

FIGURE 20-1

Adherence of fluorescein-labeled uropathogenic *Escherichia coli* to a uroepithelial cell.

Genetic Factors

Increasing evidence suggests that host genetic factors influence susceptibility to UTI. A maternal history of UTI is more often found among women who have experienced recurrent UTIs than among controls. The number and type of receptors on uroepithelial cells to which bacteria may attach are, at least in part, genetically determined. Many of these structures are components of blood group antigens and are present on both erythrocytes and uroepithelial cells. For example, P fimbriae mediate attachment of *E. coli* to P-positive erythrocytes and are found on nearly all strains causing acute uncomplicated pyelonephritis. Conversely, P blood group–negative individuals, who lack these receptors, are at decreased risk of pyelonephritis. Furthermore, nonsecretors of blood group antigens are at increased risk of recurrent UTI; this predisposition may relate to a different profile of genetically determined glycolipids on uroepithelial cells. Mutations in host genes integral to the immune response (e.g., Toll-like receptors, interferon γ receptors) may also affect susceptibility to UTI.

CLINICAL PRESENTATION

Localization of Infection

Unfortunately, available methods of distinguishing renal parenchymal infection from cystitis are neither reliable nor convenient enough for routine clinical use. Fever or an elevated C-reactive protein level often accompanies acute pyelonephritis and is found in rare cases of cystitis but also occurs in infections other than pyelonephritis.

Cystitis

Patients with cystitis usually report dysuria, frequency, urgency, and suprapubic pain. The urine often becomes grossly cloudy and malodorous and is bloody in ~30% of cases. White cells and bacteria can be detected by examination of unspun urine in most cases. However, some women with cystitis have only 10^2–10^4 bacteria per milliliter of urine, and in these instances bacteria cannot be seen in a Gram-stained preparation of unspun urine. Physical examination generally reveals only tenderness of the urethra or the suprapubic area. If a genital lesion or a vaginal discharge is evident, especially in conjunction with $<10^5$ bacteria per milliliter on urine culture, then pathogens that may cause urethritis, vaginitis, or cervicitis (e.g., *C. trachomatis*, *N. gonorrhoeae*, *Trichomonas*, *Candida*, and HSV) should be considered. Prominent systemic manifestations, such as a temperature of $>38.3°C$ ($>101°F$), nausea, and vomiting, usually indicate concomitant renal infection, as does costovertebral angle tenderness. However, the absence of these findings does not ensure that infection is limited to the bladder and urethra.

Acute Pyelonephritis

Symptoms of acute pyelonephritis generally develop rapidly over a few hours or a day and include fever, shaking chills, nausea, vomiting, abdominal pain, and diarrhea. Symptoms of cystitis are sometimes present. Besides fever, tachycardia, and generalized muscle tenderness, physical examination generally reveals marked tenderness on deep pressure in one or both costovertebral angles or on deep abdominal palpation. The range of illness severity is broad. Some patients have mild disease; in others, signs and symptoms of gram-negative sepsis predominate. Most patients have significant leukocytosis and bacteria detectable in Gram-stained unspun urine. Leukocyte casts are present in the urine of some patients, and the detection of these casts is pathognomonic. Hematuria may be demonstrated during the acute phase of the disease; if it persists after acute manifestations of infection have subsided, a stone, a tumor, or tuberculosis should be considered.

Except in individuals with papillary necrosis, abscess formation, or urinary obstruction, the manifestations of acute pyelonephritis usually respond to appropriate therapy within 48–72 h. However, despite the absence of symptoms, bacteriuria or pyuria may persist. In severe pyelonephritis, fever subsides more slowly and may not disappear for several days, even after appropriate antibiotic treatment has been instituted. Persistence of fever or of symptoms and signs beyond 72 h suggests the need for urologic imaging.

Urethritis

Of women with acute dysuria, frequency, and pyuria, ~30% have midstream urine cultures with either no growth or insignificant bacterial growth. Clinically, these women cannot always be readily distinguished from those with cystitis. In this situation, a distinction should be made between women infected with sexually transmitted pathogens (e.g., *C. trachomatis*, *N. gonorrhoeae*, or HSV) and those with low-count *E. coli* or *S. saprophyticus* infection of the urethra and bladder. Chlamydial or gonococcal infection should be suspected in women with a gradual onset of illness, no hematuria, no suprapubic pain, and >7 days of symptoms. The additional history of a recent sex-partner change, especially if the partner has recently had chlamydial or gonococcal urethritis, should heighten the suspicion of a sexually transmitted infection, as should the finding of mucopurulent cervicitis. Gross hematuria, suprapubic pain, an abrupt onset of illness, a duration of illness of <3 days, and a history of UTIs favor the diagnosis of *E. coli* UTI.

Catheter-Associated UTIs

Bacteriuria develops in at least 10–15% of hospitalized patients with short-term indwelling urethral catheters.

The risk of infection is ~3–5% per day of catheterization. *E. coli, Proteus, Pseudomonas, Klebsiella, Serratia*, staphylococci, enterococci, and *Candida* usually cause these infections. Many infecting strains display markedly broader antimicrobial resistance profiles than do organisms that cause community-acquired UTIs. Factors associated with an increased risk of catheter-associated UTI include female sex, prolonged catheterization, severe underlying illness, disconnection of the catheter and drainage tube, other types of faulty catheter care, and lack of systemic antimicrobial therapy.

Infection occurs when bacteria reach the bladder by one of two routes: migration through the column of urine in the catheter lumen (intraluminal route) or up the mucous sheath outside the catheter (periurethral route). Hospital-acquired pathogens can reach the patient's catheter or urine-collecting system on the hands of hospital personnel, in contaminated solutions or irrigants, and via contaminated instruments or disinfectants. Bacteria usually enter the catheter system at the catheter–collecting tube junction or at the drainage bag portal. The organisms then ascend intraluminally into the bladder within 24–72 h. Alternatively, the patient's own bowel flora may colonize the perineal skin and periurethral area and reach the bladder by ascending along the external surface of the catheter. Studies have shown the importance of bacterial attachment to and growth on the device's surfaces in the pathogenesis of catheter-associated UTI. Bacterial growth in biofilms on the catheter eventually produces encrustations consisting of bacteria, bacterial glycocalyces, host urinary proteins, and urinary salts. These encrustations provide a refuge for bacteria and may protect them from antimicrobial agents and phagocytes.

Clinically, catheter-associated infections usually cause minimal symptoms without fever and often resolve after withdrawal of the catheter. The frequency of upper tract infection associated with catheter-induced bacteriuria is unknown. Gram-negative bacteremia, which follows catheter-associated bacteriuria in 1–2% of cases, is the most significant recognized complication of catheter-induced UTIs. The catheterized urinary tract has repeatedly been shown to be the most common source of gram-negative bacteremia in hospitalized patients, generally accounting for ~30% of cases.

In patients catheterized for <2 weeks, catheter-associated UTIs can sometimes be prevented by use of a sterile closed collecting system, by attention to aseptic technique during catheter insertion and care, and by measures to minimize cross-infection. Other preventive approaches, including short courses of systemic antimicrobial therapy, topical application of periurethral antimicrobial ointments, use of preconnected catheter–drainage tube units, and addition of antimicrobial drugs to the drainage bag, have all been protective in at least one controlled trial but are not recommended for general use. The use of catheters impregnated with antimicrobial agents reduces the incidence of asymptomatic bacteriuria in patients catheterized for <2 weeks. Despite precautions, the majority of patients catheterized for >2 weeks eventually develop bacteriuria. For example, because of spinal cord injury, incontinence, or other factors, some patients in hospitals or nursing homes require long-term or semipermanent bladder catheterization. Measures intended to prevent infection have been largely unsuccessful in these chronically catheterized patients, essentially all of whom develop bacteriuria. If feasible, intermittent catheterization by a nurse or by the patient appears to reduce the incidence of bacteriuria and associated complications in such patients. Treatment should be provided when symptomatic infections arise, but treatment of asymptomatic bacteriuria in such patients has no apparent benefit.

DIAGNOSTIC TESTING

Determination of the number and type of bacteria in the urine is an extremely important diagnostic procedure. In symptomatic patients, bacteria are usually present in the urine in large numbers ($\geq 10^5$/mL). Since the large number of bacteria in the bladder urine is due in part to bacterial multiplication in the bladder cavity, samples of urine from the ureters or renal pelvis may contain $<10^5$ bacteria per milliliter and yet indicate infection. Similarly, the presence of bacteriuria of any degree in suprapubic aspirates or of $\geq 10^2$ bacteria per milliliter of urine obtained by catheterization usually indicates infection. In some circumstances (antibiotic treatment, high urea concentration, high osmolarity, low pH), urine inhibits bacterial multiplication, resulting in relatively low bacterial colony counts despite infection. For this reason, antiseptic solutions should not be used to wash the periurethral area before collection of the urine specimen. Water diuresis or recent voiding also reduces bacterial counts in urine.

Microscopy of urine from symptomatic patients can be of great diagnostic value. Microscopic bacteriuria, which is best assessed with Gram-stained uncentrifuged urine, is found in >90% of specimens from patients whose infections are associated with colony counts of at least 10^5/mL, and this finding is very specific. However, bacteria cannot usually be detected microscopically in infections with lower colony counts (10^2–10^4/mL). The detection of bacteria by urinary microscopy thus constitutes firm evidence of infection, but the absence of microscopically detectable bacteria does not exclude the diagnosis. When carefully sought by chamber-count microscopy, pyuria is a highly sensitive indicator of UTI in symptomatic patients. Pyuria is demonstrated in nearly all acute bacterial UTIs, and its absence calls the diagnosis into question. The leukocyte esterase "dipstick" method is less sensitive than microscopy in identifying pyuria but is a useful alternative when microscopy is not feasible. Pyuria in the absence of bacteriuria (sterile pyuria) may indicate infection with unusual agents such as *C. trachomatis*, *U. urealyticum*, or *Mycobacterium tuberculosis* or with fungi. Alternatively, sterile pyuria may be documented in noninfectious urologic conditions such as calculi, anatomic abnormality, nephrocalcinosis, vesicoureteral reflux, interstitial nephritis, or polycystic disease.

Although many authorities have recommended that urine culture and antimicrobial susceptibility testing be performed for any patient with a suspected UTI, it is more practical and cost-effective to manage women who have symptoms characteristic of acute uncomplicated cystitis without an initial urine culture. Two approaches to presumptive therapy have generally been used. In the first, treatment is initiated solely on the basis of a typical history and/or typical findings on physical examination. In the second, women with symptoms and signs of acute cystitis and without complicating factors are managed with urinary microscopy (or, alternatively, with a leukocyte esterase test). A positive result for pyuria and/or bacteriuria provides enough evidence of infection to omit urine culture and susceptibility testing and treat the patient empirically. Urine should be cultured, however, when a woman's symptoms and urine-examination findings leave the diagnosis of cystitis in question. Pretherapy cultures and susceptibility testing are also essential in the management of all patients with suspected upper tract infections and of those with complicating factors (including all men). In these situations, any of a variety of pathogens may be involved, and antibiotic therapy is best tailored to the individual organism.

UROLOGIC EVALUATION

Very few women with recurrent UTIs have correctable lesions discovered at cystoscopy or upon IV pyelography, and these procedures should not be undertaken routinely in such cases. Urologic evaluation should be performed for selected female patients—namely, women with relapsing infection, a history of childhood infections, stones or painless hematuria, or recurrent pyelonephritis. Most male patients with UTI should be considered to have complicated infection and thus should be evaluated urologically. Possible exceptions include young men who have cystitis associated with sexual activity, who are uncircumcised, or who have AIDS. Men or women presenting with acute infection and signs or symptoms suggestive of an obstruction or stones should undergo prompt urologic evaluation, generally by means of ultrasound.

℞ **Treatment:**
URINARY TRACT INFECTIONS

The following principles underlie the treatment of UTIs:

1. Except in acute uncomplicated cystitis in women, a quantitative urine culture or a comparable alternative diagnostic test should be performed to confirm infection before empirical treatment is begun, and antimicrobial sensitivity testing should be used to direct therapy.
2. Factors predisposing to infection, such as obstruction and calculi, should be identified and corrected if possible.
3. Relief of clinical symptoms does not always indicate bacteriologic cure.
4. Each course of treatment should be classified after its completion as a failure (symptoms and/or bacteriuria not eradicated during therapy or in the immediate posttreatment culture) or a cure (resolution of symptoms and elimination of bacteriuria). Recurrent infections should be classified as same-strain or different-strain and as early (occurring within 2 weeks of the end of therapy) or late.
5. In general, uncomplicated infections confined to the lower urinary tract respond to short courses of therapy, while upper tract infections require longer treatment. After therapy, early recurrences due to the same strain may result from an unresolved upper tract focus of infection but often (especially after short-course therapy for cystitis) result from persistent vaginal colonization. Recurrences >2 weeks after the cessation of therapy nearly always represent reinfection with a new strain or with the previously infecting strain that has persisted in the vaginal and rectal flora.
6. Despite increasing resistance, community-acquired infections (especially initial infections) are usually due to relatively antibiotic-sensitive strains.
7. In patients with repeated infections, instrumentation, or recent hospitalization, the presence of antibiotic-resistant strains should be suspected. Although many antimicrobial agents reach high concentrations in urine, in vitro resistance usually predicts a substantially higher failure rate.

The anatomic location of a UTI greatly influences the success or failure of a therapeutic regimen. Bladder bacteriuria (cystitis) can usually be eliminated with short courses or even single doses of antimicrobial agents. In the past, it was demonstrated that as little as a single 500-mg dose of intramuscular kanamycin eliminated bladder bacteriuria in most cases. With upper tract infections, however, single-dose therapy fails in the majority of cases, and 7- to 14-day courses are generally needed. Longer periods of treatment (2–6 weeks) aimed at eradicating a persistent focus of infection may be necessary in some cases.

ACUTE UNCOMPLICATED CYSTITIS Taken together, *E. coli* and *S. saprophyticus* cause >90–95% of cases of acute uncomplicated cystitis. Although resistance patterns vary geographically (both globally and within the United States), resistance has increased in many areas. Nevertheless, most strains are sensitive to several antibiotics. In most parts of the United States, more than one-quarter of *E. coli* strains causing acute cystitis are resistant to amoxicillin, sulfa drugs, and cephalexin; resistance to trimethoprim (TMP) and trimethoprim-sulfamethoxazole (TMP-SMX) is now approaching these levels in many areas. Substantially higher rates of resistance to TMP-SMX have been documented in some other countries, as has resistance to fluoroquinolones. Thus, knowledge of local resistance patterns is needed to guide empirical therapy.

Many have advocated single-dose treatment for acute cystitis. The advantages include less expense, ensured compliance, fewer side effects, and perhaps less intense pressure favoring the selection of resistant organisms in the intestinal, vaginal, or perineal flora. However, more frequent recurrences develop shortly after single-dose therapy than after 3-day treatment, and single-dose therapy does not eradicate vaginal colonization with *E. coli* as effectively as longer regimens. A 3-day course of TMP-SMX, TMP, norfloxacin, ciprofloxacin, or levofloxacin appears to preserve the low rate of side effects of single-dose therapy while improving efficacy (Table 20-1); thus, 3-day regimens of these drugs are currently preferred for acute cystitis. In areas where TMP-SMX resistance exceeds 20%, either a fluoroquinolone or nitrofurantoin can be used (Table 20-1). Resistance to these agents among strains causing cystitis remains low. A 3-day regimen of amoxicillin/ clavulanate was found to be significantly less effective than a 3-day regimen of ciprofloxacin in treating uncomplicated UTIs in women. Neither single-dose nor 3-day therapy should be used for women with symptoms or signs of pyelonephritis, urologic abnormalities or stones, or previous infections due to antibiotic-resistant organisms. Male patients with UTI often have urologic abnormalities or prostatic involvement and hence are not candidates for single-dose or 3-day therapy. For empirical therapy, they should generally receive a 7- to 14-day course of a fluoroquinolone (Table 20-1).

ACUTE URETHRITIS The choice of treatment for women with acute urethritis depends on the etiologic agent involved. In chlamydial infection, azithromycin (1 g in a single oral dose) or doxycycline (100 mg twice daily by mouth for 7 days) should be used. Women with acute dysuria and frequency, negative urine cultures, and no pyuria usually do not respond to antimicrobial agents.

ACUTE UNCOMPLICATED PYELONEPHRITIS In women, most cases of acute uncomplicated pyelonephritis without accompanying clinical evidence of calculi or urologic disease are due to *E. coli*. Although the optimal route and duration of therapy have not been established, a 7- to 14-day course of a fluoroquinolone is usually adequate. Neither ampicillin nor TMP-SMX should be used as initial therapy because >25% of *E. coli* strains causing pyelonephritis are now resistant to these drugs in vitro. For at least the first few days of treatment, antibiotics should probably be given intravenously to most patients, but patients with mild symptoms can be treated for 7–14 days with an oral antibiotic (usually ciprofloxacin or levofloxacin), with or without an initial single parenteral dose (Table 20-1). Patients who fail to respond to treatment within 72 h or who relapse after therapy should be evaluated for unrecognized suppurative foci, calculi, or urologic disease.

COMPLICATED URINARY TRACT INFECTIONS Complicated UTIs (those arising in a setting of catheterization, instrumentation, anatomic or functional urologic abnormalities, stones, obstruction, immunosuppression, renal disease, or diabetes) are typically due to hospital-acquired bacteria, including *E. coli*, *Klebsiella*, *Proteus*, *Serratia*, *Pseudomonas*, enterococci, and staphylococci. Many of the infecting strains are antibiotic resistant. Empirical antibiotic therapy ideally provides broad-spectrum coverage against these pathogens. In patients with minimal or mild symptoms, oral therapy with a fluoroquinolone, such as ciprofloxacin or levofloxacin, can be administered until culture results and antibiotic sensitivities are known. In patients with more severe illness, including acute pyelonephritis or suspected urosepsis, hospitalization and parenteral therapy should be undertaken. In patients with diabetes, severe outcomes are more common and should be anticipated; they include renal suppurative foci, papillary necrosis, emphysematous infection, and unusual infecting agents. Commonly used empirical regimens include imipenem alone, an extended-spectrum penicillin or cephalosporin plus an aminoglycoside, and (when the involvement of enterococci is unlikely) ceftriaxone or ceftazidime. When information on the antimicrobial sensitivity pattern of the infecting strain becomes available, a more specific antimicrobial regimen can be selected. Therapy should generally be administered for 10–21 days, with the exact duration depending on the severity of the infection and the susceptibility of the infecting strain. Follow-up cultures should be performed 2–4 weeks after cessation of therapy to demonstrate cure.

TABLE 20-1

TREATMENT REGIMENS FOR BACTERIAL URINARY TRACT INFECTIONS

CONDITION	CHARACTERISTIC PATHOGENS	MITIGATING CIRCUMSTANCES	RECOMMENDED EMPIRICAL TREATMENT[a]
Acute uncomplicated cystitis in women	*Escherichia coli, Staphylococcus saprophyticus, Proteus mirabilis, Klebsiella pneumoniae*	None	3-Day regimens: oral TMP-SMX, TMP, quinolone; 7-day regimen: macrocrystalline nitrofurantoin[b]
		Diabetes, symptoms for >7 d, recent UTI, use of diaphragm, age >65 years	Consider 7-day regimen: oral TMP-SMX, TMP, quinolone[b]
		Pregnancy	Consider 7-day regimen: oral amoxicillin, macrocrystalline nitrofurantoin, cefpodoxime proxetil, or TMP-SMX[b]
Acute uncomplicated pyelonephritis in women	*E. coli, P. mirabilis, S. saprophyticus*	Mild to moderate illness, no nausea or vomiting; outpatient therapy	Oral[c] quinolone for 7–14 d (initial dose given IV if desired); or single-dose ceftriaxone (1 g) or gentamicin (3–5 mg/kg) IV followed by oral TMP-SMX[b] for 14[d]
		Severe illness or possible urosepsis: hospitalization required	Parenteral[d] quinolone, gentamicin (± ampicillin), ceftriaxone, or aztreonam until defervescence; then oral[c] quinolone, cephalosporin, or TMP-SMX for 14 d
Complicated UTI in men and women	*E. coli, Proteus, Klebsiella, Pseudomonas, Serratia,* enterococci, staphylococci	Mild to moderate illness, no nausea or vomiting: outpatient therapy	Oral[c] quinolone for 10–14 d
		Severe illness or possible urosepsis: hospitalization required	Parenteral[d] ampicillin and gentamicin, quinolone, ceftriaxone, aztreonam, ticarcillin/clavulanate, or imipenem-cilastatin until defervescence; then oral[c] quinolone or TMP-SMX for 10–21 d

[a]Treatments listed are those to be prescribed before the etiologic agent is known; Gram's staining can be helpful in the selection of empirical therapy. Such therapy can be modified once the infecting agent has been identified. Fluoroquinolones should not be used in pregnancy. TMP-SMX, although not approved for use in pregnancy, has been widely used. Gentamicin should be used with caution in pregnancy because of its possible toxicity to eighth-nerve development in the fetus.
[b]Multiday oral regimens for cystitis are as follows: TMP-SMX, 160/800 mg q12h; TMP, 100 mg q12h; norfloxacin, 400 mg q12h; ciprofloxacin, 250 mg q12h; ofloxacin, 200 mg q12h; levofloxacin, 250 mg/d; lomefloxacin, 400 mg/d; enoxacin, 400 mg q12h; macrocrystalline nitrofurantoin, 100 mg qid; amoxicillin, 250 mg q8h; cefpodoxime proxetil, 100 mg q12h.
[c]Oral regimens for pyelonephritis and complicated UTI are as follows: TMP-SMX, 160/800 mg q12h; ciprofloxacin, 500 mg q12h; ofloxacin, 200–300 mg q12h; lomefloxacin, 400 mg/d; enoxacin, 400 mg q12h; levofloxacin, 200 mg q12h; amoxicillin, 500 mg q8h; cefpodoxime proxetil, 200 mg q12h.
[d]Parenteral regimens are as follows: ciprofloxacin, 400 mg q12h; ofloxacin, 400 mg q12h; levofloxacin, 500 mg/d; gentamicin, 1 mg/kg q8h; ceftriaxone, 1–2 g/d; ampicillin, 1 g q6h; imipenem-cilastatin, 250–500 mg q6–8h; ticarcillin/clavulanate, 3.2 g q8h; aztreonam, 1 g q8–12h.
Note: UTI, urinary tract infection; TMP, trimethoprim; TMP-SMX, trimethoprim-sulfamethoxazole.

ASYMPTOMATIC BACTERIURIA The need for treatment as well as the optimal type and duration of treatment for catheterized patients with asymptomatic bacteriuria have not been established. Removal of the catheter in conjunction with a short course of antibiotics to which the organism is susceptible probably constitutes the best course of action and nearly always eradicates bacteriuria. Treatment of asymptomatic catheter-associated bacteriuria may be of greatest benefit to elderly women, who most often develop symptoms if left untreated. If the catheter cannot be removed, antibiotic therapy usually proves unsuccessful and may in fact result in infection with a more resistant strain. In this situation, the bacteriuria should be ignored unless the patient develops symptoms or is at high risk of developing bacteremia. In these cases, use of systemic antibiotics or urinary bladder antiseptics may reduce the degree of bacteriuria and the likelihood of bacteremia.

Asymptomatic bacteriuria in noncatheterized patients is common, especially among the elderly, but has not been linked to adverse outcomes in most circumstances other than pregnancy (see below). Thus antimicrobial therapy is unnecessary and may in fact promote the emergence of resistant strains in most patients with asymptomatic bacteriuria. High-risk patients with neutropenia, renal transplants, obstruction, or other complicating conditions may require treatment when asymptomatic bacteriuria occurs. Seven days of therapy with an oral agent to which the organism is sensitive should be given initially. If bacteriuria persists, it can be monitored without further treatment in most patients. Longer-term therapy (4–6 weeks) may be necessary in high-risk patients with persistent asymptomatic bacteriuria.

TREATMENT DURING PREGNANCY In pregnancy, acute cystitis can be managed with 7 days of treatment with amoxicillin, nitrofurantoin, or a cephalosporin. All pregnant women should be screened for asymptomatic bacteriuria during the first trimester and, if bacteriuric, should be treated with one of the regimens listed in Table 20-1. After treatment, a culture should be performed to ensure cure, and cultures should be repeated monthly thereafter until delivery. Acute pyelonephritis in pregnancy should be managed with hospitalization and parenteral antibiotic therapy, generally with a cephalosporin or an extended-spectrum penicillin. Continuous low-dose prophylaxis with nitrofurantoin should be given to women who have recurrent infections during pregnancy.

PROGNOSIS

In uncomplicated cystitis or pyelonephritis, treatment ordinarily results in complete resolution of symptoms. Lower tract infections in women are of concern mainly because they cause discomfort, morbidity, loss of time from work, and substantial health care costs. Cystitis may also result in upper tract infection or in bacteremia (especially during instrumentation), but little evidence suggests that renal impairment follows. When repeated episodes of cystitis occur, they are more commonly reinfections rather than relapses.

Acute uncomplicated pyelonephritis in adults rarely progresses to renal functional impairment and chronic renal disease. Repeated upper tract infections often represent relapse rather than reinfection, and renal calculi or an underlying urologic abnormality should be vigorously sought. If neither is found, 6 weeks of chemotherapy may be useful in eradicating an unresolved focus of infection.

Repeated symptomatic UTIs in children and in adults with obstructive uropathy, neurogenic bladder, structural renal disease, or diabetes progress to renal scarring and chronic renal disease with unusual frequency. Asymptomatic bacteriuria in these groups as well as in adults without urologic disease or obstruction predisposes to increased numbers of episodes of symptomatic infection but does not result in renal impairment in most instances.

PREVENTION

Women who experience frequent symptomatic UTIs (≥3 per year on average) are candidates for long-term administration of low-dose antibiotics directed at preventing recurrences. Such women should be advised to avoid spermicide use and to void soon after intercourse. Daily or thrice-weekly administration of a single dose of TMP-SMX (80/400 mg), TMP alone (100 mg), or nitrofurantoin (50 mg) has been particularly effective. Fluoroquinolones have also been used for prophylaxis. Prophylaxis should be initiated only after bacteriuria has been eradicated with a full-dose treatment regimen. The same prophylactic regimens can be used after sexual intercourse to prevent episodes of symptomatic infection in women in whom UTIs are temporally related to intercourse. Postmenopausal women who are not taking oral estrogen replacement therapy can effectively manage recurrent UTIs with topical intravaginal estrogen cream. Other patients for whom prophylaxis appears to have some merit include men with chronic prostatitis; patients undergoing prostatectomy, both during the operation and in the postoperative period; and pregnant women with asymptomatic bacteriuria. All pregnant women should be screened for bacteriuria in the first trimester and should be treated if bacteriuria is detected.

PAPILLARY NECROSIS

When infection of the renal pyramids develops in association with vascular diseases of the kidney or with urinary tract obstruction, renal papillary necrosis is likely to result. Patients with diabetes, sickle cell disease, chronic alcoholism, and vascular disease seem peculiarly susceptible to this complication. Hematuria, pain in the flank or abdomen, and chills and fever are the most common presenting symptoms. Acute renal failure with oliguria or anuria sometimes develops. Rarely, sloughing of a pyramid may take place without symptoms in a patient with chronic UTI, and the diagnosis is made when the necrotic tissue is passed in the urine or identified as a "ring shadow" on pyelography. If renal function deteriorates suddenly in a diabetic individual or a patient with chronic obstruction, the diagnosis of renal papillary necrosis should be entertained, even in the absence of fever or pain. Renal papillary necrosis is often bilateral; when it is unilateral, however, nephrectomy may be a lifesaving approach to the management of overwhelming infection.

EMPHYSEMATOUS PYELONEPHRITIS AND CYSTITIS

These unusual clinical entities almost always occur in diabetic patients, often in concert with urinary obstruction and chronic infection. Emphysematous pyelonephritis is usually characterized by a rapidly progressive clinical course, with high fever, leukocytosis, renal parenchymal necrosis, and accumulation of fermentative gases in the kidney and perinephric tissues. Most patients also have pyuria and glucosuria. *E. coli* causes most cases, but occasionally other Enterobacteriaceae are isolated. Gas in tissues is often seen on plain films and is best confirmed and localized by CT. Surgical resection of the involved tissue in addition to systemic antimicrobial therapy is usually needed to prevent a fatal outcome in emphysematous pyelonephritis.

Emphysematous cystitis also occurs primarily in diabetic patients, usually in association with *E. coli* or other facultative gram-negative rods and often in relation to bladder outlet obstruction. Patients with this condition generally are less severely ill and have less rapidly progressive disease than those with emphysematous pyelonephritis. The patient typically reports abdominal pain, dysuria, frequency, and (in some cases) pneumaturia. CT shows gas within both the bladder lumen and the bladder wall. Generally, conservative therapy with systemic antimicrobial agents and relief of outlet obstruction are effective, but some patients do not respond to these measures and require cystectomy.

PROSTATITIS

The term *prostatitis* has been used for various inflammatory conditions affecting the prostate, including acute and chronic infections with specific bacteria and, more commonly, instances in which signs and symptoms of prostatic inflammation are present but no specific organisms can be detected. Patients with acute bacterial prostatitis can usually be identified readily on the basis of typical symptoms and signs, pyuria, and bacteriuria. To classify a patient with suspected chronic prostatitis correctly, a midstream urine specimen, a prostatic expressate, and a postmassage urine specimen should be quantitatively cultured and evaluated for numbers of leukocytes. On the basis of these studies and other considerations, patients with suspected chronic prostatitis can be categorized as having chronic bacterial prostatitis or chronic pelvic pain syndrome, with or without inflammation (Table 20-2).

ACUTE BACTERIAL PROSTATITIS

When it occurs spontaneously, this disease generally affects young men; however, it may also be associated with an indwelling urethral catheter in older men. It is characterized by fever, chills, dysuria, and a tense or boggy, extremely tender prostate. Although prostatic massage usually produces purulent secretions with a large number of bacteria on culture, vigorous massage may cause bacteremia and should be avoided. The etiologic agent can usually be identified by Gram's staining and culture of urine. In cases not associated with catheters, the infection is generally due to common gram-negative urinary tract pathogens (*E. coli* or *Klebsiella*). Initially, an intravenous fluoroquinolone is the preferred antibiotic regimen; alternatively, a third-generation cephalosporin or an aminoglycoside can be administered. The response to antibiotics in acute bacterial prostatitis is usually prompt, perhaps because drugs penetrate readily into the acutely inflamed prostate. In catheter-associated cases, the spectrum of etiologic agents is broader, including hospital-acquired gram-negative rods and enterococci. The urinary Gram stain may be particularly helpful in such cases. Imipenem, an aminoglycoside, a fluoroquinolone,

TABLE 20-2

CLASSIFICATION OF PROSTATITIS

CLASSIFICATION	CLINICAL PRESENTATION	PROSTATE	EPS	ETIOLOGIC AGENT	ANTIBIOTICS
Acute bacterial prostatitis	Acute onset of fever, chills, dysuria, urgency	Tender, tense, boggy	PMNs, bacteria	*Escherichia coli*, other uropathogens	Fluoroquinolone, other (see text)
Chronic bacterial prostatitis	Recurrent UTIs, obstructive symptoms, perineal pain	Normal	PMNs, bacteria	*E. coli*, other uropathogens	Fluoroquinolone, other (see text)
Chronic pelvic pain syndrome Inflammatory	Perineal and low-back pain, obstructive symptoms, recent NGU	Normal	↑PMNs	*Ureaplasma*? *Mycoplasma*? *Chlamydia*?	4–6 weeks of oral macrolide, tetracycline, other (see text)
Noninflammatory	Same as above	Normal	No PMNs	Unknown	None

Note: EPS, expressed prostatic secretion; NGU, nongonococcal urethritis; PMNs, polymorphonuclear leukocytes.

or a third-generation cephalosporin should be used for initial empirical therapy. The long-term prognosis is good, although in some instances acute infection may result in abscess formation, epididymoorchitis, seminal vesiculitis, septicemia, or residual chronic bacterial prostatitis. Since the advent of antibiotics, the frequency of acute bacterial prostatitis has diminished markedly.

CHRONIC BACTERIAL PROSTATITIS

This entity is now infrequent but should be considered in men with a history of recurrent bacteriuria. Symptoms are often lacking between episodes, and the prostate usually feels normal on palpation. Obstructive symptoms or perineal pain develops in some patients. Intermittently, infection spreads to the bladder, producing frequency, urgency, and dysuria. A pattern of relapsing infection in a middle-aged man strongly suggests chronic bacterial prostatitis. Classically, the diagnosis is established by culture of *E. coli*, *Klebsiella*, *Proteus*, or other uropathogenic bacteria from the expressed prostatic secretion or postmassage urine in higher quantities than are found in midstream urine. Antibiotics promptly relieve the symptoms associated with acute exacerbations but are less effective in eradicating the focus of chronic infection in the prostate. This relative ineffectiveness for long-term cure is due in part to the poor penetration of most antibiotics into the prostate. In this respect, fluoroquinolones are considerably more successful than other antimicrobial agents, but even they must generally be given for at least 12 weeks to be effective. Patients with frequent episodes of acute cystitis in whom attempts at curative therapy fail can be managed with prolonged suppressive courses of low-dose antimicrobial agents (usually a sulfonamide, TMP, or nitrofurantoin). Total prostatectomy obviously results in the cure of chronic prostatitis but is associated with considerable morbidity. Transurethral prostatectomy is safer but cures only one-third of patients.

CHRONIC PELVIC PAIN SYNDROME (FORMERLY NONBACTERIAL PROSTATITIS)

Patients who present with symptoms of prostatitis (intermittent perineal and low-back pain, obstructive voiding symptoms), few signs on examination, no bacterial growth in cultures, and no history of recurrent episodes of bacterial prostatitis are classified as having chronic pelvic pain syndrome (CPPS). Patients with CPPS are divided into inflammatory and noninflammatory subgroups based on the presence or absence of prostatic inflammation. Prostatic inflammation can be considered present when the expressed prostatic secretion and post-massage urine contain at least tenfold more leukocytes than midstream urine or when the expressed prostatic secretion contains ≥ 1000 leukocytes per microliter.

The likely etiology of CPPS associated with inflammation is an infectious agent, but the agent has not yet been identified. Evidence for a causative role of both *U. urealyticum* and *C. trachomatis* has been presented but is not conclusive. Since most cases of inflammatory CPPS occur in young, sexually active men, and since many cases follow an episode of nonspecific urethritis, the causative agent may well be sexually transmitted. The effectiveness of antimicrobial agents in this condition is uncertain. Some patients benefit from a 4- to 6-week course of treatment with erythromycin, doxycycline, TMP-SMX, or a fluoroquinolone, but controlled trials are lacking. Patients who have symptoms and signs of prostatitis but who have no evidence of prostatic inflammation (normal leukocyte counts) and negative urine cultures are classified as having noninflammatory CPPS. Despite their symptoms, these patients most likely do not have prostatic infection and should not be given antimicrobial agents.

FURTHER READINGS

De Souza RM et al: Urinary tract infection in the renal transplant patient. Nat Clin Pract Nephrol 4:252, 2008

Fihn SD et al: Clinical practice: Acute uncomplicated urinary tract infection in women. N Engl J Med 349:259, 2003

Hooton TM et al: Amoxicillin-clavulanate vs ciprofloxacin for the tresatment of uncomplicated cystitis in women. A randomized trial. JAMA 293:949, 2005

Johnson JR et al: Systematic review. Antimicrobial urinary catheters to prevent catheter-associated UTI in hospitalized patients. Ann Intern Med 144:116, 2006

Saint S et al: Catheter-associated urinary tract infection and the Medicare rule changes. Ann Intern Med 150:877, 2009

Scholes D et al: Risk factors associated with acute pyelonephritis in healthy women. Ann Intern Med 142:20, 2005

Stamm WE, Schaeffer AJ (eds): *The State of the Art in the Management of Urinary Tract Infections*. Am J Med 113(Suppl 1A):1S, 2002

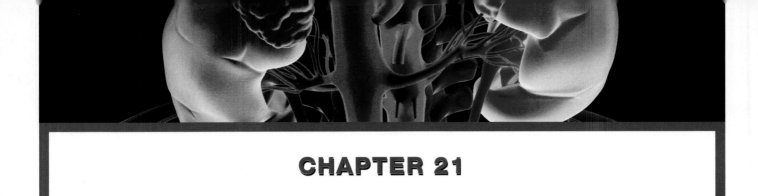

CHAPTER 21

URINARY TRACT OBSTRUCTION

Julian L. Seifter ■ Barry M. Brenner

Obstruction to the flow of urine, with attendant stasis and elevation in urinary tract pressure, impairs renal and urinary conduit functions and is a common cause of acute and chronic renal failure. With early relief of obstruction, the defects in function usually disappear completely. However, chronic obstruction may produce permanent loss of renal mass (renal atrophy) and excretory capability, as well as enhanced susceptibility to local infection and stone formation. Early diagnosis and prompt therapy are, therefore, essential to minimize the otherwise devastating effects of obstruction on kidney structure and function.

ETIOLOGY

Obstruction to urine flow can result from *intrinsic* or *extrinsic mechanical blockade* as well as from *functional defects* not associated with fixed occlusion of the urinary drainage system. Mechanical obstruction can occur at any level of the urinary tract, from the renal calyces to the external urethral meatus. Normal points of narrowing, such as the ureteropelvic and ureterovesical junctions, bladder neck, and urethral meatus, are common sites of obstruction. When blockage is above the level of the bladder, unilateral dilatation of the ureter (*hydroureter*) and renal pyelocalyceal system (*hydronephrosis*) occur; lesions at or below the level of the bladder cause bilateral involvement.

Common forms of obstruction are listed in **Table 21-1**. Childhood causes include *congenital malformations,* such as narrowing of the ureteropelvic junction and anomalous (retrocaval) location of the ureter. Vesicoureteral reflux is a common cause of prenatal hydronephrosis and, if severe, can lead to recurrent urinary infections and renal scarring in childhood. Hydronephrosis in utero may be associated with oligohydramnios and associated fetal respiratory complications. Posterior urethral valves are the most common cause of bilateral hydronephrosis in boys. Bladder dysfunction may be secondary to congenital urethral stricture, urethral meatal stenosis, or bladder neck obstruction. Prenatal obstructive uropathy may lead to decreased tubular function and decreased nephron number, which may contribute to development of hypertension and chronic kidney disease later in life. In adults, urinary tract obstruction (UTO) is due mainly to *acquired defects*. Pelvic tumors, calculi, and urethral stricture predominate. Ligation of, or injury to, the ureter during pelvic or colonic surgery can lead to hydronephrosis which, if unilateral, may remain relatively silent and undetected. *Schistosoma haematobium* and genitourinary tuberculosis are infectious causes of ureteral obstruction. Obstructive uropathy may also result from extrinsic neoplastic (carcinoma of cervix or colon) or inflammatory disorders. Retroperitoneal fibrosis, an inflammatory condition in middle-aged men, must be distinguished from other retroperitoneal causes of ureteral obstruction, particularly lymphomas and pelvic and colonic neoplasms.

248

TABLE 21-1

COMMON MECHANICAL CAUSES OF URINARY TRACT OBSTRUCTION

URETER	BLADDER OUTLET	URETHRA
Congenital		
Ureteropelvic junction narrowing or obstruction	Bladder neck obstruction	Posterior urethral valves
Ureterovesical junction narrowing or obstruction and reflux	Ureterocele	Anterior urethral valves
Ureterocele		Stricture
Retrocaval ureter		Meatal stenosis
		Phimosis
Acquired Intrinsic Defects		
Calculi	Benign prostatic hyperplasia	Stricture
Inflammation	Cancer of prostate	Tumor
Infection	Cancer of bladder	Calculi
Trauma	Calculi	Trauma
Sloughed papillae	Diabetic neuropathy	Phimosis
Tumor	Spinal cord disease	
Blood clots	Anticholinergic drugs and	
Uric acid crystals	α-adrenergic antagonists	
Acquired Extrinsic Defects		
Pregnant uterus	Carcinoma of cervix, colon	Trauma
Retroperitoneal fibrosis	Trauma	
Aortic aneurysm		
Uterine leiomyomata		
Carcinoma of uterus, prostate, bladder, colon, rectum		
Lymphoma		
Pelvic inflammatory disease, endometriosis		
Accidental surgical ligation		

Functional impairment of urine flow usually results from disorders that involve both the ureter and bladder. Causes include neurogenic bladder, often with adynamic ureter, and vesicoureteral reflux. Reflux of urine from bladder to ureter(s) is more common in children and may result in severe unilateral or bilateral hydroureter and hydronephrosis. Abnormal insertion of the ureter into the bladder is the most common cause. Vesicoureteral reflux in the absence of urinary tract infection or bladder neck obstruction usually does not lead to renal parenchymal damage and often resolves with age. Reinsertion of the ureter into the bladder is indicated if reflux is severe and unlikely to improve spontaneously, if renal function deteriorates, or if urinary tract infections recur despite chronic antimicrobial therapy. Urinary retention may be the consequence of levodopa, anticholinergic agents, and opiates. Diphenhydramine may decrease bladder emptying in the elderly patient and should be used with caution. Hydronephrosis is common in pregnancy, due both to ureteral compression by the enlarged uterus and to functional effects of progesterone.

CLINICAL FEATURES

The pathophysiology and clinical features of UTO are summarized in Table 21-2. *Pain*, the symptom that most commonly leads to medical attention, is due to distention of the collecting system or renal capsule. Pain severity is influenced more by the rate at which distention develops than by the degree of distention. Acute supravesical obstruction, as from a stone lodged in a ureter (Chap. 9), is associated with excruciating pain, known as *renal colic*. This pain is relatively steady and continuous, with little fluctuation in intensity, and often radiates to the lower abdomen, testes, or labia. By contrast, more insidious causes of obstruction, such as chronic narrowing of the ureteropelvic junction, may produce little or no pain and yet result in total destruction of the affected kidney. Flank pain that occurs only with micturition is pathognomonic of vesicoureteral reflux.

Azotemia develops when overall excretory function is impaired, often in the setting of bladder outlet obstruction, bilateral renal pelvic or ureteric obstruction, or

TABLE 21-2

PATHOPHYSIOLOGY OF BILATERAL URETERAL OBSTRUCTION		
HEMODYNAMIC EFFECTS	**TUBULE EFFECTS**	**CLINICAL FEATURES**
Acute		
↑Renal blood flow ↓GFR ↓Medullary blood flow ↑Vasodilator prostaglandins	↑Ureteral and tubule pressures ↑Reabsorption of Na$^+$, urea, water	Pain (capsule distention) Azotemia Oliguria or anuria
Chronic		
↓Renal blood flow ↓↓GFR ↑Vasoconstrictor prostaglandins ↑Renin-angiotensin production	↓Medullary osmolarity ↓Concentrating ability Structural damage; parenchymal atrophy ↓Transport functions for Na$^+$, K$^+$, H$^+$	Azotemia Hypertension ADH-insensitive polyuria Natriuresis Hyperkalemic, hyperchloremic acidosis
Release of Obstruction		
Slow ↑ in GFR (variable)	↑Tubule pressure ↓Solute load per nephron (urea, NaCl) Natriuretic factors present	Postobstructive diuresis Potential for volume depletion and electrolyte imbalance due to losses of Na$^+$, K$^+$, PO$_4^{2-}$, Mg^{2+}, and water

Note: GFR, glomerular filtration rate.

unilateral disease in a patient with a solitary functioning kidney. Complete bilateral obstruction should be suspected when acute renal failure is accompanied by anuria. Any patient with renal failure otherwise unexplained, or with a history of nephrolithiasis, hematuria, diabetes mellitus, prostatic enlargement, pelvic surgery, trauma, or tumor should be evaluated for UTO.

In the acute setting, bilateral obstruction may mimic prerenal azotemia. However, with more prolonged obstruction, symptoms of *polyuria* and *nocturia* commonly accompany partial UTO and result from impaired renal concentrating ability. This defect usually does not improve with administration of vasopressin and is therefore a form of acquired nephrogenic diabetes insipidus. Disturbances in sodium chloride transport in the ascending limb of the loop of Henle and, in azotemic patients, the osmotic (urea) diuresis per nephron lead to decreased medullary hypertonicity and, hence, a concentrating defect. Partial obstruction, therefore, may be associated with increased rather than decreased urine output. Indeed, wide fluctuations in urine output in a patient with azotemia should always raise the possibility of intermittent or partial UTO. If fluid intake is inadequate, severe dehydration and hypernatremia may develop. Hesitancy and straining to initiate the urinary stream, postvoid dribbling, urinary frequency, and incontinence are common with obstruction at or below the level of the bladder.

Partial bilateral UTO often results in *acquired distal renal tubular acidosis*, *hyperkalemia*, and *renal salt wasting*. These defects in tubule function are often accompanied by renal tubulointerstitial damage. Initially the interstitium becomes edematous and infiltrated with mononuclear inflammatory cells. Later, interstitial fibrosis and atrophy of the papillae and medulla occur and precede these processes in the cortex.

UTO must always be considered in patients with urinary tract infections or urolithiasis. Urinary stasis encourages the growth of organisms. Urea-splitting bacteria are associated with magnesium ammonium phosphate (struvite) calculi. *Hypertension* is frequent in acute and subacute unilateral obstruction and is usually a consequence of increased release of renin by the involved kidney. Chronic hydronephrosis, in the presence of extracellular volume expansion, may result in significant hypertension. *Erythrocytosis*, an infrequent complication of obstructive uropathy, is probably secondary to increased erythropoietin production.

DIAGNOSIS

A history of difficulty in voiding, pain, infection, or change in urinary volume is common. Evidence for distention of the kidney or urinary bladder can often be obtained by palpation and percussion of the abdomen. A careful rectal examination may reveal enlargement or nodularity of the prostate, abnormal rectal sphincter tone, or a rectal or pelvic mass. The penis should be inspected for evidence of meatal stenosis or phimosis. In the female, vaginal, uterine, and rectal lesions responsible for UTO are usually revealed by inspection and palpation.

Urinalysis may reveal hematuria, pyuria, and bacteriuria. The urine sediment is often normal, even

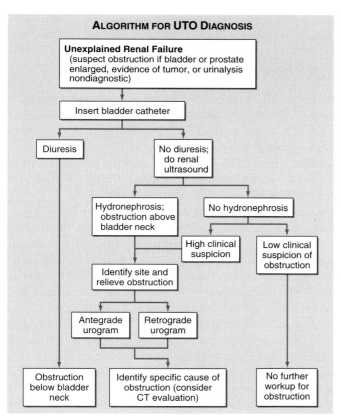

ALGORITHM FOR UTO DIAGNOSIS

Unexplained Renal Failure
(suspect obstruction if bladder or prostate enlarged, evidence of tumor, or urinalysis nondiagnostic)

↓

Insert bladder catheter

→ Diuresis

→ No diuresis; do renal ultrasound

→ Hydronephrosis; obstruction above bladder neck

→ No hydronephrosis

→ High clinical suspicion

→ Low clinical suspicion of obstruction

Identify site and relieve obstruction

Antegrade urogram | Retrograde urogram

Obstruction below bladder neck

Identify specific cause of obstruction (consider CT evaluation)

No further workup for obstruction

FIGURE 21-1

Diagnostic approach for urinary tract obstruction in unexplained renal failure. CT, computed tomography.

when obstruction leads to marked azotemia and extensive structural damage. An abdominal scout film may detect nephrocalcinosis or a radiopaque stone. As indicated in **Fig. 21-1**, if UTO is suspected, a bladder catheter should be inserted. If diuresis does not follow, then abdominal ultrasonography should be performed to evaluate renal and bladder size, as well as pyelocalyceal contour. Ultrasonography is approximately 90% specific and sensitive for detection of hydronephrosis. False-positive results are associated with diuresis, renal cysts, or the presence of an extrarenal pelvis, a normal congenital variant. Hydronephrosis may be absent on ultrasound when obstruction is associated with volume contraction, staghorn calculi, retroperitoneal fibrosis, or infiltrative renal disease. Duplex Doppler ultrasonography may detect an increased resistive index in urinary obstruction, but that finding is not specific. Ultrasound often does not allow visualization of the ureter.

In some cases, the intravenous urogram may define the site of obstruction. In the presence of obstruction, the appearance time of the nephrogram is delayed. Eventually the renal image becomes more dense than normal because of slow tubular fluid flow rate, which results in greater concentration of contrast medium. The

renal pelvis, and ureter above the obstruction. The ureter is not tortuous as in chronic obstruction. In comparison with the nephrogram, the urogram may be faint, especially if the dilated renal pelvis is voluminous, causing dilution of the contrast medium. The radiographic study should be continued until the site of obstruction is determined or the contrast medium is excreted. Radionuclide scans, though sensitive for the detection of obstruction, define less anatomic detail than intravenous urography and, like the urogram, are of limited value when renal function is poor. They have a role in patients at high risk for reaction to intravenous contrast. Patients suspected of having intermittent ureteropelvic obstruction should have radiologic evaluation while in pain, since a normal urogram is commonly seen during asymptomatic periods. Hydration often helps to provoke a symptomatic attack.

To facilitate visualization of a suspected lesion in a ureter or renal pelvis, *retrograde* or *antegrade urography* should be attempted. These diagnostic studies may be preferable to the intravenous urogram in the azotemic patient, in whom poor excretory function precludes adequate visualization of the collecting system. Furthermore, intravenous urography carries the risk of contrast-induced acute renal failure in patients with proteinuria, renal insufficiency, diabetes mellitus, or multiple myeloma, particularly if they are dehydrated. The retrograde approach involves catheterization of the involved ureter under cystoscopic control, while the antegrade technique necessitates placement of a catheter into the renal pelvis via a needle inserted percutaneously under ultrasonic or fluoroscopic guidance. While the antegrade approach may provide immediate decompression of a unilateral obstructing lesion, many urologists initially attempt the retrograde approach unless the catheterization is unsuccessful or general anesthesia is contraindicated.

Voiding cystourethrography is of value in the diagnosis of vesicoureteral reflux and bladder neck and urethral obstructions. Patients with obstruction at or below the level of the bladder exhibit thickening, trabeculation, and diverticula of the bladder wall. Postvoiding films reveal residual urine. If these radiographic studies fail to provide adequate information for diagnosis, endoscopic visualization by the urologist often permits precise identification of lesions involving the urethra, prostate, bladder, and ureteral orifices.

CT is useful in the diagnosis of specific intraabdominal and retroperitoneal causes of obstruction. The unenhanced helical CT is the preferred study to image obstructing urinary calculi in the patient with colic, and it is also useful in imaging nonobstructing calculi in the patient with hematuria. MRI may also be useful in the identification of specific obstructive causes.

℞ Treatment:
URINARY TRACT OBSTRUCTION

UTO complicated by infection requires relief of obstruction as soon as possible to prevent development of generalized sepsis and progressive renal damage. On a temporary basis, drainage is often satisfactorily achieved by nephrostomy, ureterostomy, or ureteral, urethral, or suprapubic catheterization. The patient with acute urinary tract infection and obstruction should be given appropriate antibiotics based on in vitro bacterial sensitivity and the ability of the drug to concentrate in the urine. Treatment may be required for 3–4 weeks. Chronic or recurrent infections in an obstructed kidney with poor intrinsic function may necessitate nephrectomy. When infection is not present, immediate surgery often is not required, even in the presence of complete obstruction and anuria because of the availability of dialysis, until acid-base, fluid and electrolyte, and cardiovascular status are restored. Nevertheless, the site of obstruction should be ascertained as soon as feasible, in part because of the possibility that sepsis may occur, a complication that necessitates prompt urologic intervention. Elective relief of obstruction is usually recommended in patients with urinary retention, recurrent urinary tract infections, persistent pain, or progressive loss of renal function. Benign prostatic hypertrophy may be treated medically with α-adrenergic blockers and 5α-reductase inhibitors. Mechanical obstruction may be alleviated by radiation therapy in cases of retroperitoneal lymphoma. Functional obstruction secondary to neurogenic bladder may be decreased with the combination of frequent voiding and cholinergic drugs. The approach to obstruction secondary to renal stones is discussed in Chap. 9.

PROGNOSIS

With relief of obstruction, the prognosis regarding return of renal function depends largely on whether irreversible renal damage has occurred. When obstruction is not relieved, the course will depend mainly on whether the obstruction is complete or incomplete and bilateral or unilateral, as well as whether or not urinary tract infection is also present. Complete obstruction with infection can lead to total destruction of the kidney within days. Partial return of glomerular filtration rate may follow relief of complete obstruction of 1 and 2 weeks' duration, but after 8 weeks of obstruction, recovery is unlikely. In the absence of definitive evidence of irreversibility, every effort should be made to decompress the obstruction in the hope of restoring renal function at least partially. A renal radionuclide scan, performed after a prolonged period of decompression, may be used to predict the reversibility of renal dysfunction.

POSTOBSTRUCTIVE DIURESIS

Relief of bilateral, but not unilateral, complete obstruction commonly results in polyuria, which may be massive. The urine is usually hypotonic and may contain large amounts of sodium chloride, potassium, and magnesium. The natriuresis is due in part to the excretion of retained urea (osmotic diuresis). The increase in intratubular pressure very likely also contributes to the impairment in net sodium chloride reabsorption, especially in the terminal nephron segments. Natriuretic factors may also accumulate during uremia and depress salt and water reabsorption when urine flow is reestablished. In the majority of patients this diuresis results in the *appropriate* excretion of the excesses of retained salt and water. When extracellular volume and composition return to normal, the diuresis usually abates spontaneously. Therefore, replacement of urinary losses should only be done in the setting of hypovolemia, hypotension, or disturbances in serum electrolyte concentrations. Occasionally, iatrogenic expansion of extracellular volume is responsible for, or sustains, the diuresis observed in the postobstructive period. Replacement of no more than two-thirds of urinary volume losses per day is usually effective in avoiding this complication. The loss of electrolyte-free water with urea may result in hypernatremia. Serum and urine sodium and osmolal concentrations should guide the use of appropriate intravenous replacement. Often replacement with 0.45% saline is required. In a rare patient, relief of obstruction may be followed by urinary salt and water losses severe enough to provoke profound dehydration and vascular collapse. In these patients, an intrinsic defect in tubule reabsorptive function is probably responsible for the marked diuresis. Appropriate therapy in such patients includes intravenous administration of salt-containing solutions to replace sodium and volume deficits.

FURTHER READINGS

BECKMAN TJ, MYNDERSE LA: Evaluation and medical management of benign prostatic hyperplasia. Mayo Clin Proc 80:1356, 2005

GULMI FA et al: Upper urinary tract obstruction and trauma, sections 36 and 37, in *Campbell's Urology*, 9th ed., PC Walsh et al (eds). Philadelphia, Saunders, 2007

KLAHR S: Urinary tract obstruction, in *Diseases of the Kidney*, 7th ed, RW Schrier, CW Gottschalk (eds). Boston, Little, Brown, 2001, pp 751–787

WILLIAMS B et al: Pathophysiology and treatment of ureteropelvic junction obstruction. Curr Urol Rep 8:111, 2007

ZEIDEL ML, PIRTSKHALAISHVILI G: Urinary tract obstruction, in *Brenner and Rector's The Kidney*, 7th ed, BM Brenner (ed). Philadelphia, Saunders, 2004, pp 1867–1894

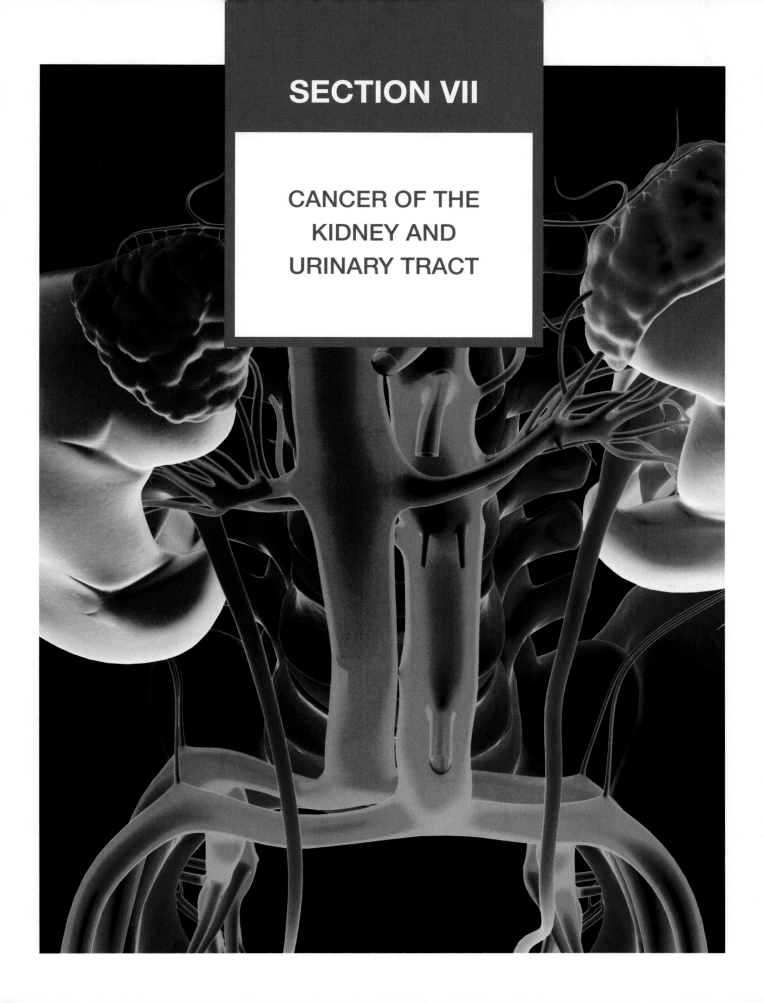

SECTION VII

CANCER OF THE KIDNEY AND URINARY TRACT

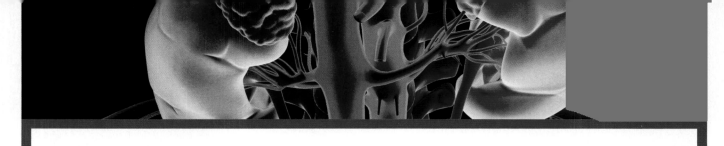

CHAPTER 22
BLADDER AND RENAL CELL CARCINOMAS

Howard I. Scher ■ Robert J. Motzer

BLADDER CANCER

A transitional cell epithelium lines the urinary tract from the renal pelvis to the ureter, urinary bladder, and the proximal two-thirds of the urethra. Cancers can occur at any point: 90% of malignancies develop in the bladder, 8% in the renal pelvis, and the remaining 2% in the ureter or urethra. Bladder cancer is the fourth most common cancer in men and the thirteenth in women, with an estimated 67,160 new cases and 13,750 deaths in the United States predicted for the year 2007. The almost 5:1 ratio of incidence to mortality reflects the higher frequency of the less lethal superficial variants compared to the more lethal invasive and metastatic variants. The incidence is three times higher in men than in women, and twofold higher in whites than blacks, with a median age at diagnosis of 65 years.

Once diagnosed, urothelial tumors exhibit poly-chronotropism—the tendency to recur over time and in new locations in the urothelial tract. As long as urothelium is present, continuous monitoring of the tract is required.

EPIDEMIOLOGY

Cigarette smoking is believed to contribute to up to 50% of the diagnosed urothelial cancers in men and up to 40% in women. The risk of developing a urothelial malignancy in male smokers is increased two- to fourfold relative to nonsmokers and continues for 10 years or longer after cessation. Other implicated agents include the aniline dyes, the drugs phenacetin and chlornaphazine, and external beam radiation. Chronic cyclophosphamide exposure may also increase risk, whereas vitamin A supplements appear to be protective. Exposure to *Schistosoma haematobium*, a parasite found in many developing countries, is associated with an increase in both squamous and transitional cell carcinomas of the bladder.

PATHOLOGY

Clinical subtypes are grouped into three categories: 75% are superficial, 20% invade muscle, and 5% are metastatic at presentation. Staging of the tumor within the bladder is based on the pattern of growth and depth of invasion: Ta lesions grow as exophytic lesions; carcinoma in situ (CIS) lesions start on the surface and tend to invade. The revised tumor, node, metastasis (TNM) staging system is illustrated in **Fig. 22-1**. About half of invasive tumors presented originally as superficial lesions that later progressed. Tumors are also rated by grade. Grade I lesions (highly differentiated tumors) rarely progress to a higher stage, whereas grade III tumors do.

More than 95% of urothelial tumors in the United States are transitional cell in origin. Pure squamous cancers with keratinization constitute 3%, adenocarcinomas 2%, and small cell tumors (with paraneoplastic syndromes) <1%. Adenocarcinomas develop primarily in

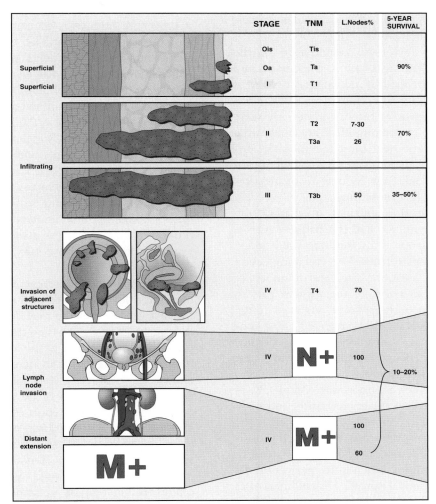

FIGURE 22-1
Bladder staging. TNM, tumor, node, metastasis.

the urachal remnant in the dome of the bladder or in the periurethral tissues; some assume a signet cell histology. Lymphomas and melanomas are rare. Of the transitional cell tumors, low-grade papillary lesions that grow on a central stalk are most common. These tumors are very friable, have a tendency to bleed, are at high risk for recurrence, and yet rarely progress to the more lethal invasive variety. In contrast, CIS is a high-grade tumor that is considered a precursor of the more lethal muscle-invasive disease.

PATHOGENESIS

The multicentric nature of the disease and high rate of recurrence has led to the hypothesis of a field defect in the urothelium that results in a predisposition to cancer. Molecular genetic analyses suggest that the superficial and invasive lesions develop along distinct molecular pathways in which primary tumorigenic aberrations precede secondary changes associated with progression to a more advanced stage. Low-grade papillary tumors that do not tend to invade or metastasize harbor constitutive activation of the receptor-tyrosine kinase-Ras signal transduction pathway and a high frequency of fibroblast growth factor receptor 3 (FGFR3) mutations. In contrast, CIS and invasive tumors have a higher frequency of *TP53* and *RB* gene alternations. Within all clinical stages, including Tis, T1, and T2 or greater lesions, tumors with alterations in *p53*, *p21*, and/or *RB* have a higher probability of recurrence, metastasis, and death from disease.

CLINICAL PRESENTATION, DIAGNOSIS, AND STAGING

Hematuria occurs in 80–90% of patients and often reflects exophytic tumors. The bladder is the most common source of gross hematuria (40%), but benign cystitis (22%) is a more common cause than bladder cancer (15%) (Chap. 3). Microscopic hematuria is more commonly of prostate origin (25%); only 2% of bladder cancers produce microscopic hematuria. Once hematuria is documented, a urinary cytology, visualization of the urothelial tract by CT or intravenous pyelogram, and cystoscopy are recommended if no other etiology is found. Screening asymptomatic individuals for hematuria increases the diagnosis of tumors at an early stage but has not been shown to prolong life. After hematuria, irritative symptoms are the next most common presentation, which may reflect in situ disease. Obstruction of the ureters may cause flank pain. Symptoms of metastatic disease are rarely the first presenting sign.

The endoscopic evaluation includes an examination under anesthesia to determine whether a palpable mass is present. A flexible endoscope is inserted into the bladder, and bladder barbotage is performed. The visual inspection includes mapping the location, size, and number of lesions, as well as a description of the growth pattern (solid vs. papillary). An intraoperative video is often recorded. All visible tumors should be resected, and a sample of the muscle underlying the tumor should be obtained to assess the depth of invasion. Normal-appearing areas are biopsied at random to ensure no field defect. A notation is made as to whether a tumor was completely or incompletely resected. Selective catheterization and visualization of the upper tracts should be performed if the cytology is positive and no disease is visible in the bladder. Ultrasonography, CT, and/or MRI may help to determine whether a tumor extends to perivesical fat (T3) and to document nodal spread. Distant metastases are assessed by CT of the chest and abdomen, MRI, or radionuclide imaging of the skeleton.

℞ Treatment: BLADDER CANCER

Management depends on whether the tumor invades muscle and whether it has spread to the regional lymph nodes and beyond. The probability of spread increases with increasing T stage.

SUPERFICIAL DISEASE At a minimum, the management of a superficial tumor is complete endoscopic resection with or without intravesical therapy. The decision to recommend intravesical therapy depends on the histologic subtype, number of lesions, depth of invasion, presence or absence of CIS, and antecedent history. Recurrences develop in upward of 50% of cases, of which 5–20% progress to a more advanced stage. In general, solitary papillary lesions are managed by transurethral surgery alone. CIS and recurrent disease are treated by transurethral surgery followed by intravesical therapy.

Intravesical therapies are used in two general contexts: as an adjuvant to a complete endoscopic resection to prevent recurrence or, less commonly, to eliminate disease that cannot be controlled by endoscopic resection alone. Intravesical treatments are advised for patients with recurrent disease, >40% involvement of the bladder surface by tumor, diffuse CIS, or T1 disease. The standard intravesical therapy, based on randomized comparisons, is bacillus Calmette-Guerin (BCG) in six weekly instillations, followed by monthly maintenance administrations for ≥1 year. Other agents with activity include mitomycin-C, interferon (IFN), and gemcitabine. The side effects of intravesical therapies include dysuria, urinary frequency, and, depending on the drug, myelosuppression or contact dermatitis. Rarely, intravesical BCG may produce a systemic illness associated with granulomatous infections in multiple sites that requires antituberculin therapy.

Following the endoscopic resection, patients are monitored for recurrence at 3-month intervals during the first year. Recurrence may develop anywhere along the urothelial tract, including the renal pelvis, ureter, or urethra. A consequence of the "successful" treatment of tumors in the bladder is an increase in the frequency of extravesical recurrences (e.g., urethra or ureter). Those with persistent disease or new tumors are generally considered for a second course of BCG or for intravesical chemotherapy with valrubicin or gemcitabine. In some cases cystectomy is recommended, although the specific indications vary. Tumors in the ureter or renal pelvis are typically managed by resection during retrograde examination or, in some cases, by instillation through the renal pelvis. Tumors of the prostatic urethra may require cystectomy if the tumor cannot be resected completely.

INVASIVE DISEASE The treatment of a tumor that has invaded muscle can be separated into control of the primary tumor and, depending on the pathologic findings at surgery, systemic chemotherapy. Radical cystectomy is the standard, although in selected cases a bladder-sparing approach is used; this approach includes complete endoscopic resection; partial cystectomy; or a combination of resection, systemic chemotherapy, and external beam radiation therapy. In some countries, external beam radiation therapy is considered standard. In the United States, its role is limited to those patients deemed unfit for cystectomy, those with unresectable local disease, or as part of an experimental bladder-sparing approach.

Indications for cystectomy include muscle-invading tumors not suitable for segmental resection; low-stage tumors unsuitable for conservative management (e.g., due to multicentric and frequent recurrences resistant to intravesical instillations); high-grade tumors (T1G3) associated with CIS; and bladder symptoms, such as frequency or hemorrhage, that impair quality of life.

Radical cystectomy is major surgery that requires appropriate preoperative evaluation and management. The procedure involves removal of the bladder and pelvic lymph nodes and creation of a conduit or reservoir for urinary flow. Grossly abnormal lymph nodes are evaluated by frozen section. If metastases are confirmed, the procedure is often aborted. In males, radical cystectomy includes the removal of the prostate, seminal vesicles, and proximal urethra. Impotence is universal unless the nerves responsible for erectile function are preserved. In females, the procedure includes removal of the bladder, urethra, uterus, fallopian tubes, ovaries, anterior vaginal wall, and surrounding fascia.

Previously, urine flow was managed by directing the ureters to the abdominal wall, where it was collected in an external appliance. Currently, most patients receive either a continent cutaneous reservoir constructed from detubularized bowel or an orthotopic neobladder. Some 70% of men receive a neobladder. With a continent reservoir, 65–85% of men will be continent at night and 85–90% during the day. Cutaneous reservoirs are drained by intermittent catheterization; orthotopic neobladders are drained more naturally. Contraindications to a neobladder include renal insufficiency, an inability to self-catheterize, or an exophytic tumor or CIS in the urethra. Diffuse CIS in the bladder is a relative contraindication based on the risk of a urethral recurrence. Concurrent ulcerative colitis or Crohn's disease may hinder the use of resected bowel.

A partial cystectomy may be considered when the disease is limited to the dome of the bladder, a margin of at least 2 cm can be achieved, there is no CIS in other sites, and the bladder capacity is adequate after the tumor has been removed. This occurs in 5–10% of cases. Carcinomas in the ureter or in the renal pelvis are treated with nephroureterectomy with a bladder cuff to remove the tumor.

The probability of recurrence following surgery is predicted on the basis of pathologic stage, presence or absence of lymphatic or vascular invasion, and nodal spread. Among those whose cancers recur, the recurrence develops in a median of 1 year (range 0.04–11.1 years). Long-term outcomes vary by pathologic stage and histology (Table 22-1). The number of lymph nodes removed is also prognostic, whether or not the nodes contained tumor.

Chemotherapy has been shown to prolong the survival of patients with invasive disease, but only when combined with definitive treatment of the bladder by radical cystectomy or radiation therapy. Thus, for the majority of patients, chemotherapy alone is inadequate to clear the bladder of disease. Experimental studies are evaluating bladder preservation strategies by combining chemotherapy and radiation therapy in patients whose tumors were endoscopically removed.

TABLE 22-1

SURVIVAL FOLLOWING SURGERY FOR BLADDER CANCER

PATHOLOGIC STAGE	5-YEAR SURVIVAL, %	10-YEAR SURVIVAL, %
T2,N0	89	87
T3a,N0	78	76
T3b,N0	62	61
T4,N0	50	45
Any T,N1	35	34

METASTATIC DISEASE The primary goal of treatment for metastatic disease is to achieve complete remission with chemotherapy alone or with a combined-modality approach of chemotherapy followed by surgical resection of residual disease, as is done routinely for the treatment of germ cell tumors. One can define a goal in terms of cure or palliation on the basis of the probability of achieving a complete response to chemotherapy using prognostic factors, such as Karnofsky Performance Status (KPS) (<80%), and whether the pattern of spread is nodal or visceral (liver, lung, or bone). For those with zero, one, or two risk factors, the probability of complete remission is 38, 25, and 5%, respectively, and median survival is 33, 13.4, and 9.3 months, respectively. Patients who are functionally compromised or who have visceral disease or bone metastases rarely achieve long-term survival. The toxicities also vary as a function of risk, and treatment-related mortality rates are as high as 3–4% using some combinations in these poor-risk patient groups.

CHEMOTHERAPY A number of chemotherapeutic drugs have shown activity as single agents; cisplatin, paclitaxel, and gemcitabine are considered most active. Standard therapy consists of two-, three-, or four-drug combinations. Overall response rates of >50% have been reported using combinations such as methotrexate, vinblastine, doxorubicin, and cisplatin (M-VAC); cisplatin and paclitaxel (PT); gemcitabine and cisplatin (GC); or gemcitabine, paclitaxel, and cisplatin (GTC). M-VAC was considered standard, but the toxicities of neutropenia and fever, mucositis, diminished renal and auditory function, and peripheral neuropathy led to the development of alternative regimens. At present, GC is used more commonly than M-VAC, based on the results of a comparative trial of M-VAC versus GC that showed less neutropenia and fever, and less mucositis for the GC regimen. Anemia and thrombocytopenia were more common with GC. GTC is not more effective than GC.

Chemotherapy has also been evaluated in the neoadjuvant and adjuvant settings. In a randomized trial, patients receiving three cycles of neoadjuvant M-VAC followed by cystectomy had a significantly better

TABLE 22-2

MANAGEMENT OF BLADDER CANCER

NATURE OF LESION	MANAGEMENT APPROACH
Superficial	Endoscopic removal, usually with intravesical therapy
Invasive disease	Cystectomy ± systemic chemotherapy (before or after surgery)
Metastatic disease	Curative or palliative chemotherapy (based on prognostic factors) ± surgery

median (6.2 years) and 5-year survival (57%) compared to cystectomy alone (median survival 3.8 years; 5-year survival 42%). Similar results were obtained in an international study of three cycles of cisplatin, methotrexate, and vinblastine (CMV) followed by either radical cystectomy or radiation therapy. The decision to administer adjuvant therapy is based on the risk of recurrence after cystectomy. Indications for adjuvant chemotherapy include the presence of nodal disease, extravesical tumor extension, or vascular invasion in the resected specimen. Another study of adjuvant therapy found that four cycles of CMV delayed recurrence, although an effect on survival was less clear. Additional trials are studying taxane- and gemcitabine-based combinations.

The management of bladder cancer is summarized in Table 22-2.

CARCINOMA OF THE RENAL PELVIS AND URETER

About 2500 cases of renal pelvis and ureter cancer occur each year; nearly all are transitional cell carcinomas similar to bladder cancer in biology and appearance. This tumor is also associated with chronic phenacetin abuse and with Balkan nephropathy, a chronic interstitial nephritis endemic in Bulgaria, Greece, Bosnia-Herzegovina, and Romania.

The most common symptom is painless gross hematuria, and the disease is usually detected on intravenous pyelogram during the workup for hematuria. Patterns of spread are like those in bladder cancer. For low-grade disease localized to the renal pelvis and ureter, nephroureterectomy (including excision of the distal ureter with a portion of the bladder) is associated with 5-year survival of 80–90%. More invasive or histologically poorly differentiated tumors are more likely to recur locally and to metastasize. Metastatic disease is treated with the chemotherapy used in bladder cancer, and the outcome is similar to that of metastatic transitional cell cancer of bladder origin.

RENAL CELL CARCINOMA

Renal cell carcinomas account for 90–95% of malignant neoplasms arising from the kidney. Notable features include resistance to cytotoxic agents, infrequent responses to biologic response modifiers such as interleukin (IL) 2, and a variable clinical course for patients with metastatic disease, including anecdotal reports of spontaneous regression.

EPIDEMIOLOGY

The incidence of renal cell carcinoma continues to rise and is now nearly 51,000 cases annually in the United States, resulting in 13,000 deaths. The male to female ratio is 2:1. Incidence peaks between the ages of 50 and 70, although this malignancy may be diagnosed at any age. Many environmental factors have been investigated as possible contributing causes; the strongest association is with cigarette smoking (accounting for 20–30% of cases). Risk is also increased for patients who have acquired cystic disease of the kidney associated with end-stage renal disease, and for those with tuberous sclerosis. Most cases are sporadic, although familial forms have been reported. One is associated with von Hippel-Lindau (VHL) syndrome, which predisposes to renal cell carcinomas, retinal hemangioma, hemangioblastoma of the spinal cord and cerebellum, and pheochromocytoma. Roughly 35% of individuals with VHL disease develop renal cell cancer. An increased incidence has also been reported for first-degree relatives.

PATHOLOGY AND GENETICS

Renal cell neoplasia represents a heterogeneous group of tumors with distinct histopathologic, genetic, and clinical features ranging from benign to high-grade malignant (Table 22-3). They are classified on the basis of morphology and histology. Categories include clear cell carcinoma (60% of cases), papillary tumors (5–15%), chromophobic tumors (5–10%), oncocytomas (5–10%), and collecting or Bellini duct tumors (<1%). Papillary tumors tend to be bilateral and multifocal. Chromophobic tumors have a more indolent clinical course, and oncocytomas are considered benign neoplasms. In contrast, Bellini duct carcinomas, which are thought to arise from the collecting ducts within the renal medulla, are very rare but very aggressive. They tend to affect younger patients.

Clear cell tumors, the predominant histology, are found in >80% of patients who develop metastases. Clear cell tumors arise from the epithelial cells of the proximal tubules and usually show chromosome 3p deletions. Deletions of 3p21–26 (where the *VHL* gene

TABLE 22-3

CLASSIFICATION OF EPITHELIAL NEOPLASMS ARISING FROM THE KIDNEY			
CARCINOMA TYPE	**GROWTH PATTERN**	**CELL OF ORIGIN**	**CYTOGENETICS**
Clear cell	Acinar or sarcomatoid	Proximal tubule	3p−
Papillary	Papillary or sarcomatoid	Proximal tubule	+7, +17, −Y
Chromophobic	Solid, tubular, or sarcomatoid	Cortical collecting duct	Hypodiploid
Oncocytic	Tumor nests	Cortical collecting duct	Undetermined
Collecting duct	Papillary or sarcomatoid	Medullary collecting duct	Undetermined

maps) are identified in patients with familial as well as sporadic tumors. *VHL* encodes a tumor-suppressor protein that is involved in regulating the transcription of vascular endothelial growth factor (VEGF), platelet-derived growth factor (PDGF), and a number of other hypoxia-inducible proteins. Inactivation of *VHL* leads to overexpression of these agonists of the VEGF and PDGF receptors, which promote tumor angiogenesis and tumor growth. Agents that inhibit proangiogenic growth factor activity show antitumor effects.

CLINICAL PRESENTATION

The presenting signs and symptoms include hematuria, abdominal pain, and a flank or abdominal mass. This classic triad occurs in 10–20% of patients. Other symptoms are fever, weight loss, anemia, and a varicocele (**Table 22-4**). The tumor can also be found incidentally on a radiograph. Widespread use of radiologic

TABLE 22-4

SIGNS AND SYMPTOMS IN PATIENTS WITH RENAL CELL CANCER	
PRESENTING SIGN OR SYMPTOM	**INCIDENCE, %**
Classic triad: hematuria, flank pain, flank mass	10–20
Hematuria	40
Flank pain	40
Palpable mass	25
Weight loss	33
Anemia	33
Fever	20
Hypertension	20
Abnormal liver function	15
Hypercalcemia	5
Erythrocytosis	3
Neuromyopathy	3
Amyloidosis	2
Increased erythrocyte sedimentation rate	55

cross-sectional imaging procedures (CT, ultrasound, MRI) contributes to earlier detection, including incidental renal masses detected during evaluation for other medical conditions. The increasing number of incidentally discovered low-stage tumors has contributed to an improved 5-year survival for patients with renal cell carcinoma and increased use of nephron-sparing surgery (partial nephrectomy). A spectrum of paraneoplastic syndromes has been associated with these malignancies, including erythrocytosis, hypercalcemia, nonmetastatic hepatic dysfunction (Stauffer syndrome), and acquired dysfibrinogenemia. Erythrocytosis is noted at presentation in only about 3% of patients. Anemia, a sign of advanced disease, is more common.

The standard evaluation of patients with suspected renal cell tumors includes a CT scan of the abdomen and pelvis, chest radiograph, urine analysis, and urine cytology. If metastatic disease is suspected from the chest radiograph, a CT of the chest is warranted. MRI is useful in evaluating the inferior vena cava in cases of suspected tumor involvement or invasion by thrombus. In clinical practice, any solid renal masses should be considered malignant until proven otherwise; a definitive diagnosis is required. If no metastases are demonstrated, surgery is indicated, even if the renal vein is invaded. The differential diagnosis of a renal mass includes cysts, benign neoplasms (adenoma, angiomyolipoma, oncocytoma), inflammatory lesions (pyelonephritis or abscesses), and other primary or metastatic cancers. Other malignancies that may involve the kidney include transitional cell carcinoma of the renal pelvis, sarcoma, lymphoma, and Wilms' tumor. All of these are less common causes of renal masses than is renal cell cancer.

STAGING AND PROGNOSIS

Two staging systems used are the Robson classification and the American Joint Committee on Cancer (AJCC) staging system. According to the AJCC system, stage I tumors are <7 cm in greatest diameter and confined to the kidney, stage II tumors are ≥7 cm and confined to the kidney, stage III tumors extend through the renal capsule but are confined to Gerota's fascia (IIIa) or involve a single hilar lymph node (N1), and stage IV disease includes tumors that have invaded adjacent organs (excluding the adrenal gland) or involve multiple lymph nodes or distant metastases. The rate of 5-year survival varies by stage: >90% for stage I, 85% for stage II, 60% for stage III, and 10% for stage IV.

℞ Treatment: RENAL CELL CARCINOMA

LOCALIZED TUMORS The standard management for stage I or II tumors and selected cases of stage III disease is radical nephrectomy. This procedure involves en bloc removal of Gerota's fascia and its contents, including the kidney, the ipsilateral adrenal gland, and adjacent hilar lymph nodes. The role of a regional lymphadenectomy is controversial. Extension into the renal vein or inferior vena cava (stage III disease) does not preclude resection even if cardiopulmonary bypass is required. If the tumor is resected, half of these patients have prolonged survival.

Nephron-sparing approaches via open or laparoscopic surgery may be appropriate for patients who have only one kidney, depending on the size and location of the lesion. A nephron-sparing approach can also be used for patients with bilateral tumors, accompanied by a radical nephrectomy on the opposite side. Partial nephrectomy techniques are being applied electively to resect small masses for patients with a normal contralateral kidney. Adjuvant therapy following this surgery does not improve outcome, even in cases with a poor prognosis.

ADVANCED DISEASE Surgery has a limited role for patients with metastatic disease. However, long-term survival may occur in patients who relapse after nephrectomy in a solitary site that can be removed. One indication for nephrectomy with metastases at initial presentation is to alleviate pain or hemorrhage of a primary tumor. Also, a cytoreductive nephrectomy before systemic treatment improves survival for carefully selected patients with stage IV tumors.

Metastatic renal cell carcinoma is highly refractory to chemotherapy and only infrequently responsive to cytokine therapy with IL-2 or IFN-α. IFN-α and IL-2 produce regressions in 10–20% of patients, but on occasion these responses are durable. IL-2 was approved on the observation of durable complete remission in a small proportion of cases.

The situation changed dramatically when two large-scale randomized trials established a role for antiangiogenic therapy in this disease as predicted by the genetic studies. These trials separately evaluated two orally administered antiangiogenic agents, sorafenib and sunitinib, that inhibited receptor tyrosine kinase signaling through the VEGF and PDGF receptors. Both showed efficacy as second-line treatment following progression during cytokine treatment, resulting in approval by regulatory authorities for the treatment of advanced renal cell carcinoma. A randomized phase 3 trial comparing sunitinib to IFN-α showed superior efficacy for sunitinib with an acceptable safety profile. The trial resulted in a change in the standard first-line treatment from IFN to sunitinib. Sunitinib is usually given orally at a dose of 50 mg/d for 4 weeks out of 6. Diarrhea is the main toxicity. Sorafenib is usually given orally at a dose of 400 mg bid. In addition to diarrhea, toxicities include rash, fatigue, and hand-foot syndrome. Temsirolimus, a mammalian target of rapamycin (mTOR) inhibitor, also has activity in previously treated patients. The usual dosage is 25 mg IV weekly.

The prognosis of metastatic renal cell carcinoma is variable. In one analysis, no prior nephrectomy, a KPS <80, low hemoglobin, high corrected calcium, and abnormal lactate dehydrogenase were poor prognostic factors. Patients with zero, one or two, and three or more factors had a median survival of 24, 12, and 5 months, respectively. These tumors may follow an unpredictable and protracted clinical course. It may be best to document progression before considering systemic treatment.

FURTHER READINGS

BLACK PC et al: Molecular markers of urothelial cancer and their use in the monitoring of superficial urothelial cancer. J Clin Oncol 24:5528, 2006

BRASSELL SA, Kamat AM: Contemporary intravesical treatment options for urothelial carcinoma of the bladder. J Natl Compr Canc Netw 4:1027, 2006

COHEN HT, McGovern FJ: Renal-cell carcinoma. N Engl J Med 353:2477, 2005

MITRA AP et al: Molecular pathways in invasive bladder cancer: New insights into mechanisms, progression, and target identification. J Clin Oncol 24:5552, 2006

MOTZER RJ et al: Sunitinib in patients with metastatic renal cell carcinoma. JAMA 295:2516, 2006

NELSON EC et al: Renal cell carcinoma: Current status and emerging therapies. Cancer Treat Rev 33:299, 2007

RINI BI et al: Renal cell carcinoma. Lancet 373:1119, 2009

SJOLUND J et al: Suppression of renal cell carcinoma growth by inhibition of Notch signaling in vitro and in vivo. J Clin Invest 118:217, 2008

SUGANO K, Kakizoe T: Genetic alterations in bladder cancer and their clinical applications in molecular tumor staging. Nature Clin Pract 3:642, 2006

WINQUIST E et al: Neoadjuvant chemotherapy for transitional cell carcinoma of the bladder: A systematic review and meta-analysis. J Urol 171:561, 2004

WOOD C et al: An adjuvant autologous therapeutic vaccine (HSPPC-96; vitespen) versus observation alone for patients at high risk of recurrence after nephrectomy for renal cell carcinoma: A multicentre, open-label, randomised phase III trial. Lancet 372:145, 2008

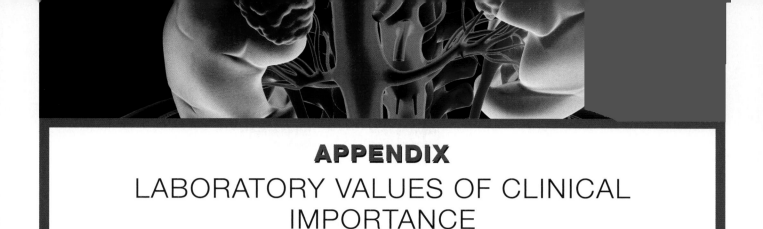

APPENDIX
LABORATORY VALUES OF CLINICAL IMPORTANCE

Alexander Kratz ■ Michael A. Pesce ■ Daniel J. Fink†

INTRODUCTORY COMMENTS

The following are tables of reference values for laboratory tests, special analytes, and special function tests. A variety of factors can influence reference values. Such variables include the population studied, the duration and means of specimen transport, laboratory methods and instrumentation, and even the type of container used for the collection of the specimen. The reference or "normal" ranges given in this appendix may therefore not be appropriate for all laboratories, and these values should only be used as general guidelines. Whenever possible, reference values provided by the laboratory performing the testing should be utilized in the interpretation of laboratory data. Values supplied in this Appendix reflect typical reference ranges in adults. Pediatric reference ranges may vary significantly from adult values.

In preparing the Appendix, the authors have taken into account the fact that the system of international units (SI, système international d'unités) is used in most countries and in some medical journals. However, clinical laboratories may continue to report values in "conventional" units. Therefore, both systems are provided in the Appendix. The dual system is also used in the text except for (1) those instances in which the numbers remain the same but only the terminology is changed (mmol/L for meq/L or IU/L for mIU/mL), when only the SI units are given; and (2) most pressure measurements (e.g., blood and cerebrospinal fluid pressures), when the conventional units (mmHg, mmH$_2$O) are used. In all other instances in the text the SI unit is followed by the traditional unit in parentheses.

---

†Deceased.

REFERENCE VALUES FOR LABORATORY TESTS

TABLE A-1

HEMATOLOGY AND COAGULATION

ANALYTE	SPECIMEN[a]	SI UNITS	CONVENTIONAL UNITS
Activated clotting time	WB	70–180 s	70–180 seconds
Activated protein C resistance (Factor V Leiden)	P	Not applicable	Ratio >2.1
Alpha$_2$ antiplasmin	P	0.87–1.55	87–155%
Antiphospholipid antibody panel			
PTT-LA (Lupus anticoagulant screen)	P	Negative	Negative
Platelet neutralization procedure	P	Negative	Negative
Dilute viper venom screen	P	Negative	Negative
Anticardiolipin antibody	S		
IgG		0–15 arbitrary units	0–15 GPL
IgM		0–15 arbitrary units	0–15 MPL
Antithrombin III	P		
Antigenic		220–390 mg/L	22–39 mg/dL
Functional		0.7–1.30 U/L	70–130%
Anti-Xa assay (heparin assay)	P		
Unfractionated heparin		0.3–0.7 kIU/L	0.3–0.7 IU/mL
Low-molecular-weight heparin		0.5–1.0 kIU/L	0.5–1.0 IU/mL
Danaparoid (Orgaran)		0.5–0.8 kIU/L	0.5–0.8 IU/mL
Autohemolysis test	WB	0.004–0.045	0.4–4.50%
Autohemolysis test with glucose	WB	0.003–0.007	0.3–0.7%
Bleeding time (adult)		<7.1 min	<7.1 min
Clot retraction	WB	0.50–1.00/2 h	50–100%/2 h
Cryofibrinogen	P	Negative	Negative
D-Dimer	P	0.22–0.74 µg/mL	0.22–0.74 µg/mL
Differential blood count	WB		
Neutrophils		0.40–0.70	40–70%
Bands		0.0–0.05	0–5%
Lymphocytes		0.20–0.50	20–50%
Monocytes		0.04–0.08	4–8%
Eosinophils		0.0–0.6	0–6%
Basophils		0.0–0.02	0–2%
Eosinophil count	WB	150–300/µL	150–300/mm^3
Erythrocyte count	WB		
Adult males		4.30–5.60 × 10^{12}/L	4.30–5.60 × 10^6/mm^3
Adult females		4.00–5.20 × 10^{12}/L	4.00–5.20 × 10^6/mm^3
Erythrocyte life span	WB		
Normal survival		120 days	120 days
Chromium labeled, half life ($t_{1/2}$)		25–35 days	25–35 days
Erythrocyte sedimentation rate	WB		
Females		0–20 mm/h	0–20 mm/h
Males		0–15 mm/h	0–15 mm/h
Euglobulin lysis time	P	7200–14400 s	120–240 min
Factor II, prothrombin	P	0.50–1.50	50–150%
Factor V	P	0.50–1.50	50–150%
Factor VII	P	0.50–1.50	50–150%
Factor VIII	P	0.50–1.50	50–150%
Factor IX	P	0.50–1.50	50–150%
Factor X	P	0.50–1.50	50–150%
Factor XI	P	0.50–1.50	50–150%
Factor XII	P	0.50–1.50	50–150%
Factor XIII screen	P	Not applicable	Present
Factor inhibitor assay	P	<0.5 Bethesda Units	<0.5 Bethesda Units

(Continued)

HEMATOLOGY AND COAGULATION

ANALYTE	SPECIMEN[a]	SI UNITS	CONVENTIONAL UNITS
Fibrin (ogen) degradation products	P	0–1 mg/L	0–1μg/mL
Fibrinogen	P	2.33–4.96 g/L	233–496 mg/dL
Glucose-6-phosphate dehydrogenase (erythrocyte)	WB	<2400 s	<40 min
Ham's test (acid serum)	WB	Negative	Negative
Hematocrit	WB		
Adult males		0.388–0.464	38.8–46.4
Adult females		0.354–0.444	35.4–44.4
Hemoglobin			
Plasma	P	6–50 mg/L	0.6–5.0 mg/dL
Whole blood	WB		
Adult males		133–162 g/L	13.3–16.2 g/dL
Adult females		120–158 g/L	12.0–15.8 g/dL
Hemoglobin electrophoresis	WB		
Hemoglobin A		0.95–0.98	95–98%
Hemoglobin A_2		0.015–0.031	1.5–3.1%
Hemoglobin F		0–0.02	0–2.0%
Hemoglobins other than A, A_2, or F		Absent	Absent
Heparin-induced thrombocytopenia antibody	P	Negative	Negative
Joint fluid crystal	JF	Not applicable	No crystals seen
Joint fluid mucin	JF	Not applicable	Only type I mucin present
Leukocytes			
Alkaline phosphatase (LAP)	WB	0.2–1.6 μkat/L	13–100 μ/L
Count (WBC)	WB	$3.54–9.06 \times 10^9$/L	$3.54–9.06 \times 10^3$/mm³
Mean corpuscular hemoglobin (MCH)	WB	26.7–31.9 pg/cell	26.7–31.9 pg/cell
Mean corpuscular hemoglobin concentration (MCHC)	WB	323–359 g/L	32.3–35.9 g/dL
Mean corpuscular hemoglobin of reticulocytes (CH)	WB	24–36 pg	24–36 pg
Mean corpuscular volume (MCV)	WB	79–93.3 fL	79–93.3 μm³
Mean platelet volume (MPV)	WB	9.00–12.95 fL	9.00–12.95 μm³
Osmotic fragility of erythrocytes	WB		
Direct		0.0035–0.0045	0.35–0.45%
Index		0.0030–0.0065	0.30–0.65%
Partial thromboplastin time, activated	P	26.3–39.4 s	26.3–39.4 s
Plasminogen	P		
Antigen		84–140 mg/L	8.4–14.0 mg/dL
Functional		0.70–1.30	70–130%
Plasminogen activator inhibitor 1	P	4–43 μg/L	4–43 ng/mL
Platelet aggregation	PRP	Not applicable	>65% aggregation in response to adenosine diphosphate, epinephrine, collagen, ristocetin, and arachidonic acid
Platelet count	WB	$165–415 \times 10^9$/L	$165–415 \times 10^3$/mm³
Platelet, mean volume	WB	6.4–11 fL	6.4–11.0 μm³
Prekallikrein assay	P	0.50–1.5	50–150%
Prekallikrein screen	P		No deficiency detected
Protein C	P		
Total antigen		0.70–1.40	70–140%
Functional		0.70–1.30	70–130%
Protein S	P		
Total antigen		0.70–1.40	70–140%
Functional		0.65–1.40	65–140%
Free antigen		0.70–1.40	70–140%
Prothrombin gene mutation G20210A	WB	Not applicable	Not present
Prothrombin time	P	12.7–15.4 s	12.7–15.4 s

(Continued)

TABLE A-1(CONTINUED)

HEMATOLOGY AND COAGULATION

ANALYTE	SPECIMEN[a]	SI UNITS	CONVENTIONAL UNITS
Protoporphyrin, free erythrocyte	WB	0.28–0.64 μmol/L of red blood cells	16–36μg/dL of red blood cells
Red cell distribution width	WB	<0.145	<14.5%
Reptilase time	P	16–23.6 s	16–23.6 s
Reticulocyte count	WB		
Adult males		0.008–0.023 red cells	0.8–2.3% red cells
Adult females		0.008–0.020 red cells	0.8–2.0% red cells
Reticulocyte hemoglobin content	WB	>26 pg/cell	>26 pg/cell
Ristocetin cofactor (functional von Willebrand factor)	P		
Blood group O		0.75 mean of normal	75% mean of normal
Blood group A		1.05 mean of normal	105% mean of normal
Blood group B		1.15 mean of normal	115% mean of normal
Blood group AB		1.25 mean of normal	125% mean of normal
Sickle cell test	WB	Negative	Negative
Sucrose hemolysis	WB	<0.1	<10% hemolysis
Thrombin time	P	15.3–18.5 s	15.3–18.5 s
Total eosinophils	WB	150–300 × 10⁶/L	150–300/mm³
Transferrin receptor	S, P	9.6–29.6 nmol/L	9.6–29.6 nmol/L
Viscosity			
Plasma	P	1.7–2.1	1.7–2.1
Serum	S	1.4–1.8	1.4–1.8
Von Willebrand factor (vWF) antigen (factor VIII:R antigen)	P		
Blood group O		0.75 mean of normal	75% mean of normal
Blood group A		1.05 mean of normal	105% mean of normal
Blood group B		1.15 mean of normal	115% mean of normal
Blood group AB		1.25 mean of normal	125% mean of normal
Von Willebrand factor multimers	P	Normal distribution	Normal distribution
White blood cells: see "leukocytes"			

[a]P, plasma; JF, joint fluid; PRP, platelet-rich plasma; S, serum; WB, whole blood.

TABLE A-2

CLINICAL CHEMISTRY AND IMMUNOLOGY

ANALYTE	SPECIMEN[a]	SI UNITS	CONVENTIONAL UNITS
Acetoacetate	P	20–99 μmol/L	0.2–1.0 mg/dL
Adrenocorticotropin (ACTH)	P	1.3–16.7 pmol/L	6.0–76.0 pg/mL
Alanine aminotransferase (AST, SGPT)	S	0.12–0.70 μkat/L	7–41 U/L
Albumin	S		
Female		41–53 g/L	4.1–5.3 g/dL
Male		40–50 g/L	4.0–5.0 g/L
Aldolase	S	26–138 nkat/L	1.5–8.1 U/L
Aldosterone (adult)			
Supine, normal sodium diet	S, P	55–250 pmol/L	2–9 ng/dL
Upright, normal sodium diet	S, P		2–5-fold increase over supine value
Supine, low-sodium diet	S, P		2–5-fold increase over normal sodium diet level
	U	6.38–58.25 nmol/d	2.3–21.0 μg/24 h
Alpha fetoprotein (adult)	S	0–8.5 μg/L	0–8.5 ng/mL
Alpha₁ antitrypsin	S	1.0–2.0 g/L	100–200 mg/dL
Ammonia, as NH₃	P	11–35 μmol/L	19–60 μg/dL
Amylase (method dependent)	S	0.34–1.6 μkat/L	20–96 U/L
Androstenedione (adult)	S	1.75–8.73 nmol/L	50–250 ng/dL

CLINICAL CHEMISTRY AND IMMUNOLOGY

ANALYTE	SPECIMEN[a]	SI UNITS	CONVENTIONAL UNITS
Angiotensin-converting enzyme (ACE)	S	0.15–1.1 μkat/L	9–67 U/L
Anion gap	S	7–16 mmol/L	7–16 mmol/L
Apo B/Apo A-1 ratio		0.35–0.98	0.35–0.98
Apolipoprotein A-1	S	1.19–2.40 g/L	119–240 mg/dL
Apolipoprotein B	S	0.52–1.63 g/L	52–163 mg/dL
Arterial blood gases			
[HCO_3^-]		22–30 mmol/L	22–30 meq/L
P_{CO_2}		4.3–6.0 kPa	32–45 mmHg
pH		7.35–7.45	7.35–7.45
P_{O_2}		9.6–13.8 kPa	72–104 mmHg
Aspartate aminotransferase (AST, SGOT)	S	0.20–0.65 μkat/L	12–38 U/L
Autoantibodies			
Anti-adrenal antibody	S	Not applicable	Negative at 1:10 dilution
Anti-double-strand (native) DNA	S	Not applicable	Negative at 1:10 dilution
Anti–glomerular basement membrane antibodies	S		
Qualitative		Negative	Negative
Quantitative		<5 kU/L	<5 U/mL
Anti-granulocyte antibody	S	Not applicable	Negative
Anti-Jo-1 antibody	S	Not applicable	Negative
Anti-La antibody	S	Not applicable	Negative
Anti-mitochondrial antibody	S	Not applicable	Negative
Antineutrophil cytoplasmic autoantibodies, cytoplasmic (C-ANCA)	S		
Qualitative		Negative	Negative
Quantitative (antibodies to proteinase 3)		<2.8 kU/L	<2.8 U/mL
Antineutrophil cytoplasmic autoantibodies, perinuclear (P-ANCA)	S		
Qualitative		Negative	Negative
Quantitative (antibodies to myeloperoxidase)		<1.4 kU/L	<1.4 U/mL
Antinuclear antibody	S	Not applicable	Negative at 1:40
Anti–parietal cell antibody	S	Not applicable	Negative at 1:20
Anti-Ro antibody	S	Not applicable	Negative
Anti-platelet antibody	S	Not applicable	Negative
Anti-RNP antibody	S	Not applicable	Negative
Anti-Scl 70 antibody	S	Not applicable	Negative
Anti-Smith antibody	S	Not applicable	Negative
Anti-smooth-muscle antibody	S	Not applicable	Negative at 1:20
Anti-thyroglobulin	S	Not applicable	Negative
Anti-thyroid antibody	S	<0.3 kIU/L	<0.3 IU/mL
B type natriuretic peptide (BNP)	P	Age and gender: specific <167 ng/L	Age and gender specific: <167 pg/mL
Bence Jones protein, serum	S	Not applicable	None detected
Bence Jones protein, urine, qualitative	U	Not applicable	None detected in 50 × concentrated urine
Bence Jones Protein, urine, quantitative	U		
Kappa		<2.5 mg/L	<2.5 mg/dL
Lambda		<50 mg/L	<5.0 mg/dL
β_2-Microglobulin			
	S	<2.7 mg/L	<0.27 mg/dL
	U	<120 μg/d	<120 μg/day
Bilirubin	S		
Total		5.1–22 μmol/L	0.3–1.3 mg/dL
Direct		1.7–6.8 μmol/L	0.1–0.4 mg/dL
Indirect		3.4–15.2 μmol/L	0.2–0.9 mg/dL
C peptide (adult)	S, P	0.17–0.66 nmol/L	0.5–2.0 ng/mL
C1-esterase-inhibitor protein	S		
Antigenic		124–250 mg/L	12.4–24.5 mg/dL
Functional		Present	Present

(Continued)

TABLE A-2 (*CONTINUED*)

CLINICAL CHEMISTRY AND IMMUNOLOGY

APPENDIX

Laboratory Values of Clinical Importance

ANALYTE	SPECIMEN[a]	SI UNITS	CONVENTIONAL UNITS
CA 125	S	0–35 kU/L	0–35 U/mL
CA 19-9	S	0–37 kU/L	0–37 U/mL
CA 15-3	S	0–34 kU/L	0–34 U/mL
CA 27-29	S	0–40 kU/L	0–40 U/mL
Calcitonin	S		
Male		3–26 ng/L	3–26 pg/mL
Female		2–17 ng/L	2–17 pg/mL
Calcium	S	2.2–2.6 mmol/L	8.7–10.2 mg/dL
Calcium, ionized	WB	1.12–1.32 mmol/L	4.5–5.3 mg/dL
Carbon dioxide content (TCO$_2$)	P (sea level)	22–30 mmol/L	22–30 meq/L
Carboxyhemoglobin (carbon monoxide content)	WB		
Nonsmokers		0–0.04	0–4%
Smokers		0.04–0.09	4–9%
Onset of symptoms		0.15–0.20	15–20%
Loss of consciousness and death		>0.50	>50%
Carcinoembryonic antigen (CEA)	S		
Nonsmokers		0.0–3.0 μg/L	0.0–3.0 ng/mL
Smokers	S	0.0–5.0 μg/L	0.0–5.0 ng/mL
Ceruloplasmin	S	250–630 mg/L	25–63 mg/dL
Chloride	S	102–109 mmol/L	102–109 meq/L
Cholesterol: see **Table A-4**			
Cholinesterase	S	5–12 kU/L	5–12 U/mL
Complement			
C3	S	0.83–1.77 g/L	83–177 mg/dL
C4	S	0.16–0.47 g/L	16–47 mg/dL
Total hemolytic complement (CH50)	S	50–150%	50–150%
Factor B	S	0.17–0.42 g/L	17–42 mg/dL
Coproporphyrins (types I and III)	U	150–470 μmol/d	100–300 μg/d
Cortisol			
Fasting, 8 A.M.–12 noon	S	138–690 nmol/L	5–25μg/dL
12 noon–8 P.M.		138–414 nmol/L	5–15 μg/dL
8 P.M.–8 A.M.		0–276 nmol/L	0–10 μg/dL
Cortisol, free	U	55–193 nmol/24 h	20–70 μg/24 h
C-reactive protein	S	0.2–3.0 mg/L	0.2–3.0 mg/L
Creatine kinase (total)	S		
Females		0.66–4.0 μkat/L	39–238 U/L
Males		0.87–5.0 μkat/L	51–294 U/L
Creatine kinase-MB	S		
Mass		0.0–5.5 μg/L	0.0–5.5 ng/mL
Fraction of total activity (by electrophoresis)		0–0.04	0–4.0%
Creatinine	S		
Female		44–80 μmol/L	0.5–0.9 ng/mL
Male		53–106 μmol/L	0.6–1.2 ng/mL
Cryoproteins	S	Not applicable	None detected
Dehydroepiandrosterone (DHEA) (adult)			
Male	S	6.2–43.4 nmol/L	180–1250 ng/dL
Female		4.5–34.0 nmol/L	130–980 ng/dL
Dehydroepiandrosterone (DHEA) sulfate	S		
Male (adult)		100–6190 μg/L	10–619 μg/dL
Female (adult, premenopausal)		120–5350 μg/L	12–535 μg/dL
Female (adult, postmenopausal)		300–2600 μg/L	30–260 μg/dL
Deoxycorticosterone (DOC) (adult)	S	61–576 nmol/L	2–19 ng/dL
11-Deoxycortisol (adult) (compound S) (8:00 A.M.)	S	0.34–4.56 nmol/L	12–158 ng/dL
Dihydrotestosterone			
Male	S, P	1.03–2.92 nmol/L	30–85 ng/dL
Female		0.14–0.76 nmol/L	4–22 ng/dL
Dopamine	P	<475 pmol/L	<87 pg/mL

(Continued)

CLINICAL CHEMISTRY AND IMMUNOLOGY

ANALYTE	SPECIMEN[a]	SI UNITS	CONVENTIONAL UNITS
Dopamine	U	425–2610 nmol/d	65–400 μg/d
Epinephrine	P		
Supine (30 min)		<273 pmol/L	<50 pg/mL
Sitting		<328 pmol/L	<60 pg/mL
Standing (30 min)		<491 pmol/L	<90 pg/mL
Epinephrine	U	0–109 nmol/d	0–20 μg/d
Erythropoietin	S	4–27 U/L	4–27 U/L
Estradiol	S, P		
Female			
Menstruating:			
Follicular phase		74–532 pmol/L	<20–145 pg/mL
Mid-cycle peak		411–1626 pmol/L	112–443 pg/mL
Luteal phase		74–885 pmol/L	<20–241 pg/mL
Postmenopausal		217 pmol/L	<59 pg/mL
Male		74 pmol/L	<20 pg/mL
Estrone	S, P		
Female			
Menstruating:			
Follicular phase		55–555 pmol/L	15–150 pg/mL
Luteal phase		55–740 pmol/L	15–200 pg/mL
Postmenopausal		55–204 pmol/L	15–55 pg/mL
Male		55–240 pmol/L	15–65 pg/mL
Fatty acids, free (nonesterified)	P	<0.28–0.89 mmol/L	<8–25 mg/dL
Ferritin	S		
Female		10–150 μg/L	10–150 ng/mL
Male		29–248 μg/L	29–248 ng/mL
Follicle stimulating hormone (FSH)	S, P		
Female			
Menstruating:			
Follicular phase		3.0–20.0 IU/L	3.0–20.0 mIU/mL
Ovulatory phase		9.0–26.0 IU/L	9.0–26.0 mIU/mL
Luteal phase		1.0–12.0 IU/L	1.0–12.0 mIU/mL
Postmenopausal		18.0–153.0 IU/L	18.0–153.0 mIU/mL
Male		1.0–12.0 IU/L	1.0–12.0 mIU/mL
Free testosterone, adult			
Female	S	2.1–23.6 pmol/L	0.6–6.8 pg/mL
Male		163–847 pmol/L	47–244 pg/mL
Fructosamine	S	<285 μmol/L	<285 μmol/L
Gamma glutamyltransferase	S	0.15–0.99 μkat/L	9–58 U/L
Gastrin	S	<100 ng/L	<100 pg/mL
Glucagon	P	20–100 ng/L	20–100 pg/mL
Glucose (fasting)	P		
Normal		4.2–6.1 mmol/L	75–110 mg/dL
Impaired glucose tolerance		6.2–6.9 mmol/L	111–125 mg/dL
Diabetes mellitus		>7.0 mmol/L	>125 mg/dL
Glucose, 2 h postprandial	P	3.9–6.7 mmol/L	70–120 mg/dL
Growth hormone (resting)	S	0.5–17.0 μg/L	0.5–17.0 ng/mL
Hemoglobin A$_{Ic}$	WB	0.04–0.06 Hb fraction	4.0–6.0%
High-density lipoprotein (HDL)			
(see **Table A-4**)			
Homocysteine	P	4.4–10.8 μmol/L	4.4–10.8 μmol/L
Human chorionic gonadotropin (hCG)	S		
Non-pregnant female		<5 IU/L	<5 mIU/mL
1–2 weeks postconception		9–130 IU/L	9–130 mIU/mL
2–3 weeks postconception		75–2600 IU/L	75–2600 mIU/mL
3–4 weeks postconception		850–20,800 IU/L	850–20,800 mIU/mL
4–5 weeks postconception		4000–100,200 IU/L	4000–100,200 mIU/mL

(*Continued*)

APPENDIX

Laboratory Values of Clinical Importance

CLINICAL CHEMISTRY AND IMMUNOLOGY

ANALYTE	SPECIMEN[a]	SI UNITS	CONVENTIONAL UNITS
5–10 weeks postconception		11,500–289,000 IU/L	11,500–289,000 mIU/mL
10–14 weeks postconception		18,300–137,000 IU/L	18,300–137,000 mIU/mL
Second trimester		1400–53,000 IU/L	1400–53,000 mIU/mL
Third trimester		940–60,000 IU/L	940–60,000 mIU/mL
β-Hydroxybutyrate	P	0–290 μmol/L	0–3 mg/dL
5-Hydroindoleacetic acid [5-HIAA]	U	10.5–36.6 μmol/d	2–7 mg/d
17-Hydroxyprogesterone (adult)	S		
Male		0.15–7.5 nmol/L	5–250 ng/dL
Female			
Follicular phase		0.6–3.0 nmol/L	20–100 ng/dL
Midcycle peak		3–7.5 nmol/L	100–250 ng/dL
Luteal phase		3–15 nmol/L	100–500 ng/dL
Postmenopausal		≤2.1 nmol/L	≤70 ng/dL
Hydroxyproline	U, 24 hour	38–500 μmol/d	38–500 μmol/d
Immunofixation	S	Not applicable	No bands detected
Immunoglobulin, quantitation (adult)			
IgA	S	0.70–3.50 g/L	70–350 mg/dL
IgD	S	0–140 mg/L	0–14 mg/dL
IgE	S	24–430 μg/L	10–179 IU/mL
IgG	S	7.0–17.0 g/L	700–1700 mg/dL
IgG_1	S	2.7–17.4 g/L	270–1740 mg/dL
IgG_2	S	0.3–6.3 g/L	30–630 mg/dL
IgG_3	S	0.13–3.2 g/L	13–320 mg/dL
IgG_4	S	0.11–6.2 g/L	11–620 mg/dL
IgM	S	0.50–3.0 g/L	50–300 mg/dL
Insulin	S, P	14.35–143.5 pmol/L	2–20 μU/mL
Iron	S	7–25 μmol/L	41–141 μg/dL
Iron-binding capacity	S	45–73 μmol/L	251–406 μg/dL
Iron-binding capacity saturation	S	0.16–0.35	16–35%
Joint fluid crystal	JF	Not applicable	No crystals seen
Joint fluid mucin	JF	Not applicable	Only type I mucin present
Ketone (acetone)	S, U	Negative	Negative
17 Ketosteroids	U	0.003–0.012 g/d	3–12 mg/d
Lactate	P, arterial	0.5–1.6 mmol/L	4.5–14.4 mg/dL
	P, venous	0.5–2.2 mmol/L	4.5–19.8 mg/dL
Lactate dehydrogenase	S	2.0–3.8 μkat/L	115–221 U/L
Lactate dehydrogenase isoenzymes	S		
Fraction 1 (of total)		0.14–0.26	14–26%
Fraction 2		0.29–0.39	29–39%
Fraction 3		0.20–0.25	20–25%
Fraction 4		0.08–0.16	8–16%
Fraction 5		0.06–0.16	6–16%
Lipase (method dependent)	S	0.51–0.73 μkat/L	3–43 U/L
Lipids: see **Table A-4**			
Lipoprotein (a)	S	0–300 mg/L	0–30 mg/dL
Low-density lipoprotein (LDL)			
(see **Table A-4**)			
Luteinizing hormone (LH)	S, P		
Female			
Menstruating:			
Follicular phase		2.0–15.0 U/L	2.0–15.0 U/L
Ovulatory phase		22.0–105.0 U/L	22.0–105.0 U/L
Luteal phase		0.6–19.0 U/L	0.6–19.0 U/L
Postmenopausal		16.0–64.0 U/L	16.0–64.0 U/L
Male		2.0–12.0 U/L	2.0–12.0 U/L
Magnesium	S	0.62–0.95 mmol/L	1.5–2.3 mg/dL
Metanephrine	P	<0.5 nmol/L	<100 pg/mL

(Continued)

CLINICAL CHEMISTRY AND IMMUNOLOGY

ANALYTE	SPECIMEN[a]	SI UNITS	CONVENTIONAL UNITS
Metanephrine	U	30–211 mmol/mol creatinine	53–367 μg/g creatinine
Methemoglobin	WB	0.0–0.01	0–1%
Microalbumin urine	U		
24-h urine		0.0–0.03 g/d	0–30 mg/24 h
Spot urine		0.0–0.03 g/g creatinine	0–30 μg/mg creatinine
Myoglobin	S		
Male		19–92 μg/L	19–92 μg/L
Female		12–76 μg/L	12–76 μg/L
Norepinephrine	U	89–473 nmol/d	15–80 μg/d
Norepinephrine	P		
Supine (30 min)		650–2423 pmol/L	110–410 pg/mL
Sitting		709–4019 pmol/L	120–680 pg/mL
Standing (30 min)		739–4137 pmol/L	125–700 pg/mL
N-telopeptide (cross linked), NTx	S		
Female, premenopausal		6.2–19.0 nmol BCE	6.2–19.0 nmol BCE
Male		5.4–24.2 nmol BCE	5.4–24.2 nmol BCE
Bone collagen equivalent (BCE)			
N-telopeptide (cross linked), NTx	U		
Female, premenopausal		17–94 nmol BCE/mmol creatinine	17–94 nmol BCE/mmol creatinine
Female, postmenopausal		26–124 nmol BCE/mmol creatinine	26–124 nmol BCE/mmol creatinine
Male		21–83 nmol BCE/mmol creatinine	21–83 nmol BCE/mmol creatinine
Bone collagen equivalent (BCE)			
5′ Nucleotidase	S	0.02–0.19 μkat/L	0–11 U/L
Osmolality	P	275–295 mosmol/kg serum water	275–295 mosmol/kg serum water
	U	500–800 mosmol/kg water	500–800 mosmol/kg water
Osteocalcin	S	11–50 μg/L	11–50 ng/mL
Oxygen content	WB		
Arterial (sea level)		17–21	17–21 vol%
Venous (sea level)		10–16	10–16 vol%
Oxygen percent saturation (sea level)	WB		
Arterial		0.97	94–100%
Venous, arm		0.60–0.85	60–85%
Parathyroid hormone (intact)	S	8–51 ng/L	8–51 pg/mL
Phosphatase, alkaline	S	0.56–1.63 μkat/L	33–96 U/L
Phosphorus, inorganic	S	0.81–1.4 mmol/L	2.5–4.3 mg/dL
Porphobilinogen	U	None	None
Potassium	S	3.5–5.0 mmol/L	3.5–5.0 meq/L
Prealbumin	S	170–340 mg/L	17–34 mg/dL
Progesterone	S, P		
Female			
Follicular		<3.18 nmol/L	<1.0 ng/mL
Midluteal		9.54–63.6 nmol/L	3–20 ng/mL
Male		<3.18 nmol/L	<1.0 ng/mL
Prolactin	S	0–20 μg/L	0–20 ng/mL
Prostate-specific antigen (PSA)	S		
Male			
<40 years		0.0–2.0 μg/L	0.0–2.0 ng/mL
>40 years		0.0–4.0 μg/L	0.0–4.0 ng/mL
PSA, free; in males 45–75 years, with PSA values between 4 and 20 μg/mL	S	>0.25 associated with benign prostatic hyperplasia	>25% associated with benign prostatic hyperplasia

TABLE A-2 (CONTINUED)

CLINICAL CHEMISTRY AND IMMUNOLOGY

ANALYTE	SPECIMEN[a]	SI UNITS	CONVENTIONAL UNITS
Protein fractions	S		
Albumin		35–55 g/L	3.5–5.5 g/dL (50–60%)
Globulin		20–35 g/L	2.0–3.5 g/dL (40–50%)
Alpha$_1$		2–4 g/L	0.2–0.4 g/dL (4.2–7.2%)
Alpha$_2$		5–9 g/L	0.5–0.9 g/dL (6.8–12%)
Beta		6–11 g/L	0.6–1.1 g/dL (9.3–15%)
Gamma		7–17 g/L	0.7–1.7 g/dL (13–23%)
Protein, total	S	67–86 g/L	6.7–8.6 g/dL
Pyruvate	P, arterial	40–130 μmol/L	0.35–1.14 mg/dL
	P, venous	40–130 μmol/L	0.35–1.14 mg/dL
Rheumatoid factor	S, JF	<30 kIU/L	<30 IU/mL
Serotonin	WB	0.28–1.14 μmol/L	50–200 ng/mL
Serum protein electrophoresis	S	Not applicable	Normal pattern
Sex hormone binding globulin (adult)	S		
Male		13–71 nmol/L	13–71 nmol/L
Female		18–114 nmol/L	18–114 nmol/L
Sodium	S	136–146 mmol/L	136–146 meq/L
Somatomedin-C (IGF-1) (adult)	S		
16–24 years		182–780 μg/L	182–780 ng/mL
25–39 years		114–492 μg/L	114–492 ng/mL
40–54 years		90–360 μg/L	90–360 ng/mL
>54 years		71–290 μg/L	71–290 ng/mL
Somatostatin	P	<25 ng/L	<25 pg/mL
Testosterone, total, morning sample	S		
Female		0.21–2.98 nmol/L	6–86 ng/dL
Male		9.36–37.10 nmol/L	270–1070 ng/dL
Thyroglobulin	S	0.5–53 μg/L	0.5–53 ng/mL
Thyroid-binding globulin	S	13–30 mg/L	1.3–3.0 mg/dL
Thyroid-stimulating hormone	S	0.34–4.25 mIU/L	0.34–4.25 μIU/mL
Thyroxine, free (fT$_4$)	S	10.3–21.9 pmol/L	0.8–1.7 ng/dL
Thyroxine, total (T$_4$)	S	70–151 nmol/L	5.4–11.7 μg/dL
(Free) thyroxine index	S	6.7–10.9	6.7–10.9
Transferrin	S	2.0–4.0 g/L	200–400 mg/dL
Triglycerides (see **Table A-4**)	S	0.34–2.26 mmol/L	30–200 mg/dL
Triiodothyronine, free (fT$_3$)	S	3.7–6.5 pmol/L	2.4–4.2 pg/mL
Triiodothyronine, total (T$_3$)	S	1.2–2.1 nmol/L	77–135 ng/dL
Troponin I	S		
Normal population, 99% tile		0–0.08 μg/L	0–0.08 ng/mL
Cut-off for MI		>0.4 μg/L	>0.4 ng/mL
Troponin T	S		
Normal population, 99% tile		0–0.1 μg/L	0–0.01 ng/mL
Cut-off for MI		0–0.1 μg/L	0–0.1 ng/mL
Urea nitrogen	S	2.5–7.1 mmol/L	7–20 mg/dL
Uric acid	S		
Females		0.15–0.33 μmol/L	2.5–5.6 mg/dL
Males		0.18–0.41 μmol/L	3.1–7.0 mg/dL
Urobilinogen	U	0.09–4.2 μmol/d	0.05–25 mg/24 h
Vanillylmandelic acid (VMA)	U, 24h	<30 μmol/d	<6 mg/d
Vasoactive intestinal polypeptide	P	0–60 ng/L	0–60 pg/mL

[a]P, plasma; S, serum; U, urine; WB, whole blood; JF, joint fluid.

TABLE A-3

TOXICOLOGY AND THERAPEUTIC DRUG MONITORING

DRUG	THERAPEUTIC RANGE		TOXIC LEVEL	
	SI UNITS	CONVENTIONAL UNITS	SI UNITS	CONVENTIONAL UNITS
Acetaminophen	66–199 µmol/L	10–30 µg/mL	>1320 µmol/L	>200 µg/mL
Amikacin				
Peak	34–51 µmol/L	20–30 µg/mL	>60 µmol/L	>35 µg/mL
Trough	0–17 µmol/L	0–10 µg/mL	>17 µmol/L	>10 µg/mL
Amitriptyline/nortriptyline (total drug)	430–900 nmol/L	120–250 ng/mL	>1800 nmol/L	>500 ng/mL
Amphetamine	150–220 nmol/L	20–30 ng/mL	>1500 nmol/L	>200 ng/mL
Bromide	1.3–6.3 mmol/L	Sedation: 10–50 mg/dL	6.4–18.8 mmol/L	51–150 mg/dL: mild toxicity
	9.4–18.8 mmol/L	Epilepsy: 75–150 mg/dL	>18.8 mmol/L	
			>37.5 mmol/L	>150 mg/dL: severe toxicity
				>300 mg/dL: lethal
Carbamazepine	17–42 µmol/L	4–10 µg/mL	85 µmol/L	>20 µg/mL
Chloramphenicol				
Peak	31–62 µmol/L	10–20 µg/mL	>77 µmol/L	>25 µg/mL
Trough	15–31 µmol/L	5–10 µg/mL	>46 µmol/L	>15 µg/mL
Chlordiazepoxide	1.7–10 µmol/L	0.5–3.0 µg/mL	>17 µmol/L	>5.0 µg/mL
Clonazepam	32–240 nmol/L	10–75 ng/mL	>320 nmol/L	>100 ng/mL
Clozapine	0.6–2.1 µmol/L	200–700 ng/mL	>3.7 µmol/L	>1200 ng/mL
Cocaine			>3.3 µmol/L	>1.0 µg/mL
Codeine	43–110 nmol/mL	13–33 ng/mL	>3700 nmol/mL	>1100 ng/mL (lethal)
Cyclosporine				
Renal transplant				
0–6 months	208–312 nmol/L	250–375 ng/mL	>312 nmol/L	>375 ng/mL
6–12 months after transplant	166–250 nmol/L	200–300 ng/mL	>250 nmol/L	>300 ng/mL
>12 months	83–125 nmol/L	100–150 ng/mL	>125 nmol/L	>150 ng/mL
Cardiac transplant				
0–6 months	208–291 nmol/L	250–350 ng/mL	>291 nmol/L	>350 ng/mL
6–12 months after transplant	125–208 nmol/L	150–250 ng/mL	>208 nmol/L	>250 ng/mL
>12 months	83–125 nmol/L	100–150 ng/mL	>125 nmol/L	150 ng/mL
Lung transplant				
0–6 months	250–374 nmol/L	300–450 ng/mL	>374 nmol/L	>450 ng/mL
Liver transplant				
0–7 days	249–333 nmol/L	300–400 ng/mL	>333 nmol/L	>400 ng/mL
2–4 weeks	208–291 nmol/L	250–350 ng/mL	>291 nmol/L	>350 ng/mL
5–8 weeks	166–249 nmol/L	200–300 ng/mL	>249 nmol/L	>300 ng/mL
9–52 weeks	125–208 nmol/L	150–250 ng/mL	>208 nmol/L	>250 ng/mL
>1 year	83–166 nmol/L	100–200 ng/mL	>166 nmol/L	>200 ng/mL
Desipramine	375–1130 nmol/L	100–300 ng/mL	>1880 nmol/L	>500 ng/mL
Diazepam (and metabolite)				
Diazepam	0.7–3.5 µmol/L	0.2–1.0 µg/mL	>7.0 µmol/L	>2.0 µg/mL
Nordazepam	0.4–6.6 µmol/L	0.1–1.8 µg/mL	>9.2 µmol/L	>2.5 µg/mL
Digoxin	0.64–2.6 nmol/L	0.5–2.0 ng/mL	>3.1 nmol/L	>2.4 ng/mL
Disopyramide	>7.4 µmol/L	2.5 µg/mL	20.6 µmol/L	>7 µg/mL
Doxepin and nordoxepin				
Doxepin	0.36–0.98 µmol/L	101–274 ng/mL	>1.8 µmol/L	>503 ng/mL
Nordoxepin	0.38–1.04 µmol/L	106–291 ng/mL	>1.9 µmol/L	>531 ng/mL
Ethanol				
Behavioral changes			>4.3 mmol/L	>20 mg/dL
Legal limit			≥17 mmol/L	≥80 mg/dL
Critical with acute exposure			>54 mmol/L	>250 mg/dL

(Continued)

TOXICOLOGY AND THERAPEUTIC DRUG MONITORING

APPENDIX

Laboratory Values of Clinical Importance

DRUG	THERAPEUTIC RANGE		TOXIC LEVEL	
	SI UNITS	CONVENTIONAL UNITS	SI UNITS	CONVENTIONAL UNITS
Ethylene glycol				
Toxic			>2 mmol/L	>12 mg/dL
Lethal			>20 mmol/L	>120 mg/dL
Ethosuximide	280–700 µmol/L	40–100 µg/mL	>700 µmol/L	>100 µg/mL
Flecainide	0.5–2.4 µmol/L	0.2–1.0 µg/mL	>3.6 µmol/L	>1.5 µg/mL
Gentamicin				
Peak	10–21 µmol/mL	5–10 µg/mL	>25 µmol/mL	>12 µg/mL
Trough	0–4.2 µmol/mL	0–2 µg/mL	>4.2 µmol/mL	>2 µg/mL
Heroin (diacetyl morphine)			>700 µmol/L	>200 ng/mL (as morphine)
Ibuprofen	49–243 µmol/L	10–50 µg/mL	>97 µmol/L	>200 µg/mL
Imipramine (and metabolite)				
Desimipramine	375–1130 nmol/L	100–300 ng/mL	>1880 nmol/L	>500 ng/mL
Total imipramine + desimipramine	563–1130 nmol/L	150–300 ng/mL	>1880 nmol/L	>500 ng/mL
Lidocaine	5.1–21.3 µmol/L	1.2–5.0 µg/mL	>38.4 µmol/L	>9.0 µg/mL
Lithium	0.5–1.3 meq/L	0.5–1.3 meq/L	>2 mmol/L	>2 meq/L
Methadone	1.3–3.2 µmol/L	0.4–1.0 µg/mL	>6.5 µmol/L	>2 µg/mL
Methamphetamine		20–30 ng/mL		0.1–1.0 µg/mL
Methanol			>6 mmol/L	>20 mg/dL
			>16 mmol/L	>50 mg/dL Severe toxicity
			>28 mmol/L	>89 mg/dL Lethal
Methotrexate				
Low-dose	0.01–0.1 µmol/L	0.01–0.1 µmol/L	>0.1 mmol/L	>0.1 mmol/L
High-dose (24 h)	<5.0 µmol/L	<5.0 µmol/L	>5.0 µmol/L	>5.0 µmol/L
High-dose (48 h)	<0.50 µmol/L	<0.50 µmol/L	>0.5 µmol/L	>0.5 µmol/L
High-dose (72 h)	<0.10 µmol/L	<0.10 µmol/L	>0.1 µmol/L	>0.1 µmol/L
Morphine	35–250 µmol/L	10–70 ng/mL	180–14000 µmol/L	50–4000 ng/mL
Nitroprusside (as thiocyanate)	103–499 µmol/L	6–29 µg/mL	860 µmol/L	>50 µg/mL
Nortriptyline	190–569 nmol/L	50–150 ng/mL	>1900 nmol/L	>500 ng/mL
Phenobarbital	65–172 µmol/L	15–40 µg/mL	>215 µmol/L	>50 µg/mL
Phenytoin	40–79 µmol/L	10–20 µg/mL	>118 µmol/L	>30 µg/mL
Phenytoin, free	4.0–7.9 µg/mL	1–2 µg/mL	>13.9 µg/mL	>3.5 µg/mL
% Free	0.08–0.14	8–14		
Primidone and metabolite				
Primidone	23–55 µmol/L	5–12 µg/mL	>69 µmol/L	>15 µg/mL
Phenobarbital	65–172 µmol/L	15–40 µg/mL	>215 µmol/L	>50 µg/mL
Procainamide				
Procainamide	17–42 µmol/L	4–10 µg/mL	>51 µmol/L	>12 µg/mL
NAPA (N-acetylprocainamide)	22–72 µmol/L	6-20 µg/mL	>126 µmol/L	>35 µg/mL
Quinidine	>6.2–15.4 µmol/L	2.0–5.0 µg/mL	>31 µmol/L	>10 µg/mL
Salicylates	145–2100 µmol/L	2–29 mg/dL	>2172 µmol/L	>30 mg/dL
Sirolimus (trough level)				
Kidney transplant	4.4–13.1 nmol/L	4–12 ng/mL	>16 nmol/L	>15 ng/mL
Tacrolimus (FK506) (trough)				
Kidney and liver				
0–2 months posttransplant	12–19 nmol/L	10–15 ng/mL	>25 nmol/L	>20 ng/mL
>2 months posttransplant	6–12 nmol/L	5–10 ng/mL		
Heart				
0–2 months posttransplant	19–25 nmol/L	15–20 ng/mL	>25 nmol/L	>20 ng/mL
3–6 months posttransplant	12–19 nmol/L	10–15 ng/mL		
>6 months posttransplant	10–12 nmol/L	8–10 ng/mL		
Theophylline	56–111 µg/mL	10–20 µg/mL	>140 µg/mL	>25 µg/mL

(Continued)

TOXICOLOGY AND THERAPEUTIC DRUG MONITORING

DRUG	THERAPEUTIC RANGE		TOXIC LEVEL	
	SI UNITS	CONVENTIONAL UNITS	SI UNITS	CONVENTIONAL UNITS
Thiocyanate				
After nitroprusside infusion	103–499 μmol/L	6–29 μg/mL	860 μmol/L	>50 μg/mL
Nonsmoker	17–69 μmol/L	1–4 μg/mL		
Smoker	52–206 μmol/L	3–12 μg/mL		
Tobramycin				
Peak	11–22 μg/L	5–10 μg/mL	>26 μg/L	>12 μg/mL
Trough	0–4.3 μg/L	0–2 μg/mL	>4.3 μg/L	>2 μg/mL
Valproic acid	350–700 μmol/L	50–100 μg/mL	>1000 μmol/L	>150 μg/mL
Vancomycin				
Peak	14–28 μmol/L	20–40 μg/mL	>55 μmol/L	>80 μg/mL
Trough	3.5–10.4 μmol/L	5–15 μg/mL	>14 μmol/L	>20 μg/mL

TABLE A-4

CLASSIFICATION OF LDL, TOTAL, AND HDL CHOLESTEROL

LDL Cholesterol, mg/dL (mmol/L)

<70 (<1.81)	Therapeutic option for very high risk patients
<100 (<2.59)	Optimal
100–129 (2.59–3.34)	Near optimal/above optimal
130–159 (3.36–4.11)	Borderline high
160–189 (4.14–4.89)	High
≥190 (≥4.91)	Very high

Total Cholesterol, mg/dL (mmol/L)

<200 (<5.17)	Desirable
200–239 (5.17–6.18)	Borderline high
≥240 (≥6.21)	High

HDL Cholesterol, mg/dL (mmol/L)

<40 (<1.03)	Low
≥60 (≥1.55)	High

Note: LDL, low-density lipoprotein; HDL, high-density lipoprotein
Source: Executive summary of the third report of the National Cholesterol Education Program (NCEP) expert panel on detection, evaluation, and treatment of high blood cholesterol in adults (adult treatment panel III). JAMA 285:2486, 2001; and Implications of recent clinical trials for the National Cholesterol Education Program Adult Treatment Panel III Guidelines: SM Grundy et al for the Coordinating Committee of the National Cholesterol Education Program. Circulation 110:227, 2004.

TABLE A-5

URINE ANALYSIS

	REFERENCE RANGE	
	SI UNITS	**CONVENTIONAL UNITS**
Acidity, titratable	20–40 mmol/d	20–40 meq/d
Ammonia	30–50 mmol/d	30–50 meq/d
Amylase		4–400 U/L
Amylase/creatinine clearance ratio [(Cl$_{am}$/Cl$_{cr}$) × 100]	1–5	1–5
Calcium (10 meq/d or 200 mg/d dietary calcium)	<7.5 mmol/d	<300 mg/d
Creatine, as creatinine		
Female	<760 μmol/d	<100 mg/d
Male	<380 μmol/d	<50 mg/d
Creatinine	8.8–14 mmol/d	1.0–1.6 g/d
Eosinophils	<100,000 eosinophils/L	<100 eosinophils/mL
Glucose (glucose oxidase method)	0.3–1.7 mmol/d	50–300 mg/d
5-Hydroxyindoleacetic acid (5-HIAA)	10–47 μmol/d	2–9 mg/d
Iodine, spot urine		
WHO classification of iodine deficiency		
Not iodine deficient	>100 μg/L	>100 μg/L
Mild iodine deficiency	50–100 μg/L	50–100 μg/L
Moderate iodine deficiency	20–49 μg/L	20–49 μg/L
Severe iodine deficiency	<20 μg/L	<20 μg/L
Microalbumin		
Normal	0.0–0.03 g/d	0–30 mg/d
Microalbuminuria	0.03–0.30 g/d	30–300 mg/d
Clinical albuminuria	>0.3 g/d	>300 mg/d
Microalbumin/creatinine ratio		
Normal	0–3.4 g/mol creatinine	0–30 μg/mg creatinine
Microalbuminuria	3.4–34 g/mol creatinine	30–300 μg/mg creatinine
Clinical albuminuria	>34 g/mol creatinine	>300 μg/mg creatinine
Oxalate		
Male	80–500 μmol/d	7–44 mg/d
Female	45–350 μmol/d	4–31 mg/d
pH	5.0–9.0	5.0–9.0
Phosphate (phosphorus) (varies with intake)	12.9–42.0 mmol/d	400–1300 mg/d
Potassium (varies with intake)	25–100 mmol/d	25–100 meq/d
Protein	<0.15 g/d	<150 mg/d
Sediment		
Red blood cells	0–2/high power field	
White blood cells	0–2/high power field	
Bacteria	None	
Crystals	None	
Bladder cells	None	
Squamous cells	None	
Tubular cells	None	
Broad casts	None	
Epithelial cell casts	None	
Granular casts	None	
Hyaline casts	0–5/low power field	
Red blood cell casts	None	
Waxy casts	None	
White cell casts	None	
Sodium (varies with intake)	100–260 mmol/d	100–260 meq/d
Specific gravity	1.001–1.035	1.001–1.035
Urea nitrogen	214–607 mmol/d	6–17 g/d
Uric acid (normal diet)	1.49–4.76 mmol/d	250–800 mg/d

Note: WHO, World Health Organization.

SPECIAL FUNCTION TESTS

TABLE A-6

RENAL FUNCTION TESTS

	REFERENCE RANGE	
	SI UNITS	CONVENTIONAL UNITS
Clearances (corrected to 1.72 m² body surface area)		
Measures of glomerular filtration rate		
Inulin clearance (CI)		
Males (mean ± 1 SD)	2.1 ± 0.4 mL/s	124 ± 25.8 mL/min
Females (mean ± 1 SD)	2.0 ± 0.2 mL/s	119 ± 12.8 mL/min
Endogenous creatinine clearance	1.5–2.2 mL/s	91–130 mL/min
Measures of effective renal plasma flow and tubular function		
p-Aminohippuric acid clearance (CI$_{PAH}$)		
Males (mean ± 1 SD)	10.9 ± 2.7 mL/s	654 ± 163 mL/min
Females (mean ± 1 SD)	9.9 ± 1.7 mL/s	594 ± 102 mL/min
Concentration and dilution test		
Specific gravity of urine		
After 12-h fluid restriction	>1.025	>1.025
After 12-h deliberate water intake	≤1.003	≤1.003
Protein excretion, urine	<0.15 g/d	<150 mg/d
Specific gravity, maximal range	1.002–1.028	1.002–1.028
Tubular reabsorption, phosphorus	0.79–0.94 of filtered load	79–94% of filtered load

MISCELLANEOUS

TABLE A-7

BODY FLUIDS AND OTHER MASS DATA

	REFERENCE RANGE	
	SI UNITS	CONVENTIONAL UNITS
Ascitic fluid		
Body fluid,		
Total volume (lean) of body weight	50% (in obese) to 70%	
Intracellular	0.3–0.4 of body weight	
Extracellular	0.2–0.3 of body weight	
Blood		
Total volume		
Males	69 mL per kg body weight	
Females	65 mL per kg body weight	
Plasma volume		
Males	39 mL per kg body weight	
Females	40 mL per kg body weight	
Red blood cell volume		
Males	30 mL per kg body weight	1.15–1.21 L/m² of body surface area
Females	25 mL per kg body weight	0.95–1.00 L/m² of body surface area
Body mass index	18.5–24.9 kg/m²	18.5–24.9 kg/m²

TABLE A-8

RADIATION-DERIVED UNITS

QUANTITY	OLD UNIT	SI UNIT	NAME FOR SI UNIT (AND ABBREVIATION)	CONVERSION
Activity	curie (Ci)	Disintegrations per second (dps)	becquerel (Bq)	$1\ Ci = 3.7 \times 10^{10}\ Bq$ $1\ mCi = 37\ mBq$ $1\ \mu Ci = 0.037\ MBq\ or\ 37\ GBq$ $1\ Bq = 2.703 \times 10^{-11}\ Ci$
Absorbed dose	rad	joule per kilogram (J/kg)	gray (Gy)	$1\ Gy = 100\ rad$ $1\ rad = 0.01\ Gy$ $1\ mrad = 10^{-3}\ cGy$
Exposure	roentgen (R)	coulomb per kilogram (C/kg)	—	$1\ C/kg = 3876\ R$ $1\ R = 2.58 \times 10^{-4}\ C/kg$ $1\ mR = 258\ pC/kg$
Dose equivalent	rem	joule per kilogram (J/kg)	sievert (Sv)	$1\ Sv = 100\ rem$ $1\ rem = 0.01\ Sv$ $1\ mrem = 10\ \mu Sv$

ACKNOWLEDGMENT

The authors acknowledge the contributions of Dr. Patrick M. Sluss, Dr. James L. Januzzi, and Dr. Kent B. Lewandrowski to this chapter in previous editions of Harrison's Principles of Internal Medicine.

FURTHER READINGS

KRATZ A et al: Case records of the Massachusetts General Hospital. Weekly clinicopathological exercises. Laboratory reference values. N Engl J Med 351(15):1548, 2004

LEHMAN HP, HENRY JB: SI units, in *Henry's Clinical Diagnosis and Management by Laboratory Methods*, 21st ed, RC McPherson, MR Pincus (eds). Philadelphia, Elsevier Saunders, 2007, pp 1404–1418

PESCE MA: Reference ranges for laboratory tests and procedures, in *Nelson's Textbook of Pediatrics*, 18th ed, RM Klegman et al (eds). Philadelphia, Elsevier Saunders, 2007, pp 2943–2949

SOLBERG HE: Establishment and use of reference values, in *Tietz Textbook of Clinical Chemistry and Molecular Diagnostics*, 4th ed, CA Burtis et al (eds). Philadelphia, Elsevier Saunders, 2006, pp 425–448

REVIEW AND SELF-ASSESSMENT*

Charles Wiener ■ Gerald Bloomfield ■ Cynthia D. Brown
■ Joshua Schiffer ■ Adam Spivak

QUESTIONS

DIRECTIONS: Choose the **one best** response to each question.

1. A 64-year-old man with congestive heart failure presents to the emergency room complaining of acute onset of severe pain in his right foot. The pain began during the night and awoke him from a deep sleep. He reports the pain to be so severe that he could not wear a shoe or sock to the hospital. His current medications are furosemide, 40 mg twice daily; carvedilol, 6.25 mg twice daily; candesartan, 8 mg once daily; and aspirin, 325 mg once daily. On examination, he is febrile to 38.5°C. The first toe of the right foot is erythematous and exquisitely tender to touch. There is significant swelling and effusion of the first metatarsophalangeal joint on the right. No other joints are affected. Which of the following findings would be expected on arthrocentesis?

   A. Glucose level of <25 mg/dL
   B. Positive Gram stain
   C. Presence of strongly negatively birefringent needle-shaped crystals under polarized light microscopy
   D. Presence of weakly positively birefringent rhomboidal crystals under polarized light microscopy
   E. White blood cell (WBC) count >100,000/μL

2. An 84-year-old man is seen by his primary care provider with symptoms of acute gouty arthritis in the first great toe and ankle on the left. He has a prior history of gout presenting similarly. His past medical history is significant for myelodysplasia, congestive heart failure, hyper-cholesterolemia, and chronic kidney disease. He is taking pravastatin, aspirin, furosemide, metolazone, lisinopril, and metoprolol XL. His baseline creatinine is 2.4 mg/dL, and uric acid level 9.3 mg/dL. His most recent complete blood count results are

2. (*Continued*)
   white blood cell count 2880/μL, hemoglobin 8.2 g/dL, hematocrit 26.2%, and platelet 68,000/μL. Which of the following medication regimens are most appropriate for the treatment of this patient?

   A. Allopurinol, 100 mg once daily
   B. Colchicine, 1 mg IV once, then 0.5 mg IV every 6 h until improvement
   C. Indomethacin, 25 mg three times daily
   D. Prednisone, 40 mg once daily
   E. Probenecid, 250 mg twice daily

3. A 46-year-old white female presents to your office with concerns about her diagnosis of hypertension 1 month previously. She asks you about her likelihood of developing complications of hypertension, including renal failure and stroke. She denies any past medical history other than hypertension and has no symptoms that suggest secondary causes. She currently is taking hydrochlorothiazide 25 mg/d. She smokes half a pack of cigarettes daily and drinks alcohol no more than once per week. Her family history is significant for hypertension in both parents. Her mother died of a cerebrovascular accident. Her father is alive but has coronary artery disease and is on hemodialysis. Her blood pressure is 138/90. Body mass index is 23. She has no retinal exudates or other signs of hypertensive retinopathy. Her point of maximal cardiac impulse is not displaced but is sustained. Her rate and rhythm are regular and without gallops. She has good peripheral pulses. An electrocardiogram reveals an axis of −30 degrees with borderline voltage criteria for left ventricular hypertrophy. Creatinine is 1.0 mg/dL. Which of the following items in her history and physical examination is a risk factor for a poor prognosis in a patient with hypertension?

*Questions and answers were taken from Wiener C, et al (eds). *Harrison's Principles of Internal Medicine Self-Assessment and Board Review*, 17th ed. New York: McGraw-Hill, 2008.

3. (*Continued*)
   A. Family history of renal failure and cerebrovascular disease
   B. Persistent elevation in blood pressure after the initiation of therapy
   C. Ongoing tobacco use
   D. Ongoing use of alcohol
   E. Presence of left ventricular hypertrophy on ECG

4. A 28-year-old female has hypertension that is difficult to control. She was diagnosed at age 26. Since that time she has been on increasing amounts of medication. Her current regimen consists of labetalol 1000 mg bid, lisinopril 40 mg qd, clonidine 0.1 mg bid, and amlodipine 5 mg qd. On physical examination she appears to be without distress. Blood pressure is 168/100, and heart rate is 84 beats/min. Cardiac examination is unremarkable, without rubs, gallops, or murmurs. She has good peripheral pulses and has no edema. Her physical appearance does not reveal any hirsutism, fat maldistribution, or abnormalities of genitalia. Laboratory studies reveal a potassium of 2.8 meq/dL and a serum bicarbonate of 32 meq/dL. Fasting blood glucose is 114 mg/dL. What is the likely diagnosis?

   A. Congenital adrenal hyperplasia
   B. Fibromuscular dysplasia
   C. Cushing's syndrome
   D. Conn's syndrome
   E. Pheochromocytoma

5. What is the best way to diagnose this disease?

   A. Renal vein renin levels
   B. 24-h urine collection for metanephrines
   C. Magnetic resonance imaging of the renal arteries
   D. 24-h urine collection for cortisol
   E. Plasma aldosterone/renin ratio

6. A patient with proteinuria has a renal biopsy that reveals segmental collapse of the glomerular capillary loops and overlying podocyte hyperplasia. The patient most likely has

   A. diabetes
   B. HIV infection
   C. multiple myeloma
   D. systemic lupus erythematosus
   E. Wegener's granulomatosis

7. A clinic patient who has a diagnosis of polycystic kidney disease has been doing research on the Internet. She is asymptomatic and has no significant family

7. (*Continued*)
   history. She asks you for screening for intracranial aneurysms. You recommend which of the following?

   A. Head CT scan without contrast
   B. CT angiogram
   C. Cerebral angiogram
   D. Magnetic resonance angiogram
   E. No further testing

8. Which of the following is the most potent stimulus for hypothalamic production of arginine vasopressin?

   A. Hypertonicity
   B. Hyperkalemia
   C. Hypokalemia
   D. Hypotonicity
   E. Intravascular volume depletion

9. A 28-year-old woman with HIV on antiretroviral therapy complains of abdominal pain in the emergency department. Laboratory data show a creatinine of 3.2 mg/dL; her baseline creatinine is 1.0 mg/dL. Urinalysis shows large numbers of white blood cells and red blood cells without epithelial cells, leukocyte esterase, or nitrites. Which test is indicated to diagnose the cause of her acute renal failure?

   A. Acid-fast stain of the urine
   B. Anti-GBM (glomerular base membrane) antibodies
   C. Renal angiogram
   D. Renal ultrasound
   E. Urine electrolytes

10. You are evaluating a 40-year-old patient admitted to the hospital with cirrhosis and an upper gastrointestinal bleed. The bleeding was treated with endoscopy and photocoagulation, and the patient is now stable. He required two units of packed red blood cells. He was briefly hypotensive upon admission but has remained stable for the past 5 days. He is becoming oliguric. Laboratory data show a creatinine of 4.0 mg/dL, whereas his baseline is 0.8–1.1 mg/dL. Sodium is 140 meq/L; BUN is 49 mg/dL. Urine sediment shows rare granular casts. His urine sodium is 50 meq/L, urine osmolality is 287 mosmol, and urine creatinine is 35 mg/dL. What is the cause of this patient's acute renal failure?

    A. Acute interstitial nephritis
    B. Acute tubular necrosis
    C. Glomerulonephritis
    D. Hepatorenal syndrome
    E. Prerenal azotemia

11. The pain associated with acute urinary tract obstruction is a result of which of the following?

    A. Compensatory natriuresis
    B. Decreased medullary blood flow
    C. Increased renal blood flow
    D. Vasodilatory prostaglandins

12. Preoperative assessment of a 55-year-old male patient going for coronary angiography shows an estimated glomerular filtration rate of 33 mL/min per 1.73 m^2 and poorly controlled diabetes. He is currently on no nephrotoxic medications, and the nephrologist assures you that he does not currently have acute renal failure. The case is due to begin in 4 h, and you would like to prevent contrast nephropathy. Which agent will definitely reduce the risk of contrast nephropathy?

    A. Dopamine
    B. Fenoldopam
    C. Indomethacin
    D. *N*-acetylcysteine
    E. Sodium bicarbonate

13. All the following forms of glomerulonephritis (GN) have associated normal serum complement C4 levels *except*

    A. lupus nephritis stage IV
    B. poststreptococcal GN
    C. hemolytic–uremic syndrome
    D. membranoproliferative GN type II
    E. endocarditis-associated GN

14. An 84-year-old female nursing home resident is brought to the emergency department due to lethargy. At the nursing home, she was found to have a blood pressure of 85/60 mmHg, heart rate 101 beats/min, temperature 37.8°C. Laboratory data are obtained: sodium 137 meq/L, potassium 2.8 meq/L, HCO_3^- 8 meq/L, chloride 117 meq/L, BUN 17 mg/dL, creatinine 0.9 mg/dL. An arterial blood gas shows PaO_2 80 mmHg, PCO_2 24 mmHg, pH 7.29. Her urine analysis is clear and has a pH of 4.5. What is the acid–base disorder?

    A. Anion-gap metabolic acidosis
    B. Non–anion-gap metabolic acidosis
    C. Non–anion-gap metabolic acidosis and respiratory alkalosis
    D. Respiratory acidosis

15. What is the most likely cause of the acid-base disorder of the patient in the preceding scenario?

15. (*Continued*)
    A. Diarrhea
    B. Diuretic use
    C. Hyperacute renal failure
    D. Hypoaldosteronism
    E. Proximal renal tubular acidosis

16. A 79-year-old male with a history of dementia is brought to the emergency department because of an 8-h history of lethargy. For the last 2 days he has been complaining of lower abdominal pain. His oral intake was normal until the last 8 h. The patient takes no medications. Temperature is normal, blood pressure is 150/90 mmHg, heart rate is 105 beats/min, and respirations are 20/min. Physical examination is notable for elevated neck veins and diffuse lower abdominal pain with normal bowel sounds. The bladder is percussed to the umbilicus, and there is an enlarged prostate. He is lethargic but responsive. Serum chemistries are notable for sodium of 128 meq/L, potassium of 5.7 meq/L, BUN of 100 mg/dL, and creatinine of 2.2 mg/dL. Two months ago his laboratory studies were normal. A Foley catheter is placed, yielding 1100 mL of urine. Which of the following statements regarding his clinical condition is true?

    A. His renal function probably will return to normal within the next week.
    B. He will need aggressive volume resuscitation over the next 24 h.
    C. He will have oliguria over the next 24 h.
    D. Immediate dialysis is indicated.
    E. Urinalysis will reveal hypertonic urine.

17. A 71-year-old woman is transferred to your hospital with new-onset renal failure requiring hemodialysis. On hospital day 1 at the outside hospital, she was admitted with a Killip class III inferior myocardial infarction. She underwent percutaneous coronary intervention on day 1 with successful angioplasty. On day 2, she spiked a fever and was started on gentamicin and a fluoroquinolone for pneumonia. A chest x-ray showed pulmonary vascular congestion on day 3, which was treated with IV loop diuretic. She complained of leg pain on day 4 which responded well to potassium repletion and ibuprofen. She is transferred to you with a urinalysis that shows 17 white blood cells, 1 red blood cell, 0 epithelial cells, no leukocyte esterase. Hansel's stain is positive for eosinophils. Serum laboratory studies show a creatinine of 4.2 mg/dL and undetectable complement levels. It is now hospital day 7. On which hospital day was her renal failure caused?

    A. 1
    B. 2

17. (*Continued*)
    C. 3
    D. 4

18. A 57-year-old man is admitted to the hospital for dehydration and confusion. In the emergency department he complained of excessive thirst and he was found to have a serum sodium of 162 meq/L and a newly elevated creatinine of 2.2 mg/dL. After receiving IV fluid, his sensorium clears and the patient relays to you that he drinks large amounts of fluid and makes about 2 L of urine each day. He has noticed that his urine output has no relation to the amount of fluid he drinks. His sodium remains elevated at 150 meq/L, and his urine osmolality returns at 80 mosmol/kg. After careful water restriction, you administer 10 μg of desmopressin intranasally and remeasure his urine osmolality. The osmolality is now 94 mosmol/kg. What is the most likely cause of his hypernatremia?

    A. Chronic hyperventilation
    B. Diabetes insipidus
    C. Excessive solute intake
    D. Gastrointestinal losses
    E. Surreptitious use of diuretics

19. What is the correct long-term treatment for the patient in the preceding scenario?

    A. Arginine vasopressin (AVP) analogues
    B. Brain imaging and, if indicated, resection
    C. Lithium carbonate
    D. Narcotics
    E. Salt restriction and diuretics

20. A 53-year-old female with long-standing depression and a history of rheumatoid arthritis is brought in by her daughter, who states that she found an empty bottle of acetylsalicylic acid by her mother's bedside. The patient is found to be confused and lethargic and is unable to provide a definitive history. What is the most likely set of laboratory values?

(SERUM, meq/L)					ROOM AIR ABG		
				SERUM CREATININE μmol/L			
Na⁺	K⁺	Cl⁻	HCO₃⁻	(mg/dL)	Po₂	Pco₂	PH
A 140	3.9	85	26	141 (1.6)	100	40	7.40
B 140	3.9	85	16	141 (1.6)	100	20	7.40
C 140	5.8	100	20	141 (1.6)	100	34	7.38
D 150	2.9	100	36	141 (1.6)	80	46	7.50
E 116	3.7	85	22	141 (1.6)	80	46	7.50

21. You are evaluating a 28-year-old man from Peru with abdominal pain. As part of the diagnostic workup, an abdominal ultrasound shows bilateral hydronephrosis and hydroureters. Which of the following conditions is least likely in this patient?

    A. Lymphoma
    B. Meatal stenosis
    C. Phimosis
    D. Retroperitoneal fibrosis

22. A 45-year-old male with a diagnosis of ESRD secondary to diabetes mellitus is being treated with peritoneal dialysis. This is being carried out as a continuous ambulatory peritoneal dialysis (CAPD). He undergoes four 2-L exchanges per day and has been doing so for approximately 4 years. Complications of peritoneal dialysis include which of the following?

    A. Hypotension after drainage of dialysate
    B. Hypoalbuminemia
    C. Hypercholesterolemia
    D. Hypoglycemia
    E. Left pleural effusion

23. While on rotation in a rural clinic, you are asked to evaluate a 70-year-old man with fever, shortness of breath, and a productive cough. You appreciate increased fremitus with egophony over the right lower lung field and make a presumptive diagnosis of community-acquired pneumonia. Blood pressure is 138/74 mmHg, heart rate 99 beats/min, temperature 38.6°C and weight 72 kg. He has a history of a nephrectomy, and he tells you that his "kidneys don't work at 100%." Before prescribing antibiotics, you would like to know his renal function. What additional data do you need in order to calculate his creatinine clearance using the Cockcroft-Gault formula?

    A. Plasma creatinine
    B. Plasma and urine creatinine
    C. Race and plasma creatinine
    D. Race, plasma creatinine, and urine creatinine

24. You are able to send the patient to the local hospital to get laboratory values drawn. His serum creatinine is 1.5 mg/dL, sodium 138 meq/L, potassium 3.8 meq/L, urine creatinine is 12 mmol. Using the Cockcroft-Gault equation, what is this patient's creatinine clearance?

    A. 27 mL/min
    B. 47 mL/min
    C. 70 mL/min
    D. 105 mL/min

25. All of these findings are consistent with a chronic unilateral urinary tract obstruction *except*

    A. anemia
    B. dysuria
    C. hypertension
    D. pain with micturition
    E. pyuria

26. A 72-year-old male develops acute renal failure after cardiac catheterization. Physical examination is notable for diminished peripheral pulses, livedo reticularis, epigastric tenderness, and confusion. Laboratory studies include (mg/dL) BUN 131, creatinine 5.2, and phosphate 9.5. Urinalysis shows 10 to 15 white blood cells (WBC), 5 to 10 red blood cells (RBC), and one hyaline cast per high-power field (HPF). The most likely diagnosis is

    A. acute interstitial nephritis caused by drugs
    B. rhabdomyolysis with acute tubular necrosis
    C. acute tubular necrosis secondary to radiocontrast exposure
    D. cholesterol embolization
    E. renal arterial dissection with prerenal azotemia

27. A 34-year-old male is brought to the hospital with altered mental status. He has a history of alcoholism. He is somnolent and does not answer questions. Physical examination reveals blood pressure 130/80, heart rate 105 beats/min, respiratory rate 24/min, and temperature 37°C (98.6°F). The remainder of the physical examination is unremarkable. Microscopic analysis of urine is shown below. Which of the following most likely will be found on further diagnostic evaluation?

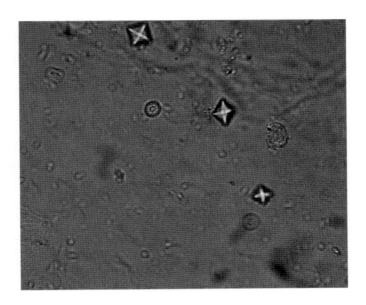

27. (*Continued*)
    A. More than 10,000 bacterial colonies on urine culture
    B. Anion-gap metabolic acidosis
    C. Hydronephrosis on ultrasound
    D. Nephrolithiasis on CT scan
    E. Positive antinuclear antibodies (ANA)

28. A 52-year-old man is found at home hypotensive and confused. In the emergency department, his blood pressure is 82/60 mmHg and his heart rate is 115 beats/min. He is confused and lethargic. Laboratory data show: sodium 133 meq/L, potassium 2.4 meq/L, chloride 70 meq/L, HCO_3^- 50 meq/L, BUN 44 mg/dL, creatinine 1.7 mg/dL. An arterial blood gas shows PO_2 of 62 mmHg, PCO_2 49 mmHg, pH 7.66. What acid-base disorder is present?

    A. Anion-gap metabolic acidosis
    B. Metabolic alkalosis
    C. Metabolic alkalosis plus respiratory acidosis
    D. Respiratory acidosis
    E. Respiratory alkalosis

29. What is the most likely cause of the acid-base disorder for the patient in the preceding scenario?

    A. Acute myocardial infarction
    B. Bartter's syndrome
    C. Cushing's disease
    D. Mineralocorticoid excess
    E. Vomiting

30. A 52-year-old diabetic patient is referred to the emergency department from the endoscopy suite. The patient has diabetes and a history of colon cancer that was removed 3 years ago. He also has hyperlipidemia, which is well controlled on atorvastatin. He presented to the endoscopy suite for a scheduled surveillance colonoscopy. Blood drawn upon arrival shows a sodium of 121 meq/L and the patient seemed disoriented. On physical examination, mucous membranes are dry and there is no axillary moisture. Serum osmolality is checked and is 270 mosmol/kg. What is the most likely cause of this patient's hyponatremia?

    A. Diabetes insipidus
    B. Hyperglycemia
    C. Hyperlipidemia
    D. Hypovolemia
    E. Syndrome of inappropriate secretion of antidiuretic hormone (SIADH)

31. You are evaluating a patient with stage 5 chronic kidney disease (CKD) who has an estimated glomerular filtration rate of 12 mL/min per 1.73 m². She has

31. (*Continued*)
    no complaints and takes all of her medications on schedule. Physical examination reveals a woman in no acute distress. There is no pericardial rub, and reflexes and mental status are intact. She has trace peripheral edema. Laboratory data show a creatinine of 6.3 mg/dL, potassium 4.8 meq/L, HCO_3^- 20 meq/L. She has known proteinuria. What is best next step in the management of this patient's CKD?

    A. Check serum blood urea nitrogen (BUN).
    B. Continue current management.
    C. Referral to the emergency department for initiation of dialysis.
    D. Renal biopsy.
    E. Urine analysis.

32. Your clinic patient presents to your office complaining of numbness and tingling in her hands and around her mouth. On physical examination, you elicit Chvostek's sign (twitching of the circumoral muscles in response to gently tapping on the facial nerve) and Trousseau's sign (carpal spasm induced by inflation of a blood pressure cuff to 20 mmHg above the patient's systolic blood pressure for 3 min). You make a presumptive diagnosis of hypocalcemia. What laboratory test is the next step in diagnosing the cause of her hypocalcemia?

    A. $1,25(OH_2)D$
    B. Ionized calcium
    C. Parathyroid hormone (PTH)
    D. Serum magnesium
    E. Thyroid-stimulating hormone

33. A 25-year-old man comes to your clinic because of a change in the color of his urine. He states that his urine has become red-tinged and has the foaminess of beer in the bowl. He has no abdominal pain or respiratory complaints. He has no cough, although he does report unintentional weight loss of 2–7 kg over the past month. He has no past medical history. In your office, you perform a urinalysis and dipstick, which shows red blood cell (RBC) casts and RBCs (including dysmorphic cells). He has no white blood cells and no bacteria. The urine dipstick is 2+, with a spot protein-to-creatinine ratio of 850. What is the next step in this patient's evaluation?

    A. Measure antineutrophilic cytoplasmic antibody levels.
    B. Cystoscopy.
    C. Initiate therapy with an angiotensin-converting enzyme (ACE) inhibitor with close follow-up.
    D. Measure urine microalbumin.
    E. Renal CT scan.

34. A 10-year-old girl complaining of profound weakness, occasional difficulty walking, and polyuria is brought to the pediatrician. Her mother is sure the girl has not been vomiting frequently. The girl takes no medicines. She is normotensive, and no focal neurologic abnormalities are found. Serum chemistries include Na^+ 142 mmol/L, K^+ 2.5 mmol/L, HCO_3^- 32 mmol/L, and Cl^- 100 mmol/L. A 24-h urine collection on a normal diet reveals Na^+ 200 mmol/d, K^+ 50 mmol/d, and Cl^- 30 mmol/d. Renal ultrasound demonstrates symmetrically enlarged kidneys without hydronephrosis. A stool phenolphthalein test and a urine screen for diuretics are negative. Plasma renin levels are found to be elevated. Which of the following conditions is most consistent with these data?

    A. Conn's syndrome
    B. Chronic ingestion of licorice
    C. Bartter's syndrome
    D. Wilms' tumor
    E. Proximal renal tubular acidosis

35. A 32-year-old patient presents to your clinic complaining of right-sided flank pain and dark urine. He states that these symptoms began about a month ago. He denies any burning on urination and has had no fevers. He has not suffered any trauma and has not been sexually active recently. On review of systems he reports early satiety and describes a burning sensation in his chest when he lies down. An ultrasound of his right flank is performed and reveals >20 cysts of varying sizes in his right kidney. Which of the following statements is true?

    A. Adult-onset polycystic kidney disease (PCKD) will lead to end-stage renal disease in 100% of patients by age 70.
    B. Aortic stenosis is present in 25% of patient with PCKD.
    C. Forty percent of patients with PCKD will have hepatic cysts by age 60.
    D. PCKD is inherited as an autosomal recessive trait in adults.
    E. There is a significantly increased risk of embolic stroke in patients with PCKD.

36. In patients with chronic renal failure, which of the following is the most important contributor to renal osteodystrophy?

    A. Impaired renal production of 1,25-dihydroxyvitamin D_3 $[1,25(OH)_2D_3]$
    B. Hypocalcemia
    C. Hypophosphatemia
    D. Loss of vitamin D and calcium via dialysis
    E. The use of calcitriol

37. A 74-year-old female sees her physician for a follow-up visit for hypertension. One week ago she was started on an oral medication for hypertension. She takes no other medications. Blood pressure is 125/80 mmHg, and heart rate is 72 beats/min. Serum chemistries reveal a sodium of 132 meq/L. Two weeks ago serum chemistries were normal. Which of the following medications most likely was initiated 1 week ago?

    A. Enalapril
    B. Furosemide
    C. Hydrochlorothiazide
    D. Metoprolol
    E. Spironolactone

38. Laboratory evaluation of a 19-year-old male who is being worked up for polyuria and polydipsia yields the following results:

    Serum electrolytes (meq/L): Na^+ 144, K^+ 4.0, Cl^- 107, HCO_3^- 25
    BUN: 6.4 mmol/L (18 mg/dL)
    Blood glucose: 5.7 mmol/L (102 mg/dL)
    Urine electrolytes (mmol/L): Na^+ 28, K^+ 32
    Urine osmolality: 195 mosmol/kg water
    After 12 h of fluid deprivation, body weight has fallen by 5%. Laboratory testing now reveals the following:
    Serum electrolytes (meq/L): Na^+ 150, K^+ 4.1, Cl^- 109, HCO_3^- 25
    BUN: 7.1 mmol/L (20 mg/dL)
    Blood glucose: 5.4 mmol/L (98 mg/dL)
    Urine electrolytes (mmol/L): Na^+ 24, K^+ 35
    Urine osmolality: 200 mosmol/kg water
    One hour after the subcutaneous administration of 5 units of arginine vasopressin urine values are as follows:
    Urine electrolytes (meq/L): Na^+ 30, K^+ 30
    Urine osmolality: 199 mosmol/kg water
    The likely diagnosis is

    A. nephrogenic diabetes insipidus
    B. osmotic diuresis
    C. salt-losing nephropathy
    D. psychogenic polydipsia
    E. none of the above

39. A 28-year-old man is diagnosed with acute myelogenous leukemia and has a white blood cell count of 168,000/μL. He initiates chemotherapy with cytarabine, etoposide, and daunorubicin. Within 24 h, his creatinine has increased from 1.0 mg/dL to 2.5 mg/dL, and he is oliguric. Pretreatment with which of the following medications may have prevented this complication?

    A. Allopurinol
    B. Colchicine

39. (Continued)
    C. Furosemide
    D. Prednisone
    E. Sodium bicarbonate

40. A 37-year-old man is brought to the emergency department by his wife from home. He was painting their garage and became unconscious. He has no past medical history. CT scan of the head is normal. Urine and serum toxicology screen, including ethanol and acetaminophen, are negative. Laboratory data show: sodium 138 meq/L, potassium 4.4 meq/L, HCO_3^- 5 meq/L, chloride 102 meq/L, BUN 15 mg/dL, calcium 9.7 mg/dL, glucose 94 mg/dL. An arterial blood gas on room air shows PaO_2 95 mmHg, PCO_2 20 mmHg, pH 7.02. A urine analysis is unremarkable. On physical examination his blood pressure is 110/72 mmHg. He is barely arousable but responds to painful stimuli. Otherwise, he has no focal abnormalities. What is the acid-base disorder?

    A. Anion-gap metabolic acidosis
    B. Anion-gap metabolic acidosis with respiratory alkalosis
    C. Non–anion-gap metabolic acidosis
    D. Respiratory acidosis

41. The "dose" of dialysis is currently defined as

    A. the counter-current flow rate of the dialysate
    B. the fractional urea clearance
    C. the hours per week of dialysis
    D. the number of sessions actually completed in a month

42. A patient with a diagnosis of scleroderma who has diffuse cutaneous involvement presents with malignant hypertension, oliguria, edema, hemolytic anemia, and renal failure. You make a diagnosis of scleroderma renal crisis (SRC). What is the recommended treatment?

    A. Captopril
    B. Carvedilol
    C. Clonidine
    D. Diltiazem
    E. Nitroprusside

43. Your patient with end-stage renal disease on hemodialysis has persistent hyperkalemia. He has a history of total bilateral renal artery stenosis, which is why he is on hemodialysis. He only has electrocardiogram changes when his potassium rises above 6.0 meq/L, which occurs a few times per week. You admit him to the hospital for further evaluation. Your laboratory evaluation, nutrition counseling, and medication adjustments have not impacted his serum

43. (*Continued*)

potassium. What is the next reasonable step to undertake for this patient?

A. Adjust the dialysate.
B. Administer a daily dose of furosemide.
C. Perform "sodium modeling."
D. Implant an automatic defibrillator.
E. Perform bilateral nephrectomy.

44. A 63-year-old male is brought to the emergency department after having a seizure. He has a history of an unresectable lung mass treated with palliative radiation therapy. He is known to have a serum sodium of 128 meq/L chronically. The patient's wife reports that on the night before admission he was somnolent. This morning, while she was trying to awaken him, he developed a generalized tonic-clonic seizure lasting approximately 1 min. In the emergency room he is unresponsive. Vital signs and physical examination are otherwise normal. Serum sodium is 111 meq/L. He is treated with 3% saline and transferred to the intensive care unit. One day later serum sodium is 137 meq/L. He has had no further seizures since admission and is awake but is barely able to move his extremities and is dysarthric. Which of the following studies is most likely to explain his current condition?

A. Arteriogram showing a vertebral artery thrombus
B. CT of the head showing metastases
C. EEG showing focal seizures
D. MRI of the brainstem showing demyelination
E. Transesophageal echocardiogram showing left atrial thrombus

45. A 25-year-old female with nephrotic syndrome from minimal-change disease is seen in the emergency department with increased right leg swelling. Ultrasound of the leg shows thrombosis of the superficial femoral vein. Which of the following is not a mechanism of hypercoagulability in this disorder?

A. Increased platelet aggregation
B. Low serum levels of protein C and protein S
C. Chronic disseminated intravascular coagulation
D. Hyperfibrinogenemia
E. Low serum levels of antithrombin III

46. It is hospital day 5 for a 65-year-old patient with prerenal azotemia secondary to dehydration. His creatinine was initially 3.6 mg/dL on admission, but it has improved today to 2.1 mg/dL. He complains of mild lower back pain, and you prescribe naproxen to be taken intermittently. By what mechanism might this drug further impair his renal function?

46. (*Continued*)

A. Afferent arteriolar vasoconstriction
B. Afferent arteriolar vasodilatation
C. Efferent arteriolar vasoconstriction
D. Proximal tubular toxicity
E. Ureteral obstruction

47. A 63-year-old male with a history of diabetes mellitus is found to have a lung nodule on chest radiography. To stage the disease further he undergoes a contrast-enhanced CT scan of the chest. One week before the CT scan, his BUN is 26 mg/dL and his creatinine is 1.8 mg/dL. Three days after the study he complains of dyspnea, pedal edema, and decreased urinary output. Repeat BUN is 86 mg/dL and creatinine is 4.4 mg/dL. The most likely mechanism of the acute renal failure is

A. acute tubular necrosis
B. allergic hypersensitivity
C. cholesterol emboli
D. immune-complex glomerulonephritis
E. ureteral outflow obstruction

48. In the patient in Question 47 the urinalysis is most likely to show

A. granular casts
B. red blood cell casts
C. urinary eosinophils
D. urinary neutrophils
E. white blood cell casts

49. A 35-year-old female presents with complaints of bilateral lower extremity edema, polyuria, and moderate left-sided flank pain that began approximately 2 weeks ago. There is no past medical history. She is taking no medications and denies tobacco, alcohol, or illicit drug use. Examination shows normal vital signs, including normal blood pressure. There is 2+ edema in bilateral lower extremities. The 24-h urine collection is significant for 3.5 g of protein. Urinalysis is bland except for the proteinuria. Serum creatinine is 0.7 mg/dL, and ultrasound examination shows the left kidney measuring 13 cm and the right kidney measuring 11.5 cm. You are concerned about renal vein thrombosis. What test do you choose for the evaluation?

A. Computed tomography of the renal veins
B. Contrast venography
C. Magnetic resonance venography
D. ^{99}Tc-labeled pentetic acid (DPTA) imaging
E. Ultrasound with Doppler evaluation of the renal veins

50. The posterior pituitary secretes arginine vasopressin (antidiuretic hormone) under which of the following stressors?

50. (*Continued*)
    A. Hyperosmolarity
    B. Hypernatremia
    C. Volume depletion
    D. A and B
    E. A and C

51. A 29-year-old man is admitted to the hospital with a severe asthma exacerbation. He is taken to the intensive care unit (ICU) and treated with continuous aerosolized β-adrenergic agonists and glucocorticoids. He requires bilevel positive airway pressure mechanical respiration. After 18 h of this therapy, his respiratory status begins to improve. He begins to complain of fatigue and myalgias in his legs. He has difficulty ambulating and on neurologic examination he has three out of five symmetric weakness in the lower extremities. On the cardiac monitor, you notice flattened T waves, ST depression, and a prolonged QT interval. What is the cause of this patient's neurologic and cardiac findings?

    A. Adrenal insufficiency
    B. ICU psychosis
    C. Medication effect
    D. Myocardial infarction with congestive heart failure
    E. Todd's paralysis

52. A 33-year-old male is brought for medical attention after completing an ultramarathon. Upon finishing he was disoriented and light-headed. His normal weight is 60 kg. Physical examination reveals a body temperature of 38.3°C (100.9°F), blood pressure of 85/60 mmHg, and heart rate of 125 beats/min. The patient's neck veins are flat, and skin turgor is poor. Laboratory studies are notable for a serum sodium of 175 meq/L. The patient's estimated free water deficit is

    A. 0.75 L
    B. 1.5 L
    C. 7.5 L
    D. 15 L
    E. 22.5 L

53. A 66-year-old woman is being treated with penicillin for mitral valve endocarditis due to *Streptococcus viridans*. She initially improved with resolution of her fever after 7 days, but now comes to the emergency room complaining of fever and rash during week 4 of her treatment. She continues to receive penicillin IV via a central line equipped with an infusion system. She has had no drainage from the site of her central line and has otherwise been feeling well until she developed a diffuse pruritic rash over her entire body, beginning on her trunk. She also has had a fever to as high as 38.3°C at home. On examination, she has an erythematous

53. (*Continued*)
    maculopapular rash over her trunk and legs. In many areas, it has coalesced to form raised plaques. She currently has a temperature of 39°C. Her laboratory values show a white blood cell count of 12,330/μL with 72% polymorphonuclear cells, 12% lymphocytes, 5% monocytes, and 11% eosinophils. Her BUN is 65 mg/dL, and creatinine is 2.5 mg/dL. At the time of her hospital discharge, the patient's BUN was 24 mg/dL and creatinine was 1.2 mg/dL. Which test is most likely to yield the diagnosis of her acute renal failure?

    A. 24-h urine protein level
    B. Antistreptolysin O titers
    C. Blood culture for aerobic and anaerobic bacteria
    D. Echocardiogram
    E. Hansel's stain for eosinophils in the urine

54. All the following are complications during hemodialysis *except*

    A. anaphylactoid reaction
    B. fever
    C. hyperglycemia
    D. hypotension
    E. muscle cramps

55. A 42-year-old man with a history of pulmonary sarcoidosis is admitted to the intensive care unit with confusion and nausea. His family reports that he has had polyuria and polydipsia for some time but it has increased dramatically in the past week. On physical examination, his mucous membranes are dry and he is orthostatic by pulse. In the emergency room, his blood glucose is 90 mg/dL. An electrocardiogram (ECG) taken at that time is shown below.

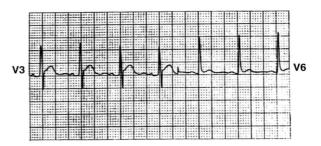

    What is the cause of this patient's symptoms?

    A. Hypercalcemia
    B. Hyperkalemia
    C. Hypocalcemia
    D. Hypokalemia

56. The patient in the preceding scenario is found to have a serum calcium of 12.1 mg/dL. Of the following

56. (*Continued*)

interventions, what therapy is most appropriate in this patient?

A. Glucocorticoids
B. Intravenous loop diuretic
C. Intravenous phosphate
D. Oral calcitriol
E. Zoledronic acid

57. You are consulting to advise on another antihypertensive agent for a patient with difficult-to-control hypertension. Despite high doses of a beta blocker, the patient remains hypertensive. The estimated glomerular filtration rate (GFR) is 75 mL/min per 1.73 m². On physical examination, there is no exophthalmos and no thyroid bruit. The great vessels are without bruit as well. Abdominal examination reveals bruits loudest in bilateral flanks as well as a left femoral bruit. Peripheral pulses are intact. An ultrasound confirms the presence of bilateral renal artery stenosis. Which medication class would *not* be a good choice to add to this patient's regimen?

A. Thiazide diuretic
B. Calcium-channel blocker
C. Angiotensin II receptor blocker
D. Central acting alpha blocker

58. Which of the following patients in need of dialysis would receive the greatest benefit from placing a peritoneal dialysis catheter rather than a hemodialysis catheter?

A. High-peritoneal transporters
B. Patients in developing countries
C. Patients older than 65
D. Patients with no residual kidney function
E. Patients with prior abdominal surgery

59. A patient with a history of Sjögren's syndrome has the following laboratory findings: plasma sodium 139 meq/L, chloride 112 meq/L, bicarbonate 15 meq/L, and potassium 3.0 meq/L; urine studies show a pH of 6.0, sodium of 15 meq/L, potassium of 10 meq/L, and chloride of 12 meq/L. The most likely diagnosis is

A. type I renal tubular acidosis (RTA)
B. type II RTA
C. type III RTA
D. type IV RTA
E. chronic diarrhea

60. The condition of a 50-year-old obese female with a 5-year history of mild hypertension controlled by a

60. (*Continued*)

thiazide diuretic is being evaluated because proteinuria was noted during her routine yearly medical visit. Physical examination disclosed a height of 167.6 cm (66 in.), weight of 91 kg (202 lb), blood pressure of 130/80 mmHg, and trace pedal edema. Laboratory values are as follows:

Serum creatinine: 106 μmol/L (1.2 mg/dL)
BUN: 6.4 mmol/L (18 mg/dL)
Creatinine clearance: 87 mL/min
Urinalysis: pH 5.0; specific gravity 1.018; protein 3+; no glucose; occasional coarse granular cast
Urine protein excretion: 5.9 g/d

A renal biopsy demonstrates that 60% of the glomeruli have segmental scarring by light microscopy, with the remainder of the glomeruli appearing unremarkable (see following figure).

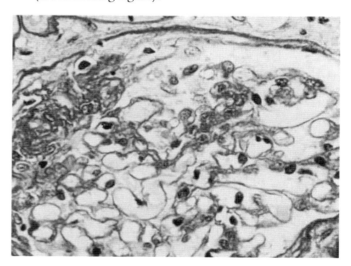

The most likely diagnosis is

A. hypertensive nephrosclerosis
B. focal and segmental sclerosis
C. minimal-change (nil) disease
D. membranous glomerulopathy
E. crescentic glomerulonephritis

61. A 20-year-old college student seeks medical attention for light-headedness. He just completed a rigorous tennis match and did not drink any water or fluids. Supine blood pressure is 110/70 mmHg, and heart rate is 105 beats/min. Upright, the blood pressure is 95/60 mmHg with a heart rate of 125 beats/min. Temperature and mental status are normal. Which of the following laboratory results is most likely in this patient?

A. Serum BUN/creatinine ratio <20
B. Serum sodium <140 meq/L

61. (*Continued*)

    C. Urine potassium <20 meq/L

    D. Urine sodium <20 meq/L

    E. Urine red blood cell casts

62. A 50-year-old male is admitted to the hospital with pneumonia. He does well after the administration of antibiotics, but his sodium is noted to rise from 140 to 154 meq/L over 2 days. He reports thirst and has had a urine output of approximately 5 L/d. Which of the following is the most appropriate next step to evaluate the patient's disorder?

    A. Measurement of serum osmolality

    B. Measurement of serum vasopressin level

    C. 24-h measurement of urinary sodium

    D. Trial of arginine vasopressin

    E. Trial of free water restriction

63. A 16-year-old female star gymnast presents to your office complaining of fatigue, diffuse weakness, and muscle cramps. She has no previous medical history and denies tobacco, alcohol, or illicit drug use. There is no significant family history. Examination shows a thin female with normal blood pressure. Body mass index (BMI) is 18 kg/m^2. Oral examination shows poor dentition. Muscle tone is normal, and neurologic examination is normal. Laboratory studies show hematocrit of 38.5%, creatinine of 0.6 mg/dL, serum bicarbonate of 30 meq/L, and potassium of 2.7 meq/L. Further evaluation should include which of the following?

    A. Urinalysis and urine culture

    B. Plasma renin and aldosterone levels

    C. Urine toxicology screen for opiates

    D. Urine toxicology screen for diuretics

    E. Serum magnesium level

ANSWERS

1. The answer is C.

(*Chap. 8*) Acute gouty arthritis is frequently seen in individuals on diuretic therapy. Diuretics result in hyperuricemia through enhanced urate reabsorption in the proximal tubule of the kidney in the setting of volume depletion. Hyperuricemia remains asymptomatic in many individuals but may manifest as acute gout. Acute gout is an intensely inflammatory arthritis that frequently begins at night. While any joint may be affected, the initial presentation of gout is often in the great toe at the metatarsophalangeal joint. There is associated joint swelling, effusion, erythema, and exquisite tenderness. A typical patient will complain that the pain is so great that they are unable to wear socks or allow sheets or blankets to cover the toes. Arthrocentesis will reveal an inflammatory cloudy-appearing fluid. The diagnosis of gout is confirmed by the demonstration of monosodium urate crystals seen both extracellularly and intracellularly within neutrophils. Monosodium urate crystals appear strongly negatively birefringent under polarized light microscopy and have a typical needle- and rod-shaped appearance. The WBC count is usually <50,000/μL with values >100,000/μL being more likely to be associated with a septic arthritis. Likewise, very low glucose levels and a positive Gram stain are not manifestations of acute gout but are common in septic arthritis. Calcium pyrophosphate dihydrate crystals appear as weakly positively birefringent rhomboidal crystals and are seen in pseudogout.

2. The answer is D.

(*Chap. 8*) In acute gouty arthritis, the initial therapy is directed against the intense inflammatory response. Typical agents include colchicine, nonsteroidal anti-inflammatory drugs (NSAIDs), and oral glucocorticoids. The choice of agent should be made in the context of the patient's comorbid conditions and medications as well as potential side effects of the medication. Oral glucocorticoids are the treatment of choice for this patient. These medications, such as prednisone, are highly effective, and there are no contraindications to the use of prednisone. Colchicine may be poorly tolerated in the elderly. In addition, renal disease and blood dyscrasias are relative contraindications to the use of the colchicine. Colchicine is usually administered orally as 0.6-mg tablets, which may be taken every 6 h until the appearance of intolerance or gastrointestinal side effects. Intravenous colchicine is rarely used except in hospitalized individuals who are unable to take oral medications. Sudden death with IV administration has been reported as well as marked bone marrow suppression, and thus this medication should not be used in this individual. NSAIDs, such as indomethacin in full anti-inflammatory doses, are effective in ~90% of individuals with acute gout, with resolution of symptoms in 5–8 days. The most effective drugs are indomethacin, ibuprofen, or diclofenac. However, given the degree of renal impairment in this patient, NSAIDs should not be used. Hypouricemic agents such as allopurinol and probenecid should not be used in acute gouty arthritis as they may worsen the acute attack. Probenecid is a uricosuric agent that is also contraindicated in this patient because of the underlying renal disease.

3. The answer is C.

(*Chap. 19*) Several factors have been shown to confer an increased risk of complications from hypertension. In the patient described here there is only one: ongoing tobacco use. Epidemiologic factors that have poorer prognosis include African-American race, male sex, and onset of hypertension in youth. In addition, comorbid factors that independently increase the risk of atherosclerosis worsen the prognosis in patients with hypertension. These factors include hypercholesterolemia, obesity, diabetes mellitus, and tobacco use. Physical and laboratory examination showing evidence of end organ damage also may portend a poorer prognosis. This includes evidence of retinal damage or hypertensive heart disease with cardiac enlargement or congestive heart failure. Furthermore, electrocardiographic evidence of ischemia or left ventricular strain but not left ventricular hypertrophy alone may predict worse outcomes. A family history of hypertensive complications does not worsen the prognosis if diastolic blood pressure is maintained at less than 110 mmHg.

4. and 5. The answers are D and E.

(Chap. 19) This patient presents at a young age with hypertension that is difficult to control, raising the question of secondary causes of hypertension. The most likely diagnosis in this patient is primary hyperaldosteronism, also known as Conn's syndrome. The patient has no physical features that suggest congenital adrenal hyperplasia or Cushing's syndrome. In addition, there is no glucose intolerance as is commonly seen in Cushing's syndrome. The lack of episodic symptoms and the labile hypertension make pheochromocytoma unlikely. The findings of hypokalemia and metabolic alkalosis in the presence of difficult to control hypertension yield the likely diagnosis of Conn's syndrome. Diagnosis of the disease can be difficult, but the preferred test is the plasma aldosterone/renin ratio. This test should be performed at 8 A.M., and a ratio above 30 to 50 is diagnostic of primary hyperaldosteronism. Caution should be made in interpreting this test while the patient is on ACE inhibitor therapy as ACE inhibitors can falsely elevate plasma renin activity. However, a plasma renin level that is undetectable or an elevated aldosterone/renin ratio in the presence of an ACE inhibitor therapy is highly suggestive of primary hyperaldosteronism. Selective adrenal vein renin sampling may be performed after the diagnosis to help determine if the process is unilateral or bilateral. Although fibromuscular dysplasia is a common secondary cause of hypertension in young females, the presence of hypokalemia and metabolic alkalosis should suggest Conn's syndrome. Thus, magnetic resonance imaging of the renal arteries is unnecessary in this case. Measurement of 24-h urine collection for potassium wasting and aldosterone secretion can be useful in the diagnosis of Conn's syndrome. The measurement of metanephrines or cortisol is not indicated.

6. The answer is B.

(Chaps. 4 and 15) A collapsing variant of focal segmental glomerulosclerosis is typically diagnostic of HIV nephropathy, which presents with proteinuria and subacute loss of renal function. Diabetes typically causes thickening of glomerular basement membrane, mesangial sclerosis, and

arteriosclerosis. Multiple myeloma causes proteinuria via deposition of light chains in the glomeruli and tubules and the development of renal amyloidosis. Microscopy shows amyloid proteins with Congo red staining. SLE causes membranous and proliferative nephritis due to immune complex deposition. Wegener's granulomatosis and microscopic polyangiitis cause pauci-immune necrotizing glomerulonephritis.

7. The answer is E.

(Chap. 16) Intracranial aneurysms are present in 5–10% of asymptomatic patients with ADPKD. Screening of all ADPKD patients is not recommended. Any presenting symptoms or a family history of subarachnoid hemorrhage or sudden death should prompt further screening with magnetic resonance angiography (MRA) or CT angiography, or consideration of cerebral angiography.

8. The answer is A.

(Chap. 6) Excretion of water is tightly regulated at the collecting duct by arginine vasopressin (AVP, formerly antidiuretic hormone). An increase in plasma tonicity is sensed by hypothalamic osmoreceptors, causing AVP secretion from the posterior pituitary. AVP binding to the collecting duct leads to insertion of water channels (aquaporin-2) into the luminal membrane, promoting water reabsorption. Serum sodium is the principal extracellular solute, and so effective osmolality is determined predominantly by the plasma sodium concentration. Plasma osmolality normally is regulated within 1–2% of normal (280 to 290 mosmol/kg). The sensitivity of the baroreceptors for AVP release is far less than that of the osmoreceptors. Depletion of intravascular volume sufficient to decrease mean arterial pressure is necessary to stimulate AVP secretion.

9. The answer is D.

(Chaps. 3 and 10) In the evaluation of azotemia, the initial diagnostic modalities are urine analysis and renal ultrasound. Renal ultrasound is important so that obstructive causes can be corrected urgently with urologic evaluation. This patient may have an obstructive nephropathy due to nephrolithiasis, as certain HIV medications can cause nephrolithiasis. Patients with nephrolithiasis can often have pyuria and hematuria. Urine electrolytes are useful to establish prerenal azotemia but should be performed only after urine analysis is unremarkable and renal ultrasound shows normal sized kidneys. Anti-GBM antibodies are an important component of the evaluation of glomerulonephritis. Angiogram is useful when renal vascular disease is suspected. (See Fig. 3-1.)

10. The answer is B.

(Chaps. 3 and 10) Acute renal failure with urine sediment showing muddy brown (granular) casts or an amorphous sediment in the absence of white blood cells, red blood cells, eosinophils or severe proteinuria has a high likelihood

of being acute tubular necrosis. This is particularly true when an episode of renal hypoperfusion (hypotension) is present. It is possible to differentiate between prerenal azotemia and acute tubular necrosis by calculating the fractional excretion of sodium (FeNa) and by measuring the BUN/creatinine ratio, urine sodium, urine osmolality, and the urine/plasma creatinine ratio (see Table 3-2). In this case, the BUN/creatinine ratio is <20, the urine sodium is >40 meq/L, urine osmolality is <350 mosmol, FeNa is 4%, and urine/plasma creatinine is <20, indicating that this is acute renal failure with tubular injury. Pyuria is present in 75% of cases of acute interstitial nephritis (AIN) and there is no proximate drug exposure to suggest AIN. Hepatorenal syndrome is excluded by the elevated urine sodium. Glomerulonephritis is unlikely given the absence of red cell casts on urine analysis and the clinical situation.

11. The answer is C.

(Chap. 21) In acute urinary tract obstruction, pain is due to distention of the collecting system or renal capsule. Acutely, there is a compensatory increase in renal blood flow when kidney function is impaired by obstruction, which further exacerbates capsular stretch. Eventually, vasodilatory prostaglandins act to preserve renal function when glomerular filtration rate has decreased. Medullary blood flow decreases as the pressure of the obstruction further inhibits the renal parenchyma from perfusing; however, the ensuing chronic renal destruction may occur without substantial pain. When an obstruction has been relieved, there is a postobstructive diuresis that is mediated by relief of tubular pressure, increased solute load (per nephron), and natriuretic factors. There can be an extreme amount of diuresis, but this is not painful.

12. The answer is E.

(Chap. 10) Radiocontrast agents cause renal injury through intrarenal vasoconstriction and through generation of oxygen radicals causing acute tubular necrosis. These medications cause an acute decrease in renal blood flow and glomerular filtration rate. Patients with chronic kidney disease, diabetes mellitus, heart failure, multiple myeloma, and volume depletion are at highest risk of contrast nephropathy. It is clear that hydration with normal saline is an effective measure to prevent contrast nephropathy. Of the other measures mentioned here, only sodium bicarbonate or N-acetylcysteine could be recommended for clinical use to reduce the risk of contrast nephropathy. Dopamine has been proven an ineffective agent to prevent contrast nephropathy. Fenoldopam, a D_1-receptor agonist, has been tested in several clinical trials and does not appear to reduce the incidence of contrast nephropathy. Although several small clinical studies have suggested a clinical benefit to the use of N-acetylcysteine, a meta-analysis has been inconclusive, and the medication should be administered well in advance of the procedure. Sodium bicarbonate begun within 1 h of the procedure has shown a significant

benefit in a single-center, randomized, controlled trial. Due to the time limitations, and based on the evidence, only sodium bicarbonate would be helpful in this patient.

13. The answer is A.

(Chap. 15) In different disease processes the complement pathway is activated either by classical pathway activation or by alternative pathway activation. If the classical pathway is activated, as in lupus nephritis, the serum complement measures of C3, C4, and CH50 are low. If the alternative pathway is activated, C3 and CH50 may be low but C4 is at normal levels. When acute GN is suspected, measurement of serum complement levels will often limit the differential diagnosis. Other conditions with normal C4 include ANCA-associated diseases. Low C4 may be seen with membranoproliferative GN types I and III. Type I disease also may be associated with cryoglobulinemia.

14. The answer is B. (Chap. 5)

The pH is <7.35; therefore, the primary process is an acidosis. The HCO_3^- is low and the P_{CO_2} is low, excluding a primary respiratory acidosis. The anion gap is normal at 12. The expected P_{CO_2} is between 24 and 16 mmHg for appropriate respiratory compensation. The P_{CO_2} in this example represents normal respiratory compensation for a metabolic acidosis.

15. The answer is A.

(Chap. 5) Metabolic acidosis occurs because of endogenous acid production or loss of bicarbonate. The anion gap is elevated in the presence of unmeasured anions (or, less commonly, a loss of unmeasured cations) and is normal with bicarbonate loss. A fall in the serum albumin of 1 g/dL from normal lowers the expected anion gap by 2.5 meq/L. The differential diagnosis for a non–anion-gap metabolic acidosis includes gastrointestinal losses, renal acidosis, and drug-induced and other less common causes. Nursing home residents are at risk for institutionally acquired diarrheas, often infectious. The urine pH is usually high in proximal renal tubular acidosis, and the patients usually younger. Defects in the renin-angiotensin system, such as hypoaldosteronism, cause hyperkalemia, not hypokalemia. This patient has no evidence of renal failure. Diuretic use will usually cause a metabolic alkalosis.

16. The answer is A.

(Chap. 21) The prognosis for the return of normal renal function is excellent in patients with acute bilateral renal obstruction, such as an obstruction that is due to prostate enlargement. With relief of the obstruction, the prognosis depends on whether irreversible renal damage has occurred. Return of GFR usually follows relief of obstruction lasting 1 to 2 weeks, provided that there has been no intercurrent infection. After 8 weeks of obstruction recovery is unlikely. Acute relief of bilateral obstruction commonly results in polyuria. An osmotic diuresis caused by excretion of retained urea and resolution of volume expansion contributes to the diuresis. The urine is hypotonic. The diuresis usually abates with resolution of normal extracellular volume, and so aggressive volume resuscitation is generally not necessary unless hypotension or overt volume depletion develops. Indications for acute hemodialysis are those for the usual complications of acute renal failure, including electrolyte disturbances, uremia, and inability to control volume.

17. The answer is A.

(Chap. 10) Atheroembolic disease can cause acute renal failure (ARF) after manipulation of the aorta or renal arteries during angiography. Cholesterol crystals embolize to the renal vasculature and lodge in small- to medium-sized vessels inciting a fibrotic reaction in the vessel wall, narrowing the lumen. Diagnostic clues to atheroembolic ARF are recent manipulation of the aorta or renal vessels, eosinophiluria, and low complement levels. The ARF usually occurs days to weeks after the inciting event. Aminoglycosides, diuretics, or nonsteroidal anti-inflammatory drugs can cause renal failure but it does not classically present with eosinophiluria or hypocomplementemia. Atheroembolic ARF is usually irreversible.

18. The answer is B.

(Chap. 6) The differential diagnosis for hypernatremia is fairly narrow as it results in a relative loss of water. Water is lost via renal or nonrenal mechanisms. The urine osmolality is a key historic piece of data. If the patient is excreting the minimum amount of maximally concentrated urine, gastrointestinal (osmotic diarrhea), insensible (skin or respiratory loss), or remote renal losses (diabetes mellitus) are the cause. This patient is excreting a large amount of dilute urine. He is not excreting >750 mosmol in his urine daily, which would suggest diuretic use. Either central or nephrogenic diabetes insipidus (DI) must be the cause. In this patient, the lack of response to desmopressin indicates nephrogenic DI.

19. The answer is E.

(Chap. 6) The patient in the preceding scenario has nephrogenic diabetes insipidus (NDI). Causes of NDI include drugs (particularly lithium carbonate), hypercalcemia, hypokalemia, papillary necrosis, or congenital disorders. Symptomatic polyuria due to NDI can be treated with a low-sodium diet and thiazide diuretics, which induce mild volume depletion and enhanced proximal reabsorption of salt and water. Narcotics may be useful in patients with gastrointestinal hypermotility and water loss as a result thereof. AVP analogues are used to treat central diabetes insipidus and would have no impact on NDI. If a patient is found to have central diabetes insipidus, brain imaging should be obtained to rule out destruction of the neurohypophysis. Lithium carbonate is a cause of NDI and should be discontinued if causing symptomatic NDI.

20. The answer is B.

(Chap. 5; N Engl J Med 338:26–34, 1998.) A respiratory alkalosis with a combined metabolic acidosis is typical of salicylate toxicity. Salicylate intoxication can result in respiratory alkalosis, mixed respiratory alkalosis and metabolic acidosis, or, less commonly, a simple metabolic acidosis. Respiratory alkalosis is caused by direct stimulation of the respiratory center by salicylate. The accumulation of lactic acid and ketoacids leads to the concomitant metabolic acidosis. The severity of the neurologic manifestations largely depends on the concentration of salicylate in the central nervous system. Therapy is directed at limiting further drug absorption by administering activated charcoal and promoting the exit of salicylate from the CNS. This can be accomplished by alkalinizing the serum, typically by means of the addition of intravenous fluids with sodium bicarbonate, with the goal of raising the serum pH to between 7.45 and 7.50. Increasing the GFR will also enhance salicylate excretion. Hemodialysis is reserved for severe cases, especially those involving fulminant renal failure.

21. The answer is D.

(Chap. 21) The level of obstruction is important when considering urinary tract obstruction. Bilateral hydronephrosis and hydroureter suggest either a systemic process or mechanical obstruction at or below the level of the uretero-vesical junctions. While retroperitoneal fibrosis can cause such a picture, it is most common among middle-aged men. In patients of reproductive age, genital tract infections can cause meatal stenosis if left untreated or if infections are recurrent. Retroperitoneal lymphomas can cause bilateral hydroureter, as can more distal obstructions like phimosis. In the developing world, one may also consider schistosomiasis and genitourinary tuberculosis.

22. The answer is B.

(Chap. 12; Rubin et al: JAMA 291:697–703, 2004.) Peritonitis is the most common serious complication of peritoneal dialysis. These patients typically present with abdominal pain, fever, and a cloudy peritoneal dialysate. Persistent or recurrent peritonitis may require the removal of the catheter. Further complications include losses of amino acids as well as albumin, which may be as much as 5–15 g/d. In addition, patients can absorb glucose through the peritoneal dialysate, resulting in hyperglycemia, not hypoglycemia. The resulting hyperglycemia can cause a hypertriglyceridemia, especially in patients with diabetes mellitus. Leakage of the dialysate fluid into the pleural space can also occur, more frequently on the right than on the left. It can be diagnosed by analysis of the pleural fluid, which typically has an elevated glucose concentration. Rapid fluid shifts are uncommon with peritoneal dialysis, and this approach may be favored for patients with congestive heart failure or unstable angina. A recent report suggested improved patient satisfaction with peritoneal dialysis compared with hemodialysis.

23. The answer is A.

(*Chap. 3*) The serum creatinine is widely used as a reflection of renal function because metabolism of creatinine from muscle varies little in the steady state and it is a freely filtered small solute. Therefore, creatinine clearance is used as a reflection of glomerular filtration rate. However, many factors such as loss of muscle from aging, chronic disease, or malnutrition can mask significant changes in creatinine clearance with small changes in serum creatinine. Two formulas, the Cockcroft-Gault formula and the MDRD (modification of diet in renal disease), are often used to calculate creatinine clearance. The Cockcroft-Gault formula requires age, lean body weight, plasma creatinine, and sex to calculate the creatinine clearance. The more cumbersome and more accurate MDRD uses plasma creatinine, sex, race, and age. Urine creatinine is not a variable in either the Cockcroft-Gault or the MDRD formulas. Race is a variable only in the MDRD equation.

24. The answer is B. (*Chap. 3*)

Creatinine clearance = [(140 − age) × lean weight (kg)]/ creatinine (mg/dL) × 72

Using the Cockcroft-Gault formula, this patient's creatinine clearance is 47 mL/min. This patient would have moderate (stage 3) renal insufficiency. This information may be important for drug dosing.

25. The answer is D.

(*Chap. 21*) Erythrocytosis can develop in an obstructive uropathy as a result of increased erythropoietin production. Anemia in kidney disease occurs as a result of progressive renal parenchymal destruction. As the kidney attempts to preserve renal function and expand blood volume, renin levels increase and can cause a secondary hypertension. Dysuria can be seen in cases of chronic urinary tract obstruction due to urinary stasis and the propensity to develop urolithiasis. Pain with micturition is a hallmark of vesicoureteral reflux, which causes a chronic functional obstructive uropathy. Pyuria is common, as is urinary tract infection. Stasis promotes the growth of bacteria and urinary tract infection.

26. The answer is D.

(*Chap. 10*) Cholesterol embolization (also known as atheroembolic renal disease) is characterized by pyuria, progressive renal failure (usually nonoliguric), and associated organ dysfunction (including bowel, pancreas, and CNS). Hypocomplementemia and eosinophiluria also may be seen. The urinalysis is not compatible with acute tubular necrosis because of the absence of granular casts.

27. The answer is B.

(*Chaps. 3 and 5*) The octahedral, or envelope-shaped, crystals are due to the presence of calcium oxalate in the urine. Calcium oxalate crystals are classically seen in ethylene glycol ingestion, which also causes a high-anion-gap metabolic acidosis. White blood cell casts indicate an upper urinary tract infection associated with a positive urine culture. Uric acid (rhomboid shapes) or struvite ("coffin lids") crystals may be seen in cases of nephrolithiasis that causes hydronephrosis. Red blood cell casts are indicative of glomerular disease, often associated with a positive ANA.

28. The answer is B.

(*Chap. 5*) The pH is high and the plasma bicarbonate is high. This is indicative of a metabolic alkalosis, not a primary acidosis. A respiratory alkalosis is not consistent with an elevated P_{CO_2}. Similarly, the P_{CO_2} is elevated appropriately to compensate for the metabolic alkalosis, excluding a primary respiratory acidosis. The respiratory compensation for a metabolic alkalosis is limited by the hypoxic drive. When the P_{CO_2} rises into the 40s and 50s, the hypoxic drive maintains a Pa_{O_2} of >55–60 mmHg, preventing further hypoventilation to additionally increase P_{CO_2}.

29. The answer is E.

(*Chap. 5*) The differential diagnosis for a metabolic alkalosis can be divided into those disorders with extracellular fluid contraction and normotension (or hypotension) and those with extracellular fluid expansion and hypertension (see Table 5-6). Cushing's disease and mineralocorticoid excess cause a metabolic alkalosis with hypertension. Patients with Bartter's syndrome are normotensive. This patient has evidence of hypovolemia with altered mental status, hypotension, and tachycardia. Myocardial infarction causing cardiogenic shock would result in an anion gap metabolic acidosis due to lactate accumulation.

30. The answer is D.

(*Chap. 6*) This patient is most likely hypovolemic from the osmotic preparation for his colonoscopy. Physical examination supports hypovolemic hyponatremia. Hyperglycemia and hyperlipidemia can cause hyponatremia, but these conditions would be associated with a high and normal plasma osmolality, respectively. SIADH is unlikely to be causing the hyponatremia if the extracellular volume status is decreased. Diabetes insipidus is a hypernatremic disorder caused by excess water loss.

31. The answer is B.

(*Chap. 12*) Commonly accepted criteria for initiating patients on maintenance dialysis include uremic symptoms, hyperkalemia unresponsive to conservative measures, persistent extracellular fluid expansion despite diuretic therapy, acidosis refractory to medical therapy, a bleeding diathesis, and a creatinine clearance <10 mL/min per 1.73 m². This patient has none of those indications. Without symptoms of uremia, an elevated BUN is not sufficient to initiate maintenance dialysis. A urine analysis is unlikely to be helpful in deciding when to initiate dialysis for this patient. Renal biopsy does not usually have a role in stage 5 disease.

32. The answer is C.

(Chap. 7) Determining the PTH level is central to the evaluation of hypocalcemia (see Table 7-2). A suppressed or "inappropriately low" PTH level in the setting of hypocalcemia establishes absent or reduced PTH secretion as the cause. Hypomagnesemia may suppress PTH secretion and contribute to hypocalcemia. In contrast, an elevated PTH should direct attention to the vitamin D axis as the cause of hypocalcemia. Thyroid-stimulating hormone levels will not elucidate the proximate cause of hypocalcemia in the absence of PTH levels. In patients with suspected nutritional deficiency, the 25(OH)D should be checked. In patients with renal insufficiency or suspected vitamin D resistance, serum 1,25(OH)$_2$D levels are informative. An ionized calcium is a better marker of the true serum calcium levels but will not assist with diagnosis. Hypomagnesemia should be repleted along with hypocalcemia when both are present.

33. The answer is A.

(Chap. 3) A key point in the diagnostic evaluation of hematuria is the presence of dysmorphic RBCs or RBC casts in the urine. This finding is strongly suspicious for glomerulonephritis. This diagnosis requires prompt evaluation and therapy to avoid irreversible renal failure. Concerning aspects of this patient's presentation for glomerulonephritis are the presence of RBC casts and >500 mg/24 h of protein in the urine. In the evaluation of proteinuria with hematuria, these features should prompt a serologic and hematologic evaluation and strong consideration of renal biopsy. A CT scan is unlikely to reveal the cause of this patient's hematuria because he has a glomerular problem. An ACE inhibitor may treat his proteinuria but will not address the underlying cause. Since it is already apparent that this patient has proteinuria, ultrasensitive testing for microalbumin is not necessary. Cystoscopy is performed when the source of bleeding is thought to be from the bladder, after renal sources have been eliminated as causes.

34. The answer is C.

(Chaps. 6 and 16) The evaluation of patients with hypokalemia should first include a consideration of redistribution of body potassium into cells such as that which occurs in alkalosis, β_2-agonist excess with refeeding syndrome and/or insulin therapy, vitamin B$_{12}$ therapy, pernicious anemia, and periodic paralysis. In periodic paralysis serum bicarbonate is normal. If the patient is hypertensive and plasma renin is elevated, renovascular hypertension or a renin-secreting tumor (including Wilms) must be considered and appropriate imaging studies must be carried out. If plasma renin levels are low, mineralocorticoid effect may be high as a result of either endogenous hormone (glucocorticoid overproduction or aldosterone overproduction as in Conn's syndrome) or exogenous agents (licorice or steroids). In a normotensive patient a high serum bicarbonate excludes

renal tubular acidosis. High urine chloride excretion makes gastrointestinal losses less likely and implies primary renal potassium loss, as may be seen in diuretic abuse (ruled out by the urine screen) or Bartter's syndrome. In Bartter's syndrome, hyperplasia of the granular cells of the juxtaglomerular apparatus leads to high renin levels and secondary aldosterone elevations. Such hyperplasia appears to be secondary to chronic volume depletion caused by a hereditary (autosomal recessive) defect that interferes with salt reabsorption in the thick ascending loop of Henle. Chronic potassium depletion, which frequently presents initially in childhood, leads to polyuria and weakness.

35. The answer is C.

(Chap. 16) Polycystic kidney diseases (PCKDs) are the most common life-threatening inherited diseases. Adult-onset disease is typically inherited in autosomal dominant fashion. It is a systemic disease caused by mutations in either the *PKD-1* or *PKD-2* gene. Phenotypic presentation is varied. Most patients are not symptomatic until middle age. Typical presentations include abdominal discomfort, hematuria, urinary tract infections, or hypertension. Most patients experience a steady decline in renal function over one to two decades following diagnosis. About 60% of patients will develop end-stage renal disease by age 70. Hypertension precedes renal failure. Risk factors for disease progression include male gender, African-American race, hypertension, and the presence of the polycystin-1 mutation. Patients are at an increased risk of subarachnoid and cerebral hemorrhage due to aneurysm formation. Cardiac abnormalities are present in 25% of patients, and most commonly include mitral valve prolapse and aortic regurgitation. Hepatic cysts are common and are found in 40% of patients by the age of 60. Renal ultrasound is the diagnostic test of choice and is 100% sensitive in patients older than 30 who have a positive family history. Treatment of PCKD is supportive; control of hypertension and close evaluation of kidney function are paramount.

36. The answer is A.

(Chap. 11; Ifudu: N Engl J Med 339:1054–1062, 1998.) Renal osteodystrophy is a common complication of chronic renal disease and the most common complication secondary to impaired renal production of 1,25(OH)$_2$D$_3$. This leads to a decreased calcium absorption in the gut as well as impaired renal phosphate excretion. The resulting hyperphosphatemia causes a secondary hyperparathyroidism. The hyperparathyroidism is subsequently worsened by hypocalcemia, which is present because of the hyperphosphatemia and the decreased enzymatic conversion of 25-hydroxyvitamin D to 1,25(OH)$_2$D$_3$. Finally, 1,25(OH)$_2$D$_3$ deficiency worsens hyperparathyroidism as the former is a direct inhibitor of parathyroid hormone secretion into the bone. The resultant decreased serum calcium concentration leads to secondary hyperparathyroidism. In addition, other causes of renal osteodystrophy include chronic metabolic acidosis resulting from dissolution of bone buffers and decalcification and the long-term administration of aluminum-containing antacids. No significant loss of vitamin D or calcium is associated with currently employed dialysis techniques, and the treatment of renal osteodystrophy often includes calcitriol.

37. The answer is C.

(Chap. 6) Diuretic-induced hyponatremia almost always is due to thiazide diuretics. It occurs mostly in the elderly. The reduction in serum sodium may be severe and cause symptoms. Loop diuretics such as furosemide cause hyponatremia far less often than do thiazide diuretics. Thiazide diuretics inhibit sodium and potassium reabsorption in the distal tubule, leading to Na^+ and K^+ depletion and AVP-mediated water retention. In contrast, loop diuretics impair maximal urinary concentrating capacity, limiting AVP-mediated water retention. Many drugs may cause hyponatremia by promoting AVP secretion or action at the collecting duct; however, metoprolol and enalapril are not significant causes of SIADH. Spironolactone is a competitive antagonist of aldosterone at the mineralocorticoid receptor. It has weak natriuretic activity and is most likely to cause hyperkalemia.

38. The answer is A.

(Chap. 6) Failure to concentrate urine despite substantial hypertonic dehydration suggests a diagnosis of diabetes insipidus. A nephrogenic origin will be postulated if there is no increase in urine concentration after exogenous vasopressin. The only useful mode of therapy is a low-salt diet and the use of a thiazide or amiloride, a potassium-sparing distal diuretic agent. The resultant volume contraction presumably enhances proximal reabsorption and thereby reduces urine flow.

39. The answer is A.

(Chap. 8) Individuals with acute leukemia and other myeloproliferative disorders are at risk for the development of tumor lysis syndrome following institution of chemotherapy. Tumor lysis syndrome results from rapid cell death with resultant increases in serum potassium, phosphate, and uric acid levels. Renal failure develops due to acute uric acid nephropathy, and pathology demonstrates deposition of uric acid crystals in the kidneys and the collecting system. The clinical picture is one of rapidly progressive renal failure, with oliguria and rapidly rising creatinine. Markedly elevated levels of serum uric acid would be expected in acute uric acid nephropathy, but hyperuricemia occurs in any cause of renal failure. A urine uric acid/creatinine ratio of >1 mg/mg confirms hyperuricemia and uric acid nephropathy as the cause of renal failure. This complication can largely be prevented by institution of allopurinol, 200–800 mg daily, prior to chemotherapy. Once hyperuricemia develops, however, efforts should be focused on

preventing deposition of uric acid in the kidney. These measures include forced diuresis with furosemide or mannitol and alkalination of the urine with sodium bicarbonate. Dialysis may be required. Colchicine is used to treat the inflammation in acute gouty arthritis but has no effects on serum uric acid levels. It has no role in the treatment of uric acid nephropathy. Prednisone may be used in the chemotherapeutic regimens of some individuals with hematologic malignancies, but does not prevent development of hyperuricemia.

40. The answer is A.

(Chap. 5) Since the pH is low, the primary process is an acidosis. A low serum bicarbonate tells us that it is a metabolic acidosis. The anion gap [Na – (Cl + HCO_3^-)] is between 8 and 12 meq/L. In this example, the anion gap is elevated to 31 meq/L. The P_{CO_2} decreases from a normal of 40 mmHg by 1 to 1.5 for each 1-meq decrease in serum bicarbonate. In this example, the serum bicarbonate has decreased by 19 meq/L (normal is 24 meq/L) and the expected P_{CO_2} is between 11.5 and 21 mmHg. This is an example of an anion-gap metabolic acidosis with appropriate respiratory compensation. Respiratory acidosis is ruled out by the low P_{CO_2}. If this patient had a concomitant respiratory alkalosis, the P_{CO_2} would be lower.

41. The answer is B.

(Chap. 12) Although the dose is currently defined as a derivation of the fractional urea clearance, factors that are also important include patient size, residual kidney function, dietary protein intake, comorbid conditions, and the degree of anabolism/catabolism. The efficiency of dialysis depends on the counter-current flow rate of the dialysate. The number of hours/sessions prescribed for a patient are derived from the dialysis dose and is individualized.

42. The answer is A.

(Chap. 18) The prognosis for patients with scleroderma renal disease is poor. In SRC patients, prompt treatment with an ACE inhibitor may reverse acute renal failure. In recent studies the initiation of ACE inhibitor therapy resulted in 61% of patients having some degree of renal recovery and not needing chronic dialysis support. The survival rate is estimated to be 80–85% at 8 years. Among patients who needed dialysis, when treated with ACE inhibitors, over 50% were able to discontinue dialysis after 3 to 18 months. Therefore, ACE inhibitors should be used even if the patient requires dialysis support.

43. The answer is A.

(Chap. 12) The potassium concentration of dialysate is usually 2.5 meq/L but may be varied depending on the predialysis serum potassium. This patient may need a lower dialysate potassium concentration. Sodium modeling is an adjustment of the dialysate sodium that may lessen the incidence of hypotension at the end of a dialysis

session. Aldosterone defects, if present, are not likely to play a role in this patient since his kidneys are not being perfused. Therefore, nephrectomy is not likely to control his potassium. Similarly, since the patient is likely anuric, there is no efficacy in utilizing loop diuretics to effect kaluresis. This patient has no approved indications for implantation of a defibrillator.

44. The answer is D.

(Chap. 6) Rapid correction (or overcorrection) of hyponatremia may lead to the development of the osmotic demyelination syndrome. The relative hypertonicity of the extracellular fluid without time for intracellular compensation or osmotic compensation causes osmotic shrinkage of brain cells and demyelination. This syndrome usually occurs in patients with chronic hyponatremia who have osmotically equilibrated the intracellular space. These patients have flaccid paralysis, dysarthria, and dysphagia. Brain MRI will show demyelination, particularly in the brainstem (central pontine myelinolysis). Head CT scans will not demonstrate these lesions. The presence of bilateral extremity with minimal cranial nerve abnormalities would make a posterior circulation stroke less likely.

45. The answer is C.

(Chap. 15) It is important to note that nephrotic syndrome with any cause can be associated with hypercoagulability. Antithrombin III and proteins C and S are lost in the urine, with concomitantly decreased serum levels. Increased platelet aggregation has been described, and hyperfibrinogenemia is thought to result from an inflammatory response and increased liver synthetic activity caused by urinary protein losses. Additionally, IgG is lost in the urine, and occasionally these patients develop low serum levels with associated immunocompromise. Chronic disseminated intravascular coagulation is not a mechanism of hypercoagulability in patients with the nephrotic syndrome.

46. The answer is A.

(Chap. 10) Nonsteroidal anti-inflammatory drugs (NSAIDs) do not alter glomerular filtration rate in normal individuals. However, in states of mild to moderate hypoperfusion (as in prerenal azotemia) or in the presence of chronic kidney disease, glomerular perfusion and filtration fraction are preserved through several compensatory mechanisms. In response to a reduction in perfusion pressures, stretch receptors in afferent arterioles trigger a cascade of events that lead to afferent arteriolar dilatation and efferent arteriolar vasoconstriction, thereby preserving glomerular filtration fraction. These mechanisms are partly mediated by the vasodilators prostaglandin E_2 and prostacyclin. NSAIDs can impair the kidney's ability to compensate for a low perfusion pressure by interfering with local prostaglandin synthesis and inhibiting these protective responses. Ureteral obstruction is not the mechanism by which

NSAID impairs renal function in this scenario. NSAIDs are not known to be proximal tubule toxins.

47. and 48. The answers are A and A.

(Chap. 10; R Solomon: Kidney Int 53:230, 1998.) Radiocontrast agents are a common cause of acute renal failure and may result in acute tubular necrosis (contrast nephropathy). It is common for patients receiving intravenous contrast to develop a transient increase in serum creatinine. These agents cause renal failure by inducing intrarenal vasoconstriction and reducing renal blood flow, mimicking prerenal azotemia, and by directly causing tubular injury. The risk of contrast nephropathy may be reduced by initiating newer isoosmolar agents and minimizing the dose of contrast. When the reduction in renal blood flow is severe or prolonged, tubular injury develops, causing acute renal failure. Patients with intravascular volume depletion, diabetes, congestive heart failure, multiple myeloma, or chronic renal failure have an increased risk of contrast nephropathy. The urine sediment is bland in mild cases, but with acute tubular necrosis, muddy brown granular casts may be seen. Saline hydration plus *N*-acetylcysteine may decrease the risk and severity of contrast nephropathy. Red cell casts indicate glomerular disease, and white cell casts suggest upper urinary tract infection. Urinary eosinophils are seen in allergic interstitial disease caused by many drugs.

TABLE 47, 48

GUIDELINES FOR USE OF INTRAVENOUS CONTRAST IN PATIENTS WITH IMPAIRED RENAL FUNCTION

SERUM CREATININE, μmol/L (mg/L)[a]	RECOMMENDATION
<133 (<1.5)	Use either ionic or nonionic at 2 mL/kg to 150 mL total
133–177 (1.5–2.0)	Nonionic; hydrate diabetics 1 mL/kg per hour × 10 h
>177 (>2.0)	Consider noncontrast CT or MRI; nonionic contrast if required
177–221 (2.0–2.5)	Nonionic only if required (as above); contraindicated in diabetics
>265 (>3.0)	Nonionic IV contrast given only to patients undergoing dialysis within 24 h

[a]Risk is greatest in patients with rising creatinine levels.
Note: CT, computed tomography; MRI, magnetic resonance imaging.

49. The answer is C.

(Chap. 18) Renal vein thrombosis occurs in 10–15% of patients with nephrotic syndrome accompanying membranous glomerulopathy and oncologic disease. The clinical manifestations can be variable but may be characterized by fever, lumbar tenderness, leukocytosis, and hematuria. Magnetic resonance venography is the most sensitive and specific noninvasive form of imaging to make the diagnosis of renal vein thrombosis. Ultrasound

with Doppler is operator dependent and therefore may be less sensitive. Contrast venography is the gold standard for diagnosis, but it exposes the patient to a more invasive procedure and contrast load. Nuclear medicine screening is not performed to make this diagnosis.

50. The answer is D.

(Chap. 6) Arginine vasopressin is a neurohormone released from the posterior pituitary gland to help maintain water balance in the body. Also known as antidiuretic hormone, vasopressin is primarily released under conditions of hyperosmolarity and volume depletion. Although sodium is the main determinant of hyperosmolarity, sodium is not the only stimulus that affects the secretion of vasopressin. Other, less potent stimuli of vasopressin release include pregnancy, nausea, pain, stress, and hypoglycemia. In addition, many drugs can cause stimulation of the inappropriate secretion of vasopressin. This hormone acts on the principal cell in the distal convoluted tubule of the kidney to cause resorption of water. This occurs through nuclear mechanisms encoded by the aquaporin-2 gene that cause water channels to be inserted into the luminal membrane. The net effect is to cause the passive resorption of water along the osmotic gradient in the distal convoluted tubule.

51. The answer is C.

(Chap. 6) β-Adrenergic agonists such as those used to treat bronchospasm are a common cause of hypokalemia. Activation of β_2-adrenergic receptors induces cellular uptake of potassium and promotes insulin secretion by pancreatic islet β cells. Clinical manifestations include fatigue, myalgias and muscular weakness. Severe hypokalemia leads to progressive weakness, hypoventilation and eventually complete paralysis. The electrocardiogram findings are common but do not correlate with the degree of hypokalemia in the serum. Todd's paralysis occurs after seizures. Neither myocardial infarction with failure nor ICU psychosis would present with objective lower extremity weakness without other, more common indicators of these conditions. Adrenal insufficiency will generally cause hyperkalemia, not hypokalemia.

52. The answer is C.

(Chap. 6) In addition to correction of hypernatremia, patients such as this who are volume depleted require restoration of extracellular fluid volume. The quantity of water required to correct a free water deficit in hypernatremic patients can be estimated from the following equation:

Water deficit = [(plasma Na − 140)/140] × total body water

Total body water is approximately 50% of lean body mass in men and 40% of lean body mass in women. In calculating the rate of water replacement, ongoing losses should be accounted for and plasma Na^+ should be lowered by no more than 0.5 meq/L an hour over the first 24 h. More rapid administration of water and normalization of

serum sodium concentration may result in a rapid influx of water into cells that have already undergone osmotic normalization. The resulting cellular edema in the central nervous system (CNS) may cause seizures or neurologic damage.

53. The answer is E.

(Chap. 17) The most likely cause of acute renal failure in this patient is allergic interstitial nephritis (AIN) due to penicillin. Many drugs can cause AIN including β-lactams, sulfonamides, fluoroquinolones, thiazide and loop diuretics, nonsteroidal anti-inflammatory drugs (NSAIDs), and cyclooxygenase-2 (COX-2) inhibitors. Most individuals have been taking the culprit drug for several weeks before the development of AIN and present with fevers, rash, and eosinophilia. This triad is present in only 10% of patients, however. Examination of the urine sediment shows hematuria and eosinophilia. Urine eosinophils can be seen with the use of a Hansel's stain. Proteinuria is usually mild except in cases where AIN is due to NSAIDs or COX-2 inhibitors, and 24-h urine collection for protein would be nonspecific. Renal imaging may suggest enlarged kidneys, and histology would show interstitial edema with infiltration of large numbers of inflammatory cells including eosinophils, lymphocytes, and polymorphonuclear leukocytes (PMNs). The main differential diagnosis is acute glomerulonephritis, but if an individual is on a culprit drug, the drug should be discontinued as an initial step. Discontinuation of the drug usually leads to complete reversal of the renal injury, although in severe cases, prednisone may be used to improve recovery. The clinical picture does not suggest relapse of endocarditis, worsening valvular dysfunction, or a new infectious process such as an infection of the central venous catheter. Thus, blood cultures and echocardiogram are not useful in this situation. Antistreptolysin O titers are elevated in cases of poststreptococcal glomerulonephritis due to group A streptococcus, but would not be elevated in *Streptococcus viridans* endocarditis.

54. The answer is C.

(Chap. 12) Hypotension is the most common complication during hemodialysis. The risk factors for developing hypotension during hemodialysis include excessive ultrafiltration, reduced intravascular volume before dialysis, impaired autonomic responses, osmolar shifts, food intake before dialysis, impaired cardiac function, and use of antihypertensive agents. The hypotension is usually managed with fluid administration and by decreasing the ultrafiltration rate. Muscle cramps are a decreasingly common complication of hemodialysis as a result of improvements in dialysis technique. Anaphylactoid reactions to the dialyzer once were common but are also decreasing in frequency with the use of newer-generation dialysis membranes. Fever is not a usual complication of hemodialysis but suggests the presence of an infection of the dialysis

access site. Blood cultures should be obtained. Hyperglycemia is a complication of peritoneal dialysis, not of hemodialysis.

55. The answer is A. (Chap. 7)
Hypercalcemia causes characteristic changes on the ECG including bradycardia, atrioventricular block, and a shortened QT interval. Symptoms of hypercalcemia depend on the severity and time course of its development. Mild hypercalcemia is usually asymptomatic. Patients may progress to complain of vague neuropsychiatric symptoms including trouble concentrating, personality changes, and depression. Severe hypercalcemia, particularly if it develops acutely, may result in lethargy, stupor, or coma. Changes on the ECG of hypokalemia would include prominent U waves and a prolonged QU interval. Hyperkalemia acutely shows prominent T waves and PR depression. Hypocalcemia causes a prolongation of the QT interval.

56. The answer is A.
(Chap. 7) In sarcoidosis, similar to other granulomatous diseases such as tuberculosis and silicosis, there is increased conversion of 25(OH)D to the potent 1,25(OH)$_2$D. 1,25(OH)$_2$D enhances intestinal calcium absorption, resulting in hypercalcemia and suppressed parathyroid hormone. Glucocorticoids decrease 1,25(OH)$_2$D production. Initial treatment for this patient should include IV fluids to restore extracellular fluid volume. Only after volume has been restored should loop diuretics be used to decrease serum calcium. Zoledronic acid is indicated if there is increased calcium mobilization from bone, as in malignancy or severe hyperparathyroidism. Intravenous phosphate is not indicated as it chelates calcium and may deposit in tissue and cause extensive organ damage if the calcium–phosphate product is >65. The mechanism of the hypercalcemia of sarcoidosis is related to excess vitamin D; therefore, calcitriol would be contraindicated.

57. The answer is C.
(Chap. 10) In bilateral renal artery stenosis (or unilateral stenosis in a patient with a single kidney), GFR is preserved by the actions of angiotensin II: afferent arteriolar vasodilatation and efferent arteriolar vasoconstriction. Angiotensin-converting enzyme inhibitors and angiotensin II receptor blockers blunt these responses and can precipitate acute renal failure in this setting. Thiazide diuretics, calcium channel blockers, or centrally acting alpha blockers are better choices for an antihypertensive agent in a patient with bilateral renal artery stenosis.

58. The answer is B.
(Chap. 12) In peritoneal dialysis, 1.5–3.0 L of dextrose-containing fluid is allowed to dwell in the peritoneum to remove toxic materials and volume. Factors such as infection, drugs, position, and exercise impact solute and water clearance. In the developed world, hemodialysis is often the preferred method for renal replacement for patients. However, in poorer countries where access to hemodialysis centers is limited, peritoneal dialysis is used more commonly. Residual renal function alters the dose of dialysis but does not impact the mode of dialysis. Moreover, patients with no residual renal function who receive peritoneal dialysis are at higher risk of uremia than patients on hemodialysis. High-transporters through the peritoneum require more frequent doses of peritoneal dialysis, potentially negating the benefit of this modality. In the developed world, the patient's age does not impact the mode of dialysis. Patients with prior abdominal surgeries often have difficulty with peritoneal dialysis catheter placement and dialysate delivery.

59. The answer is A.
(Chap. 16) This patient has a normal-anion-gap metabolic acidosis (anion gap = 12). The calculated urine anion gap ($Na^+ + K^+ - Cl^-$) is +3; thus, the acidosis is unlikely to be due to gastrointestinal bicarbonate loss. In this patient the diagnosis is type I renal tubular acidosis, or distal RTA. This is a disorder in which the distal nephron does not lower pH normally. It is associated with a urine pH >5.5, hypokalemia, and lack of bicarbonaturia. This condition may be associated with calcium phosphate stones and nephrocalcinosis. Type II RTA, or proximal RTA, includes a pH <5.5, hypokalemia, a positive urine anion gap, bicarbonaturia, hypophosphatemia, and hypercalciuria. This condition results from defective resorption of bicarbonate. Type III RTA is rare and most commonly is seen in children. Type IV RTA is also referred to as hyperkalemic distal RTA. Hyporeninemic hypoaldosteronism is the most common cause of type IV RTA and is usually associated with diabetic nephropathy.

60. The answer is B.
(Chap. 15) The characteristic pattern of focal (not all glomeruli) and segmental (not the entire glomerulus) glomerular scarring is shown. The history and laboratory features are also consistent with this lesion: some associated hypertension, diminution in creatinine clearance, and a relatively inactive urine sediment. The "nephropathy of obesity" may be associated with this lesion secondary to hyperfiltration; this condition may be more likely to occur in obese patients with hypoxemia, obstructive sleep apnea, and right-sided heart failure. Hypertensive nephrosclerosis exhibits more prominent vascular changes and patchy, ischemic, totally sclerosed glomeruli. In addition, nephrosclerosis seldom is associated with nephrotic-range proteinuria. Minimal-change disease usually is associated with symptomatic edema and normal-appearing glomeruli as demonstrated on light microscopy. This patient's presentation is consistent with that of membranous nephropathy, but the biopsy is not. With membranous glomerular nephritis all glomeruli are uniformly involved with subepithelial

dense deposits. There are no features of crescentic glomerulonephritis present.

61. The answer is D.

(Chap. 6) This patient has a reduction in extracellular fluid (ECF) volume as evidenced by the resting tachycardia and orthostatic fall in blood pressure. In response (to maintain ECF volume), there is renal arteriolar vasoconstriction that causes a decrease in the glomerular filtration rate and filtered sodium. Tubular reabsorption of sodium increases as a result of the decreased filtered load and the effects of angiotensin II. These changes result in low (<20 meq/L) urine sodium excretion. There will also be an *increase* in the ratio of BUN to creatinine because of increased BUN reabsorption. As a result of the effects of aldosterone and the avid sodium reabsorption, urine potassium will be higher than urine sodium. Sweat is hypotonic relative to serum, and so patients with excessive sweating are more likely to be hypernatremic than hyponatremic. Red blood cell casts indicate glomerular disease. Prolonged hypotension caused by ECF contraction may cause tubular injury, leading to granular or epithelial cell casts.

62. The answer is B.

(Chap. 6) The patient's polyuria and thirst with rising sodium suggest diabetes insipidus. Although primary polydipsia can present similarly with thirst and polyuria, it does not cause hypernatremia; instead, hyponatremia results from increased extracellular water. Often patients with diabetes insipidus are able to compensate as outpatients when they have ready access to free water, but once hospitalized and unable to receive water freely, they develop hypernatremia. The first step in the evaluation of diabetes insipidus is to determine if it is central or nephrogenic. This is easily accomplished through measurement of the vasopressin level. In central diabetes insipidus it is low because of a failure of secretion from the posterior pituitary gland, whereas it is elevated in nephrogenic disease, in which the kidneys are insensitive to vasopressin. After measurement of the vasopressin level, a trial of nasal arginine vasopressin may be attempted. Generally nephrogenic diabetes insipidus will not improve significantly with this drug. Free water restriction, which will help with primary polydipsia, will cause worsening hypernatremia in patients with diabetes insipidus. Serum osmolality and 24-h urinary sodium excretion will not help in the diagnosis or management of this patient at this time.

63. The answer is D.

(Chap. 16) In any patient with hypokalemia the use of diuretics must be excluded. This patient has multiple warning signs for the use of agents to alter her weight, including her age, gender, and participation in competitive sports. Her BMI is low, and the oral examination may suggest chronic vomiting. Chronic vomiting may be associated with a low urine chloride level. Once diuretic use and vomiting are excluded, the differential diagnosis of hypokalemia and metabolic alkalosis includes magnesium deficiency, Liddle's syndrome, Bartter's syndrome, and Gittleman's syndrome. Liddle's syndrome is associated with hypertension and undetectable aldosterone and renin levels. It is a rare autosomal dominant disorder. Classic Bartter's syndrome has a presentation similar to that of this patient. It may also include polyuria and nocturia because of hypokalemia-induced diabetes insipidus. Gittleman's syndrome can be distinguished from Bartter's syndrome by hypomagnesemia and hypocalciuria.

INDEX

Bold number indicates the start of the main discussion of the topic; numbers with "f" and "t" refer to figure and table pages.